W9-BIU-748

Handbook of
FAMILIES&
HEALTH

Handbook of
FAMILIES&
HEALTH

Interdisciplinary Perspectives

Editors

D. Russell Crane
Elaine S. Marshall

Brigham Young University

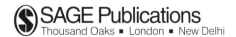
SAGE Publications
Thousand Oaks ▪ London ▪ New Delhi

For information:

Sage Publications, Inc.
2455 Teller Road
Thousand Oaks, California 91320
E-mail: order@sagepub.com

Sage Publications Ltd.
1 Oliver's Yard
55 City Road
London EC1Y 1SP
United Kingdom

Sage Publications India Pvt. Ltd.
B-42, Panchsheel Enclave
Post Box 4109
New Delhi 110 017 India

Printed in the United States of America on acid-free paper

Library of Congress Cataloging-in-Publication data

Handbook of families and health : interdisciplinary perspectives / D. Russell Crane, Elaine S. Marshall, editors.
    p. cm.
Includes bibliographical references and index.
ISBN 0-7619-3041-8 (cloth)
    1. Family—Health and hygiene. I. Crane, D. Russell. II. Marshall, Elaine S.
RA418.5.F3H36 2005
613—dc22   2005002566

05   06   07   08   09   10   9   8   7   6   5   4   3   2   1

Acquiring Editor:	Jim Brace-Thompson
Editorial Assistant:	Karen Ehrmann
Production Editor:	Sanford Robinson
Typesetter:	C&M Digitals (P) Ltd.
Copy Editor:	Diana Breti and Dan Hays
Indexer:	Julie Sherman Grayson
Cover Designer:	Ravi Balasuriya

Contents

Preface

Handbook of Families and Health: Interdisciplinary Perspectives is designed to provoke discussion of academic research, clinical thinking, and practice about the reciprocal interactions of issues related to families and health. The goal is to begin the discussion about how to understand and then assist individuals, families, and societies as they struggle with these important issues. Just as the understanding of individuals cannot be separated from understanding of their families, so it is that families cannot be understood without addressing the broader societal and public policies that affect individuals and families.

Experts from many disciplines have come together in this volume to address the common topics related to health and families. Our hope is that these contributions will be shared across the disciplines represented here as well as with those from other academic and clinical traditions. It is hoped that common themes will be identified to help advance theory, research, and practice that will help families who are dealing with these areas.

Acknowledgments

Our first debt of gratitude is to our contributors. Obviously, this project would not be possible without them. We sincerely appreciate their willingness to write for this book. They have given freely of their expertise that has been gained over years of commitment to issues of family health, as well as much personal effort and sacrifice.

We thank our many friends and colleagues at Brigham Young University (BYU). We appreciate the support of the administrative team of the School of Family Life at BYU: James Harper, director of the school, and Susanne Frost Olsen and Tom Holman, associate directors. We also thank the team at BYU College of Nursing: Holly Skelton, Janessa Johnson, Rose Ann Jarrett, and Denise Gibbons-Davis. We give special thanks to our staff, students, and friends who helped in the preparation of the manuscript: Nicolle Buckmiller, Kimberly Bond, Kirsten Lyons, Marie Roberts, Stacee Truman, and Madlyn Tanner.

Our deepest thanks to Sage Senior Editor Jim Brace-Thompson for his support for this work. His encouragement and guidance have been consistent and consistently appreciated.

Finally, we give our thanks and love to our respective spouses, Eileen and John, and our families, who made this effort possible.

Introduction

Interdisciplinary Perspectives on Families and Health: A Beginning

D. RUSSELL CRANE AND ELAINE S. MARSHALL

The *Handbook of Families and Health: Interdisciplinary Perspectives* is intended to explore the most recent topics in research, practice, and policy related to the important topic of helping families with health issues. It is truly interdisciplinary in nature, beginning with the collaboration of the coeditors, a marriage and family therapist and a nurse. The contributors represent scholars and practitioners from a wide range of disciplines, including marriage and family therapy, nursing, sociology, medicine, social work, law, human development, psychology, political science, and business.

The handbook began as an outgrowth of the 2002 biennial research conference at Brigham Young University (BYU), organized by the director of the Family Studies Center in the School of Family Life, D. Russell Crane. At these conferences, scholars from many areas of the world visit the BYU campus and discuss the latest issues in research and practice on topics that relate to families. The proceedings of the conference on "Families and Health" provided the nucleus of this book. Following literature reviews on various issues in health and families, we then invited additional scholars to broaden the perspective.

The purpose of the book is to open discussion to explore the road map for the next generation of scholars in areas related to families and health. The chapters represent the state-of-the-art thinking related to the reciprocal influences of couple, marital, and family issues on health. Some explore the specific areas of research, and others offer examples in practice. In addition, some chapters are instructional to professionals in areas of research funding and family health policy.

OUTLINE OF THE BOOK

In Part I, we discuss current specific health issues on the forefront of concerns among professionals and families, including cancer, heart disease, eating disorders, mental illness, genetically transmitted diseases, infertility, HIV/AIDS, and chronic illness. We also discuss some issues related to families of specific ethnic minorities, such as Hispanic/Latino families and African American families.

In Part II, we highlight issues of aging and caregiving. The chapters on end-of-life care and decision making are particularly relevant to families as they face the realities of aging, death, and bereavement.

Part III is concerned with policy, research, and the economics of health care. Chapters focus on learning about health policy issues and process and research methodologies applicable to the study of families and health. We offer two different approaches to research funding—one from the federal government of the United States, written by an expert at the National Institutes of Health, and the other by a senior investigator from the United Kingdom, who describes experiences with local and regional agencies. Finally, we offer an overview of health care financing in the United States.

Part IV provides examples and explorations of specific interventions to improve family health. For example, we address the role of family therapy in working with families and professionals in cases of genetically transmitted conditions. We also discuss the importance of the relationships between providers and family members in treatment planning and implementation.

We conclude with a brief overview of our observations of the state of science and practice in family health, given interdisciplinary and international perspectives. Here, we note strengths and weaknesses of this work and look into the future for "next steps." We explore what we know now and future directions for the next generation of researchers and practitioners in family health.

ORGANIZATION OF
THE CONTRIBUTIONS

The domains discussed here are not organized in order of importance. Such an effort would obviously be futile. We are concerned about all issues related to families and health, but we necessarily had to place one chapter in front of another. We hope our decisions in this regard are not taken as any signal of our regard for colleagues working in all these important areas.

No handbook can adequately cover all important issues related to families and health. We expect this book to be truly a beginning to provoke collegial discussion. In some cases, we were simply not able to secure authors in needed areas that met our time line. For example, an author on health issues of Native Americans was not able to make the expected contribution. We were also especially interested in the exploration of religion and spirituality on the health of families. Unfortunately, the author passed away just prior to completion of his manuscript. We send our condolences to the family of Dr. David B. Larson. We offer only a sampling of important topics in helping families with health issues. We did not require contributors to adhere to a standard format for the chapters. Instead, we encouraged authors to write in the way that best addressed their areas of expertise. We think this approach should enrich the ongoing discussion among the disciplines.

AUDIENCE FOR THE WORK

This is a beginning effort to include the perspective from a broad range of disciplines. It is a compilation rather than integration. To adequately address important needs of families, the next step for scholars is to do the difficult work of integration and true collaboration. We look forward to works that bring scholars together in such efforts.

The handbook is intended for readers from all areas devoted to the health of families. Just as we sought a wide range of scholars to create this book, we hope that readers from all disciplines may be enriched by the work. We expect that researchers, practitioners, and students from many disciplines will find areas to entice their interests, provoke their thinking, and expand their practice. We hope that differences and commonalities of family issues will emerge in the study of this book.

Part I

FAMILY AND HEALTH ISSUES

CHAPTER 1

Family Development in the Face of Cancer

KAREN WEIHS AND MARY POLITI

The National Cancer Institute reported that 8.9 million Americans who have had cancer were alive in 1999 (American Cancer Society, 2003). The number of cancer cases has increased while the incidence of cancer mortality has declined from 1973 to 1999 (Edwards et al., 2002). As a result, patients and families must learn to live with the chronic physical and psychosocial adjustments of a cancer diagnosis.

The majority of families mount a resilient response over time, despite the suffering that is universal for those living with cancer (Arpin, Fitch, Browne, & Corey, 1990; Grassi & Rosti, 1996; Skerrett, 1998). They report feeling closer to one another after marshaling resources to fight the disease (Lewis, Woods, Hough, & Bensley, 1989; Skerrett, 1998). Although many families report this positive response, the physical and emotional pressures during the different stages of cancer can strain family relationships, even among families who cope well with the diagnosis and its effects (Carlson, Bultz, Speca, & St.-Pierre, 2000; Halford, Scott, & Smythe, 2000; Veach & Nicholas, 1998).

Furthermore, some families of cancer patients express psychological distress as much as, if not more than, the patients (Ferrell, Ervin, Smith, Marek, & Melancon, 2002; Northouse, Mood, Templin, Mellon, & George, 2000; Omne-Ponten, Holmberg, Bergstrom, Sjoden, & Burns, 1993). Researchers have reported that one third to one half of cancer patients meet the diagnostic criteria for a wide range of disorders, including adjustment disorders, affective disorders, and anxiety disorders (Derogatis et al., 1983; Grassi & Rosti, 1996). In addition to the direct effects of cancer on families, these negative psychological changes in the patient can influence the quality of the family environment and family adjustment to cancer (Baider, Koch, Esacson, & Kaplan-DeNour, 1998; Ben-Zur, 2001; Omne-Ponten et al., 1993), resulting in decreased closeness in family relationships (Ell, Nishimoto, Morvay, Mantell, & Hamovitch, 1989).

Family environments can affect the level of the patient's and family members' distress. Cohesive family environments with low conflict include family members who are less distressed and have better coping than patients, partners, and children whose families are detached or high in conflict or both (Arpin et al., 1990; Bloom, Pendergrass, & Burnell, 1984; Lewis et al., 1989). Some research has shown that high emotional expressiveness and cohesion in family relationships predict better psychological adjustment to cancer in all family members (Giese-Davis, Hermanson, Koopman, Weibel, & Spiegel, 2000; Kayser, Sormanti, & Strainchamps, 1999; Trask et al., 2003). Other studies have demonstrated that spouses' avoidance and criticism can lead to patients' sense of diminished attractiveness or self-worth, suppression of emotions, anxiety, or depressed mood in response to cancer (Manne, 1999), and that perception of spouses' emotion-focused coping, such as inconsolable worry or avoidance, can increase both patients' and spouses' distress (Ben-Zur, 2001). When young children have cancer, maternal distress may have an impact on the later psychological adjustment of the children (Sawyer, Streiner, Antoniou, Toogood, & Rice, 1998). These findings highlight the major impact of family functioning on adjustment to cancer.

Another intriguing body of knowledge involves the prediction of higher rates of disease progression and death for cancer patients based on poorer social and familial relationships (Levy, Herberman, Lippman, D'Angelo, & Lee, 1991; Reynolds et al., 1994; Waxler-Morrison, Hislop, Mears, & Kan, 1991). These researchers show that some attributes of the family, such as low nonhousehold support (Weihs, 2001; Ell, Nishimoto, Mediansky, Mantell, & Hamovitch, 1992) or a hostile marital or partner relationship (Weihs, Enright, & Simmens, 2002), may adversely influence the course of the biologic disease process, although it is not clear whether the latter attributes are the same as those that correlate with psychosocial adjustment.

In this chapter, we discuss the impact of cancer on the family system during this threat to the family life cycle. We use theories of family development and attachment to organize information from published reports and studies as well as from our own research and clinical experience.

CANCER AS A THREAT TO THE LIFE COURSE OF THE FAMILY

Cancer threatens to separate the patient from his or her family members, both emotionally and physically. Such threats can seriously divert the life course of the family. The life course of the family is manifest in its continuity over time. It arises from its particular history and is guided toward the future by shared values and goals including the maintenance of health, personal development, productivity in education and in work, recreation, community involvement, and preservation of family integrity.

Our concept of *threat* is informed by the work of Brown and Harris (1989), who based their assessment of the magnitude of threat on the meaning of life events in the context of close relationships, personal history, and social circumstances. The meaning of a threatening situation is based on the values, plans, and goals of the family (Weber, 1947/1964). The assessment of threat in psychooncology is therefore likely to be a useful way to bring together the tangible facts about the cancer experience and their human context to study their effects on the family over time.

ATTACHMENT PROCESSES AND ADJUSTMENT TO CANCER

To understand the family's response to the cancer threat, we examined studies of human development that explain individual differences in responding to distress and separation among family members. Bowlby (1969) described such a behavioral, motivational system as the attachment system. There are three distinguishing features of the attachment system that are helpful in understanding its operation. First, the attachment behavioral system may or may not be active at any given time. Second, attachment is manifested in, but not defined by, a limited set of characteristics that arise when access to the attachment figure exceeds some individually defined limit. These characteristics include crying out or moving close to the person in whose presence one feels more secure. Children may become "clingy," and spouses may become overprotective. Finally, internal working models of family relationships are cognitive mental schemas based on prior attachment experiences, including changes in attachment relationships after cancer in prior generations or earlier in life, current interactions between the person and family member when the attachment behavioral system is activated, or both (Berman & Sperling, 1994).

Attachment processes operate throughout the life cycle, beginning with their influence on infant behavior during times of danger or threatened separation from the primary caretaker. Expressing distress and seeking closeness to a significant other triggers the complementary "caregiving response" in the person with whom an attachment relationship had been previously established. Ainsworth and colleagues (Ainsworth, Blehar, Waters, & Wall, 1978) developed an experimental procedure called the strange situation, which enabled the documentation of children's differences in the use of their parents for calming. Observations of reunion behavior after an experimental separation were used to classify differences in both the infant and the parental behavior. Children with a secure attachment were found to greet the returning parent with open arms. The parents of these children then responded promptly and appropriately so that the infant was easily calmed. Those children with an insecure attachment, however, displayed three types of behavior. Some displayed an "avoidant" style by keeping away from their mothers at the reunion, which prompted the mothers to provide less affectionate holding. Others maintained an "ambivalent" response by acting clingy and remaining distressed, which was a response to inconsistent sensitivity by their mothers. A third group of insecure infants identified later by Main and Hesse (1990) showed a "disorganized" pattern of responding. These infants were both avoidant and resistant, demonstrating more disorganized behaviors. Throughout the lifetime, these attachment and caregiving responses are mutually reinforced reciprocal patterns in an attachment relationship (Hinde, 1982), which has enduring and irreplaceable bonds (Bowlby, 1969, 1988).

Differences in individual attachment style develop out of attachment experiences in each person's life. They form the basis for the unfolding of family relational processes, which are highly relevant to psychological adjustment to many life events, including cancer. Wynne (1988) applied the findings related to attachment researchers in his epigenetic model of enduring family relational systems. His model informs our understanding of changes in family relationships in response to the cancer experience.

Wynne expanded on Bowlby's observations of a developmental hierarchy of capacities within the individual to describe development within relationships. He describes change in family systems as *epigenetic*. Epigenesis (Singer & Wynne, 1965) refers to

> events of *becoming (genesis)* [italics added] that build *upon (epi)* [italics added] the immediate preceding events. Constitutional and experiential influences recombine in each phase to create new potentialities. This determines the next phase. If the transactions at any given phase are distorted or omitted, all the subsequent phases will be altered because they build upon a different substrate. (p. 208)

We would then predict that activation of attachment relational processes in response to cancer would trigger an epigenetic sequence of development in family relational capacities. If secure attachments are activated and reinforced through sensitive responsiveness of family members to the cancer distress, then revisions of other relational capacities are likely to occur without distortion or impasse. Attachment relational processes, in Wynne's epigenetic model, are the substrate from which other family processes are developed (Wynne, 1988). Four capacities for relating within the family that arise in the epigenetic process are attachment/caregiving, communication, joint problem solving, and mutuality. Each process can be thought of as the positive side of a domain, which also has its converse. For example, separation is the converse of attachment; optimal relationship function includes fluctuations between separation and attachment behaviors. Through recursive, "circular" processes, each level of relational process influences adjacent levels. For instance, the quality of communicating shapes the security of attachment within relationships.

Communication is characterized as optimal when there is shared focusing of attention and a belief in a shared social reality. If this communicative sharing is not accomplished, then the security of attachment will not be reinforced, and eventually it will deteriorate to some derivative of insecurity or the relationship will be abolished. Families in which a member has cancer need to communicate their individual experiences of threat so that a shared understanding of needs and appropriateness of attachment and caregiving behaviors can occur.

Joint problem solving involves shared engagement in tasks that create the potential for relational growth (Wynne, 1970). Over time, roles develop as a result of the repetition of task-related transactions to accomplish tasks. Joint problem solving has been described as the bridge between relational processes and family structures, such as roles. For example, when a woman has cancer, her role often needs to shift dramatically during cancer treatment from predominantly caregiving for others to seeking care for herself. New problem-solving strategies are needed when a parent with cancer is unable to carry out his or her usual activities, such as driving children to after-school events, house cleaning, or planning a vacation.

Mutuality is the "flexible, adaptive pattern of relational continuity that incorporates change" (Wynne & Wynne, 1986, p. 385). Mutuality incorporates both distancing or disengagement and constructive reengagement as new circumstances make old ways of communicating and problem solving ineffective. A family that is able to relate with mutuality maintains its composition of membership but changes the roles that its members take in response to a new situation.

Cancer requires the family to revise its ways of relating; therefore, mutuality is a crucial determinant of the threat to the family life course from cancer. Problems related to cancer care require family members to shift roles, which must be mutually determined by the people involved. If common ground is not created, the relationship is at risk for rupture or for the development of pseudomutuality, when family composition is maintained but a secure and responsive base for relating has been lost.

Our observations of differences in family patterns of engagement, when cancer threatens to separate them from the patient, are consistent with the differences in attachment based on family relational processes described previously.

FAMILY RELATIONAL PROCESSES BASED ON ATTACHMENT

We use the word *family* to designate a group of individuals with close personal relationships whose identities develop in conjunction with one another over time. The family affects the lives of its members through the patterning and quality of relatedness more than through the number of members or its formal designations (marriage, family, intimate partnership, etc.). This definition allows us to use a common approach to "families" with varying compositions of individuals and across different cultural and ethnic groups.

Cancer threatens to separate the patient from his or her family members, both emotionally and physically. Family relational processes modulate the impact of the cancer-related threat on the life course of the family. Secure family relationships protect the family from the destructive impact of stressful life events on the psychological adjustment of family members and on the family life course. Conger and colleagues (Conger, Ge, Elder, Lorenz, & Simons, 1994; Conger, Patterson, & Ge, 1995) demonstrated that the effects of external stress on individual family members are mediated through changes in family relationships. They studied 225 Iowa families facing severe economic threat and found increased marital conflict and parental depression in some families. The same families were visited 1 year after the first contact. Increased marital conflict, documented in the previous year, predicted hostility in the parent-child relationship and depression and antisocial behavior in adolescents. A direct effect of economic stress on the outcomes of the children was not detected, supporting the notion that changes in the security of familial relationships mediate destructive effects of economic threat on adolescent psychological adjustment (Whitbeck et al., 1991). The cancer threat can act in a similar manner, with changes in relationships affecting the psychological adjustment of family members more than the cancer.

Insecure relationships are especially vulnerable to the destructive effects of threats. Individuals with insecure working models of

attachment are most at risk for prolonged distress from cancer, which is not assuaged by nonhousehold social support. The uniqueness of the cancer experience leaves patients feeling as if no one understands their terror and alienation (Bahnson, 1975). A person with insecure working models of attachment relationships may expect misunderstanding, criticism, rejection, burdensome care seeking from others, or all of these in response to his or her disclosure of distress about cancer treatments or fear of death (Levitt, Coffman, Guacci-Franco, & Loveless, 1994). He or she would therefore limit self-disclosure and requests for support (Mikulincer & Nachshon, 1991; Simpson, Rholes, & Nelligan, 1992). Such behavior may take the form of repressive coping, in which individuals minimize their distress in an attempt to conform to make other family members more comfortable or to appear more "normal." Repressive coping is thought to be a risk factor for more rapid disease progression by some investigators (Temoshok, 1985; Weihs, Enright, Simmens, & Reiss, 2000; Weinberger, 1990). It may also be expressed as depressed mood, irritability, and decreased social functioning.

A "cancer legacy" from the past may introduce distortions in otherwise secure family relationships. Cancer-related losses of relationships or painful, maladaptive interchanges during the illness of loved ones in the past may increase the sense of danger from cancer to the family (Rolland, 1994). Patients who fear that they will be a burden to their family may avoid disclosure of distress and thereby foreclose opportunities for comforting responses. Such withholding can signal family members to separate themselves from the patient, creating an avoidant pattern of relating with decreased communication about the cancer and decreased availability of joint problem solving for addressing the treatment needs of the patient.

Alternatively, increased security may develop in a family when such cancer legacies are revised during a new episode of cancer. When sensitive supportive responding is used to calm the distress of members threatened with separation or loss, a new and deeper sense of closeness and security may occur. In this way, the cancer experience is an opportunity for some families to revise the cancer legacy, feeling more secure in their ability to care for one another and actively manage the cancer treatment and its effects.

The Impact of Cancer on Family Relationships Varies with Security of Attachment

The threat of cancer to the family can best be estimated by understanding the personal and social contexts. Veach and Nicholas (1998) discussed the clinical course of cancer and its relation to three stages of family development: the newly forming family, the young family, and the aging family. The newly forming family consists of a married couple with no children struggling to become independent from their families of origins (Veach & Nicholas, 1998). The threat of cancer may challenge the new family bonds the couple has formed. In the absence of a secure attachment relationship, a partner might show emotional over-involvement, emotional withdrawal, or hostility toward the cancer patient. This response might lead one or both partners to turn to a more stable family setting, perhaps each partner's family of origin (Veach & Nicholas, 1998). Researchers have shown that newer couples experience more stress than older couples as a result of cancer diagnosis (O'Mahoney & Carroll, 1997; Skerrett, 1998).

The young family, consisting of a married couple with young children, often has the most difficulty coping with the threat of cancer (O'Mahoney & Carroll, 1997; Veach & Nicholas, 1998). Members of young families are focused on establishing stability and roles for each other. With the threat of cancer,

children often assume parental roles, and the parent-child relationships and boundaries are disrupted temporarily. During adolescence, the gradual development of familial responsibilities is crucial to maintaining a solid family environment as adolescents struggle between wanting more independence from their parents and still looking to them for support and reassurance. Thus, changes in relationships as a result of a threat can particularly affect the psychological adjustment of adolescents (Spira & Kenemore, 2000; Lewis, 1996). The quality of adolescent peer relationships can decline, their self-esteem can suffer, and their behavior problems can increase as more illness-related demands are placed on the family (Lewis, 1996).

Furthermore, children might feel guilt about their parent's diagnosis or internal conflict about caring for their parent while maintaining their own interests or both (Veach, 1999). Parents might struggle with deciding on appropriate information to share with their younger children (Sherman & Simonton, 2001), finding external resources to help with transportation and household duties relating to their children (Veach, 1999), and worrying about whether they will be able to parent their children through adulthood (Skerrett, 1998). These struggles are more difficult among families with trouble communicating or poor problem solving or both.

Finally, the aging family, consisting of an older patient with grown children, must cope with its own unique set of stressors. Grown children might not live in the patient's household or even in a nearby geographic location, and caretaking is often more difficult in the absence of some family members (O'Mahoney & Carroll, 1997; Veach, 1999). Older couples managing cancer are often at risk for relational, psychological, and health-related distress (Shields, Travis, & Rousseau, 2000). Since the caregiving response more naturally occurs among those who are securely attached (Hinde, 1982), these challenges are likely to be exacerbated in families with insecure patterns of attachment.

When a child has cancer, families must cope with maintaining family function despite disruption of their routines, much like when an adult has cancer. However, parents often try to mask their distress because they fear upsetting the sick child or because they feel guilty about the child's illness (Sawyer et al., 1998). When parents do not adequately cope with their distress, they can negatively affect the psychological adjustment of the child (Sawyer et al., 1998). As with families of adult patients, the family's use of appropriate communication about cancer, although difficult for many parents, can aid in the family's adjustment to cancer diagnosis in children (Sherman & Simonton, 2001).

The Impact on Family Relationships Varies with Clinical Course of Cancer

The clinical course of cancer affects the threat that families encounter (Rolland, 1994; Suinn & VandenBos, 1999). Each phase of the illness presents the possibility of revision in attachment style within the family and thereby the substrate for resilience or vulnerability to destructive changes in life course in response to cancer.

Researchers often discuss four phases of cancer: initial diagnosis, treatment, recovery and survival, and disease progression and recurrence (Sherman & Simonton, 2001; Veach, 1999; Veach & Nicholas, 1998). During the initial diagnosis of cancer, patients and family members often feel shock, anxiety, confusion, and fear about the uncertainty of the illness (Halford et al., 2000; Sherman & Simonton, 2001; Veach & Nicholas, 1998). Some refer to these issues as

the "existential plight" of cancer (Weisman & Worden, 1976), which takes place during the first 100 days after cancer diagnosis. During this time, families must deal with the sudden vulnerability of one of their members while also changing roles and priorities within the family structure to accommodate their new uncertainty. Some researchers have found that wives of cancer patients are often more distressed than the patients during the initial diagnosis phase, possibly because they often take on the burden of caregiving (Carlson et al., 2000).

During the second phase of cancer, the treatment phase, families must cope with the decision making about biomedical treatment, frequent medical appointments, treatment side effects (fatigue, hair loss, nausea, and pain), and further disruption in the family routine (Halford et al., 2000; O'Mahoney & Carroll, 1997; Sherman & Simonton, 2001; Veach & Nicholas, 1998). The side effects of treatment can also lead to sexual difficulties for couples (Halford et al., 2000; O'Mahoney & Carroll, 1997). The financial stress resulting from medical expenses and time off from work for both the patient and the spouse can increase distress in both parents and children (Sherman & Simonton, 2001). Despite these changes, many also feel relieved and empowered during this phase because of the active response taken to fight the disease (Sherman & Simonton, 2001; Veach & Nicholas, 1998).

The third phase of cancer has been described as the recovery and survival phase. Patients are no longer undergoing active treatment for their cancer, leaving some families feeling vulnerable and passive upon resuming daily routines (Veach & Nicholas, 1998). Many patients and family members feel a sense of uncertainty about the future and a fear of recurrence, causing them to reevaluate their roles, goals, priorities, or spiritual values or all of these (Halford et al., 2000; Sherman & Simonton, 2001).

Unfortunately, many of the psychological and physical effects of cancer can persist for several years (Halford et al., 2000), but patients and families are often left with weaker support because others may not recognize these lingering effects. Conflicts can arise between family members who wish to leave the experience behind them and those who are still struggling with the disease effects (Sherman & Simonton, 2001). The life course of the family may also be challenged during this phase with fewer external resources to help cope with the threat of cancer recurrence.

If the cancer recurs, spouses, especially husbands, experience extreme distress because they must deal with the possibility of losing their partner (Carlson et al., 2000). Existential and spiritual issues often reemerge in the family as the patient often undergoes more aggressive medical treatment (Sherman & Simonton, 2001). During this phase, the unpredictability of the illness again challenges the ongoing security of the family to defend its vital functions against the cancer intruder. Death and premature resolution of their life course is the final phase of the cancer experience for many patients and their families.

Silberfarb, Mauer, and Crouthamel (1980) report the phase of disease recurrence to be the most distressing for patients and families. Security in family relationships is crucial at later stages of disease when the family may already be severely taxed by the illness experience. If security in the family is low during remission of the cancer, the family could face recurrent disease without the ability to function together. Preservation and restoration of family function during each phase of illness are needed to prevent the deterioration of relationships as the disease progresses. This can be achieved through effective communication and attention to each family member's needs during the different phases of the illness. During the

recurrence phase, issues of identity, existential meaning, preserving quality of life, sustaining the caregivers, and confronting mortality should be addressed within the family or with a trained professional to help strengthen family function (Sherman & Simonton, 2001).

CANCER AND MARITAL RELATIONSHIPS

Marital status has been studied extensively as a predictor of cancer outcome. Results remain inconsistent, however. Some studies combining men and women show a survival advantage to being married (House, Robbins, & Metzner, 1982; Kravdel, 2001; Ren, 1997), whereas others have failed to find such effects (Murphy, Goldblatt, Thornton-Jones, & Silcocks, 1990; Neale, 1994). Studies of women with breast cancer often show no effect or negative effects of marriage on length of life (Forsen, 1991). Two separate studies reported an advantage in survival time for unmarried women with breast cancer compared to those who are married (Ell et al., 1992; Waxler-Morrison et al., 1991). It is possible that the type of cancer, the patient's gender, the racial background of the couple, or all three may explain some of the conflicting results (Kravdel, 2001; Zhu, Weiss, Schwartz, & Daling, 1994).

Marital quality has not been studied extensively as a prognostic factor for disease outcome in cancer patients, but there is evidence that the quality of the marital relationship can influence disease recovery (Burman & Margolin, 1992). Research by Weihs and Enright (2003) found that women who confide in their spouses during times of stress have a better prognosis for survival from breast cancer. In addition to physical health benefits, higher marital quality can decrease the level of patient distress in response to cancer and can lead to fewer illness-specific adjustment problems (Rodrigue & Park, 1996). Kayser and colleagues (1999) demonstrated that women with breast cancer who reported highly mutual partner relationships had better quality of life ratings and less depression than women whose partner relationships were not perceived as highly mutual. In the same group of women, symptoms of cancer, length of illness, and socioeconomic status did not have a strong effect on the women's psychosocial adaptation. Giese-Davis and colleagues (2000) found similar results in their study of marital status and relationship quality among metastatic breast cancer patients and their partners. They found that relationship quality and distress of the patient's partner were associated with the patient's mood, whereas indices of disease status were not, further demonstrating the significance of the marital relationship as the mediator of the effects of cancer on psychological functioning.

CASE EXAMPLES

Families in which insecure attachment patterns predominate would be expected to exhibit distortions such as overinvolvement, avoidance, or criticism in response to expressions of distress about cancer. Wynne's model suggests that subsequent dysfunctions of communication, problem solving, and mutuality would also occur in these families. Insecure relational processes fail to provide a "holding environment" in which the distress associated with cancer can be shared and relieved for some or all family members. The distressed person does not receive a comforting and accepting response. Others might become distressed and focused on their own strong feelings (emotional overinvolvement), they might withdraw from the distressed person ("flat" detachment), or they might become controlling or hostile toward the person expressing distress. These responses

do not promote security in the relationship. Whether they transform the meaning of the previous relationship depends on the meaning of the exchange to the family members involved.

There are many proposed strategies to help patients and family members cope with the disruption of cancer in their lives, particularly those struggling with insecure relational processes. Some strategies, such as support groups or family therapy or both, can help strengthen relationships by fostering communication and emotional expression in families. Normalizing the disruptive effect of cancer on family life is an essential component of these psychological interventions (Gonzalez, Steinglass, & Reiss, 1989). Furthermore, clinicians working with families with young children might want to ask the children to express their feelings through drawings or other nonverbal forms of communication. Clinicians can encourage the older family members to discuss the drawings with the children to help include even young family members in the illness experience (Sherman & Simonton, 2001).

In addition to enhancing family communication, during the early phases of cancer, some researchers and clinicians suggest that disengaged families should make schedules, lists, and organized routines to help restore order and create unity in the chaotic time of medical appointments, cancer treatments, and changing roles within the family (Sherman & Simonton, 2001). After treatment has ended, clinicians can encourage discussion about the different needs of each family member to maintain family cohesion. Insecure family members often avoid the topic of cancer because it reminds them of the illness-related stressors, leaving the patient feeling neglected as he or she continues to face the long-term effects of cancer (Sherman & Simonton, 2001). Therapists can address these issues in their work with the families.

The following vignette from our study of families of breast cancer patients includes the avoidant insecure relational process and demonstrates the cumulative destructive effect of inadequate attachment and caregiving exchanges. Family members may feel overwhelmed and unable to respond to their own emotions and those of the patient when asked about the cancer experience, leaving the patient feeling distressed. HK and her daughter found themselves in this situation after HK was diagnosed with breast cancer:

Patient: So what about you?

Daughter: Mom, don't ask me no questions (nervous laughter).

Patient: You have to say something. . . . How did you feel when you found out I had breast cancer?

Daughter: I don't have anything to say.

Patient: Hmm?

Daughter: I have nothing to say.

Patient: What did you think? How did you feel?

Daughter (raising voice slightly): I have nothing to say.

Patient: I think your brother should be here, I want to know how he feels.

Daughter: He'd have nothing to say.

Patient: He hasn't talked to the doctors because he hasn't been here. I'd still like to know how he feels. (No response. Long pause). Well, I feel good. So what do you have to say?

Daughter (almost yelling): I have nothing to say!

Patient: How did you feel when you found out I had breast cancer?

Daughter: Oh, I was sad (sarcastically).

This mother-daughter relationship exemplifies an insecure avoidant attachment relationship. Constricted communication about cancer prevents the reciprocal exchange of distress and caregiving. The lack of openness about the cancer increases insecurity in the mother-daughter attachment and perpetuates anxiety for both the mother and the daughter. Later in the interaction, the insecure, detached relationship style deteriorates to criticism with the threats of death engendered by cancer:

Patient: It hurts me when I am in bed.

Daughter (rolls her eyes and makes a motion with her head)

Patient: It hurts me when I sleep on it.

Daughter: So buy a new mattress!

Patient: I'll have to put money aside.

Daughter (rolls eyes again and says sarcastically): Oh, isn't that a hint!

Patient (long pause): Well, I don't really have a problem, I guess.

Daughter: Getting back and forth from the doctor's.

Patient: In the wintertime, I'll take the bus until the snow gets on the ground. So it's no problem.

Daughter: Then she'll say, (whines) 'Oh, I took the bus and it was soooo cold.'

Patient: I'll get some boots so I can walk when it's cold. I have about three more weeks left of my radiation. So it won't be that cold by then. So what else?

Daughter: Nothing, you're well now.

Patient: I'm not well. Y'all have never thought I was sick (nervous laughter). The only comments were, 'Mom, you feel all right?' I wanted [son's name] to say something, he acts like I have something contagious. I don't cook for him no more.

Daughter: He doesn't want you to?

Patient: He doesn't have time, or something.

Daughter: You do cook for him.

Patient: No, I don't. Not lately.

Again, the daughter did not respond to the patient's distress, nor was she communicative about her own stress. When the patient attempted to communicate her feelings about breast cancer, the daughter made sarcastic comments, feigned sympathy, or ignored the patient's concerns, leaving the patient feeling burdened with the need to take care of her problems alone. Early in the interaction, the patient even commented, "I just had to be strong so y'all didn't conk out. So I had to be strong." The patient seems to be saying, "I wish you would comfort me," but she only begins to communicate this feeling to her daughter. As soon as she suggests that the daughter could have been more supportive, she quickly changes the subject to her son out of fear of her daughter's criticism.

Another course is possible for families with insecure attachment styles who face cancer. The uniqueness of need, which arises

because of a malignant disease, may illicit new and more productive caregiving responses within the family. A more fruitful pattern of communicating with shared attention and meaning could then arise, feeding back to reinforce a more secure attachment. It is likely that this would occur in situations in which cancer is a novel threat, which can be responded to outside the family's usual patterns of behavior. Insecure families in which an earlier cancer experience has shaped their understanding of themselves, however, would be expected to have amplified fears as a result of the cancer diagnosis.

When disease severity is high, secure relationships may be insufficient to contain the distress. The transformation of relationships over the course of cancer is illustrated by the following family, whose secure attachments were challenged by the patient's illness:

Spouse: I don't know if I've said this to you before, but from the time you were diagnosed, I went through two changes. In the beginning, I wanted to support you. That's what I was trying to do. But afterwards, I went through a time when I truly couldn't accept it. Since the conversation we had 3 months ago, my eyes have opened up. And I hope truthfully that what you're seeing is a lot better than what it was.

Patient (nodding head): Yup.

Spouse: I was really unfair.

Patient: Majorly in denial.

Spouse: The bad part about it was, it's like I told mom and I even mentioned it to you. I found solace in beer cans, a glass of wine, a drink, a computer, every place except where I needed it and that's in the family. I was afraid to talk about it, I was afraid to face it, but I didn't think I was afraid. I just thought I was being really brave and solid.

This patient's spouse distanced himself from the patient out of fear and shock upon the initial diagnosis of cancer. The demands for emotional involvement were beyond his ability to respond, although he wanted to support the patient. After the patient confronted her spouse about his avoidance of her cancer, however, the communication and mutuality of family process allowed him to fulfill his role as a supportive family member. The couple then reported feeling closer as a result of the cancer threat.

CONCLUSION

We have described a model of relational development in families when a member has cancer. It is founded on the notion that the threat of cancer is modulated by the security of attachment, such that attachment and caregiving systems are activated in most patients and family members when cancer-related risks of separation and loss become apparent. The magnitude of threat experienced by each patient and family is the product of its particular high-risk characteristics and varies greatly from family to family. It is within this particular system that the threat of cancer arises for a particular patient.

Wynne's epigenetic model of relational processes, combined with the stage of family development and the phase of cancer, is proposed as a template for distinguishing the type of distortions potentially found in a population of cancer patients and their families. Family therapists suggest that intervention that addresses the specific level of distortion or impasse in family development may help the natural developmental processes in relationships to flourish (Hill, Fonagy, Safier, & Sargent, 2003). Further application of the epigenetic model of family relational processes is likely to be fruitful for understanding and promoting resilience in the cancer patient and his or her family.

REFERENCES

Ainsworth, M. D. S., Blehar, M. C., Waters, E., & Wall, S. (1978). *Patterns of attachment: A psychological study of the strange situation.* Hillsdale, NJ: Lawrence Erlbaum.

American Cancer Society. (2003). *Cancer facts and figures.* Retrieved August 25, 2003, from http://www.cancer.org

Arpin, K., Fitch, M., Browne, G. B., & Corey, P. (1990). Prevalence and correlates of family dysfunction and poor-adjustment to chronic illness in specialty clinics. *Journal of Clinical Epidemiology, 43,* 373-383.

Bahnson, C. B. (1975). Psychologic and emotional issues in cancer: The psychotherapeutic care of the cancer patient. *Seminars in Oncology, 2,* 293-309.

Baider, L., Koch, U., Esacson, R., & Kaplan-DeNour, A. (1998). Prospective study of cancer patients and their spouses: The weakness of marital strength. *Psycho-Oncology, 7,* 49-56.

Ben-Zur, H. (2001). Your coping strategy and my distress: Inter-spouse perceptions of coping and adjustment among breast cancer patients and their spouses. *Families, Systems, & Health, 19,* 83-94.

Berman, W. H., & Sperling, M. B. (1994). The structure and function of adult attachment. In M. B. Sperling & W. H. Berman (Eds.), *Attachment in adults* (pp. 1-30). New York: Guilford.

Bloom, J. R., Pendergrass, S. M., & Burnell, G. M. (1984). Social functioning of women with breast cancer: Validation of a clinical scale. *Journal of Psychological Oncology, 2,* 93-101.

Bowlby, J. (1969). *Attachment & loss* (2nd ed., Vol. 1). New York: Basic Books.

Bowlby, J. (1988). *A secure base.* New York: Basic Books.

Brown, G., & Harris, T. (Eds.). (1989). *Life events and illness.* New York: Guilford.

Burman, B., & Margolin, G. (1992). Analysis of the association between marital relationships and health problems: An interactional perspective. *Psychological Bulletin, 112,* 39-63.

Carlson, L. E., Bultz, B. D., Speca, M., & St.-Pierre, M. (2000). Partners of cancer patients: Part II. Current psychosocial interventions and suggestions for improvements. *Journal of Psychosocial Oncology, 18*(3), 33-43.

Conger, R., Ge, X., Elder, G., Lorenz, F., & Simons, R. (1994). Economic stress, coercive family process and developmental problems of adolescents. *Child Development, 65,* 541-561.

Conger, R., Patterson, G., & Ge, X. (1995). Parental stress and child adjustment: An across-site replication. *Child Development, 66,* 80-97.

Derogatis, L. R., Morrow, G. R., Fetting, J., Penman, D., Piasetsky, S., Schmale, A. M., et al. (1983). The prevalence of psychiatric disorders among cancer patients. *Journal of the American Medical Association, 249,* 751-757.

Edwards, B. K., Howe, H. L., Ries, L. A. G., Thun, M. J., Rosenberg, H. M., Yancik, R., et al. (2002). Annual report to the nation on the status of cancer, 1973-1999, featuring implications of age and aging on the U.S. cancer burden. *Cancer, 94,* 2766-2792.

Ell, K., Nishimoto, R., Mediansky, L., Mantell, J., & Hamovitch, M. (1992). Social relations, social support and survival among patients with cancer. *Journal of Psychosomatic Research, 36,* 531-541.

Ell, K., Nishimoto, R., Morvay, T., Mantell, J., & Hamovitch, M. (1989). A longitudinal analysis of psychological adaptation among survivors of cancer. *Cancer, 63,* 406-446.

Ferrell, B., Ervin, K., Smith, S., Marek, T., & Melancon, C. (2002). Family perspectives of ovarian cancer. *Cancer Practice, 10*(6), 269-276.

Forsen, A. (1991). Psychological stress as a risk factor for breast cancer. *Psychotherapy and Psychosomatics, 55,* 176-185.

Giese-Davis, J., Hermanson, K., Koopman, C., Weibel, C., & Spiegel, D. (2000). Quality of couples' relationship and adjustment to metastatic breast cancer. *Journal of Family Psychology, 14*(2), 251-266.

Gonzalez, S., Steinglass, P., & Reiss, D. (1989). Putting the illness in its place: Discussion groups for families with chronic medical illnesses. *Family Process, 28,* 69-87.

Grassi, L., & Rosti, G. (1996). Psychosocial morbidity and adjustment to illness among long-term cancer survivors: A six-year-follow-up study. *Psychosomatics, 37,* 523-532.

Halford, W. K., Scott, J. L., & Smythe, J. (2000). Couples and coping with cancer: Helping each other through the night. In K. B. Schmaling & T. G. Sher (Eds.), *The psychology of couples and illness: Theory, research, & practice* (pp. 135-170). Washington, DC: American Psychological Association.

Hill, J., Fonagy, P., Safier, E., & Sargent, F. (2003). The ecology of attachment in the family. *Family Process, 42,* 205-221.

Hinde, R. A. (1982). Attachment: Some conceptual and biological issues. In C. M. Parks & J. Stevenson-Hinde (Eds.), *The place of attachment in human behavior* (pp. 31-53). New York: Basic Books.

House, J. S., Robbins, C., & Metzner, H. L. (1982). The association of social relationships and activities with mortality: Prospective evidence from the Tecumseh Community Health Study. *American Journal of Epidemiology, 116*(1), 123-140.

Kayser, K., Sormanti, M., & Strainchamps, E. (1999). Women coping with cancer: The influence of relationship factors on psychosocial adjustment. *Psychology of Women Quarterly, 23,* 725-730.

Kravdel, O. (2001). The impact of marital status on cancer survival. *Social Science & Medicine, 52,* 357-368.

Levitt, M., Coffman, S., Guacci-Franco, N., & Loveless, S. (1994). Attachment relationships and life transitions: An expectancy model. In M. B. Sperling & W. H. Berman (Eds.), *Attachment in adults* (pp. 232-235). New York: Guilford.

Levy, S. M., Herberman, R. B., Lippman, M., D'Angelo, T., & Lee, J. (1991). Immunological and psychosocial predictors of disease recurrence in patients with early stage breast cancer. *Behavioral Medicine, 17*(2), 67-75.

Lewis, F. M. (1996). The impact of breast cancer on the family: Lessons learned from the children and adolescents. In L. Baider, C. L. Cooper, & A. Kaplan-DeNour (Eds.), *Cancer and the family* (pp. 271-287). New York: John Wiley.

Lewis, F. M., Woods, N. F., Hough, E. E., & Bensley, L. S. (1989). The family's functioning with chronic illness in the mother: The spouse's perspective. *Social Science and Medicine, 29,* 1261-1269.

Main, M., & Hesse, E. (1990). Parents' unresolved traumatic experiences are related to infant disorganized attachment status: Is frightened and/or frightening parental behavior the linking mechanism? In M. Greenberg, D. Cicchetti, & E. Cummings (Eds.), *Attachment in the preschool years* (pp. 161-185). Chicago: University of Chicago Press.

Manne, S. L. (1999). Intrusive thoughts and psychological distress among cancer patients: The role of spouse avoidance and criticism. *Journal of Consulting and Clinical Psychology, 67,* 539-546.

Mikulincer, M., & Nachshon, O. (1991). Attachment styles and patterns of self-disclosure. *Journal of Personality and Social Psychology, 61,* 321-331.

Murphy, M., Goldblatt, P., Thornton-Jones, H., & Silcocks, P. (1990). Survival among women with cancer of the uterine cervix: Influence of marital status and social class. *Journal of Epidemiology & Community Health, 44*(4), 293-296.

Neale, A. V. (1994). Racial and marital status influences on 10 year survival from breast cancer. *Journal of Clinical Epidemiology, 47*(5), 475-483.

Northouse, L. L., Mood, D., Templin, T., Mellon, S., & George, T. (2000). Couples' patterns of adjustment to colon cancer. *Social Science & Medicine, 50,* 271-284.

O'Mahoney, J. M., & Carroll, R. A. (1997). The impact of breast cancer and its treatment on marital functioning. *Journal of Clinical Psychology in Medical Settings, 4*(4), 397-415.

Omne-Ponten, M., Holmberg, L., Bergstrom, R., Sjoden, P., & Burns, T. (1993). Psychosocial adjustment among husbands of women treated for breast cancer: Mastectomy vs. breast-conserving surgery. *European Journal of Cancer, 29A,* 1393-1397.

Ren, X. S. (1997). Marital status and quality of relationships: The impact on health perception. *Social Science & Medicine, 44,* 241-249.

Reynolds, P., Boyd, P. T., Blacklow, R. S., Jackson, J. S., Greenberg, R. S., Austin, D. F., et al. (1994). Relationship between social ties and survival in black and white breast cancer patients. *Cancer Epidemiology, Biomarkers & Prevention, 3,* 253-259.

Rodrigue, J. R., & Park, T. L. (1996). General and illness-specific adjustment to cancer: Relationship to marital status and marital functioning. *Journal of Psychosomatic Research, 40*(1), 29-36.

Rolland, J. S. (1994). *Families, illness, and disability: An integrative treatment model.* New York: Basic Books.

Sawyer, M. G., Streiner, D. L., Antoniou, G., Toogood, I., & Rice, M. (1998). Influence of parental and family adjustment on the later psychological adjustment of children treated for cancer. *Journal of the American Academy of Child and Adolescent Psychiatry, 37*(8), 915-922.

Sherman, A. C., & Simonton, S. (2001). Coping with cancer in the family. *Family Journal: Counseling and Therapy for Couples and Families, 9*(2), 193-200.

Shields, C. S., Travis, L. A., & Rousseau, S. L. (2000). Marital attachment and adjustment in older couples coping with cancer. *Aging & Mental Health, 4,* 223-233.

Silberfarb, P. M., Mauer, L. H., & Crouthamel, C. S. (1980). Psychosocial aspects of neoplastic disease: I. Functional status of breast cancer patients during different treatment regimens. *American Journal of Psychiatry, 137*(4), 450-455.

Simpson, J., Rholes, W., & Nelligan, J. (1992). Support seeking and support giving within couples in an anxiety-provoking situation: The role of attachment styles. *Journal of Personality and Social Psychology, 62,* 434-446.

Singer, M. T., & Wynne, L. C. (1965). Thought disorder and family relations of schizophrenics: IV. Results and implications. *Archives of General Psychiatry, 12,* 201-212.

Skerrett, K. (1998). Couple adjustment to the experience of breast cancer. *Families, Systems, and Health, 16*(3), 281-298.

Spira, M., & Kenemore, E. (2000). Adolescent daughters of mothers with breast cancer: Impact and implications. *Clinical Social Work Journal, 28,* 183-195.

Suinn, R. M., & VandenBos, G. R. (1999). *Cancer patients and their families: Readings on disease course, coping, and psychological interventions.* Washington, DC: American Psychological Association.

Temoshok, L. (1985). Biopsychosocial studies on cutaneous malignant melanoma: Psychosocial factors associated with prognostic indicators, progression, psychophysiology and tumor-host response. *Social Science & Medicine, 20*(8), 833-840.

Trask, P. C., Paterson, A. G., Trask, C. L., Bares, C. B., Birt, J., & Maan, C. (2003). Parent and adolescent adjustment to pediatric cancer: Associations with coping, social support, and family function. *Journal of Pediatric Oncology Nursing, 20*(1), 36-47.

Veach, T. A. (1999). Families of adult cancer patients. *Journal of Family Psychotherapy, 10*(1), 43-60.

Veach, T. A., & Nicholas, D. R. (1998). Understanding families of adults with cancer: Combining the clinical course of cancer and stages of family development. *Journal of Counseling and Development, 76,* 144-156.

Waxler-Morrison, N., Hislop, G. T., Mears, B., & Kan, L. (1991). Effects of social relationships on survival for women with breast cancer: A prospective study. *Social Science & Medicine, 33,* 177-183.

Weber, M. (1964). *The theory of social and economic organization* (A. M. Henderson & T. Parsons, Trans.) (pp. 9-10). New York: Free Press. (Original work published 1947)

Weihs, K. L. (2001). Social support network size predicts breast cancer recurrence and mortality, after control for disease severity. *Psychosomatic Medicine, 63*(1), 153.

Weihs, K. L., Enright, T., & Simmens, S. (2002). High quality spousal or long-term partner relationships predict time to recurrence of breast cancer, after control for disease severity. *Psychosomatic Medicine, 64*(1), 107.

Weihs, K. L., Enright, T. M., Simmens, S. J., & Reiss, D. (2000). Negative affectivity, restriction of emotions and site of metastases predict mortality in recurrent breast cancer. *Journal of Psychosomatic Research, 49*(1), 59-68.

Weinberger, D. A. (1990). The construct validity of the repressive coping style. In J. L. Singer (Ed.), *Repression and dissociation implication for personality theory, psychopathology, and health* (pp. 337-386). Chicago: University of Chicago Press.

Weisman, M. D., & Worden, J. W. (1976). The existential plight in cancer: Significance of the first 100 days. *International Journal of Psychiatry in Medicine, 7,* 1-15.

Whitbeck, L., Simons, R., Conger, R., Lorenz, F., Huck, S., & Elder, G. (1991). Family economic hardship, parental support, and adolescent self-esteem. *Social Psychology Quarterly, 54,* 353-363.

Wynne, L. C. (1970). Communication disorders and the quest for relatedness in families of schizophrenics. *American Journal of Psychoanalysis, 30,* 100-114.

Wynne, L. C. (1988). An epigenetic model of family processes. In C. J. Falicov (Ed.), *Family transitions: Continuity and change over the life cycle* (pp. 81-106). New York: Guilford.

Wynne, L. C., & Wynne, A. R. (1986). The quest for intimacy. *Journal of Marital and Family Therapy, 12,* 383-394.

Zhu, K., Weiss, N. S., Schwartz, S. M., & Daling, J. R. (1994). Assessing the relationship between marital status and cancer incidence: Methodologic considerations. *Cancer Causes & Control, 5*(1), 83-87.

CHAPTER 2

Hostility, Marriage, and the Heart

The Social Psychophysiology of Cardiovascular Risk in Close Relationships

TIMOTHY W. SMITH AND KELLY M. GLAZER

Coronary heart disease (CHD) is the leading cause of death in most industrialized nations, including the United States, where it is responsible for approximately 450,000 deaths each year (American Heart Association, 2004). In the current U.S. population of healthy 40-year-old adults, approximately one third of the women and nearly one half of the men will develop CHD at some point in their life. Each year in the United States, individuals experience approximately 1 million initial or recurrent coronary events, with associated annual costs in direct medical care, disability, and lost productivity exceeding $100 billion (American Heart Association, 2004). Obviously, CHD represents a critically important health problem.

Approaches to the prevention and management of CHD have been guided by evidence of the role of modifiable risk factors. For example, smoking, high levels of cholesterol in the blood, high blood pressure, high blood glucose, obesity, and low levels of regular physical activity confer increased risk of CHD; modification of these characteristics can reduce risk and improve prognosis. These traditional risk factors, however, even when combined with unmodifiable CHD risk factors such as increasing age, male sex, and a positive family history, provide an incomplete account of the causal influences on this disease. A growing body of evidence indicates that psychosocial characteristics can confer increased risk of the onset and unfavorable course of CHD above and beyond the influence of the traditional risk factors. These include low socioeconomic status, depressive symptoms and disorders, other negative emotional traits (e.g., anxiety and pessimism), acute and chronic stress, and social isolation and conflict (Kop, 1999; Krantz & McCeney, 2002; Rozanski, Blumenthal, & Kaplan, 1999; Smith & Ruiz, 2002). The identification of psychosocial risk factors not only expands our understanding of influences on this prevalent and costly disease but also suggests additional avenues for prevention and management.

The personality trait of hostility is one of the most widely studied and well-documented of the psychosocial risk factors (Miller,

Smith, Turner, Guijarro, & Hallet, 1996; Smith, Glazer, Ruiz, & Gallo, 2004). An outgrowth of prior interest in the Type A coronary prone behavior pattern (Rosenmann, 1978; Smith, 1992), research on hostility has demonstrated that several related individual differences confer increased risk of CHD and premature mortality from all causes (Miller et al., 1996; Smith et al., 2004). As typically used in this area of research (Smith, 1994), the term *hostility* refers to three related but distinct traits, only one of which is most accurately called "hostility." Individual differences in several emotions are often studied under the label of hostility, specifically the tendency to exhibit anger, irritation, resentment, and contempt. The term hostility, however, most accurately refers to individual differences in cognition, such as cynicism, mistrust, and the tendency to attribute aggressive intent to the actions of others. Individual differences in overt aggressive behavior have also been studied in this regard, such as verbal or physical aggressiveness.

Although typically conceptualized as simply a characteristic of the person, hostility and related traits are consistently related to important interpersonal experiences. For example, hostile people report low levels of social support and high levels of conflict compared to more agreeable people (Smith, 1992). Furthermore, these features of the social context of hostility may be essential elements of the mechanisms linking these personality traits to CHD. As a result, interpersonal processes are likely to be important considerations in understanding the health consequences of hostility and designing interventions to reduce them (Smith et al., 2004).

In this chapter, we review evidence that at least some of the effects of hostility on CHD and general health involve close relationships, specifically marriage. Hostility is associated with increased exposure to conflict and reduced levels of support in marriage, and both of these interpersonal experiences

are associated with increased risk of CHD and premature mortality (Smith & Ruiz, 2002). In addition, hostile people display increased physiological reactivity during stressful marital interactions, and these responses have been implicated in the initiation and progression of CHD (Smith & Ruiz, 2002). Therefore, a comprehensive understanding of the mechanisms linking hostility and health must include an examination of the context of marriage and other close relationships. Furthermore, if anger and hostility are included in interventions intended to reduce risk of initial or recurrent cardiovascular events, then the context of relationships may prove to be a useful addition to the usual individual focus of such treatments.

PATHOPHYSIOLOGY OF CORONARY HEART DISEASE AND THE ROLE OF STRESS

Understanding the effect of psychosocial risk factors on CHD requires an understanding of the nature of the disease and the basic psychophysiological processes through which personality, emotions, and the social environment may contribute to disease development. In the following sections, we describe the nature and development of CHD and the role of psychological stress in the underlying pathophysiological processes.

Coronary Artery Disease and Manifestations of CHD

The clinical manifestations of CHD include angina pectoris, myocardial infarction, and sudden coronary death. All three of these clinical end points result from coronary artery disease (CAD) or atherosclerosis in the arteries that supply blood to the heart. Beginning as early as childhood and becoming more common and extensive with age, lipids and related cells (e.g., macrophages and foam cells) accumulate in the walls of the coronary arteries in microscopic amounts, progressing into visible fatty streaks. Inflammatory and reparative processes at these sites contribute to the further development of these lesions through continuing intracellular deposition of lipids, the proliferation of smooth muscle cells, and extracellular accumulation of lipids (Becker, de Boer, & van der Wal, 2001; Ross, 1999). Hemodynamic (i.e., increased blood pressure and associated "sheer stress" within the artery) and neuroendocrine processes (e.g., circulating catecholamines) can further damage the endothelium or lining of the coronary arteries and contribute to lesion growth.

At later stages of CAD development, these expanding lesions develop fibrous tissues and calcification and are extensive enough to encroach into the lumen or opening within the artery through which blood flows. Sufficiently advanced CAD of this type can cause myocardial ischemia (i.e., insufficient oxygen supply to the heart muscle) when the reduced supply capacity caused by narrowing of these arteries cannot match the heart's demand for oxygen during times of physical exertion or emotional stress. This ischemia is often "silent" or without symptoms but also often causes stable angina, which is chest pain of cardiac origin that regularly occurs during physical exertion or emotional arousal.

Inflammatory and hemodynamic processes can also contribute to the progression of some CAD lesions to an unstable form and precipitate the rupture of such unstable plaques. Ruptured plaques contribute to the rapid formation of blood clots (i.e., thrombi), which in turn can cause sudden and severe blockage of the coronary blood supply. The resulting ischemia can cause unstable angina (i.e., rapidly worsening cardiac chest pain), myocardial infarction (i.e., death of heart muscle due to prolonged, severe ischemia), or sudden death. Sudden cardiac death is typically caused by a severe disturbance in the

rhythm of the heart, ventricular fibrillation, that is promoted by ischemia and causes a rapid cessation of systemic circulation.

The Role of Psychological Stress

Psychological stress has a variety of immediate physiological effects that are implicated in the initiation and progression of CAD as well as in the emergence of the clinical manifestations of CHD among people with advanced CAD (Kop, 1999; Smith & Ruiz, 2002). Cardiovascular reactivity (CVR) is perhaps the most extensively studied of these mechanisms. More frequent, pronounced, and prolonged increases in blood pressure, heart rate, and other cardiovascular responses (e.g., increases in sympathetic excitation of the heart and decreased parasympathetic activity) have been identified as contributing to the initial development and progression of CAD and atherosclerosis at other sites, and several studies support this view (Kop, 1999; Rozanski et al., 1999; Smith & Ruiz, 2002). Other physiological responses to stress that may promote CAD include increases in circulating catecholamines, cortisol, and plasma lipids; activation of blood platelets; and inflammatory responses (Kop, 1999, 2003).

Among people with established CAD, psychological stress can induce myocardial ischemia both in the laboratory, as assessed by a variety of techniques, and during daily activities, as assessed through ambulatory electrocardiograph (ECG) recording (Krantz & McCeney, 2002). Transient stress-induced ischemia may result when increases in the rate and force of myocardial contractions during psychological threats or challenges create increased oxygen demand in this tissue. This stress-induced increase in the heart's demand for oxygen may exceed the available supply because blood flow to the heart muscle is limited by occlusive lesions in the coronary arteries. Transient reductions in oxygen supply may also contribute to these effects. In segments of coronary artery without lesions, psychological stress causes vasodilation, presumably to accommodate the increased oxygen demand that occurs during such episodes. At the sites of CAD lesions, however, arteries typically do not dilate and may even constrict. Other physiological responses to stress that may contribute to ischemia and the emergence of manifestations of CHD among people with advanced CAD include increases in the activation of blood platelets, coagulation and viscosity of blood, and circulating levels of proinflammatory substances (Kop, 1999; Krantz & McCeney, 2002). Hence, the psychophysiological correlates of hostility during potentially stressful circumstances could have much to do with the long-term effects of this personality trait on cardiovascular disease and general health.

ASSOCIATION OF HOSTILITY WITH CARDIOVASCULAR AND GENERAL HEALTH

In evaluating the contribution of hostility to the development of CHD, three issues are central. First, the nature and adequacy of the measures of these individual differences in emotion, cognition, and social behavior must be considered. Second, the statistical association between these measures and CHD must be evaluated. Finally, the nature of the mechanisms potentially accounting for this association must be described and tested. Hence, the evidence regarding the health consequences of hostility consists of research on these three issues.

Assessment

A variety of measures have been used to assess individual differences in anger, hostility, and aggressiveness in studies of CHD and general health. To ensure that studies in this area are indeed evaluating the health consequences of these related traits, these measures must be reliable and valid (Smith, 1992; Smith et al., 2004). The most commonly used assessments are ratings of hostile behavior during the Type A structured interview (Rosenmann, 1978), the Cook and Medley (1954) hostility (Ho) scale derived from the Minnesota Multiphasic Personality Inventory, and other self-report scales such as the Buss-Perry Aggression Questionnaire (AQ) (Buss & Perry, 1992). Behavioral ratings of hostility can be made reliably and are generally stable over time (Barefoot & Lipkus, 1994). Similarly, with some exceptions (Smith & Gallo, 2001; Smith et al., 2004), these self-report measures are internally consistent and stable over time. In most cases, evaluations of construct validity have indicated that these assessments show expected associations with measures of conceptually related constructs and smaller associations with measures of conceptually dissimilar traits (i.e., convergent and divergent or discriminant validity, respectively).

These assessments are modestly intercorrelated, however, most likely because they use different methods (e.g., behavioral ratings vs. self-report) and tap different facets or aspects of the interrelated but distinct cognitive, affective, and behavioral components of this trait domain (Barefoot & Lipkus, 1994). Individuals may characteristically display hostility during social interactions, such as structured interviews, but be unwilling or unable to accurately describe this social style on self-report instruments, especially given the negative connotation of these behaviors and the susceptibility of self-report instruments to social desirability artifacts. Furthermore, even among self-report instruments, the content varies in terms of the relative emphasis on affective, cognitive, or behavioral traits, and these characteristics differ in important ways (Costa, McCrae, & Dembroski, 1989; Gallo & Smith, 1998). Hence, the association of hostility and health may vary across types of measures used to assess this multifaceted trait, and the mechanisms linking it to health may also vary as a function of which specific emotional, cognitive, or behavioral characteristic is considered.

Associations With CHD and Longevity

Although there are some inconsistencies among studies testing the prospective relationship between hostility and subsequent CHD and premature death, this literature generally indicates a robust effect. In a quantitative review of studies published before 1996, hostility was associated with increased risk of CHD and premature mortality (Miller et al., 1996), although this effect was stronger in studies that used behavioral ratings to assess this trait than in those that used self-reports of hostility. Since that time, several studies have confirmed this association. Among initially healthy people, high scores on various self-reports and behavioral ratings of hostility have been associated with increased risk of CHD, stroke, and early mortality (Chang, Ford, Meoni, Wang, & Klag, 2002; Everson et al., 1997, 1999; Kawachi, Sparrow, Spiro, Vokonas, & Weiss, 1996; Matthews, Gump, Harris, Haney, & Barefoot, 2004; Williams et al., 2000; Williams, Nieto, Sanford, Couper, & Tyroler, 2002), although some negative findings have been reported (Eng, Fitzmaurice, Kubzansky, Rimm, & Kawachi, 2003; Sykes et al., 2002).

In recent studies of people with established CHD, various measures of hostility have been associated with recurrent coronary events and progression of CAD (Angerer et al., 2000; Chaput et al., 2002; Goodman, Quigley, Moran, Meilman, & Sherman, 1996; Mendes De Leon, Kop, de Swart, Bar, & Appels, 1996), although some studies have reported negative findings in this population (Kaufman et al., 1999; Welin, Lappas, & Wilhelmsen, 2000).

Overall, the association between hostility and the initial occurrence of CHD and longevity among initially healthy people appears to be robust, whereas the association with the course of established CHD is somewhat more variable. This may be due to a selection artifact; given the consistent association of hostility with initial disease development and CHD death, hostile people who survive the initial occurrence of CHD may be more resilient than hostile people who did not. This would make it more difficult to detect the effects of hostility on health in clinical samples with established CHD (Williams, 2000).

The statistical association between hostility and CHD incidence among initially healthy people may reflect the effects of this personality trait at any number of time points in the decades-long development of this disease. That is, hostility may affect the initiation or rate of progression of asymptomatic CAD, the progression of stable CAD to unstable and imminently dangerous forms, or the occurrence of myocardial ischemia among people with advanced disease. Studies suggest that anger, hostility, and aggressiveness may influence several of these phases of the disease process. For example, in healthy individuals, these traits are associated with ultrasound measures of endothelial dysfunction, an early indication of atherosclerosis (Harris, Matthews, Sutton-Tyrrell, & Kuller, 2003). In other ultrasound assessments of healthy people, hostility has been associated with more extensive and more rapidly progressing carotid artery disease (Julkunen, Salonen, Kaplan, Chesney, & Salonen, 1994; Matthews, Owens, Kuller, Sutton-Tyrrell, & Jansen-McWilliams, 1998). Carotid artery disease contributes to stroke, but atherosclerosis in these arteries is often accompanied by CAD. Recent developments in computed tomography scan technology have provided similar noninvasive tests of CAD through the imaging of calcium deposits that occur at lesion sites. In one study using this approach, hostility was associated with CAD (Iribarren et al., 2000), but another study reported negative findings (O'Malley, Jones, Feuerstein, & Taylor, 2000). Thus, most, but not all, of the available evidence suggests that hostility may contribute to early stages of the disease process. Other research suggests that hostility predicts the development of high blood pressure (Rutledge & Hogan, 2002), and this effect of hostility may contribute to atherosclerosis.

Several methodologies have been used to evaluate the role of hostility in later stages of CHD. For example, among CHD patients, hostility is associated with greater myocardial ischemia during laboratory stressors (Burg, Jain, Soufer, Kerns, & Zaret, 1993; Helmers et al., 1993; Rosenberg et al., 2001). Similarly, among CHD patients, experimentally induced anger can produce myocardial ischemia (Ironson et al., 1992), and episodes of anger are associated with greater ischemia during daily activities, as measured by Holter monitoring of ambulatory ECG (Gabbay et al., 1996). Among patients hospitalized for acute myocardial infarction, interviews about activities and experiences preceding the emergence of symptoms of the unfolding coronary event indicate that like smoking and heavy physical exertion, anger is significantly more common immediately before the onset of the event than during similar time periods that were not followed by acute illness (Mittleman et al., 1995; Möller et al., 1999). Hence, across these very different methods, evidence suggests that anger and hostility can contribute to the emergence of manifestations of CHD among those with advanced disease.

Mechanisms Linking Hostility and Disease

A variety of mechanisms may underlie the associations among hostility, CHD, and mortality described previously. For example, it is possible that hostile people are prone to smoking, a sedentary lifestyle, and poor diet, and that these traditional behavioral risk factors may explain the association between hostility and health. Some evidence of this mechanism has emerged in epidemiological research. Everson et al. (1997) found that the association between hostility and subsequent CHD was accounted for by the fact that hostile people displayed higher levels of these behavioral or lifestyle risk factors. In most studies, however, the association between hostility and subsequent health remains significant even when behavioral risk factors are controlled. As a result, two additional pathways have received considerable attention in research: exposure to stressors and physiological reactivity to stressors.

Hostility and Exposure to Stressors

Individual differences in hostility are consistently related to increased exposure to a variety of stressors and to lower levels of stress, buffering social support. For example, compared to people who score low on various measures of anger and hostility, hostile people report higher levels of major life stressors, minor daily stressors or hassles, job stress, and other chronic stressors (Gallo & Smith, 1999; Smith, Pope, Sanders, Allred, & O'Keefe, 1988). Furthermore, hostility is also associated with reports of reduced levels of social support and greater levels of interpersonal conflict (Hart, 1999; McCann, Russo, & Benjamin, 1997; O'Neil & Emery, 2002). In studies sampling daily experiences directly, hostility is associated with more frequent and intense negative social interactions and with less frequent and less intense positive interactions (Brondolo et al., 2003). Given their role as risk factors for CHD (Smith & Ruiz, 2002), high levels of stress and low levels of social support constitute psychosocial vulnerability to cardiovascular and other illnesses, and these risk factors may account for the association between hostility and health (Smith, 1992).

The consistent association of hostility with low support and high stress likely reflects the impact of the hostile person's characteristic style of thought and behavior on the social context. That is, by expecting mistreatment, attributing hostile intent to the actions of others, and behaving in a cold and antagonistic manner, hostile people may create or exacerbate conflict and undermine potential sources of social support. This is the premise of the transactional model of the effects of hostility on health (Smith, 1992). In this view, hostile people are exposed to greater stress and experience less support in large part because of the effects of their interpersonal style on those around them. The transactional model is an extension of the psychosocial vulnerability model in that it provides a dynamic account of the hostile person's increased exposure to stressors and other unhealthy aspects of the social environment.

Hostility and Physiological Reactivity to Stressors

Another account of the mechanisms linking hostility and health emphasizes physiological responses to stressors rather than exposure to such events. In this basic model (Williams, Barefoot, & Shekelle, 1985), hostile people are hypothesized to respond to a given social stressor (e.g., disagreement and conflict) with more pronounced increases in blood pressure, heart rate, and circulating levels of stress hormones (e.g., catecholamines and cortisol) than do nonhostile people encountering similar circumstances. As described previously, this heightened psychophysiological reactivity may initiate and hasten the development of CAD and promote the emergence of later manifestations of CHD among people with advanced CAD (Kop, 1999; Smith & Ruiz, 2002; Treiber et al., 2003).

A large body of research supports the hypothesis that hostile people respond to

social stressors with increased physiological reactivity (Smith & Gallo, 2001; Smith et al., 2004). For example, compared to people with low hostility, those high on behaviorally rated or self-reported anger, hostility, and aggressiveness have been found to display larger increases in blood pressure, heart rate, and various stress hormones in response to provocation (Miller et al., 1998; Smith, Crawford, & Green, 2001; Suarez, Kuhn, Schanberg, Williams, & Zimmermann, 1998); discussion of past anger-inducing events (Fredrickson et al., 2000); current events discussions or debates (Davis, Matthews, & McGrath, 2000; Gallo, Smith, & Kircher, 2000; Smith & Allred, 1989); and the self-disclosure of personal information (Christensen & Smith, 1993). Studies of cardiovascular and endocrine responses during typical daily activities suggest that the heightened reactivity of hostile people also occurs in "real life" situations (Benotsch, Christensen, & McKelvey, 1997; Brondolo et al., 2003; Polk, Kamarck, & Shiffman, 2002; Pope & Smith, 1990). In addition to these physiological correlates, hostility is associated with higher levels of blood lipids and larger stress-induced increases in these atherogenic substances (Finney, Stoney, & Engebretson, 2002; Suarez, Bates, & Harralson, 1998). Other psychobiologic mechanisms potentially contributing to the health effects of hostility include activation of blood platelets (Markovitz, 1998), higher concentrations of plasma homocystine (Stoney & Engebretson, 2000), and higher levels of circulating proinflammatory cytokines (Suarez, 2003a, 2003b; Suarez, Lewis, & Kuhn, 2002).

MARRIAGE AS A KEY CONTEXT FOR MECHANISMS LINKING HOSTILITY AND HEALTH

The studies reviewed previously clearly indicate that hostile people may be at greater risk of CHD because they are both exposed to more stressful experiences and have more pronounced physiological responses to such stressors. Research in our laboratory and elsewhere suggests that marriage may be an important context for both these mechanisms. As reviewed in the following sections, hostile people experience more conflict and disruption in their marriages and derive less support from this relationship. Furthermore, they exhibit larger physiological reactivity during stressful marital interactions. Other research suggests that these processes can contribute to cardiovascular disease.

General Health Consequences of Marital Difficulties

Married individuals are generally at lower risk of CHD and other causes of premature mortality than are their unmarried counterparts, presumably reflecting the beneficial effects of the social support inherent in marriage. Interestingly, this protective effect of marriage is generally stronger for men than women (Kiecolt-Glaser & Newton, 2001). Studies suggest, however, that the quality of marriage is also an important influence on health. For example, in one study of men with elevated risk factors for CHD, marital disruption (i.e., separation and divorce) was associated with increased CHD incidence (Matthews & Gump, 2002). In a study of postmenopausal women, marital strain was associated with increased risk of atherosclerosis (Gallo et al., 2003). Finally, in studies of patients with established heart disease, marital strain was associated with poor prognosis (Orth-Gomer et al., 2000).

The effects of marital strain and disruption on CHD may involve the psychophysiological pathways described previously. A variety of studies have examined the effects of stressful marital interactions on increases in heart rate, blood pressure, and circulating levels of catecholamines, cortisol, and other stress hormones (Kiecolt-Glaser & Newton, 2001; Robles & Kiecolt-Glaser, 2003). For example, discussions of topics of marital disagreement reliably evoke increases in heart rate and blood pressure, and the magnitude of these increases is a positive function of the level of negative behavior (e.g., hostility and criticism) displayed by couples during the discussion (Ewart, Taylor, Kraemer, & Agras, 1991). Similarly, negative behavior during such discussions is associated with higher circulating levels of catecholamines and other stress hormones (e.g., cortisol, growth hormone, and adrenocorticotropic hormone) (Malarkey, Kiecolt-Glaser, Pearl, & Glaser, 1994). Marital stress and negative behavior during conflict discussions are also associated with alterations in immune function (Robles & Kiecolt-Glaser, 2003), and atherosclerosis and acute coronary events are influenced by inflammation and other immune system mechanisms (Ross, 1999). Hence, just as the positive and supportive aspects of marriage may reduce the risk of CHD and other illnesses by dampening cardiovascular, neuroendocrine, and immunological responses to stress, marital disruption and strain may influence CAD and CHD by increasing the frequency and severity of these psychophysiological responses.

Hostility and Exposure to Marital Stress

Several studies have demonstrated that hostility is associated with concurrent reports of reduced marital satisfaction and support from one's spouse and with higher levels of marital conflict (Glazer, Smith, Nealey, & Hawkins, 2002a, 2002b; Smith et al., 1988). For example, in a sample of 120 young married couples, we found that husbands' and wives' scores on the anger and hostility scales of the Buss-Perry AQ were associated with lower concurrent levels of overall marital satisfaction, as assessed by the Locke-Wallace Marital Adjustment Test (MAT), and with higher levels of reported conflict with the spouse, as assessed by the Quality of Relationship Inventory. Similar associations emerged among hostility, anger, and lower reports of support from the spouse, although these effects were weaker and less consistent.

Prospective studies have also provided evidence of greater exposure to marital stress among hostile people. For example, Miller, Marksides, Chiriboga, and Ray (1995) found that individual differences in irritability were associated with marital separation, divorce, dissolution of a nonmarital relationship, and unmarried status during an 11-year follow-up period. In a sample of newlywed couples, Newton and Kiecolt-Glaser (1995) found that among husbands, higher scores on the Ho scale were associated with decreases in their own and their wives' reports of marital quality during a 3-year follow-up period. In an 18-month follow-up of our sample of young married couples, higher initial levels of wives' trait anger and hostility were associated with decreases in their own and their husbands' MAT scores. When these two related personality characteristics were analyzed together, trait anger was an independent predictor of decreases in marital satisfaction over time, but hostility was not. That is, the effects of hostility on decreases in MAT scores were due to its overlap with trait anger. Interestingly, these effects of wives' trait anger on declining marital satisfaction appeared to be mediated by husbands' reports of marital conflict. That is, the association between wives' trait anger and reductions in marital satisfaction over time was accounted for by husbands' initial descriptions of wives high in trait anger as displaying high levels of hostile and critical behavior during marital interaction.

Studies of actual marital interactions provide converging evidence of higher exposure to marital conflict among hostile people. In one of our early studies of this type, we classified husbands and wives as high versus low hostile on the basis of their Ho scale scores (Smith, Sanders, & Alexander, 1990). From a list of common topics of marital disagreement (e.g., finances, in-laws, and children), couples identified two low conflict topics and one high conflict topic. Couples first discussed a low conflict topic, followed by the high conflict topic and then the second low conflict topic. The discussions were videotaped and later coded for the levels of hostility displayed during the interaction. Couples also rated their anger before and during the conversations, the extent to which they blamed their spouse for their disagreements on the high conflict topic, and the extent to which they viewed the spouse's behavior during such discussions as intentionally causing disagreements. Couples consisting of one or more high hostile members displayed large increases in the proportion of discussion comments rated as hostile as they turned from the initial low conflict topic to the high conflict topic. During the initial low conflict discussion, all couples made approximately one hostile statement for every 10 comments, and couples consisting of two low trait hostile people maintained this low level of negativity during the remainder of the discussions. In contrast, couples with one or more hostile members increased the rate of negativity to three hostile comments for every 10 statements, and this increased level of negativity did not dissipate when they turned to the second low conflict topic.

The association between trait hostility and hostile behavior during the marital interaction task was significant for both men and women, although it was stronger for men. Similarly, the association between trait hostility and the magnitude of increases in state anger during the high conflict discussion task was stronger for men than women, as was the tendency for hostile spouses to blame and attribute hostile intent to their partner for their difficulties regarding the high conflict topic. Overall, individual differences in hostility were associated with behavioral displays of heightened marital conflict and related cognitive and affective responses, although this pattern was more apparent for men than women. Our prospective study of changes in marital satisfaction suggested that trait anger, rather than the cognitive aspects of hostility assessed by the Ho scale (e.g., cynicism and mistrust), may have been a better predictor of these responses among women. Nonetheless, the results of this behavioral interaction study are consistent with the results of studies of concurrent levels of and longitudinal changes in marital adjustment over time: Hostile people experience greater exposure to marital difficulties. As described previously, this exposure to relationship difficulties may account for at least some of the health consequences of hostility.

Hostility and Physiological Reactivity During Marital Interaction

In several studies, high levels of trait hostility have been associated with larger increases in heart rate and blood pressure during potentially stressful marital interactions. In our first study of this type (Smith & Brown, 1991), we asked couples to discuss a hypothetical problem in a local school district (i.e., which personnel to retain during a budget cutback). Half of the couples simply discussed the issue, whereas the other half did so with an incentive to influence the opinions of their spouses. Among husbands, high scores on the Ho scale were associated with greater CVR when they were attempting to influence their wives but not when they were simply discussing the issue. Wives of high hostile husbands also displayed greater CVR. In contrast, wives' levels of trait hostility were unrelated to their own or their husbands' levels of CVR. In a replication of this study (Smith & Gallo, 1999), we asked couples to discuss current events topics. Half of the couples simply discussed the issues, and half did so with

the understanding that their remarks would be evaluated for knowledge and effectiveness. Among husbands, total scores on the Buss-Perry AQ were associated with greater CVR during the high, but not low, evaluative threat discussions. Husbands' AQ scores were also positively correlated with the magnitude of their wives' cardiovascular responses during the task.

In further analyses, among the four AQ subscales (hostility, anger, verbal aggressiveness, and physical aggressiveness), hostility was the best predictor of husbands' CVR. As in the prior study, wives' AQ total scores were unrelated to their own or their husbands' cardiovascular responses during the discussion task. Hence, at least for men, hostility has been consistently associated with heightened CVR during potentially stressful marital interactions. Wives' ratings of their husbands' behavior during the discussion task indicated that in the high, but not low, threat condition, hostile husbands were perceived as more dominant and controlling than low hostile husbands. This suggests that the greater cardiovascular responses displayed by hostile husbands in the high threat condition may result from efforts to exert control or status in the discussion. Prior research in our laboratory indicates that effortful attempts to influence or control others evoke increases in heart rate and blood pressure (Smith, Ruiz, & Uchino, 2000).

The most recent study of hostility, marital interaction, and cardiovascular response in our laboratory was an effort to address some of the potential limitations of our prior work (Smith, Nealey-Moore, Uchino, & Hawkins, 2003). For example, the hypothetical problems and current events that served as the focus of the discussion tasks in prior studies do not resemble closely the topics couples typically identify as sources of conflict, thereby posing a threat to the external or "ecological" validity of our findings. Furthermore, trait hostility predicted CVR during marital interaction for husbands but not wives in two prior studies, but wives' trait anger was the best predictor of decreases in their own and their husbands' marital satisfaction in our recent prospective study (Glazer et al., 2002b). Therefore, we examined both trait anger and hostility to determine if these related but distinct personality characteristics were differentially related to CVR for men and women. We also assessed spouses' affective responses and rating of their partners' behavior during the interaction to determine if the level of unfriendliness or that of dominance or both displayed during the task paralleled the cardiovascular patterns we observed.

Toward this end, we randomly assigned 80 married couples to one of two discussion tasks. In the low conflict condition, participants took turns describing what they knew of their spouse's typical daily schedule. In the high conflict condition, we provided both spouses with a list of negative trait descriptors (e.g., lazy and selfish) and asked them to select three that described their partner. During the task, participants took turns discussing the negative characteristics that they had selected as descriptive of their spouse. Before the discussion task, participants completed measures of state anger, and after the task they completed a second state anger measure and rated their spouse's behavior during the task on the dimensions of warmth versus hostility and dominance versus submissiveness. For husbands, those high in trait hostility and participating in the high conflict discussion displayed the largest increases in blood pressure and heart rate. For example, high hostile husbands in the high conflict condition displayed larger increases in systolic blood pressure than did low hostile husbands in this condition and high hostile husbands in the low conflict task. Trait anger did not predict these responses for husbands. The high hostile husbands in the high conflict condition were rated by their spouses as

unfriendly relative to the other groups of husbands but not more controlling. Also, these husbands did not report larger increases in state anger than did the other groups of husbands.

For wives, those high in trait anger participating in the high conflict discussion displayed the largest increases in blood pressure and heart rate. Specifically, high trait anger wives displayed larger increases in systolic and diastolic blood pressure as well as heart rate than did high trait anger wives in the low conflict condition and low trait anger wives in either discussion condition. Among wives, trait hostility did not predict these cardiovascular responses. High trait anger wives in the high conflict condition reported much larger increases in state anger than did the other three groups of wives, and they were also rated by their husbands as displaying much more dominance during the interaction.

Hence, for both husbands and wives the basic personality trait by situation interactive effect that is the basis of the psychophysiological reactivity model emerged, but the specific trait involved in this pattern differed for men and women. Cognitive aspects of this domain captured by the AQ hostility subscale (e.g., cynicism, mistrust, and attributions of hostile intent) were important for men, whereas affective aspects assessed by the AQ trait anger subscale were important for women. When combined with the results of our other studies, it is clear that stressful marital interactions can evoke heightened cardiovascular reactivity from hostile men and women in a pattern consistent with the psychophysiological reactivity model, although the specific individual differences related to reactivity may differ for men and women. Furthermore, aspects of stressful marital context that evoke this heightened reactivity from characteristically hostile and angry spouses involve not only conflict and anger inducing discord but also interactions in which challenges to dominance and control are salient.

In couples for whom mistrust and antagonism are common, the maintenance of power or concerns about being subjected to its unfair use may be a significant source of stress and its physiological effects.

A MODEL OF HOSTILITY, MARITAL INTERACTION, AND PHYSIOLOGICAL REACTIVITY

From the previous sections, it is clear that characteristically hostile and angry people are exposed to greater stress in marriage, experience less support in this otherwise beneficial relationship, and respond to potentially stressful marital interactions with heightened physiological reactivity. Figure 2.1 presents a general model of the mechanisms that link these traits with psychosocial vulnerability and psychophysiological reactivity in the marital context. Although the model emphasizes the personality trait of hostility, it is also relevant to other personality traits or individual differences that have been found to (a) predict the development and course of

CHD and (b) be related to exposure to aspects of marital functioning. For example, both depression—as indexed by clinical disorders or subclinical variation in depressive symptoms—and the trait of optimism versus pessimism are related to CHD in this way (Smith & Ruiz, 2002) and have been found to predict exposure to levels of marital conflict and support (Glazer et al., 2002a, 2002b; Whisman, 2001).

The model is based on our previously described application of the concepts of interpersonal psychology (Keisler, 1996) to the study of psychosocial risk factors and the mechanisms linking them with disease (Gallo & Smith, 1999; Smith & Gallo, 1999; Smith, Gallo, & Ruiz, 2003; Smith et al., 2004). The interpersonal tradition in personality and clinical psychology (for a review, see Pincus & Ansell, 2003) is based on the assumption that personality comprises recurring patterns of interpersonal situations and interactions. The social behavior characterizing these patterns varies along two basic dimensions: dominance versus submissiveness (i.e., control) and friendliness versus hostility (i.e.,

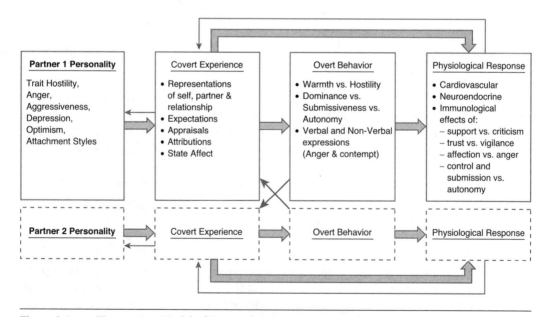

Figure 2.1   Transaction Model of Personality Processes, Marital Adaptation, and Health

warmth). Related conceptual approaches (Benjamin, 1974), however, suggest that autonomy is an additional aspect of social behavior; granting it to others is the opposite of exerting dominance, whereas asserting one's own autonomy is the opposite of submission. Finally, the interpersonal perspective maintains that the recurring patterns of interpersonal interaction that make up personality are themselves made up of transactional cycles in which elements of the initial actor's covert experience (e.g., beliefs, expectations, appraisals, and affect) influence the level of warmth, control, or autonomy in his or her overt behavior. The initial actor's overt behavior, in turn, influences or restricts the covert experience of the interaction partner, prompting this person to display overt behavior that tends to complement the initial actor's covert experience and overt behavior. For example, the initial actor's trusting expectations and feeling of fondness for the interaction partner are likely to prompt expressions of warmth and friendly cooperation. Such actions are likely to be appraised positively by the interaction partner, prompting friendly feelings and overt expressions of warmth in turn and thereby complementing the initial actor's overt behavior and confirming the initial positive expectations. In contrast, hostile beliefs and expectations are likely to prompt cold and disagreeable overt actions, likely evoking similarly unfriendly actions from others. These transactional cycles operate both within specific moment-to-moment interactions and over longer periods of multiple recurring cycles in ongoing relationships.

Figure 2.1 depicts these basic concepts in the context of mechanisms linking personality traits such as hostility to exposure to marital stress and heightened physiological reactivity to such stressful interactions. For example, trait anger and hostility are associated with negative views not only of others and relationships but also of the hostile person himor herself. Such people are likely to expect

mistreatment from others, including the spouse; appraise ambiguous actions by the spouse as hostile, controlling, threatening, or some other form of mistreatment; attribute negative intent to such actions; and experience an increase in irritation or state anger. These aspects of the hostile person's covert experience are likely to lead to low levels of expressed warmth and high levels of hostility, control, and defensiveness in their overt actions toward the spouse. Such actions, in turn, restrict the spouse's covert experience, making some interpretations and affects much more common than others. As a result, the spouse is likely to display unfriendly overt behavior in response to the initial actor. In this way, the hostile covert experiences and overt behavior of the initial actor are confirmed and complemented in a manner that makes the continuation of prior personality tendencies and relationship qualities likely. That is, hostile people continually re-create experiences in close relationships that promote the continuation of the hostile tendencies and the poor quality of their marriages (for a review of transactional elements of anger, hostility, and aggressiveness, see Smith et al., 2004). It is important to note that these processes influence not only high levels of negative experiences in close relationships (e.g., conflict, criticism, struggles for control, and mistrusting vigilance for impending mistreatment) but also low levels of positive experiences (e.g., support). Furthermore, if uninterrupted, a recurring pattern of such cycles may place the couple at risk of marital disruption (i.e., separation and divorce).

Most close relationships are characterized by at least some negative interactions. The psychophysiological reactivity model of the health effects of hostility posits that hostility and trait anger are associated with larger perturbations in cardiovascular, neuroendocrine, and immunological parameters at such times. Hostile people will interpret such events (e.g., attribute hostile intent to the partner) and respond to them in ways (e.g., effortful assertion of hostile control) that heighten such physiological responses. They also experience more frequent occurrences of such events (and fewer positive or supportive interactions) through the transaction mechanisms described previously. In this way, their greater risk of disease reflects both increased reactivity and exposure to stressors in this context as well as less frequent and pronounced physiological benefits of positive aspects of relationships.

The specific interactions involving warmth versus hostility and autonomy granting versus control, described previously and depicted in Figure 2.1, may be made more or less frequent and pronounced by various aspects of the couple's context. Their relationship history, developmental stage (e.g., level of parenting demands and caregiving for their own parents), and other sources of chronic stress (e.g., crowded and unsafe neighborhoods and high job stress) may make positive or negative marital transactional patterns more likely.

IMPLICATIONS OF THE MARITAL APPROACH TO HOSTILITY AND HEALTH

The model described previously suggests several lines of additional needed research. The specific cognitive, affective, and behavioral processes involved in maladaptive marital patterns associated with these traits should be documented further. In describing and explicating these patterns, it will be important to consider specific aspects of trait anger, hostility, and aggressiveness. For example, verbal aggressiveness is an interpersonally unfriendly and dominant style (Gallo & Smith, 1998) and may therefore be associated with marital patterns involving conflicts regarding control. In contrast, hostility reflects a more submissive form of unfriendliness and therefore may

be involved in marital patterns in which vigilance for potential mistreatment, withdrawal, and resentful submission are more common. In general, the varieties of hostile and angry personality characteristics linked to CHD are likely to be involved in similarly varied maladaptive patterns of marital interaction.

Our findings regarding cardiovascular responses to aspects of marital interaction should be replicated and extended, but such research should also examine the other physiological responses to stress that are implicated in the development of CHD, especially the inflammatory processes that are emerging as central to the development and progression of this disease. As noted previously, the model is also relevant to other CHD risk factors that are also related to marital functioning. Particularly relevant in this regard is depression because it is a robust predictor of the development and course of CHD and seems to be both a cause and a consequence of disturbed marital functioning. Protective psychosocial characteristics such as optimism may also be examined in this manner. Finally, for hostility, depression, and other individual differences linked to both CHD and marital functioning, more complete tests of the general perspective are needed in which the combined effects of the individual difference and social context are examined as predictors of CHD incidence and course.

Additional supportive findings from such research would naturally raise questions about applications to the management or prevention of CHD. Psychosocial interventions such as stress management have beneficial effects on emotional, social, and even physical outcomes among CHD patients (Dusseldorp, van Elderen, Maes, Meulman, & Kraaij, 1999; Linden, Stossel, & Maurice, 1996), although there have been notable negative results of such interventions for CHD. Several treatments for trait anger and related characteristics have been found effective (DiGiuseppe & Tafrate, 2003), and preliminary evidence suggests that they may be useful in treating anger and hostility among CHD patients (Gidron, Davidson, & Bata, 1999). A large body of research indicates that marital distress can be treated successfully with several different relatively short-term interventions, and treatments for the prevention of marital difficulties have also been found to be effective (Baucom, Shoham, Mueser, Daiuto, & Stickle, 1998). In the event that research continues to support the importance of the marital context in understanding the influence of hostility and other psychosocial risk factors on CHD, such marital interventions could be evaluated as adjuncts to traditional interventions for the management of CHD patients and for the reduction of risk prior to the onset of the disease. Until the results of intervention research of this sort are available, the existing evidence seems sufficient to support the suggestion that clinicians at least consider the marital context when evaluating these patients and planning their care.

REFERENCES

American Heart Association. (2004). *Heart and stroke statistical update*. Dallas, TX: Author.

Angerer, P., Siebert, U., Kothny, W., Muhlbauer, D., Mudra, H., & von Schacky, C. (2000). Impact of social support, cynical hostility and anger expression on progression of coronary atherosclerosis. *Journal of the American College of Cardiology, 36*(6), 1781-1788.

Barefoot, J. C., & Lipkus, I. M. (1994). The assessment of anger and hostility. In A. W. Siegman & T. W. Smith (Eds.), *Anger, hostility, and the heart* (pp. 43-66). Hillsdale, NJ: Lawrence Erlbaum.

Baucom, D., Shoham, V., Mueser, K. T., Daiuto, A. D., & Stickle, T. R. (1998). Empirically supported couple and family interventions for marital distress and adult mental health problems. *Journal of Consulting and Clinical Psychology, 66*, 53-88.

Becker, A. E., de Boer, O. J., & van der Wal, A. C. (2001). The role of inflammation and infection in coronary artery disease. *Annual Review of Medicine, 52*, 289-297.

Benjamin, L. S. (1974). Structural analysis of social behavior. *Psychological Review, 81*, 392-425.

Benotsch, E. G., Christensen, A. J., & McKelvey, L. (1997). Hostility, social support, and ambulatory cardiovascular activity. *Journal of Behavioral Medicine, 20*, 163-176.

Brondolo, E., Rieppi, R., Erickson, S. A., Bagiella, E., Shapiro, P. A., McKinley, P., et al. (2003). Hostility, interpersonal interactions, and ambulatory blood pressure. *Psychosomatic Medicine, 65*, 1003-1011.

Burg, M., Jain, D., Soufer, R., Kerns, R. D., & Zaret, B. L. (1993). Role of behavioral and psychological factors in mental stress-induced silent left ventricular dysfunction in coronary artery disease. *Journal of the American College of Cardiology, 22*, 440-448.

Buss, A. H., & Perry M. (1992). The aggression questionnaire. *Journal of Personality and Social Psychology, 63*, 452-459.

Chang, P. P., Ford, D. E., Meoni, L. A., Wang, N. Y., & Klag, M. J. (2002). Anger in young men and subsequent premature cardiovascular disease: The precursors study. *Archives of Internal Medicine, 162*(8), 901-906.

Chaput, L. A., Adams, S. H., Simon, J. A., Blumenthal, R. S., Vittinghoff, E., Lin, F., et al. (2002). Hostility predicts recurrent events among postmenopausal women with coronary heart disease. *American Journal of Epidemiology, 156*(12), 1092-1099.

Christensen, A. J., & Smith, T. W. (1993). Cynical hostility and cardiovascular reactivity during self-disclosure. *Psychosomatic Medicine, 55*, 193-202.

Cook, W. W., & Medley, D. M. (1954). Proposed hostility and pharisaic virtue scales for the MMPI. *Journal of Applied Psychology, 38*, 414-418.

Costa, P. T., Jr., McCrae, R. R., & Dembroski, T. M. (1989). Agreeableness versus antagonism: Explication of a potential risk factor for CHD. In A. Siegman & T. M. Dembroski (Eds.), *In search of coronary-prone behavior: Beyond type A* (pp. 41-63). Hillsdale, NJ: Lawrence Erlbaum.

Davis, M. C., Matthews, K. A., & McGrath, C. E. (2000). Hostile attitudes predict elevated vascular resistance during interpersonal stress in men and women. *Psychosomatic Medicine, 62*(1), 17-25.

DiGuiseppe, R., & Tafrate, R. C. (2003). Anger treatment for adults: A meta-analytic review. *Clinical Psychology, Science and Practice, 10*, 70-84.

Dusseldorp, E., van Elderen, T., Maes, S., Meulman, J., & Kraaij, V. (1999). A meta-analysis of psychoeducational programs for coronary heart disease patients. *Health Psychology, 18*, 506-519.

Eng, P. M., Fitzmaurice, G., Kubzansky, L. D., Rimm, E. B., & Kawachi, I. (2003). Anger expression and risk of stroke and coronary heart disease among male health professionals. *Psychosomatic Medicine, 65*(1), 100-110.

Everson, S. A., Kaplan, G. A., Goldberg, D. E., Lakka, T. A., Sivenius, J., & Salonen, J. T. (1999). Anger expression and incident stroke: Prospective evidence from the Kuopio ischemic heart disease study. *Stroke, 30*(3), 523-528.

Everson, S. A., Kauhanen, J., Kaplan, G., Goldberg, D., Julkunen, J., Tuomilehto, J., et al. (1997). Hostility and increased risk of mortality and myocardial infarction: The mediating role of behavioral risk factors. *American Journal of Epidemiology, 146*, 142-152.

Ewart, C. K., Taylor, C. B., Kraemer, H. C., & Agras, W. S. (1991). High blood pressure and marital discord: Not being nasty matters more than being nice. *Health Psychology, 10*, 155-163.

Finney, M. L., Stoney, C. M., & Engebretson, T. O. (2002). Hostility and anger expression in African American and European American men is associated with cardiovascular and lipid reactivity. *Psychophysiology, 39*(3), 340-349.

Fredrickson, B. L., Maynard, K. E., Helms, M. J., Haney, T. L., Siegler, I. C., & Barefoot, J. C. (2000). Hostility predicts magnitude and duration of blood pressure response to anger. *Journal of Behavioral Medicine, 23*, 229-243.

Gabbay, F. H., Krantz, D. S., Kop, W., Hedges, S., Klein, J., Gottdiener, J. S., et al. (1996). Triggers of myocardial ischemia during daily life in patients with coronary artery disease: Physical and mental activities, anger, and smoking. *Journal of the American College of Cardiology, 27*, 585-592.

Gallo, L. C., & Smith, T. W. (1998). Construct validation of health-relevant personality traits: Interpersonal circumplex and five-factor model analyses of the Aggression Questionnaire. *International Journal of Behavioral Medicine, 5*, 129-147.

Gallo, L. C., & Smith, T. W. (1999). Patterns of hostility and social support: Conceptualizing psychosocial risk factors as a characteristic of the person and the environment. *Journal of Research in Personality, 33,* 281-310.

Gallo, L. C., Smith, T. W., & Kircher, J. C. (2000). Cardiovascular and electrodermal responses to support and provocation: Interpersonal methods in the study of psychophysiological reactivity. *Psychophysiology, 37,* 289-301.

Gallo, L. C., Troxel, W. M., Kuller, L. H., Sutton-Tyrrell, K., Edmundowicz, D., & Matthews, K. A. (2003). Marital status, marital quality, and atherosclerotic burden in post-menopausal women. *Psychosomatic Medicine, 65,* 952-962.

Gidron, Y., Davidson, K., & Bata, I. (1999). The short-term effects of a hostility-reduction intervention on male coronary heart disease patients. *Health Psychology, 18,* 416-420.

Glazer, K., Smith, T. W., Nealey, J., & Hawkins, M. (2002a). *Dispositional optimism and relationship quality in married couples.* Paper presented at the International Conference on Personal Relationships.

Glazer, K., Smith, T. W., Nealey, J., & Hawkins, M. (2002b). *Hostility and marital adjustment.* Paper presented at the annual meeting of the Society of Behavioral Medicine.

Goodman, M., Quigley, J., Moran, G., Meilman, H., & Sherman, M. (1996). Hostility predicts restenosis after percutaneous transluminal coronary angioplasty. *Mayo Clinic Proceedings, 71,* 729-734.

Harris, K. F., Matthews, K. A., Sutton-Tyrrell, K., & Kuller, L. H. (2003). Associations between psychological traits and endothelial function in post-menopausal women. *Psychosomatic Medicine, 65,* 402-409.

Hart, K. E. (1999). Cynical hostility and deficiencies in functional support: The moderating role of gender in psychosocial vulnerability to disease. *Personality and Individual Differences, 27*(1), 69-83.

Helmers, K. F., Krantz, D. S., Howell, R., Klein, J., Bairey, N., & Rozanski, A. (1993). Hostility and myocardial ischemia in coronary artery disease patients: Evaluation by gender and ischemic index. *Psychosomatic Medicine, 50,* 29-36.

Iribarren, C., Sidney, S., Bild, D. E., Liu, K., Markovitz, J. H., Roseman, J. M., et al. (2000). Association of hostility with coronary artery calcification in young adults: The CARDIA study. *Journal of the American Medical Association, 283,* 2546-2551.

Ironson, G., Taylor, C. B., Boltwood, M., Bartzokis, T., Dennis, C., Chesney, M., et al. (1992). Effects of anger on left ventricular ejection fraction in coronary disease. *American Journal of Cardiology, 70,* 281-285.

Julkunen, J., Salonen, R., Kaplan, G. A., Chesney, M. A., & Salonen, J. T. (1994). Hostility and the progression of carotid atherosclerosis. *Psychosomatic Medicine, 56,* 519-525.

Kaufmann, M. W., Fitzgibbons, J. P., Sussman, E. J., Reed, J. F., 3rd, Einfalt, J. M., Rodgers, J. K., et al. (1999). Relation between myocardial infarction, depression, hostility, and death. *American Heart Journal, 138,* 549-554.

Kawachi, I., Sparrow, D., Spiro, A., Vokonas, P., & Weiss, S. T. (1996). A prospective study of anger and coronary heart disease. The Normative Aging Study. *Circulation, 94,* 2090-2095.

Kiecolt-Glaser, J., & Newton, T. (2001). Marriage and health: His and hers. *Psychological Bulletin, 127,* 472-503.

Kiesler, D. J. (1996). *Contemporary interpersonal theory and research: Personality, psychopathology, and psychotherapy.* New York: John Wiley.

Kop, W. J. (1999). Chronic and acute psychological risk factors for clinical manifestations of coronary artery disease. *Psychosomatic Medicine, 61,* 476-487.

Kop, W. J. (2003). The integration of cardiovascular behavioral medicine and psychoneuroimmunology: New developments based on converging research fields. *Brain Behavior and Immunology, 17*(4), 233-237.

Krantz, D. S., & McCeney, M. K. (2002). Effects of psychological and social factors on organic disease: A critical assessment of research on coronary heart disease. *Annual Review of Psychology, 53*(1), 341-369.

Linden, W., Stossel, C., & Maurice, J. (1996). Psychosocial interventions for patients with coronary artery disease: A meta-analysis. *Archives of Internal Medicine, 156,* 745-752.

Malarkey, W. B., Kiecolt-Glaser, J. K., Pearl, D., & Glaser, R. (1994). Hostile behavior during marital conflict alters pituitary and adrenal hormones. *Psychosomatic Medicine, 56*(1), 41-51.

Markovitz, J. H. (1998). Hostility is associated with increased platelet activation in coronary heart disease. *Psychosomatic Medicine, 60*(5), 586-591.

Matthews, K. A., & Gump, B. B. (2002). Chronic work stress and marital dissolution increase risk of posttrial mortality in men from the Multiple Risk Factor Intervention Trial. *Archives of Internal Medicine, 162,* 309-315.

Matthews, K. A., Gump, B. B., Harris, K. F., Haney, T. L., & Barefoot, J. C. (2004). Hostile behaviors predict cardiovascular mortality among men enrolled in the Multiple Risk Factor Intervention Trial. *Circulation, 109,* 66-70.

Matthews, K. A., Owens, J. F., Kuller, L. H., Sutton-Tyrrell, K., & Jansen-McWilliams, L. (1998). Are hostility and anxiety associated with carotid atherosclerosis in healthy postmenopausal women? *Psychosomatic Medicine, 60,* 633-638.

McCann, B. S., Russo, J., & Benjamin, G. A. (1997). Hostility, social support, and perceptions of work. *Journal of Occupational Health Psychology, 2*(2), 175-185.

Mendes De Leon, C. F., Kop, W. J., de Swart, H. B., Bar, F. W., & Appels, A. P. (1996). Psychosocial characteristics and recurrent events after percutaneous transluminal coronary angioplasty. *American Journal of Cardiology, 77,* 252-255.

Miller, S. B., Dolgoy, L., Friese, M., Sita, A., Lavoie, K., & Campbell, T. (1998). Hostility, sodium consumption, and cardiovascular response to interpersonal stress. *Psychosomatic Medicine, 60,* 71-77.

Miller, T. Q., Marksides, K. S., Chiriboga, D. A., & Ray, L. A. (1995). A test of the psychosocial vulnerability and health behavior models of hostility: Results from an 11-year follow-up study of Mexican Americans. *Psychosomatic Medicine, 57,* 572-581.

Miller, T. Q., Smith, T. W., Turner, C. W., Guijarro, M. L., & Hallet, A. J. (1996). A meta-analytic review of research on hostility and physical health. *Psychological Bulletin, 119,* 322-348.

Mittleman, M. A., Maclure, M., Sherwood, J. B., Mulry, R. P., Tofler, G. H., Jacobs, S. C., et al. for the Determinants of Myocardial Infarction Onset Study Investigators. (1995). Triggering of acute myocardial infarction onset by episodes of anger. *Circulation, 92*(7), 1720-1725.

Möller, J., Hallqvist, J., Diderichsen, F., Theorell, T., Reuterwall, C., & Ahlbom, A. (1999). Do episodes of anger trigger myocardial infarction? A case-crossover analysis in the Stockholm Heart Epidemiology Program (SHEEP). *Psychosomatic Medicine, 61,* 842-849.

Newton, T. L., & Kiecolt-Glaser, J. K. (1995). Hostility and erosion of marital quality during early marriage. *Journal of Behavioral Medicine, 18,* 601-619.

O'Malley, P. G., Jones, D. L., Feuerstein, I. M., & Taylor, A. J. (2000). Lack of correlation between psychological factors and subclinical coronary artery disease. *New England Journal of Medicine, 343,* 1298-1304.

O'Neil, J. N., & Emery, C. F. (2002). Psychosocial vulnerability, hostility, and family history of coronary heart disease among male and female college students. *International Journal of Behavioral Medicine, 9*(1), 17-36.

Orth-Gomer, K., Wamala, S. P., Horsten, M., Schenck-Gustafsson, K., Schneiderman, N., & Mittleman, M. A. (2000). Marital stress worsens prognosis in women with coronary heart disease: The Stockholm Female Coronary Risk Study. *Journal of the American Medical Association, 284,* 3008-3014.

Pincus, H. A., & Ansell, E. B. (2003). Interpersonal theory of personality. In T. Millon & M. J. Lerner (Eds.), *Handbook of psychology: Personality and social psychology* (Vol. 5, pp. 209-229). New York: John Wiley.

Polk, D. E., Kamarck, T. W., & Shiffman, S. (2002). Hostility explains some of the discrepancy between daytime ambulatory and clinic blood pressures. *Health Psychology, 21*(2), 202-206.

Pope, M. K., & Smith, T. W. (1990). Cortisol excretion in high and low cynically hostile men. *Psychosomatic Medicine, 53,* 386-392.

Robles, T., & Kiecolt-Glaser, J. (2003). The physiology of marriage: Pathways to health. *Physiology and Behavior, 79,* 409-416.

Rosenberg, E. L., Ekman, P., Jian, W., Babyak, M., Coleman, R. E., Hanson, M., et al. (2001). Linkages between facial expressions of anger and transient myocardial ischemia in men with coronary artery disease. *Emotion, 1*(2),107-115.

Rosenmann, R. H. (1978). The interview method of assessment of the coronary-prone behaviors in the Western Collaborative Group Study. In T. M. Dembroski, S. M. Weiss, J. L. Shields, & M. Feinleib (Eds.), *Coronary prone behavior* (pp. 55-69). New York: Springer-Verlag.

Ross, R. (1999). Atherosclerosis: An inflammatory disease. *New England Journal of Medicine, 340,* 115-126.

Rozanski, A., Blumenthal, J. A., & Kaplan, J. (1999). Impact of psychological factors on the pathogenesis of cardiovascular disease and implications for therapy. *Circulation, 99,* 2192-2217.

Rutledge, T., & Hogan, B. E. (2002). A quantitative review of prospective evidence linking psychological factors with hypertension development. *Psychosomatic Medicine, 64,* 758-766.

Smith, B. D., Crawford, D., & Green, L. (2001). Hostility and caffeine: Cardiovascular effects during stress and recovery. *Personality and Individual Differences, 30*(7), 1125-1137.

Smith, T. W. (1992). Hostility and health: Current status of a psychosomatic hypothesis. *Health Psychology, 11,* 139-150.

Smith, T. W. (1994). Concepts and methods in the study of anger, hostility, and health. In A. W. Siegman & T. W. Smith (Eds.), *Anger, hostility and the heart* (pp. 23-42). Hillsdale, NJ: Lawrence Erlbaum.

Smith, T. W., & Allred, K. D. (1989). Blood pressure responses during social interaction in high and low cynically hostile males. *Journal of Behavioral Medicine, 12,* 135-143.

Smith, T. W., & Brown, P. W. (1991). Cynical hostility, attempts to exert social control, and cardiovascular reactivity in married couples. *Journal of Behavioral Medicine, 14,* 581-592.

Smith, T. W., & Gallo, L. C. (1999). Hostility and cardiovascular reactivity during marital interaction. *Psychosomatic Medicine, 61,* 436-445.

Smith, T. W., & Gallo, L. C. (2001). Personality traits as risk factors for physical illness. In A Baum, T. Revenson, & J. Singer (Eds.), *Handbook of health psychology* (pp. 139-172). Hillsdale, NJ: Lawrence Erlbaum.

Smith, T. W., Gallo, L. C., & Ruiz, J. M. (2003). Toward a social psychophysiology of cardiovascular reactivity: Interpersonal concepts and methods in the study of stress and coronary disease. In J. Suls & K. Wallston (Eds.), *Social psychological foundations of health and illness* (pp. 335-366). Cambridge, MA: Blackwell.

Smith, T. W., Glazer, K., Ruiz, J. M., & Gallo, L. C. (2004). Hostility, anger, aggressiveness and coronary heart disease: An interpersonal perspective on personality, emotion and health. *Journal of Personality, 72,* 1217-1270.

Smith, T. W., Nealey-Moore, J., Uchino, B. N., & Hawkins, M. (2003). *Hostility, anger, and cardiovascular reactivity during marital interaction.* Paper presented at the annual meeting of the American Psychosomatic Society.

Smith, T. W., Pope, M. K., Sanders, J. D., Allred, K. D., & O'Keefe, J. L. (1988). Cynical hostility at home and work: Psychosocial vulnerability across domains. *Journal of Research in Personality, 22,* 525-548.

Smith, T. W., & Ruiz, J. M. (2002). Psychosocial influences on the development and course of coronary heart disease: Current status and implications for research and practice. *Journal of Consulting and Clinical Psychology, 70*(3), 548-568.

Smith, T. W., Ruiz, J. M., & Uchino, B. N. (2000). Vigilance, active coping, and cardiovascular reactivity during social interaction in young men. *Health Psychology, 19,* 382-392.

Smith, T. W., Sanders, J., & Alexander, J. (1990). What does the Cook and Medley Hostility Scale measure? Affect, behavior, and attributions in the marital context. *Journal of Personality and Social Psychology, 58,* 699-708.

Stoney, C. M., & Engebretson, T. O. (2000). Plasma homocysteine concentrations are positively associated with hostility and anger. *Life Sciences, 66*(23), 2267-2275.

Suarez, E. C. (2003a). Plasma interleukin-6 is associated with psychological coronary risk factor: Moderation by use of multivitamin supplements. *Brain Behavior and Immunology, 17*(4), 296-303.

Suarez, E. C. (2003b). Joint effect of hostility and severity of depressive symptoms on plasma interleukin-6 concentration. *Psychosomatic Medicine, 65*(4), 523-527.

Suarez, E. C., Bates, M. B., & Harralson, T. L. (1998). The relation of hostility to lipids and lipoproteins in women evidence for the role of antagonistic hostility. *Annals of Behavioral Medicine, 20*(2), 59-63.

Suarez, E. C., Kuhn, C. M., Schanberg, S. M., Williams, R. B., & Zimmermann, E. A. (1998). Neuroendocrine, cardiovascular, and emotional responses of hostile men: The role of interpersonal challenge. *Psychosomatic Medicine, 60*(1), 78-88.

Suarez, E. C., Lewis, J. G., & Kuhn, C. (2002). The relation of aggression, hostility, and anger to lipopolysaccharide-stimulated tumor necrosis factor (TNF)-α by blood monocytes from normal men. *Brain, Behavior, and Immunity, 16,* 675-684.

Sykes, D. H., Arveiler, D., Salters, C. P., Ferrieres, J., McCrum, E., Amouyel, P., et al. (2002). Psychosocial risk factors for heart disease in France and Northern Ireland: The Prospective Epidemiological Study of Myocardial Infarction (PRIME). *International Journal Epidemiology, 31*(6),1227-1234.

Treiber, F. A., Kamarck, T., Schneiderman, N., Sheffield, D., Kapuku, G., & Taylor, T. (2003). Cardiovascular reactivity and development of preclinical and clinical disease states. *Psychosomatic Medicine, 65*(1), 46-62.

Welin, C., Lappas, G., & Wilhelmsen, L. (2000). Independent importance of psychosocial factors for prognosis after myocardial infarction. *Journal of Internal Medicine, 247,* 629-639.

Whisman, M. (2001). The association between depression and marital dissatisfaction. In S. R. H. Beach (Ed.), *Marital and family processes in depression: A scientific foundation for clinical practice* (pp. 3-24). Washington, DC: American Psychological Association.

Williams, J. E., Nieto, F. J., Sanford, C. P., Couper, D. J., & Tyroler, H. A. (2002). The association between trait anger and incident stroke risk: The Atherosclerosis Risk in Communities (ARIC) study. *Stroke, 33*(1), 13-20.

Williams, J. E., Paton, C. C., Siegler, I. C., Eigenbrodt, M. L., Nieto, F. J., & Tyroler, H. A. (2000). Anger proneness predicts coronary heart disease risk: Prospective analysis from the Atherosclerosis Risk in Communities (ARIC) study. *Circulation, 101,* 2034-2039.

Williams, R. B., Jr. (2000). Psychological factors, health, and disease: The impact of aging and the life cycle. In S. B. Manuck, R. Jennings, B. S. Rabin, & A. Baum (Eds.), *Behavior, health, and aging* (pp. 135-151). Mahwah, NJ: Lawrence Erlbaum.

Williams, R. B., Jr., Barefoot, J. C., & Shekelle, R. (1985). The health consequences of hostility. In M. A. Chesney & R. H. Rosenman (Eds.), *Anger and hostility in cardiovascular and behavioral disorders* (pp. 173-185). New York: Hemisphere.

CHAPTER 3

Health Issues in Latino Families and Households

Barbara A. Zsembik

The Latino population in the United States continues to increase, diversify, and disperse geographically in dramatic fashion. Latinos are now the largest race/ethnic minority group in the United States, a fact not fully recognized by scholars, public officials, health practitioners, or people in the United States (Grieco & Cassidy, 2001). They are projected to constitute nearly one fourth of the total population by 2050 (24.4%), contrasting with population shares of non-Latino blacks (14.6%) and whites (50.1%) (U.S. Census Bureau, 2003, Table 15). Not only is the Latino population growth reshaping the ethnic composition of the national population but also the ethnic composition of the Latino population is changing. Recent migration streams from Caribbean basin nations have swelled, reducing the proportion of the Latino subpopulation that is of Mexican origin. The geographic distribution of Latinos has expanded substantially, ranging from the traditional regions and cities, such as the southwestern states, New York City, and Miami to new gateway cities and their suburban rings, such as Washington, D.C., Orlando, and Atlanta, and more rural destinations in the southeastern United States (Singer, 2004). It is clear that an understanding and incorporation of the Latino population into U.S. health and family research is crucial for evaluating health and well-being among U.S. families and households.

During the past decade, the national public health agenda has established the importance of research on race and ethnic disparities in health. The number of demographic studies of Latinos' health has soared recently, with most researchers established in subspecialty fields of mortality, fertility,

AUTHOR'S NOTE: I use the terms *whites* and *blacks* to refer to non-Latino whites and blacks. I use the term *black* rather than *African American* in recognition that immigrants from African Diaspora countries such as Haiti and from the African continent form an important component of the U.S. population of African descent.

aging, and health demography. This chapter integrates and appraises this proliferating literature. First, I present patterns, trends, and differentials in Latino family and household characteristics and then suggest their implications for health. Next, I review basic facts about Latino health and present common explanations for observed differences. Third, I identify, describe, and critically evaluate the major research themes and findings that characterize this body of research. I present directions in which future research is likely to go in the next decade. Finally, I consider the implications of expanding knowledge of Latino health for health disparities research and research on families and households.

CURRENT PATTERNS AND EXPLANATIONS

Latinos and Their Families and Households

The Latino population is more youthful relative to whites and blacks. Nearly one third of Latinos (29.7%) and one fourth of blacks (25.9%) are younger than the age of 15, in contrast to the 19.9% of comparably aged whites (U.S. Census Bureau, 2003, Table 13). Latinos are less likely to be in late middle or old age (19.4% compared to 37.5% among whites), when mortality rates and diagnoses of serious chronic disease increase. Cubans have an older age structure, similar to that of whites. Mexicans have the most youthful age structure, with approximately one third of its population younger than age 15 and slightly more than 15% older than age 45.

Latino culture arguably is manifest in nativity and language. As U.S. citizens, Puerto Ricans are not international migrants and do not share migration barriers experienced by Mexican, Caribbean basin, and South American populations. Yet the cultural heritage and complicated political relationship of the island with the United States render the Puerto Rican incorporation experience more comparable to that of migrants from Latin American countries. Because of their longer historical presence in the United States, Mexicans have a greater variability than Puerto Ricans and Cubans in the sizes and numbers of immigrant generations. A broader conceptualization of culture attends to the beliefs, values, and attitudes of a social group. The conceptual model of immigrant incorporation dominant among scholars and nonscholars presumes that ethnic culture is cut whole cloth from a country of origin and brought to the United States, where it withers with time lived in the United States and further weakens across successive family generations. Due to concern about culturally competent health services, practitioners are asked to understand cultural factors of family orientation (*familism*), respect (*respeto*), personalized relationships between client and provider (*personalismo*), and building trust (*confianza*) (National Alliance for Hispanic Health, 2001).

By any measure of social class, Latinos are concentrated in the lower segments of the national socioeconomic distribution. Latino adults have lower levels of education, occupational status, and income than whites and blacks (U.S. Census Bureau, 2003, Tables 40 and 47). Moreover, these resources are spread across larger family households, indicating lower per capita resource levels. Disproportionate concentration in agricultural, construction, manufacturing, and personal service occupations not only produces lower incomes but also constrains wealth accumulation and health insurance coverage. Latinos of Mexican origin are especially likely to earn lower incomes and have less than a high school education (54.2%).

The socioeconomic success across immigrant generations is less clear but appears to vary across ethnic groups (Portes & Rumbaut, 1990). The vital Cuban enclave provided opportunities to the immigrant generation and their children, and the youngest Cuban generations are now successfully transitioning into the professional classes (Zsembik, 2000). Social mobility appears highest for children of Mexican immigrants, but the third generation's successes are lower than those of their parents (Zsembik & Llanes, 1996). The Puerto Rican experience better fits the segmented assimilation model, wherein social mobility is generally constrained across all generations (Landale, Oropesa, Llanes, & Gorman, 1999; Massey, 1993; Tienda, 1989; Torres & Rodriguez, 1991), partially due to their concentration in the economically struggling northeastern metropolises. Finally, Latinos are much more likely than whites or blacks to lack any type of health insurance coverage (Hummer, Pacewicz, Wang, & Collins, 2004).

The economic and cultural characteristics of households are intertwined with their compositions and structures. Here, families are broadly defined as inclusive of families of orientation (parents and siblings), families of procreation (partners and children), kith, and other kin, such as those from extended horizontal ties (grandparents and grandchildren) and extended lateral and horizontal ties (cousins, aunts, and uncles). Although families are typically spread across multiple households, a single household is conventionally used to indicate individual families. Despite the obvious limitations of using a household as a family group, households do have some utility as a unit of analysis. First, households most often hold individual families of procreation with shared and routinized everyday activities (including resource acquisition and distribution and health-related activities) located in the household's physical space. Second, households are the conventional operational unit of public services, such as utilities and state-provided assistance programs. The broader family grouping is recognized as linking households.

Patterns in Latino family and household structures differ appreciably from those observed among whites and blacks. Latinos are more likely to live in family households (81.1% compared to 68.7% and 67.4% for whites and blacks, respectively) and less likely to live alone or with nonfamily members (U.S. Census Bureau, 2003, Table 46). Latino households tend to be larger (U.S. Census Bureau, 2003, Table 67). For example, Mexicans are most likely to live in households with five or more members (28.1%) compared to whites (9.4%) and blacks (11.3%). A larger proportion of Latino households are composed of married couples, dependent children (especially children younger than age 5), and an older adult family member. Trend data for the past several decades indicate patterns shifting toward smaller households, more unmarried adults with dependent children, and more adults living alone. Because the majority of Latinos are of Mexican origin, Latino household profiles better fit their experiences and mask the substantial differences among Latino ethnic groups. Specifically, Puerto Ricans present household structure profiles most similar to those observed among blacks, and Cuban household structures appear most similar to those of whites.

Implications for Health

Characteristics of the Latino population and their families and households bear implications for health. Larger households and families may increase exposure to communicable conditions, the benefits and detriments of social ties, and more widespread impact of an individual's health or illness. Cultural values and beliefs about families, health, and health care also affect health promotion, health risks, self-care and informal care, and use and opinions of formal medical care.

Economic characteristics of family households determine access to employer-provided and state-provided health insurance, affordability of basic needs, the ability to purchase out-of-pocket medical care, and the ability to economically survive illness and poor health episodes.

Basic Facts of Latino Health and Well-Being

There is an overwhelming consensus that blacks experience significantly higher levels of mortality and morbidity across the life course than whites, concomitant with substantial barriers to receipt of adequate amounts of sufficient quality medical care. In contrast, there is no general agreement that Latinos face significant and widespread health disparities in the United States. The profile of Latino health is more complex, revealing a mix of health disparities, health equities, and health advantages. The complexity of the profile has its origins in the wide variety of health indicators used in comparisons, the lack of comparable study samples in research, and the heterogeneity of the Latino population. Explaining the complexity poses additional challenges because the positive health outcomes of Latinos are contradictory to their socioeconomic characteristics, a relationship in stark contrast to the negative health outcomes accruing to the socioeconomically vulnerable depicted in most theoretical and empirical studies.

Mortality

Death rates, life expectancy, and cause of death collectively suggest that Latinos have a mortality advantage over whites and blacks. The U.S. Census Bureau estimated life expectancy at birth, a standard indicator of population health, and at age 85 using mortality data from the mid-1990s (Day, 1996). Among women, life expectancy at birth is

highest among Latinas (82.2 years), followed by whites (80.1 years) and blacks (74.5 years). A similar pattern is observed among Latino men (74.9 years), white men (73.6 years), and black men (64.8 years). Life expectancy at age 65 reveals a similar survival advantage among older women (Latina, 21.8 years; white, 19.4 years; and black, 17.6 years) and older men (Latino, 18.5 years; white, 15.7 years; and black, 13.6 years).

The National Center for Health Statistics (2003) has calculated cause-specific "years of potential life lost" up to age 75 for each race/ethnic group, which offer clear insight into mortality and survivorship patterns. Latinos lose fewer years of life than whites, ranking only below Asian Americans. Years of potential life lost by cause of death indicate that heart disease, cancer, and unintentional injuries are the major causes of years lost for Latinos and whites (National Center for Health Statistics, 2003). Latinos, however, lose disproportionately more years than whites due to deaths from strokes, liver disease and cirrhosis, diabetes, HIV, and homicide.

Age-adjusted death rates for the past two decades reveal lower levels of mortality among Latinos, both males and females, than all race groups except Asians (U.S. Census Bureau, 2003, Tables 110 and 111). Recent age-specific death rates show lower death rates for Latinos than whites at all ages except for Latino infants of non-Mexican origin (Arias, Anderson, Hsiang-Ching, Murphy, & Kochanek, 2003). Examination of age-sex mortality rates, however, reveals disparities. For example, Mexican men between the ages of 15 and 24 have higher mortality than comparably aged white men. Puerto Rican mortality rates for women and men between the ages of 15 and 64 exceed those of whites. There is growing consensus that the mortality and survival profile varies among Latino ethnic groups, bookended by the "disparities" profile of

Puerto Ricans and the "advantage" profile of Cubans.

Morbidity

Morbidity data are less generalizable to the Latino population because national census and survey data began to include a "Hispanic" identifier only in the late 1970s, meeting new standards for race and ethnic data collection set by the Office of Management and Budget. The number of Latinos was rarely sufficient to allow for separate analyses, and many surveys, in response, began to oversample Latinos in the mid-1990s. One data source stands as an important exception: the Hispanic Health and Nutrition Examination Survey (HHANES). It was fielded in 1982 through 1984 and sampled Mexicans in five southwestern states, Cubans in Dade County, Florida, and Puerto Ricans in selected metropolitan areas of the northeast. It continues to serve as a primary data source on the health of Latinos, despite its age and sample restriction.

Do Latinos experience health equity or advantages, with their health benefiting from the same processes that extend their lives? Do Latinos experience significant health disparities, a consequence of their location in the U.S. opportunity structure? The answer available from current data is that the Latino health profile is complexly patterned. The impact of continued migration from Latin America may undergird higher prevalence rates of serious infections, such as tuberculosis and childhood measles, associated with increases in local outbreaks. Community and clinical data have consistently indicated higher prevalence rates of adult-onset diabetes among the Mexican origin population, an observation supported by analyses made increasingly possible with oversample designs. Disability data from the 2000 U.S. Census, however, show greater levels of disability among Latinos than

whites and clear differences across Latino ethnic groups (U.S. Bureau of the Census, 2003, Tables 40 and 47). Among those between the ages of 5 and 20, 9.1% of Latinos have a disability compared to 7.4% of whites and 10.0% of blacks. Latinos' disparities increase in adulthood, rising to 25.1% of working-age Latinos relative to 16.7% of whites, and extend into old age (48.5% relative to 40.4% for whites).

Why Are Latinos Different?

Morbidity data tend to more readily reveal health disparities, which stand in contrast to the profile of health equity or advantage, the so-called epidemiological paradox, more often observed in mortality and survivorship comparisons. The *epidemiological paradox* is a term coined to describe Latinos' paradoxically lower mortality rates than those of whites—paradoxical because of the lower socioeconomic status of Latinos (Abraido-Lanza, Dohrenwend, Ng-Mak, & Turner, 1999; Cobas, Balcazar, Benin, Keith, & Chong, 1996; Hummer, Rogers, Amir, Forbes, & Frisbie, 2000; Idler & Angel, 1990; Landale, Oropesa, & Gorman, 2000; Sorlie, Backlund, Johnson, & Hogat, 1993). Health disparities are defined by Congress as disproportionately high levels of disease, functional impairments, disability, and mortality compared to levels of the general population. Explanatory frameworks developed around health differentials focus either on Latino disparities in morbidity or on Latino successes in survivorship.

Health Equities and
Health Advantages

Assuming Latinos have lower levels of material resources, any absence of a health disparity is paradoxical. One explanation for health equity and health advantage among Latinos posits that they have a healthier population composition produced by migrant selectivity. Two complementary migration streams are hypothesized to produce a healthier Latino population: migration of healthier individuals to the United States and repatriation of ailing migrants to their hometowns, a migration stream called the "salmon bias" (Abraido-Lanza et al., 1999; Markides & Coreil, 1986; Palloni & Arias, 2004; Sorlie et al., 1993). First, migrants to the United States are typically teens and young adults—groups relatively free of age-related chronic health conditions. Second, migrants tend to draw from the healthier segments of their countries of origin because the physical and psychological rigors of migration form barriers to the more vulnerable segments. Third, migrants who become ill or disabled in the United States may return to their countries of origin because they may no longer successfully compete in the U.S. labor market, need more labor-intensive personal care from family members, or prefer to rehabilitate or die "at home."

A second category of explanations for Latino health equities and advantages features the cultural determinants of health (Abraido-Lanza et al., 1999; LeClere, Rogers, & Peters, 1997; Sorlie et al., 1993). For example, research consistently shows lower levels of smoking, drinking, and drug use among immigrants (Scribner, 1996). The empirical generalization that emerged argues that cultural barriers to negative health behaviors indirectly promote better health and survivorship. High levels of ethnic group solidarity and social support are presented as a second cultural mechanism that promotes health (Balcazar, Peterson, & Krull, 1997). Social solidarity and support encourage the mutual exchange of material and nonmaterial resources that sustain health and assist in recovery. Solidarity may reinforce cultural barriers to negative health habits.

The migrant selectivity and cultural factors hypotheses are not competing explanations.

Indeed, they naturally fit together. The cultural factors explanation presents ethnic culture as originating in a Latin American country's culture and embodied in the quotidian nature of immigrant life. Therefore, a component of healthy migrant selectivity may be a selection for those with culturally based health habits.

Health Disparities

Explanations for Latino health disparities take two general forms. The first explanation attributes health disparities to a constrained access to health resources, including education, income and wealth, and insurance coverage. The second explanation questions whether acculturation in U.S. social life has a cost to health.

Latinos are likely to experience higher levels of morbidity because they are less likely to have health insurance (Andersen, Giachello, & Aday, 1986; Angel & Angel, 1996; Angel, Frisco, Angel, & Chiriboga, 2003; Lieu, Newacheck, & McManus, 1993; Schur, Albers, & Berk, 1995; Trevino, Moyer, Valdez, & Stroup-Benham, 1991). Legal and undocumented immigrants face especially high hurdles in securing insurance access (Granados, Puvvula, Berman, & Dowling, 2001). Any access to health insurance provides an opportunity for Latinos to develop a usual source of care, to seek medical care when symptoms of illness arise, and to engage in preventive medical care such as health screenings. Quality and continuity of insurance coverage also play important roles in shaping health disparities (Angel, Angel, & Markides, 2002). Movement of Latinos off and on state-provided health care (i.e., Medicaid) may disrupt therapeutic and preventive health care (Capps, 2001; Ellwood & Ku, 1998; Espenshade, Baraka, & Huber, 1997; Fix & Passel, 2002; Park, Sarnoff, Bender, & Koronbut, 2000). Moreover, it may delay medical care to a point of greater severity in the natural history of a disease or condition. Quality of coverage may limit critically needed services (e.g., oral or mental health) or price out-of-pocket expenses or deductibles beyond the income level.

Related to disparities in insurance access, lower levels of socioeconomic status also create barriers to securing basic daily health needs, such as nutrition, rest, and adequate housing. Lower levels of material resources indirectly produce health disparities through a greater vulnerability to disease risk exposures. This is a perspective found in theorizing about more structural determinants of health (House & Williams, 2001; Link & Phelan, 1995).

A second disparities explanation focuses on the processes of acculturation and appears as the other side of the health advantages-cultural coin. With acculturation, cultural barriers to negative health behaviors are removed (Cobas et al., 996; Harris, 1999; Scribner & Dwyer, 1989). Levels of drinking, smoking, and drug use will increase to those of the general population, perhaps even exceed them. Also, evidence is emerging to suggest that acculturation may play a role in Latino development of unhealthy weight levels (Gordon-Larsen, Harris, Ward, & Popkin, 2003). Among immigrants and their children, living life in two cultures produces tensions and conflicts within individuals and between generations (Shrout et al., 1992). Psychosocial stress and disorientation yields vulnerability to low self-esteem, addiction disorders, and depression (Gamst et al., 2002; Ge, Elder, Regnerus, & Cox, 2001; Harker, 2001; Kaplan & Marks, 1990; Rumbaut, 1996; Thoman & Suris, 2004). Acculturation is shaped by the sociocultural segment of society in which immigrants acculturate (Portes & Zhou, 1993). Consequently, acculturation into social groups with members of high behavioral health risk will accelerate the adoption of negative health behaviors.

MAJOR RESEARCH THEMES

The health research agenda for Latinos continues to promote basic documentation of Latino health patterns and differentials relative to whites. The major research themes observed in the demographic literature unsurprisingly are rooted in data availability and demographic subspecialty traditions. Fertility specialists took advantage of the new self-report of racial and ethnic identifiers in the 1970 census and Current Population Surveys (CPS) in the 1970s to conduct research on the reproductive health of Latinas. In the 1980s, demographic research included a significant body of research focused on race and ethnic differentials in infant mortality. Finally, demographers turned their attention to race and ethnic patterns in the demography of aging in the 1990s.

Reproductive and Sexual Health

Rapid population growth arose as a key concern of the industrialized world after World War II. The research focus quickly centered on fertility levels and differences in fertility among subpopulations as the critical engine to rapid population growth. Primarily due to census and CPS data, the field of reproductive health comprises a large literature on the demography of Latino health. Initial demographic research on Latina fertility relied on the new Hispanic identifier in the 1970 census and CPS data from the 1970s. The national-level data revealed higher numbers of children ever born among Latinos than whites or blacks, although differentials have narrowed over time and there is considerable variability in fertility among Latino ethnic groups (Bean & Tienda, 1987). For example, Cubans tend to have fertility patterns similar to those of whites: later age at first birth, longer intervals between children, and fewer children ever born. Even with similar patterns, Cuban women bear fewer children than whites over their entire reproductive period. Mexican-origin women are most likely to become mothers at earlier ages, have shorter intervals between children, and bear more children during their reproductive years. Fertility levels and patterns among Latinos of other ethnic origins are generally intermediate to these two extremes.

National fertility surveys conducted throughout the hemisphere in the 1970s, and expansion of U.S. fertility surveys (five cycles of the National Survey of Family Growth [NSFG]) provided national and international data on pregnancy and childbirth, contraceptive use, and infant health. The NSFG, however, did not sample sufficient numbers of Latinas to conduct analyses of their reproductive health until 1988. The NSFG also expanded its data collection to include younger women and unmarried women and to obtain data on sexual behaviors and reproductive and sexual attitudes. Latinas have higher levels of teenage motherhood, both intended and unintended pregnancies, and lower levels of contraceptive use. Moreover, low levels of prenatal care observed among pregnant Latinas raised practitioners' concerns about their higher risks for maternal and infant mortality and morbidity. Much research focused on understanding the mechanisms that sustained high levels of pregnancy and inadequate levels of contraceptive use and prenatal care and also on developing family planning programs to reverse them. Current census and fertility survey data continue to show higher fertility levels among Mexican-origin women, partially arising from a continued immigration of reproductive-age women from Mexico, purportedly a more pronatal culture than that of the United States. For example, preference for sons among immigrants may raise the number of children ever born as women strive to have some desired number of sons (Unger & Molina, 1997). Two extensions of this original research agenda on fertility differentials

have arisen in more contemporary research: sexual behaviors leading to sexually transmitted diseases (STDs) and prenatal care.

Pregnancy prevention programs are currently focused on teenage women to encourage young Latinas to delay parenthood until schooling is complete, reduce unintended pregnancies, and reduce abortion rates (Erickson, 1994; Jones, Darroch, & Henshaw, 2002). As pregnancy prevention became redirected toward adolescence, research on sexual behavior expanded to better understand proximate risk factors of age at first intercourse and contraceptive use. Even as the increasing use of oral contraceptives reduced the number of unintended pregnancies, rates of STDs increased alarmingly. The past decade has also been a time of rapidly rising rates of HIV/AIDS among Latino teens and, indeed, Latinos of all ages. Reproductive and sexual health research is focused on attitudes, knowledge, and practices of condom use and sexual behaviors that shape Latinos' understanding of STDs and HIV/AIDS and how to prevent them (East & Kiernan, 2001; Forrest, Austin, Valdes, Fuentes, & Wilson, 1993; Hollander, 2002; Marin, Gomez, & Hearst, 1993; Singer et al., 1990).

Adequate prenatal care is associated with better infant and maternal outcomes (Institute of Medicine, 1985). Yet fertility surveys reveal Latinas' lower levels of prenatal care, raising concern about their risk for poor maternal and infant health (U.S. Bureau of the Census, 2003, Tables 84 and 91). Only 75% of Mexican, Puerto Rican, and black women received prenatal care in the first trimester compared to 85% of white women. In contrast, 92% of Cuban women received first-trimester prenatal care. Approximately 6% of Mexican, Puerto Ricans, and black women received late or no prenatal care, in contrast to white (3.2%) and Cuban (1.3%) women. The proportion of women in all race and ethnic groups receiving prenatal care in the first trimester has increased since 1990, perhaps serving as evidence that family planning interventions have had some success.

An interesting observation arose from research on Latinas' relatively greater absence from adequate formal prenatal care regimens. Lack of prenatal care among economically vulnerable black women has been associated with poor birth outcomes. Similarly vulnerable Latinas who also receive less prenatal care, however, do not yield equally poor birth outcomes, an epidemiological paradox that forms the second major research theme.

Infant and Child Health

The U.S. infant mortality rate has declined considerably during the past half century. Research initially focused on black-white differences in an effort to document and explain significantly higher levels of infant mortality among blacks (Boone, 1989; Eberstein & Parker, 1984). Subsequently, research on ethnic differences in infant mortality began to increase substantially in the 1980s as individual states began to add a Hispanic origin item to death certificates, often specifying the ethnic national heritage (Becerra, Hogue, Atrash, & Perez, 1991; Powell-Griner, 1988; Rogers, 1984, 1989). Because Latinas receive low levels of prenatal care and are economically vulnerable, initial hypotheses predicted higher infant mortality among Latinos than whites. Evidence, however, consistently revealed rates of Latino infant mortality that were equivalent to or lower than those of whites, a phenomenon researchers called the epidemiological paradox.

The research agenda has progressed from providing basic documentation of differentials among Latino ethnic groups to developing explanations of the differences. First, significant variability among Latino ethnic groups exists. Most studies of multiple ethnic groups report that Mexicans and Cubans have lower infant mortality than whites; the Puerto Rican infant mortality rate exceeds that of whites, however (Albrecht, Clarke, Miller, & Farmer, 1996; Becerra et al., 1991; Hummer, Eberstein, & Nam, 1992; Singh & Yu, 1995). Second, a sizeable body of literature has emerged that strives to explain differences. One critical explanatory factor is nativity, with evidence consistently showing lower infant mortality among immigrants relative to native-born whites or native-born coethnics (Collins & Shay, 1994; Hummer et al., 1999). Other types of explanatory factors are socioeconomic characteristics, pregnancy, labor and delivery characteristics, birth outcomes, and cause of death. Foreign-born Latinos have higher-birth-weight infants than native-born Latinos, likely due to lower rates of smoking, drinking, and drug use among pregnant immigrant women, and thus lower infant mortality than native-born whites. Research has emerged to study whether acculturation to U.S. society adversely affects infant outcomes, narrowing Latino advantages and widening Latino disparities (Landale et al., 1999).

Birth outcomes are an important variable of interest because low birth weight and preterm births are the predominant risk factors for infant mortality (Institute of Medicine, 1985), and they vary significantly across race and ethnic groups. Cubans and Mexicans have higher or equivalent levels of healthy birth outcomes relative to whites, whereas Puerto Rican women have lower-birth-weight infants (Becerra et al., 1991; Hummer et al., 1992; Samuels, 1986). Contemporary research notes that although infant mortality rates have declined, the adverse birth outcomes of low birth weight and preterm births have increased (Guyer, Freedman, Strobino, & Sondik, 2000). Demographic studies report that the risks of low birth weight and preterm births are significantly higher for Mexicans and Puerto

Ricans, although the risk of infant mortality continues to remain paradoxically low for Mexican immigrants (Frisbie & Song, 2003).

Aging and Health

Analysis of a population's age structure, including its determinants and consequences for society, is a mainstay of demographic research. Demographic research on the causes and consequences of the aging of industrialized society increased rapidly in the mid-1980s. A significant portion of the demography of aging research agenda questioned whether increasing longevity would yield greater morbidity among older adults or spark a concomitant delay in morbidity to later ages. Another key question concerned economic issues associated with aging, retirement patterns, health care costs, and individual savings patterns (Zsembik, Drevenstedt, & McLane, 1997; Zsembik & Singer, 1990).

Census and CPS data, in addition to regional survey epidemiologic data, were used in initial studies of older Latinos that focused on living arrangements. A survey of older Latinos (Survey of Elderly Hispanics [SHE]) was fielded in 1988. Older Latinos are disproportionately absent from nursing homes and more likely than whites to live as dependents in multigenerational households (Burr & Mutchler, 1992; Worobey & Angel, 1990). Multigenerational coresidence is highest among older immigrants and among Mexican-origin and Cuban families (Zsembik, 1993, 1996). These observations sparked debate about the absence of Latinos in nursing homes and the presence in multigenerational family households. Multigenerational coresidence was found to be higher even among older Latinos in relative health, suggesting family pooling of incomes to provide better household material resources. Multigenerational coresidence was also found among the more frail older Latinos, suggesting a cultural basis for family care of older

and ill family members (Angel et al., 2003; Burr & Mutchler, 1999; Zsembik, 1993, 1996). An appreciable number of physically vulnerable older Latinos remained in their own residences, declaring a strong reluctance to enter a nursing home (Zsembik & Bonilla, 2000). Some studies raised the issues of a lack of cultural relevance and lack of eligibility for health care financing as factors deterring long-term residential care.

The next wave of research on aging and health among Latinos began the basic documentation of health, functioning, and disability among adults. Analyses of active life expectancy, the estimated time spent alive and in good health, reveal that Latinos tend to experience a longer active life expectancy than blacks but not whites (Hayward & Heron, 1999). Data on adults older than the age of 50 are more complete due to the Health and Retirement Study (HRS), the Asset and Health Dynamics Among the Oldest Old (AHEAD), and the Hispanic Established Populations for Epidemiologic Study of the Elderly (HEPESE). Latinos report higher levels of most serious medical conditions (e.g., heart disease and diabetes) and of impaired physical functioning than whites (Smith & Kington, 1997). A large number of studies report on data from the longitudinal HEPESE documenting health statuses and processes among older Mexican Americans (Peek, Ottenbacher, Markides, & Ostir, 2003). For example, physical functioning is predictive of mortality 2 years later (Markides et al., 2001). Research has begun to focus on chronic disease epidemiology and data on Latinos at midlife. Data pooled from several years (1991-1995) of the National Health Interview Survey (NHIS) reveal that near elderly Puerto Ricans report poorer health than whites, whereas Cubans report better or equivalent health than whites (Hajat, Lucas, & Kington, 2000). Also, Mexicans report fewer activity limitations than whites, but they rate their health more negatively and receive less medical care than whites. NHIS data collected after 1996 provide national-level data on several ethnic Latino groups across the life course. Puerto Ricans experience higher levels of medical conditions, functional limitations, and disability than other Latino groups at midlife, whereas Cubans retain levels of health comparable to those of whites (Zsembik, 2003a).

Demographic research has also focused on Latino disparities in health care financing as they approach and live through the older years (Angel & Angel, 1996; Angel et al., 2002, 2003; Granados et al., 2001; Lieu et al., 1993; Schur et al., 1995; Trevino et al., 1991). As a group, Latinos are less likely to have any form of health insurance than whites, and they are especially less likely to have private health insurance based in employment. Lack of health insurance is associated with less use of preventive health care, loss of a usual source of care, and little access to specialty care such as mental and oral health. Public sources of health care financing (e.g., Medicare and Medicaid) constitute a larger portion of medical expenditures among Latinos than whites, indicating their critical role in reducing Latino health care disparities (Escarce & Kapur, 2003). Economically vulnerable Latinos face serious risk of lack of health care even with public sources due to their insufficient income to pay for out-of-pocket expenses, medications, and deductibles.

ASSESSING THE RESEARCH AGENDA

Appreciation of the importance of research on Latino health has increased in a short time. Much has been accomplished in building the knowledge base through changes in sampling, data collection, and conceptual development. Researchers must continue to expand the knowledge base. Future research

is likely to extend in new directions as well as continue to elaborate on current themes.

Representative Samples

An initial observation concerns the rapid growth in generalizable knowledge during the past 20 years. There was a scarcity of generalizable knowledge about Latinos' health until the 1980s. What was known drew from community and local samples of Spanish-surnamed people residing in the southwestern United States. Censuses began to obtain self-reported ethnic identity in 1970. Vital statistics data began to assign ethnic identification in the late 1970s, although the quality of Latino ethnic identity was compromised through the 1990s by misclassification errors and the uneven adoption by states of a "Hispanic" item on certificates (Rosenberg et al., 1999). Representative surveys used in health research began to oversample Latinos and obtain self-reported "Hispanic" identity and conduct interviews in Spanish. These included the NSFG in 1988, NHIS in 1997, and the HRS and AHEAD in the early 1990s. Several representative surveys of Latinos were also fielded: HHANES in 1982 through 1984 and SHE in 1988. Subsequent waves of the NSFG and the NHIS expanded their categories of national origin to provide greater detail on Latino ethnic groups. The National Health Examination and Nutrition Study (2001) oversamples Latinos, but only Mexican-origin people can be identified.

Despite the inclusion of Latinos in data used for health research, there are two critical, perhaps competing, tasks that demographic health researchers must perform. First, as the ethnic composition of the Latino population changes with ethnic group-specific fertility rates and growing migration from countries of the Caribbean basin, data must be collected for each of these subgroups. As the Latino population becomes more ethnically diverse, however, the second critical task is how to respond to the challenge of classifying and analytically organizing the growing diversity. Latinos have appreciable rates of intermarriage with whites, blacks, and Latinos of different ethnic origins, creating multiple categories of "mixed" ethnic heritage. These individuals may not find the current ethnic categories as befitting their multiple heritages and thus opt for subgroup categories such as "other" or refuse to answer the ethnic identity item. Conventional practice is to exclude individuals in these ethnic categories from analysis because they are too heterogeneous to offer confident interpretations of patterns and trends. Thus, analytical focus is biased toward single ethnic identity individuals. The numbers of "mixed heritage" Latinos are likely to grow. Even if they constitute small numbers, they may be especially concentrated among more acculturated Latinos, a critical explanatory concept in health research.

Health Outcomes

Health research initially focused on Mexican-origin women's reproductive health and subsequently expanded to include a focus on infant health. Research on early and middle childhood and on adolescent males was and remains relatively neglected (Flores et al., 2002). Mortality studies included adult men and women, but we still know relatively little about adult health patterns and trends. Health research priorities for the Latino community tend to be skewed toward the negative health effects of behaviors often labeled as deviant: teenage childbearing, STDs and HIV/AIDS, violence, and substance abuse (Murdaugh, Hunt, Sowell, & Santana, 2004). There is a risk of "pathologizing" the Latino population with disproportionate attention to a small range of health behavior risks because the Latino

prevalence level exceeds that of whites. For example, heart disease remains the top cause of mortality among Latinos.

Basic documentation of levels, trends, and differentials of the full range of health and well-being indicators is needed, but generalizable knowledge about chronic disease epidemiology among adult women and men is sparse. Recent analyses of data pooled from the 1997 to 2000 National Health Interview surveys reveal a complex profile of disparities and advantages and differentials across ethnic groups (Zsembik, 2003; Zsembik & Fennell, in press). For example, adult Mexicans exhibit health advantages, whereas Puerto Ricans experience health disparities. Cubans and Dominicans reveal a mix of health disparities and advantages, depending on the health outcome. The effects of social determinants of health are also contingent on ethnicity. For example, worse health is associated with higher levels of socioeconomic status and acculturation among Mexicans but with lower levels of socioeconomic status and acculturation among Latinos whose origins are from Caribbean islands. The profile is contingent on location in the life course, however. Mexicans hold a health advantage in young adulthood but experience health disparities in middle and old age. The data suggest health disparities among Puerto Ricans in young adulthood, whereas older Puerto Ricans appear to be healthier than older whites. Cubans hold a health advantage in young adulthood and the absence of midlife or late-life health disparities, evidence that only Cubans are participating in the delays of morbidity until old age. Reducing disparities and promoting health are more effectively addressed by targeting specific Latino ethnic groups, focusing on health states earlier in the disablement process, and redirecting attention to ethnoracial differentials earlier in the adult life course.

Furthermore, relatively little is known about cognition across the life course among

Latinos. The phase in the life course known as early childhood has drawn attention because of new information on the social context of neural and cognitive development before age 5 (Shonkoff & Phillips, 2000). If Latino infants have a health and survival advantage at birth, does it indicate a child development advantage (Padilla, Boardman, Hummer, & Espitia, 2002)? Research also focuses on the sociocognitive health and development of middle childhood in relation to educational achievement but rarely includes adequate samples of Latino children (Flores et al., 2002). Mexican-origin children have lower prevalence levels of cognitive conditions than white children, whereas Latino children of Caribbean origin (Puerto Rican, Cuban, and Dominican) have prevalence levels equivalent to those of whites (Zsembik & Johnson, 2003). Children of all ethnic origins who are more acculturated to North America are also more likely to be diagnosed with either attention deficit disorder or a learning disability and to have activity limitation. Research on Alzheimer's disease and other causes of cognitive impairment are also the focus of the national research agenda (Stern & Carstensen, 2000). Although national-level data indicate that older Latinos have higher levels of cognitive impairment than older whites, much research is needed to understand cognitive health and changes among Latinos.

Explaining Differences, Patterns, and Trends

A final observation concerns the conceptual development of explanations of Latino health patterns. First, research consistently reveals the importance of migration status in health outcomes, often inferred as indirect evidence of ethnocultural effects on health. The best representative data on Latino health typically ascertain limited information on ethnicity and culture, generally obtaining ethnic origin for Mexican, Cuban, and Puerto Rican subpopulations, nativity, and language of interview. Conceptual and measurement work on specifying the meaning and role of culture is a needed research task. To understand the role of migration, bicultural data (e.g., Puerto Rican Infant and Maternal Health Study and the Mexican Migration Project) are needed to sort out health-selective migration. Innovative use of data from immigrant sending and receiving countries may be useful to approximate bicultural data (Frank & Hummer, 2002; Palloni & Arias, 2004). Health researchers recognize the need to validate basic health measures for Spanish-language, immigrant, and ethnic populations (Knight, Virdin, & Roosa, 1994; Pasick, Stewart, Bird, & D'Onofrio, 2001; Zsembik, 1994). Significantly more work is warranted, especially for more subjective measures and in the fields of cognitive health and mental health. Finally, continued conceptual progress will include the synthesis of multiple sets of explanatory factors, drawn from multiple subfields in demography, to provide a more sophisticated framework. Currently, demographers commonly examine the relative contributions of cultural and economic influences on health outcomes. Fusing analytic innovations from key demographic research (e.g., biodemography, immigration, life course analysis, and multilevel analysis) will enhance our understanding of the causal mechanisms of race and ethnic health disparities.

IMPLICATIONS OF LATINO HEALTH RESEARCH

Accomplishing the current research agenda on Latino health will likely impact subsequent agendas for demographic research on health and households. Demographic health research may foster development of causal models of health disparities through its general conceptual flexibility and analytical strength. Demographic research on Latino health may contribute to the development and refinement of multilevel or ecological models and health.

Health Disparities

Health disparities research is not new to demographers, who during the past 30 years have built a large literature on race and ethnic differences in health and mortality among infants, women of reproductive age, and older adults. Social scientists, epidemiologists, health service analysts, and a diversity of researchers in other intellectual traditions conceptualize and conduct health disparities research. There is substantial imprecision in defining the critical concepts and elaborating on the causal mechanisms that link them. Latino health demography provides an opportunity to link to other intellectual traditions, thus acting as a cross-disciplinary bridge for multidisciplinary research efforts.

Demographers' conceptual flexibility places them in a favorable position to develop interdisciplinary conceptual models of health disparities, drawing research themes from social inequalities, migration and transnational communities, and cultural demography. Empirical evidence of the structure of health disparities draws heavily on the experience of black Americans. Health disparities explanations best fit the most economically vulnerable but may be less useful for the African American middle class, small though it may be. Explanations of black-white health disparities tend to discount the role of culture on health beliefs, practices, and statuses, whether culture is defined as ethnic or family culture, which remain significant features in personal life (Christensen, 2003; Earls & Carlson, 2001; Foner, 1997; Mendoza & Fuentes-Affleck, 1999).

Extending explanations of black-white disparities to Latino-white comparisons entails revision to include the effects of migration and language. Empirical data frequently suggest that the Latino-white differences are dissimilar to black-white health differences. Moreover, empirical data suggest variability in health disparities across Latino ethnic groups. Latino health research is well positioned to promote a conceptual framework of health disparities that logically organizes and integrates multiple causes inclusive of biology, culture, and social inequalities. A common conceptual frame provides comparisons among a wide array of race and ethnic groups and evaluation of direct, mediating, and moderating causal pathways. The answers to the following questions would be provided: Are there common critical causal mechanisms that create and sustain health disparities? How does health quality vary within groups?

Demographers' analytical capacity to manage and evaluate a diversity of data sources provides a second disciplinary bridging opportunity. Dynamic and multilevel demographic analyses of Latino health data will further opportunity to examine the character of the causal ties among bioindicators, individual characteristics, and community features and how the causal ties change or are sustained over time. Demographers' facility in integrating and managing multiple sources of data can be extended more widely in Latino health research. Traditional national surveys, program administration records, clinical studies, and ethnographic observation can be combined to more richly describe the structure and experience of health disparities in the United States.

Research on Families and Households

Demographic research on families and households will continue to devote an increasing amount of attention to the effect on individual health of collective characteristics, such as social capital, transnational community, and neighborhood context. A better understanding of the health of Latino children will raise awareness of Latino family households as producers and consumers of health and medical resources. Each research avenue directs deeper conceptualization of more sociocultural factors associated with health.

Latino communities historically have been characterized as having high degrees of ethnic solidarity, familism, and large social networks of family and fictive kin (Fitzpatrick, 1971; Moore, 1976; Stycos, 1955). These collectivist characteristics were thought to discourage assimilation into society and thus retard immigrant social mobility (Moore, 1976). "Cultural deficiency" models gave way to structural models, which included cultural elements manifesting partly as survival strategies but emphasized barriers to high-quality education, employment, and wealth accumulation opportunities (Vega, 1990). Recent social demographic research is revisiting the character and role of cultural forces. The emergence of social capital as a positive force on health and other outcomes calls for a return to collectivist values, norms, and practices that may arise from Latino culture. For example, values of familism may promote family prevention practices, provision of health and personal care, and a more positive psychosocial orientation (Franco & Levitt, 1998). The National Institutes of Health called for an expansion of basic social science research on the meaning and measurement of sociocultural phenomena and processes and applied research on their implications for health. Research on migration and the establishment and maintenance of transnational communities has begun to study the relationship between health and social networks (Zsembik, 2003b).

A deeper appreciation for the role of Latino culture in shaping families, social capital, and health reorients health research toward the family household as a relevant unit of analysis. Health, functioning, and disability, and health and medical care use, are typically conceptualized and operationalized simply as individual-level properties. Adult-onset chronic disease and health impairments, however, largely reflect the long-term effects of lifestyles, bundles of habits shared by family households regarding diet and nutrition, exercise, substance use, and preventive care. To the extent that lifestyles have elements of family culture, they also reflect the ethnic culture in which the family is embedded. It is conventional to assume that the Latino parent or the spouse, usually women, is the first line of defense in promoting health or providing health care. In turn, caring for an ill family member carries health costs to the care provider. Accordingly, Latino households may be characterized as sharing a collective health capital. Households also function as a consumer unit, purchasing health services and products to be shared among family members. Most common are over-the-counter medications and other therapeutic products purchased in grocery stores. Private and public insurance often encompasses an entire household, either through an employee's purchase of employer-sponsored family health plans or through eligibility characteristics for state insurance programs. Knowledge of the collective health of the Latino household is relevant to public policymakers and health care planners concerned with equity issues of long-term care, demand for formal services, and family support burdens.

CONCLUSION

The amount of research on Latino health has increased markedly, especially in the past decade. Antonia Coello Novello, surgeon general between 1990 and 1993, spearheaded the National Hispanic-Latino Health Initiative. The participants listed areas of priority for the expansion of the research agenda on Latino health research, including data collection strategies and a comprehensive agenda to shape funding and research priorities (Delgado & Estrada, 1993; Gerardo, Amaro, Eisenberg, & Opava-Stitzer, 1993). We have made some progress toward accomplishing these tasks, and there is every indication that this progress will continue and even accelerate. Latino migration and fertility, and ethnic diversity among Latinos, have transformed U.S. society and will continue to influence contemporary U.S. society. Demographers' analytical focus on health disparities and success among Latinos highlights the degree to which Latinos participate in national improvements in longevity, health, and well-being.

REFERENCES

Abraido-Lanza, A. F., Dohrenwend, B. P., Ng-Mak, D. S., & Turner, J. B. (1999). The Latino mortality paradox: A test of the "salmon bias" and healthy migrant hypotheses. *American Journal of Public Health, 89*(10), 1543-1548.

Albrecht, S. L., Clarke, L. L., Miller, M. K., & Farmer, F. L. (1996). Predictors of differential birth outcomes among Hispanic groups in the United States: The role of maternal risk characteristics and medical care. *Social Science Quarterly, 7*, 407-433.

Andersen, R. M., Giachello, A. L., & Aday, L. A. (1986). Access of Hispanics to health care and cuts in services: A state-of-the-art overview. *Public Health Reports, 101*(3), 238-252.

Angel, R. J., & Angel, J. L. (1996). The extent of private and public health insurance coverage among adult Hispanics. *The Gerontologist, 36*(3), 332-341.

Angel, R. J., Angel, J. L., & Markides, K. S. (2002). Stability and change in health insurance among older Mexican Americans: Longitudinal evidence from the Hispanic established populations for epidemiologic study of the elderly. *American Journal of Public Health, 92*(8), 1264-1272.

Angel, R. J., Frisco, M., Angel, J. L., & Chiriboga, D. A. (2003). Financial strain and health among elderly Mexican-origin individuals. *Journal of Health and Social Behavior, 44*(4), 536-551.

Arias, E., Anderson, R. N., Hsiang-Ching, K., Murphy, S. L., & Kochanek, K. D. (2003). Deaths: Final data for 2001. *National Vital Statistics Reports, 52*(3).

Balcazar, H., Peterson, G. W., & Krull, J. L. (1997). Acculturation and family cohesiveness in Mexican American pregnant women: Social and health implications. *Family and Community Health, 20*, 16-31.

Bean, F. D., & Tienda, M. (1987). *The Hispanic Population of the United States.* New York: Russell Sage Foundation.

Becerra, J., Hogue, C., Atrash, H., & Perez, N. (1991). Infant mortality among Hispanics: A portrait of heterogeneity. *Journal of the American Medical Association, 265*, 217-221.

Boone, M. (1989). *Capital crime: Black infant mortality in America.* Newbury Park, CA: Sage.

Burr, J. A., & Mutchler, J. E. (1992). The living arrangements of unmarried elderly Hispanic women. *Demography, 29*(1), 93-112.

Burr, J. A., & Mutchler, J. E. (1993). Ethnic living arrangements: Cultural convergence or cultural manifestation? *Social Forces, 72*(1), 169-179.

Burr, J. A., & Mutchler, J. E. (1999). Race and ethnic variation in norms of filial responsibility among older persons. *Journal of Marriage and the Family, 61*(3), 674-687.

Capps, R. (2001). Hardship among children of immigrants: Findings from the 1999 National Survey of America's Families. In *Assessing the New Federalism*, Series B, No. 29. Washington, DC: Urban Institute.

Christensen, P. (2003). The health-promoting family: A conceptual framework for future research. *Social Science & Medicine, 59*, 377-387.

Cobas, J. A., Balcazar, H., Benin, M. B., Keith, V. M., & Chong, Y. (1996). Acculturation and low-birth weight infants among Latino women. *American Journal of Public Health, 86*(3), 394-396.

Collins, J. W., & Shay, D. K. (1994). Prevalence of low birth weight among Hispanic infants with United States-born and foreign-born mothers: The effects of urban poverty. *American Journal of Epidemiology, 139*, 184-192.

Day, J. C. (1996). *Population projections of the United States by age, sex, race, and Hispanic origin: 1995 to 2050*, U.S. Bureau of the Census, Current Population Reports P25-1130. Washington, DC: Government Printing Office.

Delgado, J. L., & Estrada, L. (1993). Improving data collection strategies. *Public Health Report, 108*(5), 540-546.

Earls, F., & Carlson, M. (2001). The social ecology of child health and well-being. *Annual Review of Public Health, 22*, 143-166.

East, P. L., & Kiernan, E. A. (2001). Risks among youth who have multiple sisters who were adolescent parents. *Family Planning Perspectives, 33*(2), 75-80.

Eberstein, I., & Parker, J. (1984). Racial differences in infant mortality by cause of death. *Demography, 21*, 309-321.

Ellwood, M. R., & Ku, L. (1998). Welfare and immigration reforms: Unintended side effects for Medicaid. *Health Affairs, 17*(3), 137-151.

Erickson, P. I. (1994). Lessons from a repeat pregnancy prevention program for Hispanic teenage mothers in east Los Angeles. *Family Planning Perspectives, 26*(4), 174-178.

Escarce, J. J., & Kapur, K. (2003). Racial and ethnic differences in public and private medical care expenditures among aged Medicare beneficiaries. *Milbank Quarterly, 81*(2), 249-275.

Espenshade, T. J., Baraka, J. L., & Huber, G. A. (1997). Implications of the 1996 Welfare and Immigration Reform Acts for U.S. immigrants. *Population and Development Review, 23*(4), 769-801.

Fitzpatrick, J. (1971). *Puerto Rican Americans: The meaning of migration to the mainland*. Englewood Cliffs, NJ: Prentice Hall.

Fix, M., & Passel, J. (2002). *The scope and impact of welfare reform's immigrant provisions*. Washington, DC: The Urban Institute.

Flores, G., Fuentes-Affleck, E., Barbot, O., Carter-Pokras, O., Claudio, L., Lara M., et al. (2002). The health of Latino children: Urgent priorities, unanswered questions, and a research agenda. *Journal of the American Medical Association, 288*(1), 82-91.

Foner, N. (1997). The immigrant family: Cultural legacies and cultural changes. *International Migration Review, 31*(4), 961-974.

Forrest, K. A., Austin, D. M., Valdes, M. I., Fuentes, E. G., & Wilson, S. R. (1993). Exploring norms and beliefs related to AIDS prevention among California Hispanic men. *Family Planning Perspectives, 25*(3), 111-117.

Franco, N., & Levitt, M. J. (1998). The social ecology of middle childhood: Family support, friendship quality, and self-esteem. *Family Relations, 47*(4), 315-322.

Frank, R., & Hummer, R. A. (2002). The other side of the paradox: The risk of low birth weight among infants of migrant and nonimmigrant households within Mexico. *International Migration Review, 36*(3), 746-766.

Frisbie, W. P., & Song, S. (2003). Hispanic pregnancy outcomes: Differentials over time and current risk factor effects. *Policy Studies Journal, 31*(2), 237-253.

Gamst, G., Dana, R. H., Der-Karabetian, A., Aragon, M., Arellano, L. M., & Kramer, T. (2002). Effects of Latino acculturation and ethnic identity on mental health outcomes. *Hispanic Journal of Behavioral Sciences, 24*(4), 479-505.

Ge, X., Elder, G. H., Regnerus, M., & Cox, C. (2001). Pubertal transitions, perceptions of being overweight, and adolescents' psychological maladjustment: Gender and ethnic differences. *Social Psychology Quarterly, 64*(4), 363-375.

Gerardo, M., Amaro, H., Eisenberg, C., & Opava-Stitzer, S. (1993). The development of a relevant and comprehensive research agenda to improve Hispanic health. *Public Health Reports, 108*(5), 546-551.

Gordon-Larsen, P., Harris, K. M., Ward, D. S., & Popkin, B. M. (2003). Acculturation and overweight-related behaviors among Hispanic immigrants to the US: The National Longitudinal Study of Adolescent Health. *Social Science & Medicine, 57*(11), 2023-2035.

Granados, G., Puvvula, J., Berman, N., & Dowling, P. T. (2001). Health care for Latino children: Impact of child and parental birthplace on insurance status and access to health services. *American Journal of Public Health, 91*(11), 1806-1808.

Grieco, E. M., & Cassidy, R. C. (2001). *Overview of race and Hispanic origin*, U.S. Bureau of the Census, Census Brief 2000. Washington, DC: Government Printing Office.

Guyer, B., Freedman, M. A., Strobino, D. M., & Sondik, E. J. (2000). Annual summary of vital statistics: Trends in the health of Americans in the 20th century. *Pediatrics, 106*(6), 1307-1318.

Hajat, A., Lucas, J. B., & Kington, R. (2000). Health outcomes among Hispanic subgroups: Data from the National Health Interview Survey, 1992-95. In *Advance data from vital and health statistics 310*. Hyattsville, MD: National Center for Health Statistics.

Harker, K. (2001). Immigrant generation, assimilation, and adolescent psychological well-being. *Social Forces, 79*(3), 969-1004.

Harris, K. M. (1999). The health status and risk behavior of adolescents in immigrant families. In D. J. Hernandez (Ed.), *Children of immigrants: Health, adjustment, and public assistance* (pp. 286-347). Washington, DC: National Academy of Sciences Press.

Hayward, M. D., & Heron, M. (1999). Racial inequality in active life among adult Americans. *Demography, 36*(1), 77-91.

Hollander, D. (2002). Poor Hispanic women who have been sterilized are unlikely to use condoms. *Perspectives on Sexual and Reproductive Health, 34*(1), 51.

House, J. S., & Williams, D. R. (2001). Understanding and reducing socio-economic and racial/ethnic disparities in health. In B. D. Smedley & S. L. Syme (Eds.), *Promoting health: Intervention strategies from social and behavioral research* (pp. 81-124). Washington, DC: National Academy Press.

Hummer, R. A., Biegler, M., de Turk, P. B., Forbes, D., Frisbie, W. P., Hong, Y., et al. (1999). Race/ethnicity, nativity, and infant mortality in the United States. *Social Forces, 77*(3), 1083-1118.

Hummer, R. A., Eberstein, I. W., & Nam, C. B. (1992). Infant mortality differentials among Hispanic groups in Florida. *Social Forces, 70*, 1055-1075.

Hummer, R. A., Pacewicz, J., Wang, S., & Collins, C. (2004). Health insurance coverage in nonmetropolitan America. In N. Glasgow, L. W. Morton, & N. E. Johnson (Eds.), *Critical issues in rural health* (pp. 197-209). Ames, IA: Blackwell.

Hummer, R. A., Rogers, R. G., Amir, S. H., Forbes, D., & Frisbie, W. P. (2000). Adult mortality differentials among Hispanic subgroups and non-Hispanic whites. *Social Science Quarterly, 81*(1), 459-477.

Idler, E., & Angel, R. (1990). Self-rated health and mortality in the NHANES-I epidemiological follow-up. *American Journal of Public Health, 80*, 446-452.

Institute of Medicine. (1995). *Preventing low birth weight.* Washington, DC: National Academy Press.

Jones, R. K., Darroch, J. E., & Henshaw, S. K. (2002). Patterns in the socioeconomic characteristics of women obtaining abortions in 2000-2001. *Perspectives on Sexual and Reproductive Health, 34*(5), 226-235.

Kaplan, M. S., & Marks, G. (1990). Adverse effects of acculturation: Psychological distress among Mexican American young adults. *Social Science & Medicine, 31*, 1313-1319.

Knight, G. P., Virdin, L. M., & Roosa, M. (1994). Socialization and family correlates of mental health outcomes among Hispanic and Anglo American children: Consideration of cross-ethnic scalar equivalence. *Child Development, 65*(1), 212-224.

Landale, N. S., Oropesa, R. S., & Gorman, B. K. (2000). Migration and infant death: Assimilation or selective migration among Puerto Ricans. *American Sociological Review, 65*, 888-909.

Landale, N. S., Oropesa, R. S., Llanes, D., & Gorman, B. K. (1999). Does Americanization have adverse effects on health? Stress, health habits, and infant health outcomes among Puerto Ricans. *Social Forces, 78*(2), 613-630.

LeClere, F. B., Rogers, R. G., & Peters, K. D. (1997). Ethnicity and mortality in the United States: Individual and community correlates. *Social Forces, 76*(1), 169-198.

Lieu, T. A., Newacheck, P. W., & McManus, M. A. (1993). Race, ethnicity, and access to ambulatory care among U.S. adolescents. *American Journal of Public Health, 83*(7), 960-966.

Link, B. G., & Phelan, J. (1995). Social conditions as fundamental causes of disease. *Journal of Health and Social Behavior, 36*(SPEISS), 80-95.

Marin, B. V. O., Gomez, C. A., & Hearst, N. (1993). Multiple heterosexual partners and condom use among Hispanics and non-Hispanic whites. *Family Planning Perspectives, 25*(4), 170-174.

Markides, K. S., Black, S. A., Ostir, G. V., Angel, R. J., Guralnik, J. M., & Lichtenstein, M. (2001). Lower body function and mortality in Mexican American elderly people. *Journal of Gerontology Series A, 56*, M243.

Markides, K. S., & Coreil, J. (1986). The health of Hispanics in the southwestern United States: An epidemiologic paradox. *Public Health Reports, 101*(3), 253-265.

Massey, D. S. (1993). Latinos, poverty, and the underclass: A new agenda for research. *Hispanic Journal of Behavioral Sciences, 15,* 449-475.

Mendoza, F. S., & Fuentes-Afflick, E. (1999). Latino children's health and the family-community health promotion model. *Western Journal of Medicine, 170,* 85-92.

Moore, J. (with Pachon, H.). (1976). *Mexican Americans.* Englewood Cliffs, NJ: Prentice Hall.

Murdaugh, C., Hunt, S., Sowell, R., & Santana, I. (2004). Domestic violence in Hispanics in the southeastern United States: A survey and needs analysis. *Journal of Family Violence, 19*(2), 107-116.

National Alliance for Hispanic Health. (2001). *A primer for cultural competency: Towards quality health services for Hispanics.* Washington, DC: Author.

National Center for Health Statistics. (2003). *Health, United States, 2003.* Hyattsville, MD: Author.

Padilla, Y. C., Boardman, J. D., Hummer, R. A., & Espitia, M. (2002). Is the Mexican American "epidemiologic paradox" advantage at birth maintained through early childhood? *Social Forces, 80*(3), 1101-1124.

Palloni, A., & Arias, E. (2004). Paradox lost: Explaining the Hispanic adult mortality advantage. *Demography, 41*(3), 385-415.

Park, S. H., Sarnoff, R., Bender, C., & Koronbut, C. (2000). Impact of recent welfare and immigration reforms on use of Medicaid for prenatal care by immigrants in California. *Journal of Immigrant Health, 2,* 5-22.

Pasick, R. J., Stewart, S. L., Bird, J. A., & D'Onofrio, C. N. (2001). Quality of data in multiethnic health surveys. *Public Health Reports, 116*(Suppl.), 223-243.

Peek, M. K., Ottenbacher, K. J., Markides, K. S., & Ostir, G. V. (2003). Examining the disablement process among older Mexican American adults. *Social Science & Medicine, 57*(3), 413-426.

Portes, A., & Rumbaut, R. G. (1990). *Immigrant America: A portrait.* Berkeley: University of California Press.

Portes, A., & Zhou, M. (1993). The new second generation: Segmented assimilation and its variants. *Annals of the American Academy of Political and Social Sciences, 530,* 74-96.

Powell-Griner, E. (1988). Differences in infant mortality among Texas Anglos, Hispanics, and blacks. *Social Science Quarterly, 69,* 452-467.

Rogers, R. (1984). Infant mortality among New Mexican Hispanics, Anglos, and Indians. *Social Science Quarterly, 65,* 876-884.

Rogers, R. (1989). Ethnic differences in infant mortality: Fact or artifact? *Social Science Quarterly, 70,* 642-649.

Rosenberg, H. M., Maurer, J. D., Sorlie, P. D., Johnson, N. J., MacDorman, M. F., Hoyert, D. L., et al. (1999). Quality of death rates by race and Hispanic origin: A summary of current research, 1999. In *Vital health statistics,* Series 2. Hyattsville, MD: National Center for Health Statistics.

Rumbaut, R. G. (1996). The crucible within: Ethnic identity, self-esteem, and segmented assimilation among children of immigrants. In A. Portes (Ed.), *The new second generation* (pp. 119-170). New York: Russell Sage Foundation.

Samuels, B. (1986). Infant mortality and low birth weight among minority groups in the United States. In *Report of the secretary's task force on black and minority health* (No. 6, pp. 33-85). Washington, DC: Department of Health and Human Services.

Schur, C. L., Albers, L. A., & Berk, M. L. (1995). Health care use by Hispanic adults: Financial vs. non-financial determinants. *Health Care Financing Review, 17*(2), 71-89.

Scribner, R. (1996). Paradox as paradigm: The health outcomes of Mexican Americans. *American Journal of Public Health, 86*(3), 303-306.

Scribner, R. S., & Dwyer, J. H. (1989). Acculturation and low birth weight among Latinos in the Hispanic HANES. *American Journal of Public Health, 79*, 1263-1267.

Shonkoff, J. P., & Phillips, D. A. (Eds.); National Research Council & Institute of Medicine, Commission on Behavioral and Social Sciences and Education, Board on Children, Youth, and Families. (2000). *From neurons to neighborhoods: The science of early childhood development.* Washington, DC: National Academy Press.

Shrout, P. E., Canino, G. J., Brid, H. R., Rubio-Stipec, M., Bravo, M., & Burnham, M. A. (1992). Mental health status among Puerto Ricans, Mexican Americans, and non-Hispanic whites. *American Journal of Community Psychology, 20*, 729-752.

Singer, A. (2004). *The rise of new immigrant gateways.* Washington, DC: Brookings Institute.

Singer, M., Flores, C., Davison, L., Burke, G., Castillo, Z., Scanlon, K., et al. (1990). SIDA: The economic, social, and cultural context of AIDS among Latinos. *Medical Anthropology Quarterly, 4*(1), 72-114.

Singh, G. K., & Yu, S. M. (1995). Infant mortality in the United States: Trends, differentials, and projections, 1950 through 2010. *American Journal of Public Health, 85*, 957-964.

Smith, J. P., & Kington, R. (1997). Demographic and economic correlates of health in old age. *Demography, 34*(1), 159-170.

Sorlie, P. D., Backlund, E., Johnson, N. J., & Hogat, E. (1993). Mortality by Hispanic status in the United States. *Journal of the American Medical Association, 270*(20), 2464-2468.

Stern, P. C., & Carstensen, L. L. (Eds.); National Research Council, Commission on Behavioral and Social Sciences and Education, Board on Behavioral, Cognitive, and Sensory Sciences. (2000). *The aging mind: Opportunities in cognitive research..* Washington, DC: National Academy Press.

Stycos, J. M. (1955). *Family and fertility in Puerto Rico: A study of the lower income group.* New York: Columbia University Press.

Thoman, L.V., & Suris, A. (2004). Acculturation and acculturative stress as predictors of psychological distress and quality-of-life functioning in Hispanic psychiatric patients. *Hispanic Journal of Behavioral Sciences, 26*(3), 293-312.

Tienda, M. (1989). Puerto Ricans and the underclass debate: Evidence for structural explanations of labor market performance. *Annals of the American Academy of Political and Social Science, 501*, 105-119.

Torres, A., & Rodriguez, C. E. (1991). Latino research and policy: The Puerto Rican case. In E. Melendez, C. B. Rodriguez, & J. B. Figeroa (Eds.), *Hispanic in the labor force: Issues and policy* (pp. 247-263). New York: Plenum.

Trevino, F. M., Moyer, M. E., Valdez, R. B., & Stroup-Benham, C. A. (1991). Health insurance coverage and utilization of health services by Mexican Americans, mainland Puerto Ricans, and Cuban Americans. *Journal of the American Medical Association, 265*(2), 233-238.

Unger, J. B., & Molina, G. B. (1997). Desired family size and son preference among Hispanic women of low socioeconomic status. *Family Planning Perspectives, 29*(6), 284-287.

U.S. Census Bureau. (2003). *Statistical abstract of the United States, 2003.* Washington, DC: Government Printing Office.

Vega, W. A. (1990). Hispanic families in the 1980s: A decade of research. *Journal of Marriage and the Family, 52*(4), 1015-1024.

Worobey, J. L., & Angel, R. J. (1990). Poverty and health: Older minority women and the rise of the female-headed household. *Journal of Health and Social Behavior, 31*(4), 370-383.

Zsembik, B. A. (1993). Determinants of living alone among older Hispanics. *Research on Aging, 15,* 449-464.

Zsembik, B. A. (1994). Ethnic and socio-demographic correlates of the use of proxy respondents: The National Survey of Hispanic Elderly People, 1988. *Research on Aging, 19,* 401-414.

Zsembik, B. A. (1996). The preference for co-residence among older Latinos. *Journal of Aging Studies, 10,* 69-81.

Zsembik, B. A. (2000). The Cuban ethnic economy and labor market outcomes of Latinos in metropolitan Florida. *Hispanic Journal of Behavioral Sciences, 22,* 223-236.

Zsembik, B. A. (2003a, May). *Health disparities among Latinos.* Paper presented at the annual meeting of the Population Association of America, Minneapolis, MN.

Zsembik, B. A. (2003b, August). *Transnationalism and health among Puerto Ricans.* Paper presented at the annual meeting of the American Sociological Association, Atlanta, GA.

Zsembik, B. A., & Bonilla, Z. (2000). Eldercare and the changing family in Puerto Rico. *Journal of Family Issues, 21,* 652-674.

Zsembik, B. A., Drevenstedt, G., & McLane, C. P. (1997). Economic well-being among older Latinos. *International Journal of Sociology and Social Policy, 17,* 34-56.

Zsembik, B. A., & Fennell, D. (in press). Ethnic variation in health and the determinants of health among Latinos. *Social Science & Medicine.*

Zsembik, B. A., & Johnson, A. (2003, May). *Functional health among school-age Latino children.* Paper presented at the annual meeting of the Population Association of America, Minneapolis, MN.

Zsembik, B. A., & Llanes, D. (1996). Generational differences in educational achievement among Mexican Americans. *Social Science Quarterly, 77,* 363-375.

Zsembik, B. A., & Singer, A. (1990). The problem of defining retirement among minority populations: The Mexican Americans. *The Gerontologist, 30*(6), 749-757.

CHAPTER 4

Identifying Patterns of Managing Chronic Conditions

Family Management Styles

JANET A. DEATRICK, MELISSA A. ALDERFER,
GEORGE KNAFL, AND KATHLEEN KNAFL

A report by the Institute of Medicine (IOM) (Institute of Medicine, 2001; Weihs, Fisher, MacBaird, & the National Working Group on Family-Based Interventions in Chronic Disease, 2002) includes two recommendations for intervention research that targets families with chronically ill members. First, family assessment should be included in clinical trials of interventions so that subgroup analysis can determine the types of families for whom the intervention is most successful. Second, interventions should deemphasize a one-size-fits-all intervention philosophy. That is, interventions should be tailored to the specifics of the illness as well as the family's lifestyle, culture, and level of need. Optimally, such assessments and interventions would take into account not only general family processes but also the family processes related specifically to health issues or disease management.

Typologies, multidimensional classification systems that summarize dimensions of family processes, hold promise for meeting the challenges posed by the IOM. Typologies allow for the classification of families into "types" based on patterns of family processes. Families of different types may respond differently to interventions; thus, using such assessment methods may help identify those for whom interventions are most effective. Similarly, knowing the pattern of family process, or the family type, may be helpful in tailoring the intervention to meet specific needs of the family. The potential of this approach, however, is largely untapped.

The main purpose of this chapter is to guide the reader to explore typologies. Although not meant to be an exhaustive discussion, this article (a) describes the importance of family typologies in the family sciences; (b) reviews two major family typologies, including Family Management Styles

AUTHOR'S NOTE: The authors acknowledge support from the National Institute of Nursing Research/ National Institutes of Health (NR08048) in preparation of this chapter.

(FMS) and the family typology developed in the California Health Project (Fisher, Chesla, et al., 2000; Fisher, Gudmundsdottir, et al., 2000; Knafl & Deatrick, 2003); and (c) explores implications of family typologies for family sciences, particularly descriptive and intervention research.

NATURE AND IMPORTANCE OF FAMILY TYPOLOGIES

Whereas common assessment techniques describe individuals on single dimensions, empirical typologies integrate data across family members and across domains of family life to reflect a broader and more integrated picture of the family. They preserve the functional unit of the family through identifying a profile of scores (quantitative) or a specific constellation of themes and subthemes (qualitative) (Filsinger, 1990; Fisher, Chesla, et al., 2000). In other words, family typologies capture patterns of family process and allow for differentiation of family types based on emergent differences in family processes. These types may be defined based on the degree to which they engage in specific behaviors (quantitative) or the kind of processes in which they engage (qualitative). To the degree that analytic procedures are selected appropriately, both quantitative and qualitative typologies can be used to study families (Ayres, Kavanaugh, & Knafl, 2003; Sandelowski, 1996a).

A wide variety of typologies have been developed to guide the family sciences. They typically focus on either general family processes or disease management (Knafl & Deatrick, 2003). Before examining specific examples of both quantitative and qualitative typologies and their implications for tailoring family interventions, we discuss how to justify using typologies, their innate logic, and the procedures (general and specific) for generating them.

Quantitative Typologies

Justification

Quantitative or numerical typologies can be used in a variety of ways in planning, implementing, and evaluating intervention research. They can be used to inform the design of the study, to assess subjects before an intervention, to plan the content of an intervention, and to select or create sensitive outcome measures.

Numerical typologies can be generated from variables that are distributed so as to have two or more modes (multimodal data), each mode being a type. A set of types are referred to as the typology (Cattell, 1966). As such, the typology has systemic support and is a natural versus artificial way to classify phenomena. Once types have been identified, the typology embodies more information (new properties) than the original profile of scores. Within the typology, each type can be considered in terms of a case or prototype, which may have some overlap with other types. (Because of the continuous nature of variables comprising types or typologies of disease management, their boundaries often overlap, and membership in a type may be a matter of degree.)

Over time, quantitative typologies can be clarified or enhanced or both through additional research. For instance, patient scores can be added to or deleted from the profile to change or expand the description of the underlying types.

Logic

As contrasted to the Galilean approach to scientific investigation that measures the covariation among variables (e.g., factor analysis and multiple regression), typologies represent individuals or families and are based on an Aristotelian approach, which examines similarities among members of the sample and groups together those who

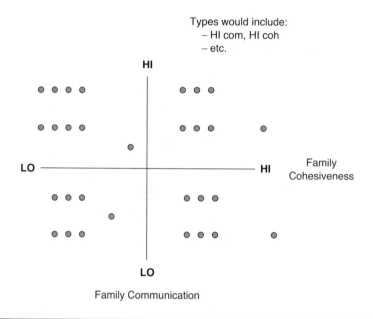

Figure 4.1   Hypothetical representation of a cluster analysis identifying family types

appear to share a common profile across a number of variables (Filsinger, 1990). Each individual or family is classified as belonging to a type, sharing the same basic profile across a number of variables, which become domains or profile scores in the typology.

Clustering Procedures

The schematic representation of a cluster analysis in Figure 4.1 illustrates the Aristotelian approach to scientific investigation. The scores of each individual or family are plotted in relation to one another in space. In these specific examples, family cohesion and communication are considered simultaneously. The dense set of data points surrounded by regions of relative sparsity illustrates the emerging clusters or types. In this hypothetical data set, for example, there are families high in communication and cohesiveness, families low in both, and families high in one but low in the other. Of course, in practice, cluster analysis is a much more complex statistical procedure.

The results of cluster analyses differ depending on the method that is used (Borgen, 1987). Exploratory methods identify clusters and assign patients to types or subgroups. For instance, Ward's exploratory method is a hierarchical agglomerative procedure that begins with each case defined as a single cluster; cases are then grouped and regrouped until the variance among cases within each cluster reaches a defined minimum level (Fisher, Chesla, et al., 2000; Fisher, Gudmundsdottir, et al., 2000).

Confirmatory methods validate the exploratory typology. How many clusters with parallel profiles are identified? Are a majority of the families assigned to these clusters? Are a high percentage of cases assigned to the same cluster in both exploratory and confirmatory phases? Average linkage is also an agglomerative or grouping method but uses different criteria to define when minimal within-cluster variance has been achieved. When using K means, the investigator must specify the number of desired groups beforehand, calculate an initial set of values that identifies each of the clusters and assign cases to them, recalculate the values that define the clusters, and reassign cases following the new specifications. Iterations continue until no cases are relocated to other clusters (Borgen, 1987; Filsinger, 1990; Lorr, 1983).

To validate clusters, investigators are advised to run several different cluster analysis procedures to determine if they achieve basically the same results. If different techniques uncover similar cluster structures, those clusters may truly exist in some form. The typology may also be replicated by separately clustering two or more different data sets or by splitting one data set into two parts and analyzing the two parts separately, searching for similar results. The challenge is to construct a typology with empirical clustering techniques and to identify a number of groups whose profiles vary in meaningful patterns.

Once the cluster of types has been identified, the investigator first classifies the family members or families using a profile of scores (Fisher, 2000, Summer). Second, the investigator examines the relationship between type or subgroup membership and other variables of interest. Can patients from one type or subgroup be differentiated significantly from patients of other types, based on additional comparisons, in ways that validate the typology and add to its meaning? Finally, the investigator names and describes each type.

Issues to Consider in the Development of Quantitative Typologies

When designing studies to generate numerical typologies, certain issues related to the sample, procedure, and variable selection need to be addressed. Often, cluster analysis is used to search for underlying types and to group people together who possess similar characteristics (same basic profile across variables) (Filsinger, 1990; Lorr, 1983). The patients or families in the sample must therefore represent all types in the population; thus, oversampling is needed. The procedure for the study must include specification, a priori, of the basis for the cluster formation, the types of clusters anticipated, and the criteria for combining cases into clusters. Because variables are used in further analyses to create typologies, it is extremely important that they are conceptually clear and make sense for the particular issue being investigated. The actual number of variables is not rigidly prescribed. Once obtained, however, the investigator must evaluate the clusters for relevance or utility or both (Michel & Allred, 1996).

Examples of Quantitative Typologies

The logic of typologic thinking is not a new notion in family studies (Filsinger, 1990; McCubbin, Thompson, Pirner, & McCubbin, 1988). For example, as far back as 1945, Burgess and Locke described two types of marriages: institutional and companionship. Typologies were formed from logical possibilities of cross-tabulation of variables, such as Olson, Sprenkle, and Russell's (1979) circumplex model. Others were formed through cluster analysis and were created to identify a set of common or shared profiles that summarize all or most of the families in the sample, such as Moos's (Moos & Moos, 1976) typology based on the Family Environment Scale. Methods of assessment used to form family typologies included semistructured and unstructured interviews (Kantor & Lehr, 1975), single self-report scales (Lavee & Olson, 1993), and observer ratings of interaction (Gottman, 1979). Perhaps the most well-researched quantitative typology related to health issues was developed by Fisher and colleagues through the California Family Health Project (CFHP).

California Family Health Project. CFHP linked health (RAND Health Survey), different family types, and well-being of family members (Family Life Scales; Fisher &

Ransom, 1995; Fisher, Ransom, & Terry, 1993; Fisher et al., 1998; Fisher, Terry, & Burge, 1992).

The investigators in the CFHP identified four broad domains of family life previously linked to health as a basis for their typology: structure/organization, emotion management, worldview, and problem solving. Data were gathered from 164 husbands and 152 wives (11 wives with extreme scores were dropped from the analysis) using self-report scales, ratings of couple interaction, and ratings of family interaction obtained during 12 hours of intensive family assessment (73 total variables). A subset of 11 family variables was empirically selected to represent the four domains in the cluster analysis.

Cluster analysis identified four coherent and meaningful family types that discriminated 97% of the adult family members on the basis of several self-reported health measures (Fisher & Ransom, 1995): balanced, traditional, disconnected, and emotionally strained. All 11 family variable components significantly differentiated the four family types for husbands and wives. Significant differences were also found among the four family types on 10 demographic and other family variables. Both husbands and wives from balanced and traditional families reported higher health scores than spouses from disconnected and emotionally strained families.

The investigators created a descriptive narrative for each family type using a profile derived from the mean scores of all families in each of the four types. As is the goal of all typologies, this family typology looked beyond each of the 11 family scores to extract meaning from the whole family profile. Fisher and colleagues compared their family types to those proposed by other researchers (Table 4.1). They commented on the similarity of the four family types to those described in the literature and particularly on the similarity with the work of Reiss

(1981) because of his influence during the planning of this project. The largest difference is Lavee and Olson's (1993) "vitalized" and "conflicted" types, which represent extremes on almost all scores and do not match any of the types shown in Table 4.1 (Fisher & Ransom, 1995).

Further Validation. Fisher and Ransom (1995) also applied this typology to a study of adolescent health, including three adolescent health indices (physical health, emotional health, and alcohol abstinence). Adolescents from traditional and disconnected families had higher and lower health scores, respectively.

Fisher also replicated these family types in a French sample in Quebec, Canada (Fisher, et al., 1998), including 1,085 families. Revisions were made in the family scales so they were valid for this cultural group. All respondents were classified into family types that paralleled the original typology. Family profile variables significantly distinguished family types.

In addition, Fisher used three of the four family domains in research on individuals with Alzheimer's disease and their caregivers. Measures appropriate for the domains as well as this population and their caregivers were used to study the family caregiving systems and the health of 136 adult offspring who were involved in care (Fisher & Lieberman, 1994). Family characteristics associated with offspring health consistently predicted health over time. Family emotional management variables predicted a reduction in offspring health scores over time.

The typology generated in CFHP refers to statistically robust family processes in culturally diverse samples. Next, we discuss a project by Fisher and colleagues that focuses on individual disease management within the context of the family in culturally diverse samples to understand how this program of research informs future application of

Table 4.1 Comparison of Family Typologies

	Family Type				
California Health Project; Fisher, Nakell, Terry, and Ransom (1992); Fisher, Ransom, Terry, Lipkin, and Weiss (1992); Fisher, Terry, and Burge (1992); Fisher et al. (1993); and Fisher and Ransom (1995)	Openness to external world, role flexibility, personal separateness coupled with family commitment (balanced)	Inward looking, highly organized, somewhat closed, religious, child-centered (traditional)	Low coherence, externally oriented, uncommitted (disconnected)	Constricted, aversive, actively conflicted, tense (emotionally strained)	
Kantor and Lehr (1975) Two-generation families	Open	Closed	Random (extreme)		
Reiss (1981) Two-generation families	Environment-sensitive	Consensus-sensitive	Distance-sensitive		
Fitzpatrick (1979) Community based couples	Independent	Traditional	Separate		
Lavee and Olson (1993) Couples presenting for marital enrichment or therapy	Balanced	Traditional			
Fals-Stewart, Schafer, and Birchler (1993) Typology of distressed couples			Disengaged	High conflict	
Fisher's (1977) overview		Internalized	Externally focused	Constricted	

SOURCE: Fisher and Ransom (1995, p. 176).

typologies in tailoring interventions with families who have members with chronic conditions.

San Francisco Family Diabetes Project (Chesla, Skaff, Bartz, Mullan, & Fisher, 2000; Fisher, Chesla, et al., 2000; Fisher, Gudmundsdottir, et al., 2000). Given their success in relating general family process types to health outcomes, Fisher and colleagues decided to explore a typology of disease management styles among European Americans and Latino adults diagnosed with type 2 diabetes. For this study, five domains were created: biologic and physical indicators, general health and functional status indicators, emotional tone indicators, diabetes quality of life indicators, and behavioral indicators. Data were collected from 192 adults with diabetes and their spouses, and analysis was completed in two steps. First, a series of exploratory and confirmatory cluster analyses were conducted using the standardized values of the 11 profile variables. Wards's method indicated a five-cluster solution was the best fit. The mean score profile was plotted for each of the five patient clusters, and each patient was assigned membership to a cluster. Average linkage and K means replicated Wards's method statistically, so the results of Wards's method were presented as the results. (See Table 4.2 for a brief description of the five disease management status [DMS] clusters: balanced, problematics, coasters, discouraged, and distressed). Second, the resulting typology, "disease management status," was validated for external validity by three groups of variables (demographics, patient, and family). Standard scores profiles for 18 comparison variables were graphed for each type. After a review of the mean type profiles, a consensus narrative was developed for each type, incorporating differences among the types based on the analysis of the comparison variables to clarify and enhance their description.

Differences were noted between the two ethnic groups regarding style. More European Americans were classified as coasters and more Latinos were classified as distressed. (Of course, these differences may also be due to the socioeconomic differences in this sample.) The researchers also compared how patients and family members resolve disagreements about disease management based on ethnicity and patient gender (Fisher, Chesla, et al., 2000; Fisher, Gudmundsdottir, et al., 2000).

In one part of the study unrelated to developing the typology, patients and family members were studied regarding how they resolve disagreements about disease management. Latino couples were rated as significantly more emotionally close, less avoidant, less hostile toward each other, and as having less dominant patients than European Americans; they achieved significantly less problem resolution and were more frequently off task than European American couples, however, particularly those with female patients (Fisher, Chesla, et al., 2000; Fisher, Gudmundsdottir, et al., 2000).

They also determined the relationship between the four domains of the typology (not the types) and self-care practices of Latinos and European American patients (Fisher, Chesla, et al., 2000). For European American patients, two domains of the typology (family worldview and family emotion management) as well as gender were related to disease management. For Latino patients, another domain of the typology (family structure/organization) and gender were related to disease management.

Finally, in a qualitative study, Chesla and colleagues (2000) described and contrasted personal explanatory models for this sample. Subjects understood diabetes and how it worked in three identifiable disease models: experiential, biomedical, or psychosocial. Although they made comparable assessments about cause, seriousness, and effectiveness of treatments, Latinos used an experiential disease model and more European Americans used a biomedical disease model. Significantly more European Americans reported changes in exercise and spontaneity, and more Latinos reported changes in fatigue and mood. Chesla and colleagues concluded that understanding the personal models of diabetic patients is crucial for the design of research and clinical interventions with diverse populations. If they had not looked beyond assessments of the cause of the disease, its seriousness, or the efficacy of various treatments, the European Americans may have appeared to be much like the Latinos. When they studied how Latinos and European Americans understood the disease process and experienced its impact on daily life, however, differences were highlighted. The results were not compared to or used with those of the quantitative typology study.

In summary, five coherent, statistically replicable, and conceptually meaningful types are included in this typology of disease management behaviors. The DMS is conceptualized to focus on patient functioning,

(Text continues on page 72)

Table 4.2 Comparison of Fisher et al.'s (2000) Disease Management Types With Similarities in Family Management Styles Themes and Subthemes

Fisher et al.'s (2000) Disease Management Type	Knafl et al.'s (1994, 1996) Family Management Styles (Parental Themes) (n and % at First Data Collection Point)	Notes
Balanced (n = 64, 33%) Cognitive (None) Motivation: higher scores on self-efficacy (None)	Thriving (n = 15, 22.7%) Definition of the situation Child identity-normal Illness view: life goes on Management mind-set-confident Parental mutuality-yes	Fisher: best and most uniformly positive DMS scores with no notable high or low spikes in their profiles; both ethnic groups and genders; Hb_{A1C} and body mass index (BMI) relatively low in comparison to others; good general health
Behavioral Role function: not inhibited by diabetes; well-balanced approach to diabetes care Management: problems—diet, physical activity, exercise; behavioral management (exercise, sweats) excellent compared to others; followed diet; no major management problems	Management behaviors Parenting philosophy: accommodative Management approach: proactive	Knafl: thriving and accommodating children significantly higher social competence than children in the Enduring, Struggling. or Floundering management styles
Emotional consequences Emotional tone: good Quality of life: satisfaction with disease management; view of future with diabetes: good quality of life with satisfaction with diabetes management and optimistic view of future with diabetes	Perceived consequences Family focus: disease not in the foreground Future expectations: no future dread	
Problematics (n = 11, 6%) Cognitive (None) (None) Motivation: poor (None)	Floundering (n = 7, 10.6%) Definition of the situation Child identity: normal/tragic Illness view: variable Management mind-set: burden/inadequate Parental mutuality: usually no	Fisher: small group of patients; general health poor; both ethnic groups and both genders; suggested personal, behavioral, social, or economic difficulty that affected profile
Behavioral Role function: poor functioning Management: problems—diet, physical activity, exercise; poor diet; highest	Management behaviors Parenting philosophy: usually missing/inconsistent Management approach: usually reactive	Knafl and Deatrick: ignorantly lower satisfaction with family functioning than those in the other styles; ill child behavioral and social adjustment significantly lower than those

(Continued)

Table 4.2 (Continued)

Fisher et al.'s (2000) Disease Management Type	Knafl et al.'s (1994, 1996) Family Management Styles (Parental Themes) (n and % at First Data Collection Point)	Notes
use of alcohol of any type, which may explain very high scores on carbohydrate ratio; low physical activity		in Thriving FMS; most oldest children in the sample; overrepresented by families of children with diabetes
Emotional consequences Emotional tone: poor Quality of life: satisfaction with disease management; view of future with diabetes: low	Perceived consequences Family focus: disease usually in foreground Future expectations: usually dread future	
Coasters (n = 63, 34%) Cognitive (None) (None) Motivation: low; adequate knowledge but "coasting along" with signs of low motivation and disease management burnout (None)	Accommodating (n = 13, 19.7%) Definition of the situation Child identity: usually normal Illness view: usually life goes on Management mind-set: mothers confident Parental mutuality: usually yes	Fisher: average to low average range of functioning (exercise, physical activity, diet) without particular deficits or strengths; general health, quality of life, and emotional tone in high midrange; more Euro-Americans; both genders equally presented; highest level of education, which parallels ethnicity; somewhat older and had diabetes somewhat longer
Behavioral Role function: average to low Management: problems—diet, physical activity, exercise; average to low without particular deficits or strengths without particular deficits or strengths	Management behaviors Parenting philosophy: usually accommodative Management approach: usually proactive	
Emotional consequences Emotional tone: high midrange Quality of life: satisfaction with disease management; view of future with diabetes: high midrange	Perceived consequences Family focus: disease not in the foreground Future expectations: usually no future dread	
Discouraged (n = 29, 16%) Cognitive (None) (None) Motivation: lowest trust in practitioner (diabetes care not too useful) (None)	Enduring (n = 18, 27.3%) Definition of the situation Child identity: normal, tragic Illness view: variable Management mind-set: confident, burdensome Parental mutuality: usually yes	Fisher: equal proportions from both ethnic groups; on comparison scores, second lowest scores on family closeness, highest scores on separate spouse activities

Fisher et al.'s (2000) Disease Management Type	Knafl et al.'s (1994, 1996) Family Management Styles (Parental Themes) (n and % at First Data Collection Point)	Notes
Behavioral 　Role function: social role (family) and general health problems; high scores on social isolation 　Management: problems-diet, physical activity, exercise: considerably overweight; high + spike on BMI 　Exercise and dietary management in midrange	Management behaviors 　Parenting philosophy: accommodative, proactive 　Management approach: usually proactive	
Emotional consequences 　Emotional tone: very poor 　Quality of life: satisfaction with disease management; view of future with diabetes: very poor diabetes quality of life	Perceived consequences 　Family focus: disease comes in and out of foreground 　Future expectations: usually dreads future	
Distressed (*n* = 20, 11%) 　Cognitive 　(None) 　(None) 　Motivation: lowest level of diabetes self-efficacy 　(None)	Struggling (*n* = 13, 19.7%) 　Definition of the situation 　　Child identity: variable 　　Illness view: variable 　　Management mind-set: mothers burden, fathers confident 　　Parental mutuality: usually no	Fisher: both genders; more Latino than Euro-American; highest level of economic distress; youngest in sample; poorest education
Behavioral 　Role function 　Management: problems—diet, physical activity, exercise: otherwise moderate profile of scores on exercise and diet	Management behaviors 　Parenting philosophy: usually accommodative 　Management approach: usually proactive	
Emotional 　Emotional tone: notable psychological depression distress (high spike on anxiety) 　Quality of life: satisfaction with disease management; view of future with diabetes: notably lack of satisfaction with diabetes care and control, and pessimism about diabetes management in future (high spike on two diabetes quality of life scores)	Perceived consequences 　Family focus: disease usually in foreground for mothers, not usually for fathers 　Future expectations: usually mothers dread future, fathers usually do not	

although data were also obtained from spouses or partners. The types distinguish one another on comparison variables, suggesting their usefulness for providing a heuristic framework for tailoring interventions. Investigators cautioned that the 18 comparison variables need to be more fully integrated into a description of the types and new comparison variables need to be tested, including perceptions of other family members.

Qualitative Typologies

Justification

Qualitative methods can be used at various points in planning, implementing, and evaluating family intervention research (Morse, Hutchinson, & Penrod, 1998; Rosenblatt & Fisher, 1993; Sandelowski, 1996b). Like quantitative typologies, qualitative typologies can be used to construct meaningful intervention protocols, inform the design of the study, and select or create sensitive outcome measures. In particular, qualitative family typologies have potential for providing the actual content of interventions and for tailoring interventions, contributing data on family type and the style of managing illness-related work.

Like quantitative typologies, each type can be considered in terms of a case or prototype, which can be clarified or enhanced or both through additional research. Overlap with other types within the typology may occur because a subtheme may be common to more than one type. The unique combination of attributes, however, is what comprises the typology.

Logic

Although many different qualitative approaches exist, analytic procedures relevant to qualitative typologies include the following: noting patterns of themes and subthemes, seeing plausibility, and clustering. These procedures are all a means of ascertaining "what goes with what" (Miles & Huberman, 1994, p. 245).

Qualitatively developed "clusters" are groups of attributes that enable us to conceptualize families that have similar patterns of characteristics. In the case at hand, we are clustering attributes of families expressed as themes and subthemes to systematically describe aspects of family process and disease management.

General Procedure

Although many different qualitative approaches exist, Miles and Huberman (1994) outlined aggregation and comparison tactics that are basic to qualitative clustering. As descriptive codes, categories, or themes are inductively created, used, and revised, they are named and defined. A conceptual structure, which may be prespecified or evolve, must provide the basis for the definitions of codes, categories, or themes. For instance, qualitative family researchers often use symbolic interactionism to provide a set of assumptions and major conceptual components (defining, management, and consequence themes). As such, the framework provides a "yoke" for the analytic process forming the structure for the subthemes, which can than be cross-classified. (See conceptual components and themes in Table 4.3.) Qualitative researchers call this *pattern coding*, which is a way of grouping codes into a smaller number of sets, themes, or constructs (Miles & Huberman, 1994) to elaborate an integrated schema, which is at a higher level of abstraction for cross-case analysis.

Miles and Huberman (1994) noted that many attributes may be relevant to complex clusters of phenomena. They recommended proceeding using a "case-by-attribute (theme) matrix" (Figure 4.2), which lists cases as rows and inductively derived attributes (theme) as

Table 4.3 Parental Themes: Family Management Styles and Related Subthemes

Conceptual Component	Themes	Family Management Styles				
		Thriving	Accommodating	Enduring	Struggling	Floundering
Defining	Child Identity	Normal	Usually normal	Normal, tragic	Variable	Tragic, problem
	Illness View	Life goes on	Usually life goes on	Variable	Variable	Serious, hateful
	Management mind-set	Confident	Mothers confident	Confident, burdensome	Mothers burden, fathers confident	Burden, inadequate
	Parenting mutuality	Yes	Usually yes	Usually yes	Usually no	Usually no
Management	Parenting philosophy	Accommodative	Usually accommodative	Accommodative, protective	Usually accommodative	Usually missing/ inconsistent
	Management approach	Proactive	Usually proactive	Usually proactive	Usually proactive	Usually reactive
Perceived consequences	Family focus	No	No	Variable	Usual mothers, unusual fathers	Usually yes
	Future expectations	Positive outlook	Usually positive outlook	Variable outlook	Mothers usually negative outlook	Negative outlook
		Favorable illness course Diminishing impact	Favorable illness course Diminishing impact	Illness course and impact	Unfavorable illness course and escalating impact; fathers usually positive	Unfavorable illness course Escalating impact

Theme	Case 1	Case 2
Manage		
Proactive		X
Reactive	X	
Parenting		
Normalize		X Case 1 and 2 would be different types
Protect	X	

Figure 4.2   Hypothetical representation of a qualitative matrix identifying family types

columns. The rows of the matrix can then be rearranged so that the cases are grouped that have similar subattributes (subthemes). After the clusters are named, a column can then be added that labels the group of cases and their subattributes. Thus, as in Figure 4.2, Cases 1 and 2 are different types because their general managing and parenting are described by different subthemes. Creating and naming different types recontextualizes the data and adds understanding and richness to their descriptive properties (Ayres et al., 2003).

Example of Qualitative Typologies

As for quantitative typologies, qualitative typologies summarize various attributes of the family. Guided by a preset or data-based conceptual structure, the major themes and subthemes are inductively derived and used to classify families or cases into types.

Initial Development of Family Management Styles. FMS is an inductively derived typology of family styles for managing children's chronic conditions. Knafl, Deatrick, and colleagues have theoretically and empirically developed this midrange theory during the past 20 years through a series of qualitative and analytical research projects with school-aged children who have chronic conditions

(Craft-Rosenberg & Dennehy, 2003; Deatrick & Knafl, 1990; Knafl, Breitmayer, Gallo, & Zoeller, 1994; Knafl & Deatrick, 1990; Knafl, Deatrick, & Kirby, 2000).

Available research in the late 1980s and the conceptual perspective of symbolic interactionism (family as the expert in its own situation) provided the basis for the major interactive components of the original FMS framework. FMS initially was conceptualized in a concept analysis as an overarching construct encompassing multiple management styles sensitized by a symbolic interactionist perspective (Mishel, 1998). Three interactive components were isolated as important: the definition of the situation, management behaviors, and sociocultural factors. Definition of the situation was the subjective meaning of what family members identified as important elements of their situation. Management behaviors were efforts directed toward caring for the illness and adapting family life to illness-related demands. Sociocultural context was defined as factors that shaped how the family defined and managed the situation.

Knafl and colleagues (1994) used the FMS framework to study 63 families in which there was a child with a chronic illness. They called this the Defining and Managing Childhood Chronic Illness (DMCI) study. Results included a typology of five distinct FMSs (thriving, accommodating, enduring, struggling, and floundering) reflecting a continuum of difficulty that families experienced in managing a child's chronic illness. The five styles were based on how components of the framework are manifested across families and include considerable specification of the defining and managing components of the framework by identifying their themes and subthemes. Eleven major themes (8 based on data from parents, and 3 based on data from ill children) were common across the major components of the model. The themes were common to all 63 families studied and reflected what the families believed were important elements of how the illness was managed and incorporated into family life. In addition, subthemes were developed that reflected variation across families with regard to how a particular theme was manifested. The sociocultural component did not differentiate FMSs, but it provided contextual information on the family's interactions with the larger social system, including health care and school. The study examined child and family correlates of various FMSs. Family correlates included satisfaction with family functioning, and child correlates included behavioral and social competence (Knafl, Breitmayer, Gallo, & Zoeller, 1996). Ill children in the thriving families had significantly higher social competence than those in the enduring, struggling, or floundering families. Parents in the floundering families expressed a lower satisfaction with family functioning than did parents with other styles; in addition, the ill children's behavioral and social adjustment was significantly lower than that in thriving families.

Recent Development of the Model. To further validate and specify the major components of the model, results of 46 studies (55 articles) published between 1988 and 1998 addressing family response to a childhood chronic conditions were reviewed. The results of the analyses were used to verify and refine both the eight parental themes from the DMCI study and the FMS framework as a whole (Knafl & Deatrick, 2003). (See Table 4.3 for the resulting model.)

The review of the literature indicated, as it had for the prior DMCI study, that sociocultural context, a major component of the original FMS model, was more appropriately conceptualized as perceived influences on management rather than a major dimension of the framework. Moreover, the literature differentiated parents' perceptions of how the illness had changed family life or family members or both from other aspects of their definition of the situation, suggesting

that it would be appropriate to include "perceived consequences" as a distinct component of the framework. The eight defining, managing, and perceived consequence subthemes that were identified in the DMCI study were also further refined. On the basis of available research, however, no changes were made on the level of the five styles (Knafl & Deatrick, 2003).

FMS still emphasizes the configuration formed across major components: individual family members' definitions, management behaviors, and perceptions of consequences. For instance, families with a thriving FMS define their child as essentially normal, their life as going on despite the illness, and the family as confident in its management mind-set and sharing mutual views about the children, the illness, and illness management. These families manage using an accommodative parenting philosophy and a proactive management approach. Finally, their perceived consequences include maintaining a family focus and future expectations that involve a positive outlook, a favorable disease course, and a diminishing impact of the condition. Families with a floundering FMS define their child's identify as tragic and problematic, the illness as serious and hateful, their management mind-set as burden and themselves as inadequate, and the family as having discrepant views about the children, the illness, and illness management. These families manage without a consistent parenting philosophy and with a reactive management approach. Lastly, their perceived consequences include focus on the illness and difficulty maintaining focus on family life and future expectations, which include a negative outlook, an unfavorable disease course, and an escalating disease impact.

FMS accounts for cognitive, behavioral, and emotional components of disease management for the family as a unit (See Tables 4.2 and 4.3; Figures 4.3 and 4.4). FMS organizes and systematizes how families manage the treatment regimen and how they

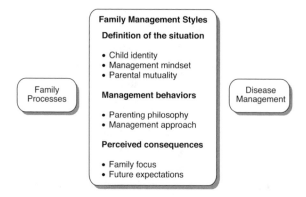

Figure 4.3 Family Management Styles (FMS) –midpoint between family functioning and disease management

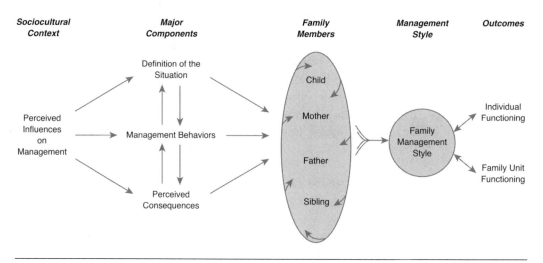

Figure 4.4 Family Management Style Framework

incorporate the illness into family life. As such, FMS describes a midpoint between family functioning and disease management and provides a possible nexus for tailoring clinical interventions to the psychosocial profile of the illness within family life.

IMPLICATIONS FOR FAMILY SCIENCES

Family typologies offer an integrated approach for assessing FMS, tailoring interventions, and measuring outcomes for clinical practice and research with families of children with chronic conditions (Fisher, Chesla, et al., 2000; Fisher, Gudmundsdottir, et al., 2000; Weihs et al., 2002). Implications for use of qualitative and quantitative approaches, nature of outcomes, foundational elements for family disease management typologies, and how to use the typologies in intervention research are discussed here. Future research is needed, however, to further develop the identification, testing, and use of typologies in family research. This research can use the rich understandings currently available in the family science literature.

Methods

The merits of both quantitative and qualitative approaches to typology formulation are noteworthy. Qualitative methods were used in each approach, in fact, to add narrative descriptions and explanatory models, thereby providing clear exemplars for clinicians and researchers (Chesla et al., 2000). Cluster analysis may not only be helpful in quantitative typology formation but also provide important links between qualitative and quantitative paradigms (Fisher, Kokes, Ransom, Phillips, & Rudd, 1985).

Foundational, Conceptual Components

Major conceptual components for the Fisher typology and the Knafl typology (see Table 4.2) include cognitive/definition of the situation, behavioral and management behaviors, and emotional consequences and perceived consequences. Furthermore, remarkable similarity exists between the attributes of Fisher and Knafl types: balanced and thriving, problematics and floundering, coasters and accommodating, discouraged and enduring, and distressed and struggling. Outcomes from both Fisher and Knafl typologies are similar in nature; that is, satisfaction with overall functioning increases with more positive styles and decreases with less positive styles. Influences of socioeconomic status, age, and education were not as apparent in Knafl's work as they were in that of Fisher. Although certain trends were exhibited in Knafl's data, no significant differences existed among FMSs over time for these parameters. Further research with larger data sets may identify such differences.

Typologies focused on both family processes and disease management may offer the most assistance because they acknowledge important aspects of the situation. In fact, remarkable similarity between two disparate programs of research described in this article may speak to important foundational elements of the family typologies selected for analysis.

Scientists design theory-based interventions (McHenry, Allen, Mishel, & Braden, 1993; Mishel, 1981, 1988, 1991, 1997) based on midrange theories and use manualized protocols to guide the process and content of interventions. These protocols also typically list clinical considerations that may be used to individualize the intervention, including issues identified in past research and clinical practice that may variously apply to the population at risk. Manualized interventions have many formats. The state of the art now dictates that careful attention is placed on the overall goals, specific objectives, and corresponding expected behaviors. This enables impartial reviewers to measure the adherence of the therapist to what is planned and the competence of the therapist to meeting the goals and objectives of the session. Such manuals also provide guidance during training of therapists.

Use in Intervention Research

Family typologies can be used to further develop manualized protocols. Depending on the design of the study, families can be assessed to determine their type before or after they are selected or randomized into the study. Then, an overall protocol can be constructed and tested with points of individualization based on the family type.

Typologies such as FMS may be used to give further suggestions to the therapist on how to work with the family, what clinical examples to use with the family, and the nature of the projected clinical considerations. For instance, a family classified as thriving according to the FMS may not be as realistic about future issues that will most likely occur related to the child's condition. This can sensitize the therapist to understanding the nature of the family's reluctance to view the future as being potentially problematic, and that it may be more acceptable to start with current successes and back into anticipatory guidance for the future. Families who are classified as floundering according to the FMS, however, may not readily appreciate suggestions for proactive management strategies until their distress is acknowledged.

Although the same strategies may be devised using good clinical skills, those strategies are generally not included in the manual, except in general clinical considerations (Nezu, Nezu, Friedman, Faddis, & Houts, 1998). If they are included in alternative scripts, examples to use with the families, or in clinical considerations, they will most likely be more effective and be able to be replicated with the next family who is similarly situated. Adherence and competence ratings will also be strengthened because raters will better

understand exactly what is expected of the interventions.

Family typologies can also be used to measure which family styles are best matched to the intervention and to measure the overall effectiveness of the intervention. The mixed results of much intervention research may not be due to the ineffectiveness of the design and implementation of the intervention. Rather, the issue may be the lack of fit with the intervention to particular styles of defining and managing illness situations as well as the particular consequences of that situation. Measuring family styles before and after an intervention will assist the investigative team to better understand the effectiveness of the intervention both for individual families and for all the families engaged in the intervention.

REFERENCES

Ayres, L., Kavanaugh, K., & Knafl, K. (2003). Within-case and across-case approaches to qualitative data analysis. *Qualitative Health Research, 13*(6), 871-883.

Borgen, F. H. B. (1987). Applying cluster analysis in counseling psychology research. *Journal of Counseling Psychology, 34,* 456-468.

Burgess, W. W., & Locke, H. J. (1945). *The family: From the institution to companionship.* New York: American Book.

Cattell, R. B. (Ed.). (1966). *Handbook of multivariate experimental psychology.* Chicago: Rand McNally.

Chesla, C. A., Skaff, M. M., Bartz, R. J., Mullan, J. T., & Fisher, L. (2000). Differences in personal models among Latinos and European Americans: Implications for clinical care. *Diabetes Care, 23*(12), 1780-1785.

Craft-Rosenberg, M., & Dennehy, E. (2003). Further refinement of the Family Management Style framework. *Journal of Family Nursing, 9*(3), 232-256.

Deatrick, J., & Knafl, K. (1990). Management behaviors: Day-to-day adjustments to childhood chronic conditions. *Journal of Pediatric Nursing, 5*(1), 15-22.

Fals-Stewart, W., Schafer, J., & Birchler, G. R. (1993). An empirical typology of distressed couples that is based on the Areas of Change Questionnaire. *Journal of Family Psychology, 7,* 307-321.

Filsinger, E. E. (1990). Empirical typology, cluster analysis, and family-level measurement. In T. W. Draper & A. C. Marcos (Ed.), *Family variables: Conceptualization, measurement, and use.* Newbury Park, CA: Sage.

Fisher, L. (1977). On the classification of families: A progress report. *Archives of General Psychiatry, 34,* 424-433.

Fisher, L., Chesla, C. A., Skaff, M. A., Gilliss, C., Kanter, R. A., Lutz, C. P., et al. (2000a). Disease management status: A typology of Latino and Euro-American patients with type 2 diabetes. *Behavioral Medicine, 26,* 53-66.

Fisher, L., Gudmundsdottir, M., Gilliss, C., Skaff, M., Mullan, J., Kanter, R., et al. (2000b). Resolving disease management problems in European-American and Latino couples with type 2 diabetes: The effects of ethnicity and patient gender. *Family Process, 39,* 403-416.

Fisher, L., Kokes, R., Ransom, D., Phillips, S., & Rudd, P. (1985). Alternative strategies for creating "relational" family data. *Family Process, 24,* 213-224.

Fisher, L., & Lieberman, M. A. (1994). Alzheimer's disease: The impact of the family on spouses's offspring, and in-laws. *Family Process, 33,* 305-325.

Fisher, L., Nakell, L. C., Terry, H. E., & Ransom, D. C. (1992). The California Health Project: III. Couple emotion management and adult health. *Family Process, 31,* 269-288.

Fisher, L., & Ransom, D. C. (1995). A typology of families in relation to adult health. *Family Process, 34,* 161-182.

Fisher, L., Ransom, D. C., & Terry, H. E. (1993). The California Family Health Project: VII. Summary and integration of findings. *Family Process, 32,* 69-86.

Fisher, L., Ransom, D. C., Terry, H. E., Lipkin, M., Jr., & Weiss, R. (1992). The California Family Health Project: I. Introduction and a description of adult health. *Family Process, 31,* 231-250.

Fisher, L., Soubhi, H., Mansi, O., Paradis, G., Gauvin, L., & Potvin, L. (1998). Family process in health research: Extending a family typology to a new cultural context. *Health Psychology, 17,* 1-9.

Fisher, L., Terry, H. E., & Burge, S. (1992). The California Health Project: IV. Family structure/organization and adult health. *Family Process, 31,* 399-419.

Fitzpatrick, M. A. (1979). *A typological approach to enduring relationships: The derivation and test of a model.* Unpublished manuscript.

Gottman, J. M. (1979). *Marital interactions: Experimental investigations.* New York: Academic Press.

Institute of Medicine. (2001). *Health and behavior: The interplay of biological, behavioral, and societal influences.* Washington, DC: National Academy Press.

Kantor, D., & Lehr, W. (1975). *Inside the family: Toward a theory of family process.* San Francisco: Jossey-Bass.

Knafl, K., Breitmayer, B., Gallo, A., & Zoeller, L. (1994). *Final report: How families define and manage a child's chronic illness,* No. NR01594. Bethesda, MD: National Institutes of Health, National Institute of Nursing Research.

Knafl, K., Breitmayer, B., Gallo, A., & Zoeller, L. (1996). Family response to childhood chronic illness: Description of management styles. *Journal of Pediatric Nursing, 11,* 315-326.

Knafl, K., & Deatrick, J. (1990). Family management style: Concept analysis and development. *Journal of Pediatric Nursing, 5*(1), 4-14.

Knafl, K., & Deatrick, J. (2003). Further refinement of the Family Management Style Framework. *Journal of Family Nursing, 9,* 232-256.

Knafl, K., Deatrick, J., & Kirby, A. (2000). Normalization promotion. In M. Craft-Rosenberg & R. J. Dennehy (Eds.), *Nursing interventions for childbearing and childrearing families* (pp. 373-388). Thousand Oaks, CA: Sage.

Lavee, Y., & Olson, D. H. (1993). Seven types of marriage: Empirical typology based on ENRICH. *Journal of Marital and Family Therapy, 19,* 325-340.

Lorr, M. (1983). *Cluster analysis for social scientists*. San Francisco: Jossey-Bass.

McCubbin, H. I., Thompson, A. I., Pirner, P. A., & McCubbin, M. (1988). *Family types and strengths: A life cycle and ecological perspective*. Edina, MN: Burgess International Group.

McHenry, J., Allen, C., Mishel, M., & Braden, C. J. (1993). Uncertainty management for women receiving treatment for breast cancer. In S. Funk, E. Tournquist, M. Champagne, & R. Wiese (Eds.), *Key aspects of caring for the chronically ill: Hospital and home*. New York: Springer.

Michel, Y., & Allred, C. (1996). Studying multidimensional constructs through cluster analysis. *Western Journal of Nursing Research, 18*(1), 102-107.

Miles, M. B., & Huberman, A. M. (1994). *An expanded sourcebook: Qualitative data analysis*. Thousand Oaks, CA: Sage.

Mishel, M. (1981). The measurement of uncertainty in illness. *Nursing Research, 30*, 258-263.

Mishel, M. (1988). Uncertainty in illness. *Image: Journal of Nursing Scholarship, 20*, 225-232.

Mishel, M. (1991). Uncertainty in gynecological cancer: A test of mediating functions of mastery and coping. *Nursing Research, 5*, 167-171.

Mishel, M. (1997). Uncertainty in acute illness. *Annual Review of Nursing Research, 15*, 57-89.

Mishel, M. (1998). Methodological studies: Instrument development. In P. Brink & M. Wood (Eds.), *Advanced design in nursing research* (pp. 235-282). Thousand Oaks, CA: Sage.

Moos, R. H., & Moos, B. S. (1976). A typology of family social environments. *Family Process, 15*, 357-371.

Morse, J., Hutchinson, S., & Penrod, J. (1998). From theory to practice: The development of assessment guides from qualitatively derived theory. *Qualitative Health Research, 8*(3), 329-340.

Nezu, A., Nezu, C., Friedman, S., Faddis, S., & Houts, P. (1998). *Helping cancer patients cope*. Washington, DC: American Psychological Association.

Olson, D. H., Sprenkle, D. H., & Russell, C. S. (1979). Circumplex model of marital and family systems: I. Cohesion and adaptability dimensions, family types, and clinical applications. *Family Process, 18*, 3-28.

Reiss, D. (1981). *The family's construction of reality*. Cambridge, MA: Harvard University Press.

Rosenblatt, P. C., & Fisher, L. R. (1993). Qualitative family research. In P. B. Boss & W. J. Doherty (Eds.), *Sourcebook of family theories and methods: A contextual approach* (pp. 167-177). New York: Plenum.

Sandelowski, M. (1996a). One is the liveliest number: The case orientation of qualitative research. *Research in Nursing and Health, 19*(6), 525-529.

Sandelowski, M. (1996b). Focus on qualitative methods: Using qualitative methods in intervention studies. *Research in Nursing and Health, 19*(4), 359-364.

Weihs, K., Fisher, L., MacBaird, M., & the National Working Group on Family-Based Interventions in Chronic Disease. (2002). Families, health and behavior. *Families, Systems, and Health, 20*(1), 7-46.

CHAPTER 5

Chronic Disease and African American Families

SHARON WALLACE WILLIAMS AND
PEGGYE DILWORTH-ANDERSON

Chronic disease affects more than 100 million Americans and is the leading cause of death and disability in the United States (National Academy on an Aging Society, 1999). Chronic disease increases with age, and rates and types of chronic disease vary within and between racial and ethnic groups. Chronic diseases, such as heart disease, diabetes, obesity, and stroke, are among the most prevalent, costly, and preventable of all health problems. Every year, 7 of 10 Americans who die, or more than 1.7 million people, die of a chronic disease. Medical costs for people with chronic diseases account for more than 70% of the $1 trillion spent annually on health care in the United States (Centers for Disease Control and Prevention [CDC], 2004a). The prolonged course of chronic illness and disability results in extended pain and suffering. It also results in decreased quality of life for millions of Americans and their families (Marks, 2003; National Academy on an Aging Society, 1999).

Diabetes is one chronic condition that varies by race, with African American, American Indian, and Hispanic adults more likely to have diabetes than whites. African Americans and American Indians are also more likely than whites to have hypertension. Poorly controlled diabetes and hypertension are positively associated with a host of negative health outcomes, including stroke and end stage renal disease.

The CDC (2004b) reports that African American women are also more likely to die of breast cancer than are women of any other racial or ethnic group. In addition, African Americans are almost twice as likely to experience strokes as white Americans (Gillum, 1999; Sacco, 2003). The prevalence of both fatal and nonfatal strokes is greater among African Americans, and recovery is slower (Horner, Swanson, Bosworth, & Matchar, 2003; Howard, Howard, Katholi, Oil, & Huston, 2001). In addition, a large percentage of older African Americans live in the "stroke belt" region (North Carolina, South Carolina, Georgia, Alabama, Mississippi, Arkansas, Tennessee, and Louisiana) of the southeastern United States. This region has the highest incidence and mortality of stroke in the entire United States. Strokes and other health disparities exist throughout the life course and at all socioeconomic levels, although stroke is more common at the low end of the socioeconomic status (SES) spectrum (Hughes & Thomas, 1998; Williams, 2002).

Individuals with a chronic disease or disability or both typically manage their disease within the larger context of the family. Family serves as the key social influence in sustaining disease management in chronic conditions. Active involvement of spouses and adult children is related to successful intervention outcomes for older adults (Rolland, 1994; Sarkisian, Brown, Norris, Wintz, & Mangione, 2003). The critical role of families in the management of chronic disease is evident but has neither been well researched nor well described in the literature. The family network and the family's system of beliefs, both organized within historical context, influence how individuals and family members identify and manage chronic disease over time (Fisher et al., 2000; Pescosolido, 1991).

Families, regardless of race and ethnicity, face similarities such as the need for information about the chronic disease and integration of the disease into family life. Racial and culture differences faced by families affect resources available to the family and family organization. This chapter focuses on chronic disease and ways in which African American families manage and are affected by management of chronic disease. Similarities and differences among African American, Native American, Indian, whites, Asian, and Hispanic families who have a family member with a chronic illness are highlighted.

Although there is no single accepted definition of race, in this chapter, we use the definition of race as a socially and historically constructed system of categorization (Williams, 1997) to conceptualize African American families in a social and historical context. Researchers are beginning to recognize the influence of race and cultural factors (e.g., values, customs, rituals, language, and ways of behaving) on how families give care to members with a chronic disease (Dilworth-Anderson, Goodwin, & Williams, 2004; Freeman, 2003). For example, Cox and Monk (1993) and Clark and Huttlinger (1998) found that cultural values and norms govern familial relationships and the care of elderly family members among Hispanics. Furthermore, Hennessy and John (1996) found that caregiving among American Indians was regarded as a reflection of their cultural ethos of interdependency and reciprocity. In this chapter, we examine structural and cultural components of family helping networks of African Americans and compare structural and cultural similarities and differences between African American families and other racial and ethnic families who have a member with a chronic disease.

Although structure and culture are intertwined and confounded with race and ethnicity, we attempt to separately examine structural and cultural similarities and differences among racial and ethnic groups. Structural characteristics, such as family network and health care access, and cultural characteristics, such as cultural beliefs, family support, and cohesion, are highlighted. Although chronic disease can affect the family at any point during the family life course, this chapter focuses on families with an older adult who has a chronic disease.

CHRONIC DISEASE

Management of chronic diseases is time-consuming and requires monitoring, adjusting, and reacting to daily demands. Management of all chronic diseases is not the same. Rolland (1984, 1987, 1994) offered a psychosocial typology of illness to classify chronic illness. The typology distinctions include onset and course of the chronic disease to examine the relationship between chronic illness and family life. The onset of disease is divided into acute and gradual, with stroke being an example of an acute onset and Parkinson's disease representing a gradual onset.

Course of disease is further divided into a progressive, constant, and relapsing typology. Progressive chronic diseases are conceptualized to be continually symptomatic and to increase in severity. Incurable cancers, Alzheimer's disease, and AIDS are examples of progressive chronic conditions. Rolland stated that the family cannot settle in when managing a progressive disease because a new stage of the progressive disease continuously approaches. Such a disease is hypothesized to lead to increasing strain and caregiving tasks for the family. In comparison to a progressive illness, within a constant course (e.g., brain injury and spinal cord injury with paralysis), an initial event occurs, but then the condition stabilizes. Families faced with such a chronic condition care for a family member typically with a clear-cut deficit that is stable and predictable. Rolland asserted that such a chronic disease is relatively less burden for the family than dealing with progressive conditions because there is not the continually worsening of the condition. The third type of course, relapsing or episodic, can be the most psychosocially challenging for the family. Such a relapsing or episodic course (e.g., asthma, multiple sclerosis, and rheumatoid arthritis) is associated with alternation of stable periods (stable level or absence of symptoms) and periods of flare-up or exacerbations. It is thought that the ongoing uncertainty can produce strain and pose a threat to families' efforts to normalize family life.

Although African American families may have to integrate and manage any one of many chronic diseases into the family system, they are more likely to care for older family members who have hypertension, diabetes, stroke, heart disease, and end stage renal disease (Freeman & Payne, 2000; Geronimus, Bound, Waidmann, Colen, & Steffick, 2001; Gornick & Eggers, 1996). The incidence of these chronic diseases is influenced by race and ethnicity (Clark & Dunbar, 2003; Tarver-Carr et al., 2002).

CHRONIC DISEASE AND THE FAMILY

Although there are differences and disparities regarding chronic disease and the family, it is known that family members are typically involved in providing or monitoring care for family members regardless of race. The family, as the vehicle or system of care throughout the life course of an individual, functions as a source of information, beliefs, and meanings. Individuals with a chronic illness or disability or both manage their disease within the larger context of the family (Fisher et al., 2000; Pescosolido, 1991). The family caregiving network is typically defined by who provides care (spouse, daughter, etc.), the type of caregivers (primary, secondary, or tertiary), and size (the number of people who provide care). Most caregiving networks (85-90%) are family caregiving networks. Friends, neighbors, and formal helpers are involved but usually in secondary roles, and more often when family members are not available. The family helps to define the illness, navigate the medical system, and make medical choices (Ballard-Reisch & Letner,2003; Pescosolido, 1991; Turner, 1996; Wicks, 1997).

A large body of research speaks to the importance of the social support provided by the family caregiving network and the positive association between social support and health outcomes for older adults and their caregivers (Glass, Matchar, Belyea, & Feussner, 1993; Grant, Elliott, Weaver,

Bartolucci, & Giger, 2002; Knapp & Hewison, 1998). Social support provided by family caregivers is typically conceptualized as instrumental, emotional, or informational social support. Social support is also conceptualized in terms of perceived versus received support. Provision of tasks, such as help with activities of daily living, is conceptualized as instrumental social support, whereas emotional support provides the sense that one is loved and cared for, and informational support usually involves giving health-related information (Campbell & McDaniel, 2001).

Management of chronic disease consists of the required daily activities to manage the chronic condition and produce optimal outcomes (Clark, 2003; Glasgow, Strycker, Toobert, & Eakin, 2000; Riley, Glasgow, & Eakin, 2001). Effective disease management strategies include adherence to medication regimen, monitoring and maintenance of risk factors such as adequately controlled blood pressure and blood glucose levels (if diabetic), making lifestyle changes often related to smoking, and dietary and physical activity management. Management of chronic illness has been shown to be improved by applying the "chronic care model" to the longitudinal management of patients. According to this model (Wagner, 1998; Wagner, Austin, & Korff, 1996; Wagner et al., 2001), a key element of improved chronic illness care is self-management by an activated patient (i.e., one who takes responsibility as a partner in his or her care). Much of the literature on improved chronic care management describes how health system redesign can foster and support self-management (Bodenheimer, Wagner, & Grumbach, 2002). The critical role of families in support of self-management is evident but has neither been well researched nor well described in the literature on the chronic care model.

Prevention and management of chronic disability and disease typically focus on the individual patient. Research on diabetes has begun to examine how the family is actively involved in day-to-day disease management tasks. For example, in adults with diabetes, treatment, adherence, illness adaptation, and blood sugar control were improved with higher levels of family support (Fisher et al., 1998; Silliman, Bhatti, Khan, Dukes, & Sullivan, 1996; Trief et al., 2003). Fisher and colleagues (1998) conducted several studies on the family context of the management of diabetes. They argued for the inclusion and examination of family members as the primary social context of disease management. Similar findings have been documented in heart failure (Clark & Dunbar, 2003), osteoarthritis (Martire et al., 2003), and Alzheimer's disease (Mittleman, Ferris, Shulman, Steinberg, & Levin, 1996). Social support from the family is also positively related to stroke outcomes (Glass et al., 2000; Tsouna-Hadjis, Vemmos, Zakopoulos, & Stamatelopoulos, 2000).

Social ecology and systems perspectives examine family-level variables and other levels (health care providers, community, media, and policy) connected to the family to understand disease management and interventions (Fisher et al., 1998). The ABC-X model and resource frameworks (resource development, African American resource development, and health promoting family model) are also used to conceptualize and understand families and their relationship to disease management. Resource theories focus on resources such as economic (education, income, and wealth), social (family, neighborhood, and social support), and emotional or physical outcomes (mental well-being and general health). Stress and coping models (Lazarus & Folkman, 1984; Pearlin, Mullan, Semple, & Skaff, 1990) concentrate more on the family's ability to cope with the chronic disease and also on various coping mechanisms. The stress and coping models also consider resources, typically conceptualized as mediators of stressors and well-being outcomes.

CHRONIC DISEASE AND AFRICAN AMERICAN FAMILIES

Structural Characteristics

Although the nuclear family is the traditional family structure, ethnic and racial families, particularly African American families, are more likely to have extended and single-parent family structures. In nuclear families, the spouse is typically the primary helper, whereas in single-parent and extended family households an adult child is more likely to be the primary helper. The structure of the family is related to the number of available helpers within the family caregiving network. The structure is also associated with race, gender, and available resources. Older African Americans, particularly older women, are more likely to live alone. Consequently, they are more likely to live in poverty. Fisher and colleagues (2000) found that for Latino families, family structure and organization were related to better disease management for adults with type 2 diabetes, whereas for European American families, family structure and organization were not associated with disease management.

Socioeconomic status is also strongly related to resources such as access to health care. Paradoxically, when low income levels are associated with receipt of Medicaid, greater access to health care is documented. Medicaid appears to facilitate access to paid services by connecting poorer individuals, who are not able to purchase services, with formal health services. Researchers (Bass & Noelker, 1987; Headen, 1993; Li, Edwards, & Morrow-Howell, 2004) have also documented that the care recipient's receipt of Medicaid is related to the use of formal

support. Access, however, does not necessary equate to better or even adequate care. Extensive evidence shows that even when controlling for SES, African Americans and other minorities do not receive the same level of care as whites. Thus, both race and SES (Institute of Medicine, 2002) can help explain equality of care or lack of it in the health care systems in the United States.

Racism and racial prejudice are a reality in the history, cultural memory, and current experience of many African Americans and other people of color (Freeman & Payne, 2000). As a result of these and other long-standing structural and personal discrimination experiences, African Americans and other minorities often express distrust toward the health care system (Corbie-Smith, Thomas, & St. George, 2002; Doescher, Saver, Fiscella, & Franks, 2004). Lillie-Blanton, Brodie, Rowland, Altman, and McIntosh (2000) documented that 64% of African American adults believed they received poorer quality health care than whites. It has been documented that fewer resources are used in caring for seriously ill African Americans than for whites, such as less use of analgesia for those dying from cancer and fewer referrals for the most sophisticated heart procedures (Bonham, 2001; Freeman & Payne, 2000; Institute of Medicine, 2003; Krakauer, Crenner, & Fox, 2002). Barriers to obtaining expensive high-tech treatment have also been documented, and some African Americans believe that limited financial and insurance resources will lead to decreased medical care (Blackhall et al., 1999; Krakauer, et al., 2002).

Individuals without insurance are more likely to access health care at later stages of illness and most often in crisis situations. Also, follow-up with health care systems is more sporadic. Even with the same level of insurance, minorities often have poorer outcomes. Racial injustice (Freeman & Payne,

2000), socioeconomic factors (Zuvekas & Taliaferro, 2003), and poor communication between patients, especially minority patients, and physicians have been cited as reasons for poorer outcomes (Ashton et al., 2003). Karter and colleagues (2002) documented in a sample of patients with diabetes that the incidence of end stage renal disease was higher for minorities, but they found similar or lower levels relative to whites for other complications.

Related to low SES and other historical factors, many low-income minorities live in communities with high levels of crime and violence and often lower levels of available high-quality food and well-stocked pharmacies (Bowles & Kington, 1998). Similarly, the safety of neighborhood streets (community-level variable) and the extent to which they are kept free of dumped materials are likely to influence physical activity because residents may choose to remain indoors rather than walk or engage in other forms of physical activity (Sherwood & Jeffery, 2000; Stahl et al., 2001). Such environmental constraints are closely tied to management of chronic disease in terms of available physical activity, nutrition, and obtaining medication.

Similar to Hispanic family caregivers, African American family caregivers typically use low levels of formal support (Cox & Monk, 1993; Miller & Guo, 2000). Formal support is help provided by professionals, paid helpers, or companies that provide caregiving help. It is assistance governed by contractual rather than affiliative norms (Eustis & Fischer, 1991; Miller, McFall, & Campbell, 1994). Operationalization of formal support often influences use of some specific services, including home health, adult day care, formal support groups, transportation services, and referral services. It is generally affirmed that the use of formal support can reduce some of the physical and mental stressors associated with providing care (Mui, Choi, & Monk, 1998; Zarit,

Gaugler, & Jarrott, 1999). Several researchers, however, have found that the use of formal support is positively associated with institutional placement for the care recipient. It has been suggested that this positive association indicates that formal support may be employed too late to be helpful in terms of lessening stress and other challenges of caregiving (Gottlieb & Johnson, 2000; Miller & McFall, 1991).

Cultural Characteristics

The formation of family structures has traditionally been fostered by cultural values and norms, including interdependence of family and community members and expected reciprocity among family members (Franklin, 1997). Family structures are sometimes created as a response to lack of access to formal services outside the family due to general racial discrimination and historical practices that prohibited African Americans from using certain goods and services available to other members of society (Franklin, 1997; Katz, 1993). Some have suggested that African American informal networks have served as social service systems, welfare systems, and community-based intervention systems (Burton & Dilworth-Anderson, 1991; Franklin, 1997; Katz, 1993).

In African American families with extended structure, the literature shows that a more varied family composition is included in providing care and support. Grandchildren and nieces and nephews are part of the family network of care. Research findings show that kin caregivers to dependent older African Americans consist of an array of family members, such as adult children, spouses, nieces, nephews, in-laws, and grandchildren (Dilworth-Anderson, Williams, & Cooper, 1999a, 1999b; Haley et al., 1995; Young & Kahana, 1995). Nonkin caregivers consist of friends and neighbors who provide care to the dependent elderly. Lawton, Rajagopal,

Brody, and Kleban (1992) reported that the quality of care to older people in African American families did not vary by relationship to the caregiver. Luckey (1994) found that roles and tasks performed by grandchildren, nieces, or nephews assisted the elderly as well as the primary caregivers interacting with formal services. Sharing living arrangements and pooling financial resources are ways in which African American networks have traditionally provided and continue to provide care to members (Franklin, 1997). Caregiving networks among African Americans, therefore, have addressed both simple and complex problems of family and community members. African American caregivers are often documented as resilient with low levels of depression or strain or both and with high levels of resiliency. It would be inaccurate, however, to assert that African American caregivers are a homogeneous group or that care is given with little emotional cost (Williams, Dilworth-Anderson, & Goodwin, 2003).

Research speaks to the importance of social support and its association with better long-term self-management and better health outcomes (Kaplan & Toshima, 1990; Uchino, Caioppo, & Kiecolt-Glaser, 1996). Higher levels of support are related to better management of diabetes (Glass et al., 1993; Grant et al., 2002; Whitfield, 2004). This relationship, however, appears to be influenced or confounded by gender. One study demonstrated that female spouses provided meals to meet dietary restriction of husbands, whereas women with diabetes were more likely to prepare two sets of meals—one for the family and a separate meal for themselves (MacLean, 1991).

The model of social-environmental support related to disease self-management (Glasgow & Eakin, 1998; Glasgow et al., 2000) examines eight levels of "psychosocial environmental support" physician and health care team, family and friends, personal actions, neighborhood, community, media and policy, community organizations, and workplace. The model also examines the perceived importance of each resource in managing illness. The model has consistently shown that physician and health care team support is most important for management of disease. This model needs to be tested with diverse populations.

Although earlier research (Hatch, 1991; Martin & Martin, 1978) documented that African American families have large and extended cohesive networks to provide support to needy members, an emerging body of literature reports that researchers can no longer assume that these large and extended networks still exist in African American families (Ajrouch, Antonucci, & Janevic, 2001; Barnes, Mendes DeLeon, Bienias, & Evans, 2004; Jarrett & Burton, 1999; McDonald & Armstrong, 2001; Roschelle, 1997). Jarrett and Burton (1999) and Roschelle (1997), in particular, suggest that characteristics such as age distribution, education, and living arrangements of those in the network can influence the type of support given and received. Roschelle also suggested that unlike in the past, more African American families will begin to rely on varied combinations of support that include the family and formal services. These findings show that the size and strength of the kin network are being challenged by the needs of multiple generations in the family coupled with declining resources in the network to address the needs of family members (Dilworth-Anderson & Burton, 1999). Other findings on social support networks document that the informal networks of Asian Americans consist of both family and friends and are similar in size to those of other racial and ethnic groups (Youn, Knight, Jeong, & Benton 1999). Phillips, de Ardon, Komnenich, Killeen, and Rusinak (2000), however, found that Mexican American caregivers had smaller social networks than non-Hispanic white caregivers.

Families help with emotional and instrumental support. Emotional support, such as encouragement and advice, and instrumental support, such as preparing different foods or preparing foods differently, are documented as helpful. Also helpful is adoption of a "we" concept of ownership of disease by the family, particularly the spouse. Such a focus is associated with new routines, such as "family exercise" or "family fitness" activities, and smoking cessation efforts. Family routines and rituals to enhance treatment adherence are beneficial to the family member with the chronic disease and may improve the health of the other participating family members (Fiese & Wamboldt, 2000). In a review of social support and chronic disease, Gallant (2003) concluded that evidence shows that the relationship between family support and diet and exercise may be stronger than the family support and medication adherence link.

It is important for health care providers and researchers to be aware of a patient's cultural beliefs about the cause (Turner, 1996) and fatalism of disease. It is also critical that providers and researchers are aware of stigma attached to disease. This is particularly relevant for HIV/AIDS, epilepsy, and, to a lesser extent, cancer (Turner, 1996). Beliefs vary by race and culture (Klonof & Landrine, 1994; Nelson, Geiger, & Mangione, 2002). For example, dementia is defined and perceived differently among diverse cultural groups. Some cultural groups view it as normal aging, whereas others may perceive it as imbalance in spiritual harmony in the body (Dilworth-Anderson & Gibson, 2002).

Nelson and colleagues (2002) found that Spanish-speaking Latinos and Asian women had higher levels of fatalistic beliefs regarding cancer than white and African American women. It has also been documented that whereas many whites focus on self-reliant or individualistic views or both and social organization around the nuclear family, more Hispanic and African Americans are documented with a focus on the extended family unit rather than the individual or nuclear family unit (Lim et al., 1996). Research also documents that African Americans perceive family members as protectors against physicians, whereas Hispanics are more likely to perceive family members as liaisons. Such health beliefs and perceptions are associated with the likelihood of changing behaviors, such as dietary and physical activity changes (Chernoff, 2001). Given the previous examples, health care providers need to consider how cultural factors such as language, perceptions, beliefs, and values of diverse groups help shape the manner in which health is defined and addressed culturally.

Sociohistorical evidence suggests that it is through a strong sense of family cohesion and connectedness that African American families have been able to support sick family members (Franklin, 1997; Martin & Martin, 1978). In a study of family competence and adjustment to disability in a sample of African American families, Ashton and McCowan (1995) found that family cohesion was positively related to adjustment. They also inferred that the strong family cohesion among African American families contributed to available family members assisting in managing tasks and adjustment to chronic disease. Syrjala, Chapko, Vitaliano, Cummings, and Sullivan (1993) suggested that families high in cohesion may mobilize the resources necessary to adjust to health challenges (bone marrow transplant in their study). Research also suggests that strong cultural values and beliefs about helping and giving support encourage cohesiveness among African American families (Dilworth-Anderson et al., 1999a, 1999b; Jarrett & Burton, 1999; Taylor & Chatters, 1986).

Whereas social support and family cohesion (connectedness or sense of closeness of family members) are positively related to better management and outcomes, the opposite is true for family conflict and strain.

Nagging and critical behavior are found to be unhelpful (Trief et al., 2003). Negative critical or hostile relationships have stronger influence than positive or supportive relationships (Campbell & McDaniel, 2001). Fisher and colleagues (2000) concluded that in general, the following family characteristics have demonstrated consistently negative relationships with chronic disease outcomes: low family cohesion, high family conflict, too rigid or too permeable generation boundaries, low levels of family organization, hostile family affiliative tone, low marital satisfaction, criticalness, lack of clear communication, and low spouse involvement.

BIDIRECTIONALITY OF CHRONIC DISEASE

Most of the previous discussion focused on how the family helps to manage disease, but it is important to remember the bidirectionality of the chronic disease on the family. Family members influence and are influenced by the health of their members. In fact, the primary caregiver, usually a spouse or adult child, has been described as the hidden patient (Medalie, 1994). The spouse is typically the most affected by the disease and management of the disease. Providing care can increase or lead to depressive or anxiety symptoms (Cannuscio et al., 2002).

Other costs to providing care include other emotional, physical, or financial burden or all three. Family members who are unsupported in their efforts may be at risk for emotional or physical problems or both.

The degree of support to family members varies. Although approximately 25% of primary caregivers provide care alone (Dilworth-Anderson et al., 1999a, 1999b), another 25% provide care with a second helper, and the other 50% of primary helpers have two or more helpers within the family helping network.

It is import to remember that the family's ability to support the patient, balance demands, and integrate the chronic disease or illness into family life affects the patient's quality of life. Family-based interventions hold promise for preventing and relieving distress for family members and for the member of the family with the chronic disease (Mitrani, Prado, Feaster, Robinson-Batista, & Szapocznik, 2003). Such intervention is based on the thesis that the potential solution lies within the collective resources of an individual's social network.

CONCLUSION

Health care and health management of chronic disease are a family responsibility, not just that of the individual and health care provider (Witt, Brawer, & Plumb, 2002). A more complete understanding of the family context of chronic illness self-management has important implications for the design of interventions that aim to enhance self-management behavior and for the health and well-being of individuals with chronic illness (Gallant, 2003). These issues have particular critical application in African American families.

REFERENCES

Ajrouch, K. J., Antonucci, T. C., & Janevic, M. R. (2001). Social networks among blacks and whites: The interaction between race and age. *Journal of Gerontology, 56,* S112-S118.

Ashton, C. M., Haidet, P., Paterniti, D. A., Collins, T. C., Gordon, H. S., O'Malley, K., et al. (2003). Racial and ethnic disparities in the use of health services: Bias, preferences, or poor communication. *Journal of General Internal Medicine, 18,* 146-152.

Ashton, R. J., & McCowan, C. J. (1995). Perception of family competence and adaptation to illness among African Americans with disabilities. *Journal of Rehabilitation, 61,* 27-32.

Ballard-Reisch, D. S., & Letner, J. A. (2003). Centering families in cancer communication research: Acknowledging the impact of support, culture, and process on client/provider communication in cancer management. *Patient Education and Counseling, 50,* 61-66.

Barnes, L. L., Mendes DeLeon, C. F., Bienias, J. L., & Evans, D. A. (2004). A longitudinal study of black-white differences in social resources. *Journal of Gerontology, 59,* S146-S153.

Bass, D. M., & Noelker, L. S. (1987). The influence of family caregivers on elders' use of in-home services. *Journal of Health and Social Behavior, 28,* 184-196.

Blackhall, L. J., Frank, G., Murphy, S. T., Michel, V., Palmer, J. M., & Azen, S. P. (1999). Ethnicity and attitudes towards life sustaining technology. *Social Science and Medicine, 48,* 1779-1789.

Bodenheimer, T., Wagner, E. H., & Grumbach, K. (2002). Improving primary care for patients with chronic illness: The chronic care model, Part 2. *Journal of the American Medical Association, 288,* 1909-1914.

Bonham, V. L. (2001). Race, ethnicity, and pain treatment: Striving to understand the causes and solutions to the disparities in pain treatment. *Journal of Law, Medicine & Ethics, 29,* 52-68.

Bowles, J., & Kingston, R. S. (1998). The impact of family function on health of African American elderly. *Journal of Comparative Family Studies, 29,* 337-349.

Burton, L. M., & Dilworth-Anderson, P. (1991). The intergenerational roles of aged black Americans. *Marriage and Family Review, 16,* 311-322.

Campbell, T. L., & McDaniel, S. H. (2001). Behavioral medicine in family practice. *Clinics in Family Practice, 3,* 1-16.

Cannuscio, C. C., Jones, C., Kawachi, I., Colditz, G. A., Berkman, L., & Rimm, E. (2002). Reverberations of family illness: A longitudinal assessment of informal care giving and mental health status in the Nurses' Health Study. *American Journal of Public Health, 92,* 1305-1311.

Centers for Disease Control and Prevention. (2004a, January). *The burden of chronic disease and the future of public health.* Retrieved May 25, 2004, from http://www.cdc.gov

Centers for Disease Control and Prevention. (2004b, June). *Racial and ethnic approaches to community health: 2010: Addressing disparities in health 2004.* Retrieved June 25, 2004, from http://www.cdc.gov/nccdphp/aag/pdf/aag_reach2004.pdf

Chernoff, R. (2001). Nutrition and health promotion in older adults [Special issue]. *Journal of Gerontology, 56,* 47-53.

Clark, M., & Huttlinger, K. (1998). Elder care among Mexican American families. *Clinical Nursing Research, 7,* 64-81.

Clark, N. M. (2003). Management of chronic disease by patients. *Annual Review of Public Health, 24,* 289-313.

Clark, P. C., & Dunbar, S. B. (2003). Preliminary reliability and validity of family care climate questionnaire for heart failure. *Families, Systems & Health, 21,* 281-291.

Corbie-Smith, G., Thomas, S. B., & St. George, D. M. (2002). Distrust, race, and research: A national perspective. *Archives of Internal Medicine, 162,* 2458-2463.

Cox, C., & Monk, A. (1993). Hispanic culture and family care of Alzheimer's patients. *Health and Social Work, 18,* 92-101.

Dilworth-Anderson, P., & Burton, L. (1999). Critical issues in understanding family support and older minorities. In T. Miles (Ed.), *Full-color aging: Facts, goals, and recommendations for America's diverse elders* (pp. 93-105). Washington, DC: Gerontological Society of America.

Dilworth-Anderson, P., & Gibson, B. (2002). The cultural influence of values, norms, meanings, and perceptions in understanding dementia in ethnic minorities. *Alzheimer's Disease and Associated Disorders, 16,* S56-S63.

Dilworth-Anderson, P., Goodwin, P., & Williams, S. W. (2004). Can culture help explain the physical health effects of care giving over time among African American caregivers? *Journal of Gerontology: Social Science, 59,* S138-S145.

Dilworth-Anderson, P., Williams, S. W., & Cooper, T. (1999a). Family care giving to elderly African Americans: Caregiver types and structures. *Journal of Gerontology, 54,* S237-S241.

Dilworth-Anderson, P., Williams, S. W., & Cooper, T. (1999b). The contexts of experiencing emotional distress among family caregivers to elderly African-Americans. *Family Relations, 48,* 391-396.

Doescher, M. P., Saver, B. G., Fiscella, K., & Franks, P. (2004). Preventive care. Does continuity count? *Journal of General Internal Medicine, 19,* 632-637.

Eustis, N. M., & Fischer, L. R. (1991). Relationships between home care clients and their workers: Implications for quality of care. *The Gerontologist, 31,* 447-456.

Fiese, B., & Wamboldt, F. S. (2000). Family routines and asthma management: A proposal for family-based strategies to increase treatment adherence. *Families, Systems & Health, 18,* 405-418.

Fisher, L., Chesla, C. A., Bartz, R. J., Gilliss, C., Skaff, M. A., Sabogal, F., et al. (1998). The family and type 2 diabetes: A framework for intervention. *The Diabetes Educator, 24,* 599-607.

Fisher, L., Chesla, C. A., Skaff, M. A., Gillis, C., Kanter, R. A., Lutz, C. P., et al. (2000). Disease management status: A typology of Latino and Euro-American patients with type 2 diabetes. *Behavioral Medicine, 26*(2), 53-66.

Franklin, D. (1997). *Ensuring inequality: The structural transformation of the African American family.* New York: Oxford University Press.

Freeman, H. P. (2003). Commentary on the meaning of race in science and society. *Cancer Epidemiology, Biomarkers and Prevention, 12,* 232s-236s.

Freeman, H. P., & Payne, R. (2000). Racial injustice in health care. *New England Journal of Medicine, 342,* 1045-1046.

Gallant, M. P. (2003). The influence of social support on chronic illness self-management: A review and directions for research. *Health Education & Behavior, 30,* 170-195.

Geronimus, A. T., Bound, J., Waidmann, T. A., Colen, C. G., & Steffick, D. (2001). Inequality in life expectancy, functional status, and active life expectancy across selected black and white populations in the United States. *Demography, 38,* 227-251.

Gillum, R. F. (1999). Stroke mortality in blacks: Disturbing trends. *Stroke, 30,* 1711-1715.

Glasgow, R. E., & Eakin, E. G. (1998). Issues in diabetes self-management. In S. A. Shumaker, E. B. Schron, J. K. Ockene, & W. L. McBee (Eds.), *The Handbook of Health Behavior Change* (pp. 435-461). New York: Springer.

Glasgow, R. E., Strycker, L. A., Toobert, D. J., & Eakin, E. (2000). A social-ecologic approach to assessing support for disease management: The chronic illness resource survey. *Journal of Behavioral Medicine, 23,* 559-583.

Glass, T. A., Dym, B., Greenberg, S., Rintell, D., Roesch, C., & Berkman, L. F. (2000). Psychological intervention in stroke: Families in Recovery From Stroke Trial (FIRST). *American Journal of Orthopsychiatry, 70,* 169-181.

Glass, T. A., Matchar, D. B., Belyea, M. J., & Feussner, J. R. (1993). Impact of social support on outcome in first stroke. *Stroke, 24,* 64-70.

Gornick, M. E., & Eggers, P. W. (1996). Effects of race and income on mortality and use of services among Medicare beneficiaries. *New England Journal of Medicine, 335,* 791-799.

Gottlieb, B. H., & Johnson, J. (2000). Respite programs for caregivers of persons with dementia: A review with practice implications. *Aging and Mental Health, 4,* 119-129.

Grant, J. S., Elliott, T. R., Weaver, M., Bartolucci, A., & Giger, J. (2002). Telephone intervention with family caregivers of stroke survivors after rehabilitation. *Stroke, 33,* 2060-2065.

Haley, W. E., West, C. A., Wadley, V. G., Ford, G. R., White, F. A., Barrett, J. J., et al. (1995). Psychological, social, and health impact of care giving: A comparison of black and white dementia family caregivers and noncaregivers. *Psychology and Aging, 10,* 540-552.

Hatch, L. R. (1991). Informal support patterns of older African American and white women. *Research and Aging, 13,* 144-170.

Headen, A. E., Jr. (1993). Economic disability and health determinants of the hazard of nursing home entry. *Journal of Human Resources, 28,* 80-110.

Hennessy, C. H., & John, R. (1996). American Indian family caregivers' perceptions of burden and needed support services. *Journal of Applied Gerontology, 15,* 275-293.

Horner, R. D., Swanson, J. W., Bosworth, H., & Matchar, D. B., for the VA Acute Stroke (VAST) Study Team. (2003). Effects of race and poverty on the process and outcome of inpatient rehabilitation services among stroke patients. *Stroke, 34,* 1027-1031.

Howard, G., Howard, V. J., Katholi, C., Oli, M. K., & Huston, S. (2001). Decline in U.S. stroke mortality: An analysis of temporal patterns by sex, race, and geographic region. *Stroke, 32,* 2213-2220.

Hughes, M., & Thomas, M. E. (1998). The continuing significance of race revisited: A study of race, class, and quality of life in America, 1972 to 1996. *American Sociological Review, 63,* 785-795.

Institute of Medicine. (2002). *Unequal treatment: Confronting racial and ethnic disparities in health care.* Washington, DC: National Academy Press.

Institute of Medicine. (2003). *Describing death in America: What we need to know.* Washington, DC: National Academy Press.

Jarrett, R. L., & Burton, L. M. (1999). Dynamic dimensions of family structure in low-income African American families: Emergent themes in qualitative research. *Journal of Comparative Family Studies, 30,* 177-187.

Kaplan, R. M., & Toshima, M. T. (1990). The functional effects of social relationships on chronic illnesses and disability. In B. R. Sarason, I. G. Sarason, & G. R. Pierce (Eds.), *Social support: An interactional view* (pp. 427-453). New York: John Wiley.

Karter, A. J., Ferrara, A., Liu, J. Y., Moffet, H. H., Ackerson, L. M., & Selby, J. V. (2002). Ethnic disparities in diabetic complications in an insured population. *Journal of the American Medical Association, 287,* 2519-2527.

Katz, M. B. (1993). *The "underclass" debate: Views from history.* Princeton, NJ: Princeton University Press.

Klonoff, E., & Landrine, H. (1994). Culture and gender diversity in commonsense beliefs about the causes of six illnesses. *Journal of Behavioral Medicine, 17,* 407-418.

Knapp, P., & Hewison, J. (1998). The protective effects of social support against mood disorder after stroke. *Psychology Health Medicine, 3,* 275-283.

Krakauer, E. L., Crenner, C., & Fox, K. (2002). Barriers to optimum end of life care for minority patients. *Journal of the American Geriatrics Society, 50,* 182-190.

Lawton, M. P., Rajagopal, D., Brody, E., & Kleban, M. H. (1992). The dynamics of care giving for demented elders among black and white families. *Journal of Gerontology: Social Science, 47,* S156-S164.

Lazarus, R., & Folkman, S. (1984). *Stress, appraisal, and coping.* New York: Springer.

Li, H., Edwards, D., & Morrow-Howell, N. (2004). Informal care giving networks and use of formal services by inner-city African American elderly with dementia. *Families in Society, 85,* 55-62.

Lillie-Blanton, M., Brodie, M., Rowland, D., Altman, E., & McIntosh, M. (2000). Race, ethnicity, and the health care system: Public perceptions and experiences. *Medical Care Research and Review, 57,* 218-235.

Lim, Y. M., Luna, I., Cromwell, S. L., Phillips, L., Russell, C. K., & de Ardon, E. T. (1996). Towards a cross-cultural understanding of family care giving burden. *Western Journal of Nursing Research, 18,* 252-266.

Luckey, I. (1994). African American elders: The support network of generational kin. *Families in Society: The Journal of Contemporary Human Services, 75,* 82-89.

MacLean, H. M. (1991). Patterns of diet related self-care in diabetes. *Social Science and Medicine, 32,* 689-696.

Marks, J. S. (2003). *The burden of chronic disease and the future of public health.* Retrieved May 25, 2004, from http://www.cdc.gov

Martin, E. P., & Martin, J. M. (1978). *The black extended family.* Chicago: University of Chicago Press.

Martire, L. M., Schulz, R., Keefe, F. J., Starz, T. W., Osial, T. A., Jr., Dew, M. A., et al. (2003). Feasibility of dyadic intervention for management of osteoarthritis: A pilot study with older patients and their spousal caregivers. *Aging & Mental Health, 7,* 53-60.

McDonald, K., & Armstrong, E. (2001). De-romanticizing black intergenerational support: The questionable expectation of welfare reform. *Journal of Marriage and the Family, 63,* 213-223.

Medalie, J. H. (1994). The caregiver as the hidden patient: Challenges for medical practice. In E. Kahana, D. E. Biegel, & M. L. Wykle (Eds.), *Family Care Giving Across the Lifespan* (pp. 312-330). Thousand Oaks, CA: Sage.

Miller, B., & Guo, S. (2000). Social support for spouse caregivers of persons with dementia. *Journal of Gerontology: Social Sciences, 55B,* S163-S172.

Miller, B., & McFall, S. (1991). The effect of caregiver's burden on change in frail older persons' use of formal helpers. *Journal of Health and Social Behavior, 32,* 165-179.

Miller, B., McFall, S., & Campbell, R. T. (1994). Changes in sources of community long-term care among African American and white frail older persons. *Journal of Gerontology, 49,* S14-S24.

Mitrani, V. B., Prado, G., Feaster, D. J., Robinson-Batista, C., & Szapocznik, J. (2003). Relational factors and family treatment engagement among low-income, HIV-positive African American mothers. *Family Process, 42,* 31-45.

Mittleman, M. S., Ferris, S. H., Shulman, E., Steinberg, G., & Levin, B. (1996). A family intervention to delay nursing home placement of patients with Alzheimer's disease: A randomized controlled trail. *Journal of the American Medical Association, 276,* 1725-1731.

Mui, A. C., Choi, N. G., & Monk, A. (Eds.). (1998). *Long-term care and ethnicity.* Westport, CT: Auburn House.

National Academy on an Aging Society. (1999). *Chronic conditions: A challenge for the 21st century.* Washington, DC: Author.

Nelson, K., Geiger, A. M., & Mangione, C. M. (2002). Effect of health beliefs on delays in care for abnormal cervical cytology in a multi-ethnic population. *Journal of General Internal Medicine, 17,* 709-716.

Pearlin, L., Mullan, J., Semple, S., & Skaff, M. (1990). Caregiving and the stress process: An overview of concepts and their measures. *The Gerontologist, 30,* 583-594.

Pescosolido, B. (1991). Illness careers and network ties: A conceptual model of utilization and compliance. *Advances in Medical Sociology, 2,* 161-184.

Phillips, L. R., de Ardon, E. T., Komnenich, P., Killeen, M., & Rusinak, R. (2000). The Mexican American caregiving experience. *Hispanic Journal of Behavioral Sciences, 22*(3), 296-305.

Riley, K. M., Glasgow, R. E., & Eakin, E. G. (2001). Resource for health: A social-ecological intervention for supporting self-management of chronic conditions. *Journal of Health Psychology, 6,* 693-705.

Rolland, J. (1984). Toward a psychosocial typology of chronic and life-threatening illness. *Family Systems Medicine, 2,* 245-263.

Rolland, J. S. (1987). Chronic illness and the life cycle: A conceptual framework. *Family Process, 26,* 203-221.

Rolland, J. S. (1994). *Families, illness and disability: An integrative treatment model.* New York: Basic Books.

Roschelle, A. R. (1997). *No more kin: Exploring race, class, and gender in family networks.* Thousand Oaks, CA: Sage.

Sacco, R. L. (2003). Preventing stroke among blacks: The challenges continue. *Journal of the American Medical Association, 289,* 3005-3007.

Sarkisian, C. A., Brown, A. F., Norris, K. C., Wintz, R. L., & Mangione, C. M. (2003). A systematic review of diabetes self-care interventions for older, African American, or Latino adults. *Diabetes Educator, 29,* 467-479.

Sherwood, N. E., & Jeffery, R. W. (2000). The behavioral determinants of exercise: Implications for physical activity interventions. *Annual Review of Nutrition, 20,* 21-44.

Silliman, R. A., Bhatti, S., Khan, A., Dukes, K. A., & Sullivan, L. M. (1996). The care of older persons with diabetes mellitus: Families and primary care physicians. *Journal of the American Geriatric Society, 44,* 1314-1321.

Stahl, T., Rutten, A., Nutbeam, D., Bauman, A., Kannas, L., Abel, T., et al. (2001). The importance of the social environment for physically active lifestyle—Results from an international study. *Social Science and Medicine, 52,* 1-10.

Syrjala, K. L., Chapko, M. K., Vitaliano, P. P., Cummings, C., & Sullivan, K. M. (1993). Recovery after allogenic marrow transplantation: Prospective study of predictors of long-term physical and psychological functioning. *Bone Marrow Transplant, 11,* 199-217.

Tarver-Carr, M. E., Powe, N. R., Eberhardt, M. S., LaVeist, T. A., Kington, R. S., Coresh, J., et al. (2002). Excess risk of chronic kidney disease among African-American versus white subjects in the United States: A population-based study of potential explanatory factors. *Journal of the American Society of Nephrology, 13,* 2363-2370.

Taylor, J. T., & Chatters, L. M. (1986). Patterns of informal support to elderly black adults: Family, friends, and church members. *Social Work, 31,* 432-438.

Trief, P. M., Sandberg, J., Greenberg, R. P., Graff, K., Castronova, N., Yoon, M., et al. (2003). Describing support: A qualitative study of couples living with diabetes. *Families, Systems & Health, 21,* 57-67.

Tsouna-Hadjis, E., Vemmos, K. N., Zakopoulos, N., & Stamatelopoulos, S. (2000). First-stroke recovery process: The role of family social support. *Archives of Physical and Medical Rehabilitation, 81,* 881-887.

Turner, D. C. (1996). The role of culture in chronic illness. *American Behavioral Scientist, 39,* 717-728.

Uchino, B. N., Caioppo, J. T., & Kiecolt-Glaser, J. K. (1996). The relationship between social support and physiological processes: A review with emphasis on underlying mechanisms and implications for health. *Psychology Bulletin, 119,* 488-531.

Wagner, E. H. (1998). Chronic disease management: What will it take to improve care for chronic illness? *Effective Clinical Practice, 1,* 1-4.

Wagner, E. H., Austin, B. T., & Korff, M. V. (1996). Organizing care for patients with chronic illness. *Milbank Quarterly, 74,* 511-544.

Wagner, E. H., Glasgow, R. E., Davis, C., Bonomi, A. E., Provost, L., McCulloch, D., et al. (2001). Quality improvement in chronic illness care: A collaborative approach. *Journal of the Joint Commission on Health Care Quality, 27,* 63-80.

Whitfield, K. (2004). *Closing the gap.* Washington, DC: Gerontological Society of America.

Wicks, M. N. (1997). A test of the Wicks family health model in families coping with chronic-obstructive pulmonary disease. *Journal of Family Nursing, 3,* 189-212.

Williams, D. (1997). Race and health: Basic questions, emerging directions. *Annals of Epidemiology, 7,* 322-333.

Williams, D. R. (2002). Racial/ethnic variations in women's health: The social embeddedness of health. *American Journal of Public Health, 92,* 588-597.

Williams, S. W., Dilworth-Anderson, P., & Goodwin, P. (2003). Caregiver role strain: The contribution of other roles and available resources in African American women. *Aging and Mental Health, 7,* 103-112.

Witt, D., Brawer, R., & Plumb, J. (2002). Cultural factors in preventive care: African Americans. *Primary Care Clinical Office Practice, 29,* 487-493.

Youn, G., Knight, B. G., Jeong, H., & Benton, D. (1999). Differences in familism values and caregiving outcomes among Korean, Korean American, and white American caregivers. *Psychology and Aging, 14,* 355-364.

Young, R. F., & Kahana, E. (1995). The context of caregiving and well-being outcomes among African and Caucasian Americans. *The Gerontologist, 35,* 225-232.

Zarit, S. J., Gaugler, J. E., & Jarrott, S. E. (1999). Useful services for families: Research findings and directions. *International Journal of Geriatric Psychiatry, 14,* 165-181.

Zuvekas, S. H., & Taliaferro, G. S. (2003). Pathways to access: Health insurance, the health care delivery system, and racial/ethnic disparities, 1996-1999. *Health Affairs, 22,* 139-153.

CHAPTER 6

The Pain and the Promise of Unfilled Dreams: Infertile Couples

Lynn Clark Callister

Susannah loved being married, and she and her husband, Greg, had high hopes for their future together, including the desire to have a large family. She said, "When we made the decision to start trying to get pregnant, my life suddenly became more complicated."

After being diagnosed with polycystic ovarian syndrome, Susannah said, "I was devastated. Although [the doctor] quickly went on to explain options available to help me conceive, I honestly don't remember anything else. Greg and I went home and had to deal with our first major shock. I was really upset. All of my life I had planned on getting married and having children of my own. It never crossed my mind that I might not ever be able to [get pregnant]. I had known couples with infertility problems, but I never imagined it happening to me.

OVERVIEW

Susannah and Greg are typical of many infertile couples. The infertility experience represents the pain and the promise of often unfulfilled dreams. Infertility is a lonely place for individuals and couples because "infertility is often a silent and solitary crucible, since it is not visible, life-threatening, or disfiguring" (Carroll et al., 2000, p. 286). Infertility is defined as the inability to conceive after 1 year of unprotected intercourse or the inability to carry a pregnancy to a live birth (Leiblum, Aviv, & Hamer, 1997). Interest in and research devoted to infertility are evidenced by the fact that listings on the Medline database for biomedical research numbered more than 1,166 articles published during 2004 in professional journals alone and in an international survey (Adashi, Cohen, & Hamberger, 2000).

It is estimated that 10% to 15% of couples of childbearing age are infertile, and this number is increasing, especially among younger women (American Society for Reproductive Medicine [ARSM], 1998). Overall, approximately one in four couples will experience infertility, and it is estimated

Table 6.1   Infertility Risk Factors

Men	Women
Age	Age
Exposure to chemicals	Endometriosis
Exposure to heat	Heredity
Sexually transmitted infections	Polycystic ovary syndrome
Smoking	Sexuality
Prescription drug use	Sexually transmitted infections
Variocele	Smoking
Surgery of reproductive organs	Premature menopause
Cancer treatment	Surgery of reproductive organs
	Cancer

SOURCE: Adapted from the American Society of Reproductive Medicine (http://www.asrm.org) and Focus on Fertility (http://www.focusonfertility.org).

that one third of women experience at least one episode of infertility during their reproductive years (Jenkins & Corrigan, 2004). Female fertility declines with age, which means that with each year there is a possibility of decreased conception (U.S. Department of Health and Human Services, 2004).

Men and women each account for 40% of infertility, and in 20% both partners are potentially infertile or the cause of the inability to conceive is unknown. Male and female risk factors for infertility are summarized in Table 6.1 (American Infertility Association, 2004). Infertility affects more than 6.1 million women and their partners in the United States. It is estimated that 7.7 million women will be infertile in the United States by 2025 (ASRM, 2004a). Secondary infertility, or the inability to become pregnant or carry a pregnancy to term after the birth of one or more biological children, is estimated to affect more than 3 million Americans (National Infertility Association, 2004a). Infertility affects those from all socioeconomic levels and racial, ethnic, and cultural groups. It is estimated that 50% of infertile couples achieve pregnancy within 2 years of infertility treatment.

The cover story of *U.S. News and World Report*, titled "Miracle Babies: How Science Is Helping Childless Couples Beat the Odds" (Mulrine, 2004), emphasized that childless couples are trying assisted reproductive technology (ART) in record numbers. Rates of success with ART are discouragingly low, with in vitro fertilization having a 26% success rate per transfer, zygote intrafallopian transfer a 30% success rate per transfer, and frozen embryo transfer a 16% success rate (Angard, 1999). National data on the success of ART are available for 384 fertility clinics throughout the United States (Centers for Disease Control and Prevention, 2001). Most health insurance policies do not cover ART, and exorbitant costs are prohibitive and often limit treatment to only those with considerable financial means.

THEORETICAL FRAMEWORK AND ASSUMPTIONS

The theoretical framework guiding this chapter is Lazarus's model used to explore stress responses and coping mechanisms in infertile couples (Lazarus & Folkman, 1984). It is essential that a biopsychosocial framework guide research and practice because infertility has a profound effect on the biological, psychological, and social aspects of the individual and the family (Engel, 1977, 1980). Three assumptions are associated with this review of infertility. First, it is assumed that becoming a biological parent is a valued and primary role in society. Second, the word *couple* refers to heterosexual couples living in a committed relationship who may use ART. The third assumption, as articulated by Jordan and Revenson (1999, p. 342), is that "every facet of a couple's psychosocial functioning is affected by the experience of infertility, from shared beliefs about the importance of parenting to the couple's identity to endless discussion of decisions regarding treatment to acceptance of the medical outcome."

CULTURE AND INFERTILITY

Sociocultural context is an important consideration in the meaning of and responses to infertility. For example, in developing nations such as Nigeria, the major cause of infertility is sexually transmitted infection. Infertile couples often seek treatment from faith healers. Women are often blamed for infertility, and men may divorce their wives or engage in polygyny or both in an effort to have children. Adoption in this culture is generally not socially acceptable, and there are medical, ethical, and legal implications to infertility treatment (Araoye, 2003). In traditional Chinese culture, women are honored for bearing a son, and even in the face of the one-child policy, having a child is extremely important (Chang & Kuo, 2000; Kartchner & Callister, 2003; Lee & Chin, 1996; Lee & Kuo, 2000). According to a Chinese proverb, "There are three ways one can dishonor one's parents, with childlessness being the foremost" (Lee & Sun, 2000, p. 153). In Japan, an infertile woman is referred to as an *umazume*, and in Korea she is referred to as a *suknyu*, both of which mean a woman made of stone. A Vietnamese woman who is infertile may be designated as *gai doc khon con*, or the poison woman without children.

Childbearing is one of the most important mitzvahs (*mitzvoth*) among Orthodox Jews (Callister, Semenic, & Foster, 1999; Semenic, Callister, & Feldman, 2004). There are rituals associated with infertility in Jewish couples, including the recitation of the following words associated with ancient scripture (Cardin, 1999):

> To everything there is a season: a time to embrace and a time to stand back; a time to sow and a time to reap; a time to laugh and a time to weep; a time to hold on and a time to let go. Our time to sow has ended; our time to let go has begun. (p. 133)

In Mexican society, the infertile woman may be viewed as incomplete, having a curse bestowed for some misdeed. In addition to the use of traditional healers, one coping mechanism is to pray to the virgin of Guadalupe, who is perceived as a survivor of great suffering. Among Native Americans, couples may use traditional healing measures or ceremonies to ensure a pregnancy (St. Hill, Lipson, & Meleis, 2003).

The importance of fertility among Muslim women is exemplified by the social pressure on newly married women to become pregnant as soon as possible, especially to have sons. Infertile women (*aquer*) may be stigmatized, divorced, or forced to agree to polygyny. In our study, one Muslim woman said, "Life would be nothing without children" (Khalaf & Callister, 1997, p. 380), and another Muslim woman explained that "people usually start asking you after the first month of marriage whether you 'save anything inside your abdomen,' meaning 'are you pregnant yet?' So is the nature of life" (p. 380).

STRESSES OF INFERTILITY

The stresses of diagnosis and treatment of infertility are multiple and complex, often referred to as a roller coaster of emotions. Both devastating failure and the hope for success are experienced (Bashford, 1999; Hart, 2002), as are often emotionally and physically exhausting experiences (Carroll et al., 2000; Eugster & Vingerhoets, 1999; Gibson & Myers, 2000; Lee, Sun, Chao, & Chen, 2001; Wiczyk, 2000). Carroll et al. note that "couples frequently report high levels of stress, a loss of hope, and feelings of frustration related to the use of complex reproductive technology, the medicalization of intimacy, invasive procedures, surgeries, and potent drugs with problematic side effects"(p. 286).

Triggers for stress and depression include medical appointments that interfere with life schedule, scheduled intercourse instead of spontaneous lovemaking, baby showers or birthday parties for young children, and trying to maintain positive marital relationships while experiencing intensive treatment (American Infertility Association & Organon Pharmaceuticals, 2004a). Decreases in marital satisfaction and adjustment have been documented (Leiblum et al., 1998). Anger, tension, depression, anxiety, guilt, and frustration are emotions fueled by the infertility experience (Anderson, Sharpe, Rattray, & Irvine, 2003; Lukse & Vacc, 1999; Merari, Cherit, & Modan, 2002).

Gender Differences in Stress and Coping

The largest body of infertility literature focuses on gender differences in stress levels for the infertile couple. Women may carry the burden because "fertility testing involves more complicated, uncomfortable, and humbling medical procedures for women . . . and their treatment is more invasive and more costly than treatment for male infertility. . . . Her life may be more disrupted than her partner's" (Jordan & Revenson, 1999, p. 343; Halman, Andrews, & Abbey, 1993; Phipps, 1993).

In a prospective longitudinal study conducted in the United Kingdom, the emotional distress of infertile couples was measured. Scores on the Hospital Anxiety and Depression Scale did not decrease over time (Anderson et al., 2003). Women had significantly greater infertility-related concerns, such as life satisfaction, sexuality, self-blame, self-esteem, and avoidance of friends, compared to their male partners.

In a study of 120 Taiwanese couples seeking ART, emotional responses to infertility differed according to education levels, duration and number of treatments, and the number of existing children. Women experienced more emotional disturbance associated with infertility than did their partners. In addition, responses had a significantly negative correlation with positive reappraisal. Infertile women adopted more coping behaviors to deal with the challenges of treatment for infertility (Hsu & Kuo, 2002).

There are also differences in responses depending on the cause of infertility, identified in an East Indian study of 120 infertile couples. Anxiety levels were significantly higher in the partner with the fertility problem. If the male partner was infertile and manifest effects on his personality and social behavior, the woman often became depressed (Dhaliwal, Gupta, Gopalan, & Kulhara, 2004).

The male infertility experience has been explicated by Petok (2004), who suggests that factors contributing to the gender disparity in response to infertility include men not being reminded on a monthly basis of infertility, the man often being assessed for infertility after the woman, and diagnostic procedures being more complicated and invasive for women. Culturally, media images are not as frequent or visible about fathering as they are about mothering, and few men's magazines focus on fathering. In addition, the expectation for men is that they should be strong and emotionally detached. Continuing a genetic line and family name is often extremely important for men.

Although infertility is stressful to both husbands and wives, some researchers have concluded that gender differences in responses to infertility may be striking (Busch, 2001; Gibson & Myers, 2000; Lee, Sun, & Chao, 2000; Phipps, 1993). A meta-analysis was done of gender differences in coping with infertility using the Ways of Coping Checklist (Folkman, Lazarus, Dunkel-Schetter, DeLongis, & Gruen, 1986). Women used three of the eight dimensions significantly more than their male partners: seeking social support, escape avoidance, planful problem solving, and positive reappraisal. These researchers concluded that there may be more similarities than differences in ways of coping between men and women. In a meta-analysis of gender differences associated with the infertility experience, women used social support as a coping strategy more often than men (Jordan & Revenson, 1999). This is supported by the work of Hsu and Kuo (2002). High levels of agreement between spouses help couples successfully manage the impact of infertility (Hidalgo, Caleffi, Baron, Mattana, & Chaves, 2004; Peterson, Newton, & Rosen, 2003).

Susannah described her perceptions of what Greg was experiencing as follows:

> I could tell that he was suffering too. I'm not really sure of his emotional experience during this time. I knew that he hurt just as bad as I did, and he cried with me, but he always seemed to be strong for me. Whenever I would try to convey to him my deep worry, he would tell me not to worry and everything would be fine. This answer was helpful for me, but it caused him to bottle up his fears. As time went on, I began to notice a

change in him. His drive to succeed, be productive, and to excel all seemed to fade. This only made me even more worried. I didn't know how to help him.

Following infertility treatment, Susannah said,

> You can imagine my surprise and great relief when I had a positive pregnancy test. Results in hand, I walked into our apartment and found Greg waiting for me to get home. When I told him, he was so excited. Even now, the image of his face is so vivid. I felt as though a heavy burden had been lifted off of my shoulders. My hope had been renewed and I was very happy.

Losses Experienced by Infertile Couples

Multiple losses experienced by infertile couples include loss of sexual identity; loss of the childbearing and child-rearing experience and the elusive child they never were able to conceive; loss of the parental identity; loss of close relationships with a spouse, extended family members, and friends; loss of health; loss of status or prestige; loss of a sense of personal control; loss of genetic legacy; loss of a grandparenting relationship; loss of a sense of spirituality and hope for the future; and loss of feelings of self-worth (Carroll et al., 2000, p. 286; Gibson & Myers, 2000; Gonzales, 2000; Hart, 2002; Imeson & McMurray, 1996; Johnston, 1994; National Infertility Association, 2004b; Reed, 2001; Sherrod, 2004).

Living With the Responses of Others: Feelings of Alienation

Often, others, including well-meaning extended family members, may assume that a couple is childless by choice. Comments may include, "So when are you going to start a family? You two aren't getting any

Table 6.2 Myths About Infertility

Infertility isn't a physical problem. . . . It's all in your head.

Infertility is not very treatable.

Infertility is a female problem.

Exercise more faith in God and you'll get pregnant.

If you can just relax, you can get pregnant.

Adopt a baby and then you'll get pregnant.

Maybe you're doing something wrong.

SOURCE: From Domar and Kelly (2002), Rutter (1996), and Wiczyk (2000).

younger" (National Infertility Association, 2004c). Others may offer "helpful" suggestions for the couple suffering with infertility. Myths associated with infertility often shared with infertile couples by others are shown in Table 6.2 (Domar & Kelly, 2002; Rutter, 1996; Wiczyk, 2000).

RESPONSES TO INFERTILITY: PHASES OF THE INFERTILITY EXPERIENCE

Responses to infertility may be categorized into phases, although responses are not orderly or consecutive. The couple may feel emotional highs and lows with hopefulness that a particular ART intervention will help and they will become pregnant, only to face disappointment one more time. In addition, spouses may be in different places emotionally and cognitively, which increases the dissonance between them.

STAGES OF GRIEF IN INFERTILE COUPLES

Providing personal views of treatment failure, Brown (2002) and Langdrige, Connolly, and Sheeran (2000) remind us that many infertile couples experience multiple failures month after month, treatment after treatment. One woman wrote the following about her experience with infertility: "Childlessness goes on and on. I see no end and I can't come to terms with what may never be. I feel empty, unwhole, angry, fearful, bitter, and lonely" (Kerr, Balen, & Brown, 1999, p. 935).

Stages of grief may include the following:

Denial: "This can't be happening to me" or "At first I tried to block out all emotion. All I wanted to do was sleep."

Isolation: "We'll keep this to ourselves. No one else can understand our pain."

Anger: Spouses may feel anger toward themselves, as indicated by the response, "If only I had worn better protective equipment when I played sports," because men are more likely to express verbal anger. Anger may be expressed toward the significant other or even other people, including other couples who seem to become pregnant whenever they want. Anger may also be expressed toward the physician and other members of the infertility team, such as, "That stupid doctor doesn't know what he's doing. That's the problem."

Unworthiness: There may be feelings of guilt or unworthiness as individuals blame themselves, such as "I don't know what I've done wrong" or "God must be punishing me for having an abortion when I was sixteen."

Depression: Feelings of a lack of control and a sense of powerlessness may contribute to depression. As one woman expressed, "Feelings of isolation and loneliness flooded over me as I listened to other women talk about their experiences of pregnancy and childbirth. How I wanted to share in their lively conversations. In the past few years I had spent endless days feeling sorry for myself. I had had enough tests, temperature taking, charting, and graphing to last a lifetime" (Zimmerman, 1992, p. 27). There is a need for couples to somehow generate a sense that they are active participants rather than "passive victims of the medical system" (Daniluk, 2001, p. 131). It is helpful for couples to set reasonable limits on the pursuit of infertility treatment so that they have a better sense of control in their lives. Developing such limits involves an exploration of their values, needs, and resources (Daniluk, 2001).

Severe grief: "I will never know what it feels like to bear a child." Infertility is a painful emotional experience generating a severe grief response (Barber, 2000; Gonzalez, 2000; Hart, 2002; Juo, Lee, Wang, & Lee, 1998; Reed, 2001; Rutter, 1996).

Healing grief: "I feel so empty, but the pain is less hurtful now."

Resolution phase: "Having faith in God's plan for me is probably the only thing that I hang on to" or "It's time to move on." It is challenging to reframe their experience when, despite exhaustive effort, couples remain childless. There may be some residual anger that needs to be resolved (Daniluk, 2001).

Susannah spoke of attending church when another couple with a child sat next to them:

They placed the baby right next to me. At that point the tears started flowing. I eventually had to bury my head in my husband's shoulder and cry. All around me were expectant mothers and little babies. They seemed to jump out at me everywhere I went.

COPING WITH INFERTILITY

Coping with infertility is often challenging because "infertility can be conceptualized as a chronic, unpredictable, and (personally or medically) uncontrollable stressor that may exceed the couple's coping resources" (Jordan & Revenson, 1999, p. 345). Carroll et al. (2000) noted the following (see also Johnson, 1996; Kirkman & Rosenthal, 1999; Lee, Chang, & Chen, 1997):

Coping strategies include distancing themselves from reminders of infertility (such as avoidance of families with children), instituting measures for regaining control, acting to increase feelings of self-worth in other areas of their lives such as achieving professional success, trying to find meaning in infertility, or sharing the burden with others. (p. 286)

One woman said (Christensen, 1996),

I built an emotional wall around myself, trying to shut out the pain. The wall provided a buffer that protected me for a time, from anyone or anything that reminded me that I had no children. However, the more I closed others out and focused on myself, the more the pain became magnified. It was a sad and lonely life, and as the walls grew higher and thicker, I grew even more discouraged and depressed. (p. 52)

Decision making about ART is anxiety producing. "Couples confronted by infertility are also challenged with sorting through a technically complex and potentially costly decision-making process surrounding possible treatment alternatives" (Carroll et al., 2000, p. 286; Slade, Emery, & Lieberman, 1997; Thomas & Rausch, 2002). Couples report that they often have difficulty accessing current information about treatment options and reliable statistics that provide essential information on the probabilities of a successful outcome (Daniluk, 2001).

A study examining the emotional impact of infertility-related stress found that men and women in couples who had equal levels of social infertility stress reported higher levels of marital adjustment compared to those couples experiencing more dissonance. Couples who reported similar needs for parenthood also had significantly higher levels of marital satisfaction. Incongruence in stress and the need to become a parent was significantly associated with depression in women but not men (Peterson et al., 2003). Incongruence has also been identified in the desire for twin gestations in individuals who are a part of an infertile couple (Kalra, Milad, Klock, & Grobman, 2003).

Richly descriptive data were generated from a Canadian qualitative study of infertile couples who had undergone diagnosis and treatment for a mean of 5 years (Daniluk, 2001). The first theme as treatment was initiated was "the beginning: It's only a matter of time." One study participant said,

> I'm not a control freak but it's one area of my life that I thought I'd always have control over. You know, I was on the pill for 5 years before we started trying to have a baby . . . 5 years when I thought I was in control of my fertility. When I didn't get pregnant it came as quite a shock. (p. 125)

The second theme described being in the middle of infertility treatment, "Work hard enough and you'll get what you want," demonstrated by the following comment (Daniluk, 2001):

> They were very optimistic. . . . The numbers that they quote are often very high so you leave thinking, "Well, I'm gonna be the whatever, the 15% to 25%" . . . so it's always an upbeat sort of thing and you leave thinking, "Yes, this is gonna work, this is gonna be the month." And it doesn't happen. (p. 125)

The final theme at the culmination of infertility treatment, "When enough is enough," was expressed as follows (Daniluk, 2001):

> We used to talk about being like the guinea pig on the wheel in the cage. Once you get on, how do you get off? Every move you make you go faster and the wheel doesn't end. Eventually you have to find a way of just jumping off in midflight to stop it. (p. 128)

Infertile women who become pregnant with the help of ART often have to make heartbreaking decisions about multifetal reduction (MFR). Collopy (2004) identified themes including the presence of infertility as a barrier to contemplating hyperfertility, multiple-birth pregnancy as another form of loss for infertile women, and the lasting effects for having made the decision. These women felt such a sense of irony because they had been desperate to conceive and now were making a decision about destroying a life. They described feelings of desperation that the risks of multiple implantations did not "sink in." A similar study on 11 couples who elected to undergo MFR after infertility treatment found that moral and ethical dilemmas were the most difficult aspect of their experience (Maifield, Hahn, Titler, & Mullen, 2003).

The circumstance of infertile couples who become pregnant after infertility treatment only to experience fetal loss is particularly poignant and has been documented by Freda and Semelsberger (2003, p. ix) in interviews with women who had this experience. Themes included "back to square one," "a struggle between hope and hopelessness," and "running out of time." One woman said,

> We'd been through so much already, so much disappointment, so much crying and pain just to become pregnant. Then the miscarriage. It was the most heart-wrenching experience I've ever been through. But the most frustrating part for me is that we can't be like normal couples who can just go to bed one night and start to conceive another baby. Why them and not us? I might never get pregnant again. (p. ix)

Another woman described her experience of perinatal loss after infertility (National Infertility Association, 2004d):

> My dear husband and I have faced reoccurring miscarriages that have been so overwhelming. We have no children and now

no hopes or dreams. I wish I could have this weight off my shoulder. We feel like we constantly live in rainy days and are just waiting for the sun to shine.

Susannah experienced perinatal loss at 14 weeks and described how she felt when an ultrasound confirmed the loss:

The room was absolutely silent. We were in shock. Minutes before we were going to have a baby. All of a sudden, here we were in a darkened room, not understanding what had just happened or what we should do next. I can't remember ever hurting as bad as I did that day. The pain I felt was so intense that it still brings back very strong emotions when I think about it. Greg and I laid in our bed and cried together. All I could think about was, "Why? Why me? Why us?" I couldn't stop the tears from flowing. Even after I thought surely there couldn't be another tear in my body, there were still many. One minute I felt I must have done something wrong, and the next I just felt like I was broken and unworthy of my husband. Why was it that teenagers and drug addicts are able to get pregnant so easily, but I wasn't? Did I not deserve to be a mother?

SOCIAL SUPPORT AND INFERTILITY

Social support is one of the most significant variables buffering adjustment to fertility diagnosis, moderating stress (Amir, Horesh, & Lin-Stein, 1999). Boivin, Scanlan, and Walker (1999) reported that infertile individuals relied on their significant other and extended family members when they were distressed. Other researchers have reported that social support results in greater marital satisfaction and quality, sexual satisfaction, enhanced feelings of self-worth, and psychological well-being. Social support mediates interpersonal conflict, stress, and feelings of loneliness (Abbey, Andrews, & Halman, 1995; Amir et al., 1999; Boivin et al., 1999; Jirka, Schuett, & Foxall, 1996). Social support makes a difference for infertile couples, as evidenced by the story of Donna and Joseph, who underwent numerous infertility treatments including surgery and suffered a miscarriage (American Infertility Association & Organon Pharmaceuticals, 2004b):

Throughout their struggle, Donna and Joseph talked about things openly, allowing friends and family to offer words and prayers of support. "You feel it when everyone really wants it for you and prays for you," Donna said, "It kept us positive that it was going to happen."

Donna did become pregnant and gave birth to a daughter. Sixty people attended a baby shower, a celebration of the couple's 4-year struggle.

An electronic support group for infertile couples is proving to be a helpful coping strategy (Epstein, Rosenberg, Grant, & Hemenway, 2002). Benefits of participation identified in a survey of 589 participants in Internet support groups sponsored by a nonprofit international infertility organization included education, empowerment, and the diminishment of feelings of depression. This forum can also be inappropriately used for escape avoidance, however. The American Fertility Organization (2004) offers an online discussion group, and quality Web sites that provide information and support for infertile couples are summarized in Table 6.3. For example, one Web site offers an infertility support group, surrogacy support group, and an adoption support group (Society for Assisted Reproductive Technology, 2004). Chat groups are found on the RESOLVE Web site, with topics such as "Survival Strategies: Balancing Infertility, Marriage, and Life," "Unexplained Infertility," and "Shared Risks" (National Infertility

Table 6.3   Infertility Web Sites

Web Site	Organization
http://www.advancedfertility.com	Advanced Fertility Center of Chicago
http://www.theafa.org	American Fertility Association
http://www.asrm.com	American Society for Reproductive Medicine
http://www.focusonfertility.org	Focus on Fertility
http://www.inciid.org	International Council on Infertility Information Dissemination
http://www.child.org.uk	National Infertility Support Network (CHILD)
http://www.fertilityplus.org	Fertility Plus
http://www.resolve.org	RESOLVE: National Infertility Association
http://www.sart.org	Society for Assisted Reproductive Technology
http://www.4woman.gov	U.S. Department of Health and Human Services Office on Women's Health

Table 6.4   Breaking the Cycle of Stress

Find a support group.

Seek professional emotional help, including couples therapy.

Investigate complementary therapies.

Pamper yourself.

Keep a journal.

Take a "vacation" from treatment.

Reconnect with your partner.

Maintain healthy habits, including diet and exercise.

SOURCE: Adapted from the American Fertility Association (2004), the American Society of Reproductive Medicine (http://www.asrm.org), Bashford (1999), Focus on Fertility (http://www.focusonfertility.org), Hsu and Kuo (2002), Johnson (1996), Lukse and Vacc (1999); and Sherrod (2004).

Association, 2004e). It should be noted that only 2% of 197 infertility-related Web sites met the standards for quality and accountability (Okamura, Bernstein, & Fidler, 2002).

Infertile couples who wanted to adopt a child but instead enrolled in a program preparing them to be foster parents were found to differ in their responses to the program from couples with children. Infertile couples had feelings of a deep emotional loss resulting from their inability to have a child (Bevc, Jerman, Ovsenik, & Ovsenik, 2003). Suggested coping strategies on the American Fertility Association and the Focus on Fertility Web sites are summarized in Table 6.4.

IMPLICATIONS FOR CLINICAL PRACTICE

The importance of psychosocial support and interventions by health care providers for infertile couples cannot be overemphasized. It should be implemented in conjunction with ART counseling. As expressed by Stotland (2002), infertility and ART involve

Table 6.5   Signs Indicating Counseling Is Needed

Persistent feelings of sadness, guilt, or worthlessness

Social isolation

Loss of interest in usual activities and relationships

Depression

Agitation and anxiety

Increased mood swings

Constant preoccupation with infertility

Marital discord

Difficulty concentrating and remembering

Increased use of alcohol and drugs

Change in appetite, weight, or sleep patterns

Thoughts about suicide or death

Difficulty with scheduled intercourse

SOURCE: Adapted from the American Society for Reproductive Medicine (http://www.asrm.org).

the most intimate body parts and the most poignant hopes and profound disappointments. Issues include reactions to the infertility diagnosis, gender differences in stress and coping, and parenting following successful ART (Schmidt, Holstein, Boivin, Sangren, et al., 2003; Schmidt, Holstein, Boivin, Tjorhnhoj-Thomsen, et al., 2003).

Brucker and McKenry (2004) examined the relationship between support from health care providers (HCPs) and psychological adjustment in 120 men and women experiencing infertility. For women, perceived support from HCPs did not predict levels of stress, depression, or anxiety. For men, greater levels of perceived support from HCPs predicted lower levels of stress and anxiety. HCPs have the opportunity to provide needed support not only to assist in conception but also to assist in better psychological adjustment to the infertility diagnosis. Signs that suggest the need for professional counseling for those who are infertile are summarized in Table 6.5 (American Society for Reproductive Medicine, 2004b).

Savitz-Smith (2003) summarized the literature on counseling infertile couples. Types of counseling include implications, support,

and therapeutic. Implications counseling explores with people how any proposed treatment would affect them, their family, and any child born as a result of treatment. Support counseling provides emotional support at any time before, during, or after treatment. Therapeutic counseling focuses on the effects, consequences, and resolution of treatment and infertility (Bagshawe & Taylor, 2003). Sherrod (2004) identified the recommendations for clinical practice with infertile couples listed in Table 6.6. Providing opportunities for couples to share their perceptions and reflect on the meaning of their experiences is essential (Daniluk, 2001).

RESEARCH RECOMMENDATIONS

Studies with larger sample sizes should be performed. Prospective longitudinal studies that differentiate those with different infertility diagnoses would be appropriate. Research on study participants who have received extensive infertility treatment and those who have discontinued treatment is recommended. More data are needed on the infertility experience in different cultural and

Table 6.6   Counseling Infertile Couples

Awareness/advice: Do not speak inappropriately or uninformed about infertility. Do not perpetuate false hopes. Present a realistic picture of treatment options and their success rates. Do not offer advice unless it is asked for. A listening ear may be the most effective intervention. Remember that adoption is expensive, complicated, and lengthy and may not meet the needs of an individual or couple to have a biological child.

Blame/balance: Remember that infertility affects couples, not just individuals. The causes of infertility are varied, but in a majority of cases a couple has done nothing "wrong." Help couples financially by being accurate in all charges for various procedures and providing information on insurance coverage and other potential ways that treatment may be paid for. Help couples establish a balance regarding each partner's limits in the process of trying to conceive (Hart, 2002). Do not assume that the male partner does not care. Although there are gender differences in emotional responses, both partners "feel" the experience (Busch, 2001; Gibson & Myers, 2000; Hart, 2002).

Competence/compassion: Remember that procedures are painful. Respond with sensitivity. Welcome and encourage the woman's partner who can offer support during procedures. Reduce the couple's anxiety and pain as you prepare for procedures. Refer the couple to local support groups, such as RESOLVE (Bashford, 1999). Help couples find ways to relieve their stress, including taking a break from infertility treatment (Sherrod, 2004).

---

ethnic groups. Research on those who are voluntarily childless and have had either a vasectomy or tubal ligation but now desire to have a child is important. Issues related to couples who experience secondary infertility after successfully bearing children are another potential area of research that should be explored. Outcomes evaluation of psychosocial interventions with infertile couples is recommended.

Reflecting on her experiences with infertility, the perinatal loss of three unborn children, and the removal of a ruptured fallopian tube because of a tubal pregnancy, Susannah said,

> My only hope comes from knowing that I still have the ability to perhaps have a baby. It is not guaranteed, and I have been trying to prepare myself for the possibility that it may never happen in this life. I think I am still in the stage where I believe we will be counted in the group of couples who are able to conceive with treatment. It is too painful to think about the other outcome.

REFERENCES

Abbey, A., Andrews, F. M., & Halman, L. J. (1995). Provision and receipt of social support and disregard: What is their impact on the marital life quality of infertile and fertile couples? *Journal of Personality and Social Psychology, 68*(3), 455-469.

Adashi, E. Y., Cohen, J., & Hamberger, L. (2000). Public perception on infertility and its treatment: An international survey. *Human Reproduction, 15,* 330-334.

American Fertility Association. (2004). *Considering treatment: Infertility risk assessment.* Retrieved February 15, 2005, from http://www.americaninfertility.org

American Infertility Association & Organon Pharmaceuticals. (2004a). *Breaking the cycle of stress and sadness.* Retrieved October 23, 2004, from http://www.focusonfertility.org/cope_sadstress.htm

American Infertility Association & Organon Pharmaceuticals. (2004b). *Real life stories: Dreams do come true.* Retrieved October 23, 2004, from http://www.focusonfertility.org/cope_reallifestory.htm

American Society for Reproductive Medicine. (1998). *Fact sheet: In vitro fertilization.* Birmingham, AL: Author.

American Society for Reproductive Medicine. (2004a). *Fertility and sterility.* Retrieved February 15, 2005, from http://asrm.org

American Society for Reproductive Medicine. (2004b). *Infertility: An overview.* Retrieved February 15, 2005, from http://asrm.org

Amir, M., Horesh, N., & Lin-Stein, T. (1999). Infertility and adjustment in women: The effects of attachment style and social support. *Journal of Clinical Psychology in Medical Settings, 6*(4), 463-479.

Anderson, K. M., Sharpe, M., Rattray, A., & Irvine, D. S. (2003). Distress and concerns in couples referred to a specialist infertility clinic. *Journal of Psychosomatic Research, 54*(4), 353-355.

Angard, N. T. (1999). Diagnosis infertility: Karen and Matthew. *Association of Women's Health, Obstetric, and Neonatal Nursing Lifelines, 3*(3), 22-29.

Araoye, M. O. (2003). Epidemiology of infertility: Social problems of the infertile couples. *Western African Journal of Medicine, 22*(2), 190-196.

Bagshawe, A., & Taylor, A. (2003). ABC's of subfertility counseling. *British Medical Journal, 327,* 1038-1040.

Barber, D. (2000). A fertile field. *Nursing Standard, 14*(26), 77-78.

Bashford, R. A. (1999). Psychological aspects of infertility. *Clinical Nurse Specialist Spectrum, 4*(4), 62-72.

Bevc, V., Jerman, J., Ovsenik, R., & Ovsenik, M. (2003). Experiencing infertility—Social work dilemmas in child adoption procedures. *Collegium Antropologicum, 27*(2), 445-460.

Boivin, J., Scanlan, L. C., & Walker, S. M. (1999). Why are infertile patients not using psychosocial counseling? *Human Reproduction, 14*(5), 1384-1391.

Brown, C. J. (2002). Managing treatment failures: A patient's view. *Human Fertility: Journal of the British Fertility Society, 5*(4), 199-202.

Brucker, P. S., & McKenry, P. C. (2004). Support from health care providers and the psychological adjustment of individuals experiencing infertility. *Journal of Obstetric, Gynecologic, and Neonatal Nursing, 33*(5), 597-603.

Busch, S. (2001). Chasing a miracle: Why infertile women continue to stay in treatment. *Association of Black Nursing Faculty Journal, 12,* 116-123.

Callister, L. C., Semenic, S., & Foster, J. C. (1999). Cultural and spiritual meanings of childbirth: Orthodox Jewish and Mormon women. *Journal of Holistic Nursing, 17*(3), 280-295.

Cardin, N. B. (1999). *Tears of sorrow, seeds of hope.* Woodstock, VT: Jewish Lights.

Carroll, J. S., Robinson, W. D., Marshall, E. S., Callister, L. C., Olsen, S. F., Dyches, T. T., et al. (2000). The family crucibles of illness, disability, death, and other losses. In D. C. Dollahite (Ed.), *Strengthening our families* (pp. 278-292). Salt Lake City, UT: Bookcraft.

Centers for Disease Control and Prevention. (2001). *Assisted reproductive technology success rates: 2001.* Retrieved October 23, 2004, from http://www.cdc.gov/reproductivehealth/ART01/nation.htm

Chang, S. Y., & Kuo, B. J. (2000). Psychosocial responses among couples undergoing first time and repeat cycles of IVF-ET treatment. *Nursing Research (Taiwan), 8,* 190-201.

Christensen, J. M. (1996). I yearned for a baby. *Ensign, 27*(8), 52-53.

Collopy, K. S. (2004). "I couldn't think that far": Infertile women's decision making about multifetal reduction. *Research in Nursing and Health, 27,* 75-86.

Daniluk, J. C. (2001). "If we had it to do over again. . . . " Couples' reflections on their experiences of infertility treatments. *Family Journal: Counseling and Therapy for Couples and Families, 9*(2), 122-133.

Dhaliwal, L. K., Gupta, K. R., Gopalan, S., & Kulhara, P. (2004). Psychological aspects of infertility due to various causes—A prospective study. *International Journal of Fertility and Women's Medicine, 49*(1), 44-48.

Domar, A. D., & Kelly, A. L. (2002). *Conquering infertility.* New York: Penguin.

Engel, G .L. (1977). The need for a new medical model: A challenge for biomedicine. *Science, 196,* 129-136.

Engel, G. L. (1980). The clinical application of the biopsychosocial model. *American Journal of Psychiatry, 137*(5), 535-544.

Epstein, Y. M., Rosenberg, H. S., Grant, T. V., & Hemenway, B. A. N. (2002). Use of the Internet as the only outlet for talking about infertility. *Fertility and Sterility, 78*(3), 507-514.

Eugster, A., & Vingerhoets, A. J. J. (1999). Psychological aspects of in-vitro fertilization: A review. *Social Science and Medicine, 48,* 575-589.

Folkman, S., Lazarus, R. S., Dunkel-Schetter, C., DeLongis, A., & Gruen, R. (1986). The dynamics of a stressful encounter: Cognitive appraisal, coping, and encounter outcomes. *Journal of Personality Sociology and Psychology, 50,* 992-1003.

Freda, M. C., & Semelsberger, C. F. (2003). *Miscarriage after infertility.* Minneapolis, MN: Fairview Press.

Gibson, D. M., & Myers, J. E. (2000). Gender and infertility: A relational approach to counseling women. *Journal of Counseling and Development, 4,* 400-410.

Gonzales, L. O. (2000). Infertility as a transformational process: A framework for psychotherapeutic support of infertile women. *Issues in Mental Health Nursing, 21,* 619-633.

Halman, L. J., Andrews, F. M., & Abbey, A. (1993). Gender differences and perceptions about childbearing among infertile couples. *Journal of Obstetric, Gynecologic, and Neonatal Nursing, 23*(7), 593-600.

Hart, V. A. (2002). Infertility and the role of psychotherapy. *Issues in Mental Health Nursing, 23*(11), 31-41.

Hidalgo, M. P., Caleffi, L., Baron, A., Mattana, E., & Chaves, M. L. (2004). Cohesion and adaptability among individuals under treatment for infertility. *Psychological Reports, 94*(1), 55-65.

Hsu, Y., & Kuo, B. (2002). Evaluations of emotional reactions and coping behaviors as well as correlated factors for infertile couples receiving assisted reproductive technologies. *Journal of Nursing Research, 10*(4), 291-302.

Imeson, M., & McMurray, A. (1996). Couples' experiences of infertility: A phenomenological study. *Journal of Advanced Nursing, 24,* 1014-1022.

Jenkins, J., & Corrigan, L. (2004). Current thinking on management of infertility. *Clinical Pulse, 5,* 20-23.

Jirka, J., Schuett, S., & Foxall, M. J. (1996). Loneliness and social support in infertile couples. *Journal of Obstetric, Gynecologic, and Neonatal Nursing, 25*(1), 55-60.

Johnson, C. L. (1996). Regaining self-esteem: Strategies and interventions for the infertile woman. *Journal of Obstetric, Gynecologic, and Neonatal Nursing, 25,* 291-295.

Johnston, G. P. (1994). *The wish, the wait, the wonder.* New York: HarperCollins.

Jordan, C., & Revenson, T. A. (1999). Gender differences in coping with infertility: A meta-analysis. *Journal of Behavioral Medicine, 22*(4), 341-358.

Juo, B. J., Lee, S. H., Wang, Y. M., & Lee, M. S. (1998). Association of traditional attitudes toward childbirth and grief responses among infertile couples. *Chung Shan Medical Journal, 9,* 89-99.

Kalra, S. K., Milad, M. P., Klock, S. C., & Grobman, M. A. (2003). Infertility patients and their partners: Differences in the desire for twin gestation. *Obstetrics and Gynecology, 102,* 152-155.

Kartchner, R., & Callister, L. C. (2003). Giving birth: Voices of Chinese women. *Journal of Holistic Nursing, 21*(2), 100-116.

Kerr, J., Balen, A., & Brown, C. (1999). The experiences of couples in the United Kingdom who have had infertility treatment. *Human Reproduction, 14,* 934-938.

Khalaf, I., & Callister, L. C. (1997). Cultural meanings of childbirth: Muslim women living in Jordan. *Holistic Nursing, 15*(4), 373-388.

Kirkman, M., & Rosenthal, D. (1999). Representations of reproductive technology in women's narratives of infertility. *Women and Health, 29*(2), 17-36.

Langdrige, D., Connolly, K., & Sheeran, P. (2000). Reasons for wanting a child: A network analytic study. *Journal of Reproductive and Infant Psychology, 18*(4), 321-338.

Lazarus, R. S., & Folkman, S. (1984). *Stress, coping and appraisal.* New York: Springer.

Lee, S. H., & Kuo, B. J. (2000). Chinese traditional childbearing attitudes and infertile couples in Taiwan. *Image: The Journal of Nursing Scholarship, 32,* 54.

Lee, T. Y., Chang, S. P., & Chen, C. C. (1997). The comparison of distress, stress, and coping strategies on infertile couples. *Nursing Research (Taiwan), 5*(5), 425-438.

Lee, T. Y., & Chin, G. C. (1996). The perceived stressors for infertile women in one medical center in southern Taiwan. *Nursing Research (Taiwan), 4*(2), 186-193.

Lee, T .Y., & Sun, G. H. (2000). Psychosocial response of Chinese infertile husbands and wives. *Archives of Andrology, 45*(3), 149-154.

Lee, T. Y., Sun, G. H., & Chao, S. C. (2000). The effect of an infertility diagnosis on the distress, marital and sexual satisfaction between husbands and wives. *Human Reproduction, 16*(8), 1762-1767.

Lee, T. Y., Sun, G. H., Chao, S. C., & Chen, C. C. (2001). Development of the coping scale for infertile couples. *Archives of Andrology, 45*(3), 149-154.

Leiblum, S. R., Aviv, A., & Hamer, R. (1997). Life after infertility treatment: A long term investigation of marital and sexual function. *Human Reproduction, 13*(12), 3569-3574.

Lukse, M. P., & Vacc, N. A. (1999). Grief, depression, and coping in women undergoing infertility treatment. *Obstetrics and Gynecology, 9*(2), 245-251.

Maifield, M., Hahn, S., Titler, M. G., & Mullen, M. (2003). Decision making regarding multifetal reduction. *Journal of Obstetric, Gynecologic, and Neonatal Nursing, 32*(3), 357-369.

Merari, D., Cherit, A., & Modan, B. (2002). Emotional reactions and attitudes prior to in vitro fertilization: An interspouse study. *Psychology and Health, 17*(5), 629-640.

Mulrine, A. (2004, September 27). Miracle babies: How science is helping childless couples beat the odds. *U.S. News and World Report,* 60-67.

National Infertility Association. (2004a). *Secondary infertility*. Retrieved February 15, 2005, from http://www.resolve.org/main/national/treatment/diagnosis/2nd infertility.jsp

National Infertility Association. (2004b). *Hidden no more: The hidden aspects of infertility*. Retrieved February 15, 2005, from http://www.resolve.org/main/national/trying/whatis/hidden.jsp

National Infertility Association. (2004c). *Managing family and friends*. Retrieved February 15, 2005, from http://www.resolve.org/main/national/coping/talk/family/family.jsp

National Infertility Association. (2004d). Retrieved February 15, 2005, from http://www.resolve.org

National Infertility Association. (2004e). Retrieved October 23, 2004, from http://www.resolve.org

Okamura, K., Bernstein, J., & Fidler, A. T. (2002). Assessing the quality of infertility resources on the World Wide Web: Tools to guide clients through the maze of fact and fiction. *Journal of Midwifery and Women's Health, 47*(4), 264-268.

Peterson, B. D., Newton, C. R., & Rosen, K. H. (2003). Examining congruence between partners' perceived infertility-related stress and its relationship to marital adjustment. *Family Process, 42*(1), 59-70.

Petok, W. D. (2004). *Male infertility: Family building magazine*. Retrieved October 23, 2004, from http://www.resolve.org

Phipps, S. A. (1993). A phenomenological study of couples' infertility: Gender influence. *Holistic Nurse Practitioner, 7*(2), 44-56.

Reed, S. A. (2001). Medical and psychological aspects of infertility and assisted reproductive technology for primary health care providers. *Military Medicine, 166*, 1018-1026.

Resolve: The National Infertility Association. (2004). *Infertility myths and facts*. Retrieved October 23, 2004, from http://www.resolve.org/main/national/coping/demystify/mythfact.jsp

Rutter, M. (1996, Spring). Families without children. *This People, 38*, 41, 43, 45-46, 49, 51.

Savitz-Smith, J. (2003). Couples undergoing infertility treatment: Implications for counselors. *Family Journal, 11*(4), 383-387.

Schmidt, L., Holstein, B. E., Boivin, J., Tjorhnhoj-Thomsen, T., Balaabjerg, J., Hald, F., et al. (2003a). High ratings of satisfaction with infertility treatment are common: Findings from the Copenhagen Multi-Centre Psychosocial Infertility Research Programme. *Human Reproduction, 18*(12), 2638-2646.

Schmidt, L., Holstein, B. E., Boivin, J., Sangren, H., Tjornhoj-Thomsen, T., Blaabjerg, J., Hald, F., et al. (2003b). Patients' attitudes to medical and psychosocial aspects of care in fertility clinics. *Human Reproduction, 18*(3), 628-637.

Semenic, S., Callister, L .C., & Feldman, P. (2004). Giving birth: The voices of Orthodox Jewish women living in Canada. *Journal of Obstetric, Gynecologic, and Neonatal Nursing, 33*(1), 80-87.

Sherrod, R. A. (2004). Understanding the emotional aspects of infertility. *Journal of Psychosocial Nursing, 42*(3), 40-47.

Slade, P., Emery, J., & Lieberman, B. A. (1997). A prospective longitudinal study of emotions and relationships in in-vitro fertilization treatment. *Human Reproduction, 12*, 183-190.

Society for Assisted Reproductive Technology. (2004). *ASRM patient fact sheet.* Retrieved February 15, 2005, from http://www.sart.org

St. Hill, P., Lipson, J. G., & Meleis, A. I. (2003). *Caring for women cross-culturally.* Philadelphia: F. A. Davis.

Stotland, N. L. (2002). Psychiatric issues related to infertility, reproductive technologies, and abortions. *Primary Care: Clinics in Office Practice, 29*(1), 13-26.

Thomas, V., & Rausch, D. T. (2002). Evaluating psychosocial factors and psychological reactions to infertility treatment. *Journal of Couple Relationship Therapy, 1*(2), 33-49.

U.S. Department of Health and Human Services (2004). *Fertility awareness and infertility.* Retrieved February 15, 2005, from http://www.4woman.gov

Wiczyk, H. (2000). Infertility: A modern workup. *Female Patients, 25*(8), 72-78.

Zimmerman, S. (1992). Would I ever be a mother? *Ensign, 23,* 27-28.

CHAPTER 7

Eating Disorders and the Family

A Biopsychosocial Perspective

MARGO D. MAINE

Eating disorders are more common than many other serious and debilitating illnesses, such as schizophrenia and Alzheimer's disease, but receive much less attention in the health care system and far less money for research, treatment, and prevention. It is estimated that 5 million people in the United States suffer from eating disorders, whereas Alzheimer's disease afflicts 4.5 million and schizophrenia 2.2 million (Powers & Bannon, 2004). Once considered to be characteristic of upwardly mobile, Caucasian adolescent females in technologically advanced nations such as the United States and Western Europe, today the effects of rapid globalization have made eating disorders a worldwide condition. Appearing in every economic, racial, and ethnic stratum of U.S. culture and in at least 40 countries worldwide, clinical eating disorders, body image despair, severe dieting, and weight preoccupation are no longer restricted to certain high-risk groups in limited geographic localities. This growing list includes places as unlikely as Nigeria, India, China, South Korea, South Africa, the former Soviet Union, and Mexico (Gordon, 2001).

Descriptions of eating disorders have been part of the psychiatric literature for centuries; eating too much, too little, or not at all and various forms of purging have long been a means for expression of pain or protest. Since the earliest detailed writings, the family has been considered an important variable in the development and progression of these conditions (Agras et al., 2004). Today, clinical eating disorders, pathogenic weight control, and body image concerns are of epidemic proportion, especially in young women. In light of the number of lives and families affected by these serious conditions, understanding the role of the family in the illness and recovery process, informed by a biopsychosocial perspective, is critical.

FACTS ABOUT EATING DISORDERS

Ninety percent of those suffering anorexia nervosa or bulimia nervosa are women. The American Psychiatric Association (2000) estimates that between 0.5% and 3.7% of young women in the United States will have

Table 7.1   Diagnostic Criteria for Eating Disorders

Anorexia nervosa

Refusal to maintain body weight at or above a minimally normal weight for height and age
Weight loss to 85% of the expected body weight for height and age or failure to gain weight during growth period resulting in weight less than 85% of expected
Intense fear of gaining weight despite being underweight
Disturbance in how weight and shape are experienced and undue influence of weight and shape on self-evaluation
Denial of seriousness of low weight
Amenorrhea (missed three or more cycles or only has period when receiving hormonal treatment)
    Types: Restricting or Binge Eating-Purging

Bulimia nervosa

Recurrent periods of binge eating (eating an abnormally large amount of food in a discrete period of time and feeling unable to stop or to control the amount eaten)
Recurrent inappropriate compensatory behavior to avoid weight gain, such as self-induced vomiting; misuse of laxatives, diuretics, enemas, or other medications; fasting; excessive exercise
Binge-purge cycles occurring, on average, twice a week for 3 months or longer
Self-evaluation unduly influenced by weight and shape
Behavior does not occur exclusively in periods of anorexia nervosa
    Types: Purging (uses self-induced vomiting or laxatives, diuretics, and enemas) or
    Non-Purging (uses other compensatory behaviors, such as fasting or exercise)

Eating Disorder Not Otherwise Specified

Atypical anorexia: key signs of anorexia present but does not meet all criteria (still menstruates or has not had significant weight loss)
Atypical bulimia: all criteria met except frequency or duration of symptoms
Use of inappropriate compensatory behaviors after eating normal amounts of food
Binge eating disorder: recurrent binging without purging, repeatedly chewing and spitting out food without swallowing

anorexia nervosa in their lifetime, and between 1.1% and 4.2% will have bulimia nervosa. At least one third of those treated in eating disorder clinics are diagnosed as Eating Disorder Not Otherwise Specified (EDNOS), sharing some but not all the features of these diagnoses (Patrick, 2002). Less data are available on these cases, despite their prevalence. Table 7.1 provides the diagnostic criteria (American Psychiatric Association, 1994).

Among psychiatric conditions, anorexia nervosa has the highest morbidity, with an estimated 10% mortality rate at 10 years of symptom duration (Sullivan, 2002) and 20% at 20-year follow-up (American Psychiatric Association, 2000). Anorexia is the leading cause of death for young women aged 15 to 24 years, with a general mortality rate 12 times the expected rate and a suicide rate

75 times greater (Sullivan, 1995). Less is known about the mortality associated with bulimia nervosa due to both the potential long-lasting medical consequences and diagnostic limitations. For example, as many as half of those with anorexia will develop bulimic symptoms but still be diagnosed with anorexia (Patrick, 2002). Even less is known about those diagnosed as EDNOS, although their symptoms, treatment needs, and outcome may be just as serious. The incidence of eating disorders in males has increased; in fact, the number of males with bulimia nervosa now surpasses the number of females with anorexia nervosa (Powers & Spratt, 1994). Males also account for 25% of the cases of binge eating disorder, a provisional diagnosis in the *Diagnostic and Statistical Manual of Mental Disorders* of the American

Psychiatric Association (American Psychiatric Association, 1994). Also of concern, the age of incidence has expanded to younger children (American Academy of Pediatrics, 2003) and to adults.

SUBCLINICAL EATING DISORDERS

Subclinical eating disorders are an additional health issue impacting families today. This term is used to describe those who may be symptomatic sporadically or whose symptoms do not quite meet the criteria for a full-blown clinical eating disorder, although some may later progress to full syndrome eating disorders (Shisslak, Crago, & Estes, 1995).

Although estimates of the incidence of subclinical eating disorders are inconsistent, two comprehensive studies provide compelling data regarding the common use of pathogenic weight control techniques in teenagers, whose bodies are still developing and growing. A study of more than 80,000 9th and 12th graders in the United States revealed that 56% of 9th-grade females and 28% of males are engaged in unsafe dieting practices, including skipping meals, ingesting diet pills or laxatives, inducing vomiting, smoking cigarettes (for the purpose of affecting their weight and food intake), and binge eating. Among 12th graders, 57% of females and 31% of males practice dangerous dieting, with Hispanic and Native American students reporting the highest rates. Research indicates that positive self-esteem, emotional well-being, school achievement, and family connectedness serve to protect teens from these dangerous dieting behaviors (Croll, Neumark-Sztainer, Story, & Ireland, 2002).

The Centers for Disease Control and Prevention (CDC) reports epidemic rates of weight loss attempts in high school students. In its extensive study of teenage diet-related behaviors, the CDC reports that 46% are trying to lose weight, 44% are actively dieting, and 60% are exercising to lose or avoid gaining weight. The breakdown by gender shows that although both sexes are troubled by weight concerns, girls are engaging in dangerous dieting much more than boys (CDC, 2002).

Subclinical eating disorders appear to be as endemic among adult women as they are among teens and young adults. Although hard data on adult eating disorders are absent, there is compelling information about the extent of dieting and body image concerns, both of which are precursors to clinical eating disorders. For example,

- Forty-three million adult women in the United States are dieting to lose weight at any given time; another 26 million are dieting to maintain their weight (Gaesser, 2002)
- Body image dissatisfaction in midlife has increased dramatically, more than doubling from 25% in 1972 to 56% in 1997 (Garner, 1997)
- Comparable levels of dieting and disordered eating are found across young and elderly age groups (Hetherington & Burnett, 1994)
- When asked what bothered them most about their bodies, a group of women aged 61 to 92 years identified weight as their greatest concern (Clarke, 2002)
- A major research project found that more than 20% of the women aged 70 or older were dieting, even though higher weight poses a very low risk for death at that age, and weight loss may actually be harmful (Berg, 2001)
- In 2003, one third of inpatient admissions to a specialized treatment center for eating disorders were older than age 30 years (W. Davis, personal communication, 2004)
- Sixty percent of adult women have engaged in pathogenic weight control, 40% are restrained eaters, 40% are overeaters, only 20% are instinctive eaters, 50% say their eating is devoid of pleasure and causes them to feel guilty, and 90% worry about their weight (Waterhouse, 1997)

Far less research is available on the prevalence of subclinical eating disorders among adult men, but the problem appears to be growing (Eliot & Baker, 2001; Hoerr, Bokram, Lugo, Bivins, & Keast, 2002; O'Dea & Abraham, 2002).

With adults of all ages experiencing such conflicts about their weight, shape, appearance, and appetite, creating a family environment resistant to eating disorders may be an elusive goal.

CULTURE-BOUND ILLNESSES

The increased prevalence of eating disorders in recent decades and the changing incidence patterns suggest the limitations of a medical model and the importance of a biopsychosocial framework to understand their origins and solutions. These illnesses appear in technologically advanced, Westernized nations and in those that are rapidly changing due to the impact of globalization. Although social changes always create stress, those associated with globalization may impact women disproportionately, increasing the risk for body image and eating problems. Culturally transformative trends, such as sophisticated and fast-growing economies and rapid technological and market changes, exert an enormous effect on the status of women, introducing a powerful global consumer culture, with expectations about appearance and beauty as well as dramatic revisions in women's social role (Gordon, 2001).

With greater access to education, increased involvement in the workplace, and the accompanying gender equity issues, women's lives and family roles are in a period of unprecedented transformation. In addition, the significant differences in today's Western diet, filled with prepared foods higher in calories and fat, and the sedentary lifestyle of the West are factors that have led to an increase in obesity. The body reality and the beauty ideal are in conflict, raising a myriad of issues for women of all ages (Gordon, 2001).

The fast-paced life inherent in current postmodern culture emphasizes adaptation, achievement, and appearance, leaving little time to reflect on these new roles and expectations. Instead of identifying, verbalizing, or describing their complex emotions, needs, and appetites, contemporary women are taught to translate these into the language of fat. Given little permission for negative feelings, and surrounded by a sociocultural environment that has labeled fat as bad, "feeling fat" is now the cover for all discomfort, anger, disappointment, and other "bad" feelings (Friedman, 1997). Unfortunately, globalization has made the language of fat universal for women.

A dramatic example of the impact of globalization and media images on attitudes and behaviors regarding food and women's bodies occurred in Fiji after television was introduced. With startling speed, strong Fijian traditions and values were overturned, and women adopted the language of fat. Historically, this island culture had valued large female bodies for their strength and contribution to the family and community life and had celebrated and enjoyed food long associated with rich traditions and meanings. Eating disorders were basically nonexistent there in 1995, but after less than 3 years of limited exposure to Western network television, they were rampant. Whereas there was little talk about dieting or weight in 1995, by 1998 11% used self-induced vomiting, 29% were at risk for eating disorders, 69% had dieted to lose weight, and 74% felt "too fat" (Becker, 2002).

The Fiji experience demonstrates the importance of sociocultural influences in the factors that contribute to eating disorders. These are truly culture-bound, biopsychosocial illnesses.

BIOGENETIC CONTRIBUTIONS

Although specialists agree that eating disorders seem to run in families, the explanations for this differ. According to a review of genetic studies, the lifetime risk to develop an eating disorder is 6% for those who have a first-degree relative who has suffered from them. The risk is only 1% for those without this shared familial background (Gorwood, Bouvard, Mouren-Simeoni, Kipman, & Ades, 1998). Although some theorists and researchers believe this points to a significant genetic loading for eating disorders, the susceptibility to eating disorders surpasses sheer genetic influences. Even those writing about the genetic contributions to eating disorders state that "genetics loads the gun. The environment pulls the trigger" (Bulik, 2004).

Although the research on the genetic contributions to eating disorders is in infancy, consensus is that genetics most likely impose indirect effects, creating a vulnerability to eating disorders. Personality characteristics, such as perfectionism, obsessionality, anxiety, sensitivity to criticism, and a family history of depression, anxiety, or addiction, have genetic roots and place an individual at risk. The social environment and psychosocial stressors will either prevent or exacerbate the effect of these risk factors. These include family functioning and communication patterns; parent-child relationships; teasing; body preoccupation; and stressful events, such as loss, illness, or abuse (Fishman, 2004).

Just as people with high risk of alcohol addiction due to genetics will only become addicted if the environment provides and endorses alcohol use, living in a culture that glorifies thinness and dieting, promotes the language of fat, and objectifies women's bodies can catalyze risk factors to blossom into full-blown eating disorders.

THE ROLE OF THE FAMILY

Although modern explanations of the etiology of eating disorders view these as multi-determined conditions, the tendency to blame families has been a recurrent theme (Russell, 2001). Starting with the description of anorexia nervosa in 1874, William Gull warned that family involvement in treatment was not necessarily helpful. He referred to friends and family members as "the worst attendants" when addressing the patients' malnutrition and poor health (Gull, 1874). Others wrote of the "curative influence of isolation," stressing that parental involvement would actually block the progression of treatment (Silverman, 1997). Also in the 1870s, Lasegue conceptualized the anorexic's food refusal as symbolic of other intrafamilial conflicts. As part of the French bourgeoisie, he noted the power of food refusal when rich and appetizing food was so available, showing a deep sensitivity to the meaning of food in a family and culture (Brumberg, 1989). A century later, Hilde Bruch, one of the first U.S. psychiatrists to write about eating disorders, expressed more compassion for the families, noting how painful it is for parents to watch their child suffering and be unable to help (Bruch, 1978).

Research in the 1970s and 1980s focused on family dysfunction and viewed eating disorder families as more disturbed than others (Kog & Vandereycken, 1989); this research suffered from many design and sampling problems, however, obscuring the validity of these findings (Kog & Vandereycken, 1985). A number of clinicians and researchers have found consistent differences between families with anorexic members and those with bulimic members. The anorexic family type tends to be more rigid in its organization, more avoidant of conflict, and more interdependent, whereas the bulimic family tends to be disorganized, chaotic, and hostile (Davis,

Shuster, Blackmore, & Fox, 2004). Other literature indicates that families with eating-disordered members have fostered poor or insecure attachment processes (Ward, Ramsay, Turnbull, Benedettinni, & Treasure, 2000).

Research on family functioning has inherent flaws because families are constantly interacting and changing, so observations or conclusions reflect only that point in time. Therefore, it is impossible to determine if the family issues or dynamics are a cause of the eating disorder or a consequence of the illness process (Polivy & Herman, 2002). Family problems, be they specific attitudes to the body, weight, and appearances or broader interactional patterns, most likely have a greater impact on members with the personality characteristics mentioned previously as biogenetic risk factors. That is, family risk factors will place members who are highly anxious, overly eager to please others, perfectionist, and obsessive at greater risk for clinical eating disorders (Davis et al., 2004). A biopsychosocial approach rejects a linear approach to causation, reduces the blame of both the family and the individual, and better reflects the dynamic nature of family functioning.

The Family as Cultural Mediator

The family is the bridge between the larger social context and the individual's predispositions, vulnerabilities, and psychosocial development. The family mediates or translates the culture's dominant messages to its members, creating its own variation, mirror, or rejection of them.

Some families wholeheartedly adopt the culture's emphasis on appearance, weight, and body image as critical aspects of the self. This may result in weightism (bias against larger people based on their size), misinformation about dieting and nutrition, and excessive exercise in the guise of health, creating risks for eating disorders to emerge. In other words, the degree to which

the family also translates emotions into the language of fat creates additional risk that a vulnerable family member will develop an eating disorder.

A number of studies demonstrate the importance of the family's beliefs and practices related to the body in the development of eating disorders. Laliberte, Boland, and Leichner (1999) reported that a family focus on appearance and achievement is a much more powerful predictor of disturbed eating than general family variables, such as cohesion, conflict, and emotional constraint. Mothers of eating-disordered daughters express more concerns about weight and shape (Woodside et al., 2002), and mothers of girls with disordered eating are more critical of their daughters' bodies than are mothers of healthy girls (Hill & Franklin, 1998).

In general, research and the clinical literature have stressed the mother's dieting and appearance concerns, but contemporary fathers also contribute to their children's body image, self-esteem, and eating problems (Maine, 2004). When fathers emphasize weight control and appearance, daughters are much more likely to be dissatisfied with their bodies, to self-induce vomiting, and to engage in other unhealthy dieting behaviors (Dixon, Gill, & Adair, 2003).

According to one study, the strongest predictor of bulimia for college women is a pattern of negative family comments about appearance and the need to diet (Crowther, Kichler, Sherwood, & Kunhert, 2002). Similar findings are reported in an elementary school population. Smolak, Levine, and Schermer (1999) report that weight loss attempts and negative body esteem are correlated to parents' comments about the child's weight as well as complaints about their own size and shape.

This research suggests that parents contribute to disordered eating through both direct comments and their modeling. Fostering a home environment that emphasizes physical appearance and attractiveness, thinness, dieting, and exercise to reach the ideal shape negatively affects children, especially girls. A poor body image, preoccupation with shape and size, and dieting are all precursors to clinical eating disorders. A variable as simple as frequent family meals, however, may serve to protect some young people from developing unhealthy eating patterns. Neumark-Sztainer, Wall, Story, and Fulkerson (2004) reported that teens enjoying more frequent family meals, a positive atmosphere at meals, and a more structured meal environment are less apt to engage in disordered eating. The impact is greater on girls than boys.

The influence of the family on attitudes toward the self, the body, and eating is significant, be it positive or negative. Contemporary families must also process the many messages about the increased rates of both child and adult obesity. Unfortunately, education and prevention attempts to date have tended to be scare tactics rather than comprehensive, integrated approaches targeted to individual needs; in turn, they may create or intensify body preoccupation, stigmatize people whose bodies do not fit the cultural ideal, and encourage unhealthy attempts to lose weight that may lead to eating disorders (Berg, 2001). As weightism and efforts as drastic as cosmetic plastic surgery and gastric bypass surgery to control weight increasingly become the norm, eating disorders, both clinical and subclinical, will remain a significant problem for families and an increasing public health issue.

Systems Theory and Eating Disorders

Families struggling with eating disorders often experience much shame and guilt, and they desperately search for easy answers to avoid these negative feelings and to help their loved one recover. A systems approach offers no simple solutions, but it also avoids blaming the individual or family for the dilemmas they are experiencing because it locates the illness in the system rather than in individuals. Systems theory, simply stated, suggests that the whole is greater than the sum of its parts and promotes the understanding of families struggling with eating disorders (Maine, 2004).

Family systems theorists (Minuchin, Rosman, & Baker, 1978; Palazzoli, 1978, 1988; Dare & Eisler, 1997; Fishman, 2004) describe the family as a cybernetic, dynamic system with all parts affecting each other through interactions, interconnections, and constant feedback. These components include the individual's physical, biochemical, and psychological functioning; vulnerabilities due to early development and psychological experiences; family functioning and organization; multigenerational family patterns; developmental stressors on the individual; and pressures from outside the family. In systems theory, there are no simple A-causes-B relationships; instead, everything is related to everything else. No part has complete control over another, although all parts influence each other.

Due to the dramatic impact of an eating disorder, it is remarkably easy to view the identified patient as the victim of a disturbed family or as a master manipulator desperate for attention and power (Lackstrom & Woodside, 1998). Over time, families develop rigid patterns that may make one person look like the villain when in fact all family members, as well as forces outside the family, have contributed. Systems theories place the symptoms and the family's response to them into a broader social context and a nonlinear biopsychosocial model.

Systemic Approaches to Eating-Disordered Families

In the 1970s and 1980s, clinicians at the Philadelphia Child Guidance Clinic, led by Salvatore Minuchin, and in Italy at the Milan group, led by Mara Selvini-Palazzoli, identified common patterns of enmeshment, blurred family boundaries, and avoidance of conflict in eating-disordered families. The two groups used different strategies, but both intended to change the family interactional patterns to promote recovery. Both groups were also treating young anorexic patients and their families.

In structural family therapy, Minuchin and colleagues view anorexic families as similar to psychosomatic families, sharing three essential ingredients:

- A psychologically vulnerable child
- A family interactional style of enmeshment, overprotectiveness, rigidity, and lack of conflict resolution
- The importance of the sick child's role to the family's pattern of avoidance and to the reinforcement of the symptoms for the child

Interventions target the problematic patterns and can have a powerful impact, sometimes using family meals to change the patterns of interaction between the child and family and reporting a success rate of 80% (Minuchin et al., 1978).

Intensive structural therapy (Fishman, 2004) is an outgrowth of the psychosomatic family model. This approach incorporates a broader social context and influences outside the family; in essence, it further contextualizes the nature of the illness. In light of these other influences, therapy may involve parties such as friends, coworkers, or social service agencies. Intensive structural therapy also recognizes that some forces in the individual's life and social context actually serve to maintain the problems, and it identifies and addresses these "homeostatic maintainers."

In Milan systems therapy (Palazzoli, 1978, 1988), the family is viewed as a homeostatic system that will respond negatively to direct pressures to change. Instead of direct interventions, the emphasis is on interviewing the family to help them become aware of their own interactional patterns and to challenge their beliefs about themselves and their family interactions. The therapist develops a hypothesis about the functions of the symptoms and uses indirect methods to avoid resistance. Like structural family therapy, this approach is widely used in the treatment of eating disorders, although less research has been done on its effectiveness.

The Maudsley method, another interactional systems model, incorporates appreciation of both genetic and sociocultural influences on the family and individual. Again, in contrast to a medical model, the illness is viewed as existing outside of the individual but resulting in symptoms, such as starvation, that deeply affect the person and family and must be addressed (Dare & Eisler, 1997). Interventions vary depending on the age of the patient, but with younger patients, families are very active in symptom management. This approach involves three phases of treatment: refeeding the patient, negotiations for a new pattern of relationship, and adolescent issues and termination, all with a noncritical stance toward the patient and family and a focus on improving relationships and restoring the patient's normal developmental progression (Russell, 2001).

Feminist family therapy is not a separate technique but a conceptual approach or sensibility that can be incorporated into other approaches. The basic premise is that women's position in modern culture puts them in conflict with their own needs. Pressured to be nurturers and caretakers and to conform to strictly defined cultural norms regarding appearance and beauty, women are at risk to develop eating disorders. Treatment must address issues of power and oppression, including the need for partnership and collaboration in the therapeutic relationship (Herscovici, 2002; Root, Fallon, & Freidrich, 1986). The therapeutic technique is less important than the attitude and beliefs about gender and its role in the development of eating disorders.

These systemic approaches inform much of the clinical work with individuals and families suffering from eating disorders. In general, treatment of these conditions is multimodal, with individual therapy, nutritional counseling, medication, group therapies, expressive arts, and even residential treatment or hospitalization occurring simultaneously. Consequently, it is difficult to separate the effect of one approach from that of the others and to truly isolate the benefits of family therapy. Effective biopsychosocial treatment, however, must appreciate the family's role and need for help, especially when the identified patient is still dependent on the family environment. With adult patients, exploration of contributing family dynamics is critical, but direct involvement should be individually determined. Sometimes, treatment involves the family of origin, or it may involve the individual's current family or close relationships. Very little research is available on adult eating disorders.

Additional Stressors for Eating Disorder Families

Chronic or life-threatening illness always creates significant stress for families, but that caused by eating disorders, when a member is refusing food or purging what is eaten and is in denial of this obvious physical illness, may be particularly challenging. Family members, especially parents, tend to blame themselves or the identified patient for the problem, to feel anxious and desperate due to the potential health risks, and to develop rigid ways of interacting and dealing with the illness. The identified patient responds similarly, and unhealthy interactional patterns may become fixed and entrenched (Maine, 2004).

The families of patients with eating disorders have very specific concerns and needs, as indicated by research (Winn, Perkins, Murray, Murphy, & Schmidt,

2004). Often, the services needed to treat these conditions are not available locally, and the family may need to move or to send the ill member away for treatment. Alternatively, families may have to patch together components of multidisciplinary care, sometimes without the help of professionals experienced with the treatment of eating disorders. Community support groups for family members may also be unavailable, except in larger metropolitan areas. Insurance issues are very prominent because policies may specify sites for treatment excluding specialized programs for eating disorders, or they may not pay for the range of services or level of care needed. This creates tremendous anxiety and hardship, sometimes requiring families to go into debt or to seek legal action to ensure that their loved one has the opportunity to recover. If the patient is no longer a minor, regulations regarding confidentiality and consent may limit family's involvement and information, potentially increasing the anxiety and the dysfunction of the family's interactions.

The medical community still suffers from a lack of awareness of signs, symptoms, treatment needs, and the recovery process related to eating disorders; consequently, it may be ineffective in its diagnosis and treatment and is not always a reliable resource for families. Desperate for information to guide their efforts to support the patient, families often have little access to basic psychoeducational information on the effects, management, or progression of eating disorders, especially if they do not have a computer and the skills to find such information. Finally, the stigma regarding mental health issues remains a problem for many families, limiting their ability to seek help. This often results in a shared anxiety, perceived inadequacy, and depression enveloping the entire family. Thus, the illness challenges the family's resources and may contribute to its dysfunction.

SUMMARY

Given the incidence and gravity of clinical and subclinical eating disorders, the changing demographics, and the globalization of these problems, they must be viewed as a potential threat to the health and well-being of all families today. They are as grave a public health issue as obesity and are more frequent than conditions such as Alzheimer's disease and schizophrenia, but they receive less attention and less funding. Efforts to prevent these disorders must include family interventions and education about the direct and indirect contributions of the family environment on attitudes toward weight, food, body image, and health. Our knowledge of eating disorder families is based primarily on families with young anorexic members; much more investigation is needed, examining the other diagnostic categories (bulimia and EDNOS) and across the life span. We must also fund research on family resilience to eating disorders and innovative outreach programs that will help parents to understand how to manage their own issues regarding appearance, food, and body preoccupation. Families need help to create an environment that encourages emotional resilience, positive body image, and a healthy approach to eating and exercise. They also need to understand the risk factors inherent in their family histories and functioning as well as the individual risks in light of their children's personalities and coping styles.

Individuals and families afflicted by eating disorders need compassion and understanding to counteract their blame, shame, and guilt. We must provide more access to information, services, and support groups to families at all points in the illness process. Because adults also suffer from these conditions, treatment options must be more flexible to meet their needs. For example, most adult women cannot consider leaving their families and their responsibilities for any protracted period of time, making outpatient options and convenient treatment packages critical. Finally, insurance, managed care, and third-party payers must also incorporate a biopsychosocial view of treatment needs, provide the appropriate and best care, and support family therapy as an important part of the treatment process.

Eating disorders also have implications for public policy. For example, we must develop an approach to the increase in obesity that is tailored to individual risk, lifestyle, and health factors instead of inflammatory scare tactics that help to create disordered eating and body dissatisfaction. Furthermore, training of all medical providers, mental health professionals, and educators in the diagnosis and progression of eating disorders is essential because most have very little experience with or information about the broad spectrum of eating disorders. They maintain old biases that these problems are limited to young, upper-middle-class Caucasian women and fail to screen young children, adults, men, and patients of different ethnicities, ages, and classes. Due to the frequency of subclinical eating disorders, all health care providers should incorporate questions about dieting, weight management, exercise, and body image in their assessments and provide education and resources to those who are struggling or at risk. Primary care providers, mental health clinicians, and health educators must provide support and education for eating-disordered women in their role as mothers to create healthy home environments and role models for their children. Helping professionals must also develop an awareness of how the war on obesity, the cultural expectations for beauty and appearance, and the dieting mentality resonate in us as clinicians and affect our ability to recognize and treat these issues effectively.

Most important, we must empower families to recognize their positive role in the prevention and recovery of eating disorders. Parents sometimes doubt their ability to compete with negative forces in the cultural environment, such as the standards of beauty and the epidemic of dieting and body image despair. When all is said and done, "It takes a family . . . to effectively care for the fierce and enervating problem of eating disorders and to transform the problem for the long term" (Fishman, 2004, p. 263). Families are instrumental in the prevention and the recovery process; health care providers, mental health clinicians, and public policy should respect, encourage, and amplify the family's unique and potentially positive influence in addressing this serious public health problem.

REFERENCES

Agras, W. S., Brandt, H. A., Bulik, C. M., Dolan-Sewell, R., Fairburn, C. G., Halmi, K. A., et al. (2004). Report of the National Institutes of Health workshop on overcoming barriers to treatment research in anorexia nervosa. *International Journal of Eating Disorders, 35*(4), 509-521.

American Academy of Pediatrics. (2003). Identifying and treating eating disorders; Policy statement. *Pediatrics, 111*(1), 204-211.

American Psychiatric Association. (1994). *Diagnostic and statistical manual of mental disorders* (4th ed.). Washington, DC: Author.

American Psychiatric Association. (2000, January). Practice guideline for the treatment of patients with eating disorders [Revision]. *American Journal of Psychiatry, 157*(1, Suppl.), 1-39.

Becker, A. E. (2002, April). *Sociocultural issues. Plenary session I.* Paper presented at the International Conference on Eating Disorders, Boston.

Berg, F. (2001). *Women afraid to eat.* Hettinger, ND: Healthy Weight Network.

Bruch, H. (1978). *The golden cage: The enigma of anorexia nervosa.* Cambridge, MA: Harvard University Press.

Brumberg, J. J. (1989). *Fasting girls: The history of anorexia nervosa.* New York: Plume.

Bulik, C. M. (attributed by Powers, P. S.) (2004, November). *Biological, psychodynamic, and cultural factors in eating disorders: Translations to clinical practice.* Paper presented at the 14th annual Renfrew Center Foundation Conference for Professionals, Philadelphia.

Centers for Disease Control and Prevention. (2002). Youth risk behavior surveillance: U.S., 2001. *Morbidity and Mortality Report, 51,* SS-4.

Clarke, L. H. (2002). Older women's perceptions of ideal body weights: The tensions between health and appearance motivations for weight loss. *Ageing and Society, 22,* 751-773.

Croll, J., Neumark-Sztainer, D., Story, M., & Ireland, M. (2002). Prevalence and risk and protective factors related to disordered eating. *Journal of Adolescent Health, 31*(2), 166-175.

Crowther, J. H., Kichler, J. C., Sherwood, N., & Kunhert, M. E. (2002). The role of family factors in bulimia nervosa. *Eating Disorders: The Journal of Treatment and Prevention, 10,* 141-151.

Dare, C., & Eisler, I. (1997). Family therapy for anorexia nervosa. In D. M. Garner & P. E. Garfinkel (Eds.), *Handbook of treatment for eating disorders* (2nd ed., pp. 307-324). New York: Guilford.

Davis, C., Shuster, B., Blackmore, E., & Fox, J. (2004). Looking good: Family focus on appearance and the risk for eating disorders. *International Journal of Eating Disorders, 35,* 136-144.

Dixon, R. S., Gill, J. M. W., & Adair, V. A. (2003). Exploring paternal influences on the dieting behaviors of adolescent girls. *Eating Disorders: The Journal of Treatment and Prevention, 11*(1), 39-50.

Eliot, A. O., & Baker, C. W. (2001). Eating disordered adolescent males. *Adolescence, 36*(143), 535-543.

Fishman, H. C. (2004). *Enduring change in eating disorders; Interventions with long-term results.* New York: Brunner-Routledge.

Friedman, S. S. (1997). *When girls feel fat: Helping girls through adolescence.* Vancouver, British Columbia, Canada: Salal.

Gaesser, G. (2002). *Big fat lies: The truth about weight and your health.* Carlsbad, CA: Gurze.

Garner, D. M. (1997, February). Survey says: Body image poll results. *Psychology Today,* 1-12.

Gordon, R. (2001). Eating disorders East and West: A culture-bound syndrome unbound. In M. Nasser, M. A. Katzman, & R. A. Gordon (Eds.), *Eating disorders and cultures in transition* (pp. 1–23). New York: Taylor & Francis.

Gorwood, P., Bouvard, M., Mouren-Simeoni, M. C., Kipman, A., & Ades, J. (1998). Genetics and anorexia nervosa: A review of candidate genes. *Psychiatric Genetics, 8,* 1-12.

Gull, W. W. (1874). Anorexia nervosa (apepsia, hysterica, anorexia hysterica). *Transactions of the Clinical Society of London, 7,* 222-228.

Herscovici, C. R. (2002). Eating disorders in adolescence. In F. Kaslow (Series Ed.) and J. Magnavita (Vol. Ed.), *Comprehensive handbook of psychotherapy: Vol. 1. psychodynamic/object relations* (pp. 133-159). New York: John Wiley.

Hetherington, M. M., & Burnett, L. (1994). Ageing and the pursuit of slimness: Dietary restraint and weight satisfaction in elderly women. *British Journal of Clinical Psychology, 33,* 391-400.

Hill, A. J., & Franklin, J. A. (1998). Mothers, daughters, and dieting: Investigating the transmission of weight control. *British Journal of Clinical Psychology, 37,* 3-13.

Hoerr, S. L., Bokram, R., Lugo, B., Bivins, T., & Keast, D. R. (2002). Risk for disordered eating relates to both gender and ethnicity for college students. *Journal of the American College of Nutrition, 21*(4), 307-314.

Kog, E., & Vandereycken, W. (1985). Family characteristics of anorexia nervosa and bulimia: A review of the research literature. *Clinical Psychology Review, 5,* 159-180.

Kog, E., & Vandereycken, W. (1989). Family interaction in eating disorder patients and normal controls. *International Journal of Eating Disorders, 8,* 11-23.

Lackstrom, J. B., & Woodside, D. B. (1998). Families, therapists and family therapy in eating disorders. In W. Vandereycken & P. J. V. Beumont (Eds.), *Treating eating disorders: Ethical, legal and personal issues* (pp. 106-126). New York: New York University Press.

Laliberte, M., Boland, F. J., & Leichner, P. (1999). Family climates: Family factors specific to disturbed eating and bulimia nervosa. *Journal of Clinical Psychology, 55,* 1021-1040.

Maine, M. (2004). *Father hunger: Fathers, daughters and the pursuit of thinness.* Carlsbad, CA: Gurze.

Minuchin, B. L., Rosman, B. L., & Baker, L. (1978). *Psychosomatic families: Anorexia nervosa in context.* Cambridge, MA: Harvard University Press.

Neumark, D., Wall, M., Story, M., & Fulkerson, J. A. (2004). Are family meal patterns associated with disordered eating behaviors among adolescents? *Journal of Adolescent Health, 35*(5), 350-359.

O'Dea, J. A., & Abraham, S. (2002). Eating and exercise disorders in young college men. *Journal of the American College of Health, 50*(6), 273-278.

Palazzoli, M. S. (1978). *Self–starvation: From individual to family therapy in the treatment of anorexia nervosa.* New York: Jason Aronson.

Palazzoli, M. S. (1988). The cybernetics of anorexia nervosa. In M. Selvini (Ed.), *The work of Mara Selvini Palazzoli* (pp. 213-227). Northvale, NJ: Jason Aronson.

Patrick, L. (2002). Eating disorders: A review of the literature with emphasis on medical complications and clinical nutrition. *Alternative Medicine Review, 7*(3), 184-202.

Polivy, J., & Herman, P. C. (2002). Causes of eating disorders. *Annual Review of Psychology, 53,* 187-213.

Powers, P. S., & Bannon, Y. (2004). The last word: Meeting the challenge of eating disorders. *Eating Disorders: The Journal of Treatment and Prevention, 12,* 91-95.

Powers, P. S., & Spratt, E. (1994). Males compared to females with eating disorders: 15 years of clinical experience. *Eating Disorders: The Journal of Treatment and Prevention, 2,* 197-214.

Root, M. P. P., Fallon, P., & Friedrich, W. N. (1986). *Bulimia: A systems approach to treatment.* New York: Norton.

Russell, G. (2001). Foreword. In J. Lock, D. Le Grange, W. S. Agras, & C. Dare (Eds.), *Treatment manual for anorexia nervosa* (pp. xi-xiii). New York: Guilford.

Shisslak, C. M., Crago, M., & Estes, L. S. (1995). The spectrum of eating disturbances. *International Journal of Eating Disorders, 18*(3), 209-219.

Silverman, J. A. (1997). Charcot's comments on the therapeutic role of isolation in the treatment of anorexia nervosa. *International Journal of Eating Disorders, 21,* 295-298.

Smolak, L., Levine, M. P., & Schermer, F. (1999). Parental input and weight concerns among elementary school children. *International Journal of Eating Disorders, 25,* 263-271.

Sullivan, P. (2002). Course and outcome of anorexia nervosa and bulimia nervosa. In C. G. Fairburn & K. D. Brownell (Eds.), *Eating disorders and obesity* (2nd ed., pp. 226-232). New York: Guilford.

Sullivan, P. F. (1995). Mortality in anorexia nervosa. *American Journal of Psychiatry, 152,* 1073-1074.

Ward, A., Ramsay, R., Turnbull, S., Benedettinni, M., & Treasure, J. (2000). Attachment patterns in eating disorders: Past and present. *International Journal of Eating Disorders, 28,* 370-376.

Waterhouse, D. (1997). *Like mother, like daughter: How women are influenced by their mother's relationship with food and how to break the pattern.* New York: Hyperion.

Winn, S., Perkins, S., Murray, J., Murphy, R., & Schmidt, U. (2004). A qualitative study of the experience of caring for a person with bulimia nervosa. Part 2: Carers' needs and experiences of services and other support. *International Journal of Eating Disorders, 36*(3), 269-279.

Woodside, D. B., Bulik, C. M., Halmi, K. A., Fichter, M. M., Kaplan, A., Berrettini, W. H., et al. (2002) Personality, perfectionism, and attitudes toward eating in parents of individuals with eating disorders. *International Journal of Eating Disorders, 31,* 290-299.

CHAPTER 8

Families and Major Mental Illness

KIM T. MUESER

The family plays an important role in everyday life and is the source of much personal gratification. Families can also be the source of significant stress and frustration. Professional perspectives on the role of the family in major mental illnesses, such as schizophrenia, bipolar disorder (manic depression), and major depression, have changed dramatically during the past several decades. Whereas families were once thought to be the primary cause of mental illnesses such as schizophrenia, the tide has shifted, and families are now understood to be critical to the long-term management and recovery of these disorders. Although family interventions for major mental illness continue to lag in their implementation in routine clinical settings, abundant research has shown that family treatment programs that focus on collaboration and shared decision making significantly improve the outcome of these disorders.

This chapter begins with a discussion of the dynamic interplay between the effect of mental illness on the family and the effect of stress in the family environment on the course of mental illness. A heuristic model is briefly described that integrates the influence of familial and illness-related factors on the course of mental illness, which has direct implications for family interventions designed to improve the outcome of the illness. Next, the general goals of family intervention for major mental illness are described, followed by a summary of different models of family intervention for this population. Because different models of family intervention share many common components, these shared features are highlighted, and clinical recommendations for family work are summarized. To provide readers with a more in-depth understanding of family intervention, more detailed description is provided for one of the most widely used family intervention programs, behavioral family therapy for psychiatric disorders. Next, research on family intervention for major mental illnesses is summarized. The chapter concludes with a discussion of the dissemination of family intervention programs, strategies for overcoming obstacles to implementing this evidence-based practice, and future directions for clinical practice and research.

MENTAL ILLNESS
AND THE FAMILY

The development of a mental illness in a loved one can have a devastating effect on the family because their hopes and expectations for the individual's future are often dashed. Not surprisingly, a major effect of mental illness on the family is the creation of high levels of stress. Although this stress can have a negative effect on everyone in the family, the effects are especially pernicious for the person with mental illness and can contribute to a more severe course of the illness. Each of these factors is considered in more detail here.

Mental Illness and Family Burden

Numerous first-person accounts by family members attest to the impact of the mental illness on relatives' emotional well-being, their time, and their financial standing (Backlar, 1994; Swados, 1991). Major mental illnesses often lead to unpredictable (and sometimes bizarre) behavior, mood shifts, and cognitive difficulties. All these symptoms of mental illness can make the person more unpredictable and more difficult to live with. Common emotional reactions include anxiety, depression, guilt, embarrassment, frustration, and anger (Lefley, 1996; Oldridge & Hughes, 1992). When the mental illness has a profound effect on the loved one's personality and future potential, its development can also be associated with a grieving process as a parent, sibling, spouse, or even child experiences the "loss" of a loved one (Miller, Dworkin, Ward, & Barone, 1990).

Feelings of anxiety are common among relatives of people with schizophrenia-spectrum disorders because these illnesses often lead to unpredictable and occasionally violent behavior directed at family members (Steadman et al., 1998). The behavior of individuals with psychoses can be perplexing

to family members who struggle to understand their relatives but cannot grasp their way of thinking. The negative symptoms of schizophrenia, such as social withdrawal, apathy, and anhedonia, can be especially frustrating for relatives, who may have difficulty understanding the person's mental illness and believe that he or she is capable of doing more to help himself or herself (Weisman, Nuechterlein, Goldstein, & Snyder, 1998).

Individuals with mood disorders, such as major depression or bipolar disorder, can also have a major impact on their loved ones. Research has shown that living with an individual with depression is associated with inducing depression in the partner (Coyne et al., 1987), indicating that depression may be somewhat contagious. During periods of mania with bipolar disorder, relatives may be drawn into a whirlwind of energy, typically characterized by a mixture of euphoria and irritability, with many problems related to grandiosity, unrealistic plans, and inflated self-esteem. These mood swings can be difficult to understand and perplexing in the same way that the psychotic symptoms of schizophrenia may be confusing to relatives (Mueser, Webb, Pfeiffer, Gladis, & Levinson, 1996).

Major mental illnesses often have a major impact on the ability of people to take care of their basic living needs (e.g., cooking, laundry, and shopping), and family members often fulfill these needs. Families of people with severe mental illnesses frequently report spending large amounts of time and significant amounts of money helping their relative (Clark, 1994). Thus, time (which represents an opportunity cost) and money expenditures can affect the financial resources of families with a mentally ill member. These effects are amplified by the fact that people with a major mental illness often have difficulty working and therefore bring little money to the household other than disability income. This problem can be especially great when an individual who was previously a wage earner for the family develops a mental illness.

The net result of the emotional, time, and financial costs of coping with a major mental illness in the family is that many relatives experience significant burden in caring for a loved one with mental illness (Baronet, 1999). Although the burden of care may be significant, it should not overshadow the fact that many families with a mentally ill member also experience significant gratifications in their relationships (Bulger, Wandersman, & Goldman, 1993). Aside from the enjoyment of a loved one's company, and the mutual sharing in personal successes, having a mental illness in a member sometimes draws families closer and leads members to develop a greater appreciation for one another than they had previously.

Family Stress and the Course of Major Mental Illness

As previously described, the challenge of coping with a family member with a major mental illness can be formidable and lead to a significant burden among the relatives. A common consequence of this burden of care is high levels of family stress. Although stress can have an untoward effect on everyone's lives, its effects on the person with mental illness can be far greater. Extensive research shows that environmental stress can provoke symptom exacerbations in major mental illnesses, leading to a deterioration in functioning (Bebbington & Kuipers, 1992; Breslau & Davis, 1985). Stresses are typically categorized into two kinds: life events (e.g., the death of a loved one, a move, and the birth of a child) and interpersonal conflict (e.g., having a relationship with another person marked by high levels of criticism, hostility, or intrusiveness).

From a family perspective, stress arising from conflict in interpersonal relationships is especially significant. Research has shown that stress in the family, as characterized by excessive criticism, hostility, or emotional overinvolvement of relatives in the life of a person with a major mental illness, greatly increases the chances of relapses and rehospitalizations (Butzlaff & Hooley, 1998). Furthermore, the relationship between higher levels of family conflict and increased vulnerability to relapse and rehospitalization does not appear to be due to client characteristics that are independently predictive of rehospitalization (Leff & Vaughn, 1985).

Although family stress can worsen the course of mental illness, the nature of this stress is understandable. Family members are often at a loss for how to cope with a family member's mental illness, and they may resort to excessive criticism or other efforts to control that member's behavior (Greenley, 1986). The result is often a vicious cycle of tension and conflict in the family. Caring for a loved one with a major mental illness is burdensome and stressful to family members, who may then respond by increasing their efforts to control the family member, resulting in increased tension and paradoxically an increased risk of relapse and worse functioning. As the family member with mental illness deteriorates in functioning, this increases the burden of care on family members, who may then respond with even more desperate attempts to control their relative's behavior. Alternatively, some families become overwhelmed and give up supporting their loved one, which can lead to housing instability and homelessness (Caton, Shrout, Eagle, Opler, & Felix, 1994). A major goal of family intervention for major mental illness is to break this cycle of burden, stress, and a deteriorating course of mental illness.

FAMILY INTERVENTION FOR MAJOR MENTAL ILLNESS

Historically, the development of family intervention models for major mental illness underwent a significant evolution during the past 40 years. Throughout the early and mid-20th century, it was widely believed in the scientific community that families were either responsible or played an important role in the etiology of disorders such as schizophrenia (Bateson, Jackson, Haley, & Weakland, 1956; Fromm-Reichman, 1948). For this reason, professionals did not look to family members as potential collaborators but, rather, as culprits in causing mental illness. The result was that professional work with families was largely eschewed, and when it was conducted, the aim was to address those family dynamics believed to be responsible for the psychiatric illness.

In the 1960s and 1970s, several developments led to the abandonment of psychogenic theories of major mental illness (Mueser & Glynn, 1999). First, research confirmed that there were significant biological factors involved in mental illness, such as genetic vulnerability and the dramatic effects of medications on symptoms, that made theories of the family etiology of mental illness untenable. Second, studies of family interaction patterns suggested that disrupted communication was more likely the result of having a relative with a mental illness than a cause of the illness. Third, family intervention models based on theories of the family as the cause of mental illness were unsuccessful in improving outcomes.

In addition to the lack of support for psychogenic theories of major mental illness, two other trends influenced the development of family intervention programs for this population. First, family members who were dismayed at the poor treatment their relatives often received in the mental health system, and who resented being kept in the dark regarding their relatives' illness and how to treat it, began to unite into a family advocacy movement, as exemplified by organizations such as the National Alliance for the Mentally Ill. This movement, which has now taken hold worldwide, has provided forceful advocacy for better mental health treatment, more respect and collaboration from mental health professionals, and help in decreasing the burden of care that often falls on the shoulders of family members (Hatfield & Lefley, 1987). These efforts highlighted the plight of family members, who are charged with managing a severe mental illness of a relative at home with little knowledge and few resources to achieve this task. Second, as previously described, research conducted primarily in the 1960s and 1970s firmly demonstrated that family stress could precipitate relapses and rehospitalizations (Butzlaff & Hooley, 1998). This created interest in developing interventions that might decrease family stress, thereby improving the course of the mental illness. Thus, family intervention models evolved with the primary focus on increasing the burden of care in family members while also decreasing family stress.

Specific Family Intervention Programs for Major Mental Illness

In the 1970s and 1980s, a variety of different models of family intervention were developed and empirically validated. The initial focus of most of these models was on the treatment of schizophrenia, although several of them have been adapted for other disorders as well. Despite differences in the treatment models for major mental illness, effective programs share more in common than they differ. Table 8.1 summarizes the common principles and goals of family intervention programs for mental illness.

Specific family intervention programs differ along a number of dimensions, such as theoretical orientation, modality (individual family work vs. multiple family groups), and locus of treatment (the clinic or home). Anderson, Reiss, and Hogarty (1986) developed a family systems-based approach oriented toward understanding the impact of schizophrenia on the family and helping the relatives rally around the treatment of a

Table 8.1   Principles and Goals of Family Intervention for Major Mental Illness

1. Involve everyone possible in family work, including the client and nonfamily significant others.

2. Establish a mutually respectful, long-term collaborative relationship between the treatment team and the family.

3. Educate the family about the nature of mental illness and the principles of its treatment to promote their acceptance of it and their ability to manage it successfully (e.g., avoiding relapses and rehospitalizations).

4. Reduce stress in the family by facilitating better communication and problem-solving skills.

5. Reduce the burden of care for the illness on the family, and improve the client's self-sufficiency.

6. Avoid blame and focusing on the past in favor of developing a future orientation based on hope and shared goals.

7. Strive to improve the functioning of all family members, not just the client.

8. Work with family members to help the client develop a personal vision of recovery from mental illness (e.g., meaningful involvement in work or school, close relationships, rewarding leisure and recreational activities, and independence).

loved one. The model developed by Kuipers, Leff, and Lam (2002) is an eclectic approach, focusing primarily on educating family members about the nature of schizophrenia, and using different strategies to reduce stressful communication between family members, including both individual family work and involvement of families in support groups. Neither of these models has been adapted for other major mental illnesses, although considering the overlap in functional impairment between schizophrenia and other serious mental disorders, these approaches could readily be modified accordingly.

Three other models of family intervention have a predominantly behavioral orientation. Barrowclough and Tarrier (1992) focus on teaching family members information about schizophrenia, helping them develop relapse prevention plans, and helping them solve practical problems. The behavioral family therapy model (Falloon, Boyd, & McGill, 1984; Miklowitz & Goldstein, 1997; Mueser & Glynn, 1999) provides education about mental illness and its treatment, communication skills training, and teaches problem-solving skills. This intervention was initially developed as a home-based intervention (Falloon et al., 1985), although research has shown that it is also effective when delivered

in the clinic (Randolph et al., 1994). McFarlane (2002) has developed a multifamily group intervention that provides education and teaches problem-solving skills in the context of multiple-family group meetings. Both the behavioral family therapy and McFarlane's multiple-family group intervention were initially developed for schizophrenia but have been adapted for other major mental illnesses.

Behavioral family therapy has been the most widely studied model of family intervention for major mental illness, with applications to a wide range of different disorders, including schizophrenia, bipolar disorder, major depression, anxiety disorders, and substance use disorders (Falloon, Held, Coverdale, Roncone, & Laidlaw, 1999; Mueser & Glynn, 1999). Because the general model has broad-scale applicability, and a detailed treatment manual including all necessary resources exists (Mueser & Glynn, 1999), a more detailed description about this program is provided next.

Behavioral Family Therapy

Behavioral family therapy (BFT) is a social learning approach to collaborating with families aimed at providing them with the information and skills necessary to manage a mental illness in a loved one. BFT focuses on improving family members' understanding of mental illness and its treatment, enhancing skills for communicating and solving problems, and working collaboratively toward goals. The information and skills are taught using skills training methods, such as modeling, role playing, feedback, and home practice assignments. A detailed explication of the program is provided by Mueser and Glynn (1999).

Logistics. BFT can be conducted either in the home or in the clinic, depending on the ease of engaging family members and the therapist's flexibility to travel. Some advantages of home-based treatment are that it is easier to engage more family members, cancellations are minimized, and the therapist gains valuable information about the environment in which family members live. A disadvantage is that additional travel time is required for the therapist, which may reduce the overall efficiency of the approach. In many situations, it is possible to work out a compromise with the family in which some sessions are done at home and others at the clinic.

Session length is typically 1 hour, with sessions initially scheduled weekly for approximately 3 months, followed by every other week for approximately 6 months and monthly for several months thereafter. The length of sessions and their frequency can be modified based on the individual circumstances of the family. For example, some clients may have difficulty attending to information for a 1-hour period and may require a break or shorter sessions. Some families may find it difficult to meet weekly and may find it easier to have longer meetings every other week. For some families, a 9- or 1-month course of BFT is sufficient to equip them with the necessary information or skills to manage the illness. Other families, such as those facing multiple stresses including severe poverty or having more than one significantly impaired family member, may require longer

periods of more intense BFT to learn the requisite skills. Some families benefit from ongoing sessions without formally terminating the treatment, with sessions often conducted biweekly or monthly.

The therapist should attempt to engage in treatment as many family members as possible but settle for working with whoever is willing to participate. Whenever possible, the client should participate with at least one other family member, preferably the one with whom the client has the most contact. Therapists should try to directly engage all family members with regular contact (weekly or biweekly contact) and inform members who are reluctant to participate that they are free to join the sessions at a later time (i.e., an "open door" policy).

In some family situations, it is helpful to involve more family members in the psychoeducational component of BFT and to work more intensively with a smaller group of family members to help them develop better communication and problem-solving skills. For example, if the client lives with his or her parents and has occasional contact with siblings, the therapist might consider including all the family members in the educational sessions about mental illness while focusing the communication and problem-solving training on just the client and his or her parents. In addition, the relative emphasis on these three components of BFT may be altered depending on the specific needs of the family. For example, families who have relatively little contact with the client may benefit primarily from learning more about the nature of schizophrenia and its treatment. Family members who have regular contact with the client, but who experience relatively few problems, may benefit from more emphasis on education and communication skills training, with less time spent on problem-solving training (e.g., a client who lives in a state hospital and sees his or her parents on a weekly basis). In general, the full BFT program is most appropriate for clients who have weekly contact with family members, especially for clients who live at home.

Engagement. Engaging the family is the single most critical step of treatment because without it, the therapist can go no further. Engagement can be broken down into three specific steps: emphasizing the importance of family work to the client, engaging the willingness of relatives to participate in BFT, and conducting an orientation meeting with the client and relatives to set positive expectations for their participation in BFT.

Clients are often skeptical about involving their family in treatment, and thus the therapist must explain the advantages of family work and how the BFT program works. BFT can be described as a time-limited program aimed at teaching basic information, decreasing stress through improved communication, and helping family members solve problems together in a cooperative manner. The therapist should present participation in BFT as a strong recommendation of the treatment team and not simply a possible treatment option.

Clients who express concerns about participating in BFT generally express one of two types of reservations. First, clients may be afraid that sessions will be stressful and involve significant family conflict. This concern can be addressed by explaining that BFT is a program aimed at helping families learn new positive skills for working together, and that it is oriented to the future, not digging up the past. Therefore, family sessions are not stressful, and the therapist ensures that there is a good working environment conducive to learning new information and skills. Second, clients may be reluctant to participate because they do not want to burden their relatives with more involvement in their treatment. These clients are often aware that their psychiatric illness has affected their family, and they are eager to spare them more grief. This concern can be addressed by explaining that

BFT is aimed at not just helping the client but also helping everyone in the family, including relatives. Thus, by participating in BFT, clients are helping reduce stress and burden on their relatives.

After the client agrees to participate in BFT, the therapist asks him or her to identify the closest family member with whom the topic of BFT can be broached. Some clients prefer to bring it up with their relatives, but many others are happy for the therapist to do it on their behalf. Similar to when describing BFT to clients, the therapist should explain that participation in BFT is a strong treatment recommendation from the client's team. When describing BFT, the therapist can explain the nature of the program in ways similar to how it was presented to the client. Family members in particular see value in the goals of working together to prevent relapses and rehospitalizations, learning more about the psychiatric illness, and learning how to support the client in becoming as self-sufficient as possible. During conversations with family members, the therapist may learn about other concerns of family members and should explain how those concerns will be addressed in BFT. BFT is often described briefly in a telephone contact with a relative and then in more detail in an in-person meeting, although many other possibilities exist.

One useful concept for engaging the relatives is to explain that a goal of BFT is to make the family extended members of the client's treatment team. This can have a powerful effect on family members because it connotes respect and a desire to collaborate with them as well as an understanding of the importance of their perspectives. Many relatives readily agree to participate in BFT after listening to a description of the program. The most common obstacle experienced in engaging relatives is burnout. Relatives may feel they have already invested huge amounts of time and energy in helping their ill family member, and they may feel frustrated and a sense of futility at the prospect of more work. With such family members, it is most helpful for the therapist to first empathize with the challenges the relative has faced and to then discuss the possibility of trying some sessions of BFT and agreeing to stop at a designated point to reevaluate whether the family sessions appear to be useful.

Once the client and one or more family members have agreed to participate in BFT, an orientation meeting is scheduled to review how BFT works and to begin planning the first meetings. At this meeting, the therapist gives all the family members an orientation sheet, which reviews the logistics of the program and the core components and also summarizes expectations of the family members and what the family members can expect of the therapist (Mueser & Glynn, 1999). The therapist reviews the sheet and answers any questions from family members. After the orientation session is completed, the therapist arranges individual meetings with each family member and schedules the first family session devoted to psychoeducation.

Assessment. The purpose of the individual assessments with each family member is to solidify a therapeutic relationship with each person; to understand their perceptions of the family, including its strengths and weaknesses; and to help members set personal goals for the BFT. Individual assessment includes a review of the family member's living situation, family history, understanding of the mental illness, perceptions of what helps and worsens the illness, and personal goals. Individual assessments are not pathology based but instead include a focus on family strengths, which can be capitalized on by the therapist when helping the family help the member with the mental illness.

In addition to the individual family interviews, the therapist conducts ongoing assessments of the family based on observations

of how members communicate with one another (Do they argue frequently? Are they sarcastic or hostile to one another? Is there a high level of tension during family interactions?). Similarly, the therapist observes how family members work on problems together, which is informative when conducting communication and problem-solving training. Individual family assessment meetings are usually quite relaxed, relatively informal, and quite naturally involve deviations from the standard questions included in the interview. These interviews usually require approximately 1 hour to complete.

Psychoeducation. Psychoeducation involves teaching people about the family member's specific mental illness and its management in a lively, interactive style that encourages all members, including the client, to share their observations and experiences in a free and open manner. Between three and five sessions are typically spent teaching educational material to the family, with handouts used to guide the teaching process. The therapist frequently pauses to ask questions about the material and to help family members identify specific examples in which information may apply to their own experiences. Table 8.2 identifies educational topics that may be discussed in these sessions.

One powerful technique for educating families about a mental illness is to denote the client as the "expert" and to request his or her assistance in teaching relatives about the experience of the illness. Denoting the client as the expert gives the client a unique and respected status in the family. The client need not acknowledge that he or she has the psychiatric disorder in question to accept the role of the expert. When clients do not accept their diagnosis, rather than trying to persuade them, the therapist can explain that it is simply a term used to describe a group of symptoms that often occur together. The therapist can then adopt alternative language

Table 8.2 Topics for Psychoeducational Sessions

Basic facts about mental illness
Bipolar disorder
Major depression
Obsessive compulsive disorder
Posttraumatic stress disorder
Schizoaffective disorder
Schizophrenia
Antipsychotic medications
Antidepressant medications
Mood-stabilizing medications
Sedative and hypnotic medications
Stress vulnerability model
Role of the family
Drug and alcohol use
A guide to effective communication

Reproducible educational handouts are available in Mueser and Glynn (1999).

for referring to the disorder in ways that the client finds more acceptable, such as "these kinds of problems," "a nervous condition," or "just a disorder." The client's experience with the mental illness is then elicited in the process of explaining the nature of the disorder and its treatment. The following is an example of how the therapist can explain hallucinations using the client's expertise to illustrate it:

Therapist: One common symptom of schizophrenia is hallucinations. Hallucinations are seeing, hearing, feeling, smelling, or tasting something when nothing around the person actually caused that sensation. The most common kind of hallucination is auditory hallucinations or hearing voices. When people have auditory hallucinations, they are often heard through their ears and sound just like a regular voice even though no one is actually talking. Joe, have you ever had hallucinations?

Joe (the client): Sometimes I hear these guys calling me names. Or I hear people talking about me.

Therapist: I see. What's that like?

Joe: It's distracting because I start listening to the voices. It also gets me down. I don't like it.

Therapist: Yes, it's common for people to feel distracted and upset when they hear voices. Darlene? Did you know Joe hears voices?

Darlene (the mother): Yes, I thought he's heard voices and sometimes he's talked about it. But I always thought that he heard the voices just inside his head. I didn't realize that they sounded like they came through his ears.

Joe: Yes, they sound just like regular voices, except they're usually putting me down.

Throughout the psychoeducational sessions, it is critical for the therapist to create an accepting atmosphere in which all family members can talk openly and express their opinions, and different perspectives can be acknowledged. Because at this point in treatment family members usually do not have well-developed problem-solving skills, therapists should acknowledge differences in opinions and perspectives without pushing to resolve them. Sometimes, family members may want to resolve family differences, and in those circumstances the therapist can step in and point out that these differences may be addressed in the problem-solving component of BFT.

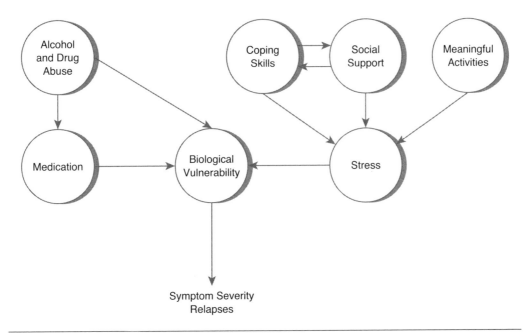

Figure 8.1   Stress-vulnerability model of major mental illness. This model proposes that major mental illnesses are caused by biological vulnerability, which interacts with stress in the environment. The stress-vulnerability model suggests the course of major mental illness can be improved by taking medications; avoiding alcohol and drug use; reducing stress; improving coping; increasing social support; and getting involved in meaningful activities, such as work, school, or fulfilling parenting responsibilities.

The session that addresses the nature of the client's mental illness is aimed at establishing it as a disease, describing its prevalence, how the illness is diagnosed, common symptoms, and associated impairments. Educating families about medication involves focusing on those medications that the client is currently prescribed, explaining the benefits of medication (e.g., symptom reduction and prevention of relapses) and their side effects, and correcting misconceptions about medication (e.g., the belief that they are addictive). Problems with medication adherence are common in major mental illnesses (Amdur, 1979; Coldham, Addington, & Addington, 2002), and the importance of taking medication is emphasized. When adherence is a problem, strategies are discussed for increasing the regularity of taking medication, such

as building in the taking of medications into the client's daily routine (Azrin & Teichner, 1998) and involving relatives in monitoring medication adherence.

When describing the stress-vulnerability model of mental illness (Figure 8.1), the therapist explains that the illness has a biological basis, which can be influenced by both biological and social factors. Medication can reduce biological vulnerability (thereby reducing risk of relapse), whereas drugs and alcohol can increase vulnerability (thereby increasing risk of relapse). Stress can also increase biological vulnerability, whereas effective coping skills and good social support can reduce the negative effects of stress. Thus, the stress-vulnerability model provides a conceptual framework to the family for the management of mental illness.

The educational topic on the role of the family addresses how family members can play a positive role by helping monitor the client's illness, encouraging medication adherence, decreasing stress, increasing coping skills, and helping the client pursue his or her personal goals. The educational handout on drugs and alcohol discusses the interactions between commonly abused substances and the symptoms and course of mental illness. When clients have special problems related to drug and alcohol abuse, additional educational sessions are conducted to educate the family about substance abuse and to motivate them to address these problems later in BFT if the client continues to use substances (Mueser & Fox, 2002). More educational handouts specifically focused on the topic of substance abuse and severe mental illness can be found in Mueser, Noordsy, Drake, and Fox (2003). Finally, the educational topic on communication skills highlights the importance of good communication (e.g., minimization of stress and facilitation of problem solving) and describes strategies for communicating effectively.

Communication Skills Training

Not all families need communication skills training, but for some it is an essential prerequisite to problem solving. Without effective communication, family members cannot discuss and cooperatively solve problems. An indication that the family may benefit from communication skills training is the presence of a high level of tension during family interactions; for example, members frequently raise their voices, call each other names, or express themselves in irritable or intrusive ways. In such circumstances, family members may benefit from three to six sessions of communication skills training.

Training is oriented toward teaching more effective and less stressful communication strategies. A premium is placed on encouraging communication that is direct, brief, behaviorally specific (when possible), and makes clear verbal statements about feelings (when appropriate). The therapist explains to family members that good communication is helpful in all walks of life, especially in close relationships with other people. In times of stress or when facing pressing problems, good communication can be easily lost, resulting in conflict and strife.

Communication skills training is taught using the principles of social skills training (Bellack, Mueser, Gingerich, & Agresta, 2004). These steps include the following:

1. Establish a rationale for learning the skill ("Why might it be helpful to be able to express positive feelings to other people?").

2. Break the skill into component steps, and discuss each step.

3. Demonstrate the skill in a role play.

4. Discuss family members' observations of the therapist's demonstration of the skill.

5. Engage a family member in a role play of the skill.

6. Obtain specific, positive feedback from family members about that person's role play.

7. Elicit or provide corrective feedback for how the skill could be done even better.

8. Engage the person in another role play (when appropriate and feasible).

9. Provide suggestions for improved performance, conduct another role play (if appropriate), and obtain positive and corrective feedback about it.

10. Assign homework to practice the skill.

Each family member is engaged in practicing the skill and providing feedback to other members about their performance. Role plays are tailored to actual situations that family members have experienced or situations they may experience in the future.

Table 8.3 Communication Skills Taught in Behavioral Family Therapy

Expressing positive feelings

Look at the person who pleased you.
Tell him or her exactly what he or she did to please you—be specific.
Tell him or her the feeling it gave you—be precise.

Making a positive request

Look at the person to whom you are making a request.
Tell him or her exactly what you are requesting—be specific.
Tell him or her how it would make you feel if the request were met—be precise.

Expressing negative feelings

Look at the person who displeased you.
Tell him or her exactly what he or she did to displease you—be specific.
Tell him or her the feeling it gave you—be precise.
Make a positive request for change, if possible.

Active listening

Look speaker in eye.
Nod head.
Ask clarifying questions.
Paraphrase what you have heard.
Wait until the speaker finishes before responding.

Compromise and negotiation

Look at the person.
Explain your viewpoint.
Listen to the other person's viewpoint.
Repeat back what you heard.
Suggest a compromise (more than one may be necessary).

Requesting a time-out

Indicate that the situation is stressful.
Tell the person that it is interfering with constructive communication.
Say that you must leave temporarily.
State when you will return, and be willing to problem solve.

Up to six specific communication skills are taught. Each skill is broken down into several components, with role-play instruction and feedback oriented toward particular components but addressing other aspects of social skill as well (e.g., nonverbal paralinguistic skills such as eye contact and voice volume). The specific skills and their component steps are summarized in Table 8.3. These skills cover the basics of social interaction, including listening to other people, expressing positive feelings, making requests, expressing negative feelings, compromising with others, and leaving a stressful situation.

Effective basic communication skills facilitate good problem solving because they keep bad temper in check and facilitate good will.

Problem-Solving Training

Problem-solving training involves teaching a standard set of steps for solving problems between people. Problem-solving training is aimed at provoking a frank but constructive discussion about how to deal with a problem or work toward achieving a desired goal. Collaboration on the steps of problem solving includes (a) talking about and agreeing on a definition of the goal, (b) brainstorming possible solutions to the problem or goal, (c) evaluating the advantages and disadvantages of each solution, (d) selecting the best solution or combination of solutions, (e) making a plan for how to implement the solution (e.g., consider who will do what, what resources are needed, and when different parts of the plan will be implemented), and (f) setting up a time to follow up the plan and to troubleshoot as necessary.

Family problem solving is conducted by electing a chairperson to lead the problem-solving session. A secretary may also be identified to keep track of the different steps of problem solving, including possible solutions and their advantages and disadvantages, if this function is not performed by the chairperson. The chairperson's role is not to solve the problem but, rather, to lead the family in using the steps of problem solving to address the problem or goal.

Problem-solving training is taught by the therapist by first explaining the rationale and steps behind problem solving and then assuming the role of the chairperson in solving problems with family members. Gradually over time, the therapist hands over to the family the responsibility of running problem-solving discussions as their skills develop and they are able to conduct independent problem solving. Families are given homework assignments to practice solving problems on their own, and during sessions they discuss difficulties they have experienced using the method. Simple problems can often be solved in a single session. Complex problems may require multiple problem-solving efforts either to overcome major problems that are encountered or because many steps are required to achieve the desired outcome.

A wide variety of problems can be addressed through problem solving, such as agreeing on household responsibilities, planning leisure and recreation pursuits, dealing with problematic symptoms, finding new places to meet friends, and dealing with drug and alcohol abuse. Problem-solving training is generally conducted for at least 5 or 6 sessions and often more than 15 sessions. Although the goal is for family members to become self-sufficient in solving problems, some families require ongoing meetings with the therapist to deal with problems. Such meetings can be either scheduled (e.g., monthly) or provided on an as-needed basis. Families in which the client has extremely severe symptoms, multiple members have psychiatric disorders, substance abuse, or cognitive impairment, or who face harsh economic conditions or health problems may benefit from maintenance problem-solving meetings.

RESEARCH ON FAMILY INTERVENTION FOR MAJOR MENTAL ILLNESS

During the past 25 years, extensive research has been conducted evaluating the effectiveness of family intervention programs for people with major mental disorders, including many randomized controlled trials. The majority of these programs have focused on the treatment of schizophrenia or schizoaffective disorder, although a growing body of research also documents the beneficial effects on bipolar disorder, major depression, and other severe psychiatric illnesses. Most of these studies have evaluated different models of family intervention sharing the core components of family work summarized in Table 8.1.

Research on family intervention can be summarized by several key findings that are consistent across multiple studies (Dixon, McFarlane, et al., 2001; Falloon et al., 1999; Pilling et al., 2002; Pitschel-Walz, Leucht, Bäuml, Kissling, & Engel, 2001). First, family intervention is effective at reducing clients' relapses and rehospitalizations, with research indicating that the risk of relapse following family intervention is reduced by approximately one half compared to that of clients not receiving family intervention. Second, family therapy programs that are longer tend to have better outcomes than brief family intervention programs. For example, the most effective family intervention programs usually last between 9 months and 2 years, whereas much more limited benefits accrue in programs that are 3 months or less in duration. Third, family intervention programs tend to produce modest benefits in terms of client functioning, such as reduced symptoms and improved functioning (e.g., social or vocational functioning). Fourth, family intervention is associated with reduced burden and distress among relatives and other caregivers. Finally, because of the effects of family intervention on reducing relapses and rehospitalizations, research indicates that family therapy is cost-effective and results in a net savings in total health care costs (Cardin, McGill, & Falloon, 1986; Tarrier, Lowson, & Barrowclough, 1991).

Whereas the majority of research has examined the effects of family intervention programs provided by mental health professionals, more limited research has evaluated the effects of family educational programs conducted by relatives of people with major mental illnesses. These programs typically provide 4 to 16 weeks of educational sessions, aimed primarily at caregivers but not the family member with the mental illness, and focus on a combination of information about mental illness and its management and social support (Burland, 1998). Preliminary research on these programs indicates that they provide benefits to caregivers in terms of increased knowledge and self-confidence in the management of mental illness and decreased burden of care (Dixon et al., 2004; Dixon, Stewart, et al., 2001; Solomon, Draine, Mannion, & Meisel, 1996).

Although research provides strong support for family therapy programs for people with major mental illnesses, many questions remain to be answered. For example, most studies on schizophrenia and bipolar disorder have focused on families in which the offspring has a major mental illness, and the relatives are caregivers. Less research has evaluated the effectiveness of these models when working with other family constellations, such as siblings and spouses of an individual with major mental illness, despite the significant burden of care often experienced by these relatives (Clausen, 1986; Mannion, Mueser, & Solomon, 1994; Moorman, 1992).

Another unresolved question concerns the timing of family intervention programs. Although it may be assumed that family therapy programs are most effective when delivered soon after the onset of a major mental illness, research addressing this question has produced conflicting results (Leavey et al., 2004; Linszen et al., 1996; Linszen & Dingemans, 2002). In addition, it is unknown how family programs need to be adapted to address the specific and different needs of a family coming to grips with the reality of a relative who has recently developed a major mental illness compared to a family who has been struggling with the illness for years. Early in the course of the mental illness, families often experience significant challenges learning to accept the psychiatric illness, developing realistic expectations for their relative, and learning how to partner with the treatment team in the management of the illness (Edwards & McGorry, 2002). Later, families often experience significant burnout from the stress of long-term caregiving, and these challenges may lead to a sense of hopelessness and helplessness that immobilizes the family from working together to help the client improve his or her life (Baronet, 1999).

Another future direction for research on family intervention concerns the question of how treatment models need to be modified to address co-occurring disorders that often occur with a major mental illness. For example, approximately half of all individuals with a major mental illness have a substance use disorder (abuse or dependence) at some time in their lives, and such disorders greatly complicate and worsen the outcome of the mental illness (Mueser et al., 2000; Regier et al., 1990). Similarly, research has shown that many individuals with major mental illnesses have co-occurring posttraumatic stress disorder, which is also associated with worsening of the mental illness (Mueser, Rosenberg, Goodman, & Trumbetta, 2002). Research has begun to address the challenge of treating substance use problems in individuals with a major mental illness, but this research is still in its infancy (Barrowclough, 2003; Barrowclough et al., 2001; Mueser & Fox, 2002). Work has yet to be conducted on family intervention with individuals with major mental illness and co-occurring posttraumatic stress disorder, although individual and group treatment approaches for this problem have been developed and are being evaluated (Harris, 1998; Mueser, Rosenberg, Jankowski, Hamblen, & Descamps, 2004; Rosenberg, Mueser, Jankowski, Salyers, & Acker, 2004).

Family intervention programs have been developed and tested in a variety of different cultures, but the nature and need for adaptations of these models remain to be determined from many cultures. Clearly, family intervention needs to be informed by an understanding of the culture to which the family belongs (Lefley, 1987), and work must be conducted within that family's cultural context (McGoldrick, Giordano, & Pearce, 1996). Extensive work has been conducted on families in U.S., British, and several European cultures, and some research has also been conducted in China. The need for and nature of cultural adaptation of family intervention programs for individuals living in Third World nations, where major mental illnesses are frequently underdetected and undertreated, remain to be determined. Family interventions in these cultures may be especially important because in many cases the family may be the only care providers available to the individual (Institute of Medicine, 2001).

SUMMARY

Major mental illnesses, such as schizophrenia, bipolar disorder, and major depression, have a dramatic effect on afflicted individuals and their loved ones, and the effective management of these disorders is truly a "family affair." Family intervention programs have been developed that are aimed at helping caregivers and clients work collaboratively with mental health professionals to improve the course of these disorders and help individuals and their relatives achieve personal and shared goals. Research supports the effectiveness of these programs in terms of both improving client outcomes and decreasing stress on the family. Collaborative family work is an important tool in clinicians' armamentarium for working with people with major mental illnesses.

REFERENCES

Amdur, M. (1979). Medication compliance in outpatient psychiatry. *Comprehensive Psychiatry, 20,* 339-346.

Anderson, C. M., Reiss, D. J., & Hogarty, G. E. (1986). *Schizophrenia and the family.* New York: Guilford.

Azrin, N. H., & Teichner, G. (1998). Evaluation of an instructional program for improving medication compliance for chronically mentally ill outpatients. *Behaviour Research and Therapy, 36,* 849-861.

Backlar, P. (1994). *The family face of schizophrenia.* New York: Tarcher/Putnam.

Baronet, A. M. (1999). Factors associated with caregiver burden in mental illness: A critical review of the research literature. *Clinical Psychology Review, 19,* 819-841.

Barrowclough, C. (2003). Family intervention for substance misuse in psychosis. In H. L. Graham, A. Copello, M. J. Birchwood, & K. T. Mueser (Eds.), *Substance misuse in psychosis: Approaches to treatment and service delivery* (pp. 227-243). Chichester, UK: Wiley.

Barrowclough, C., Haddock, G., Tarrier, N., Lewis, S., Moring, J., O'Brien, R., et al. (2001). Randomized controlled trial of motivational interviewing, cognitive behavior therapy, and family intervention for patients with comorbid schizophrenia and substance use disorders. *American Journal of Psychiatry, 158,* 1706-1713.

Barrowclough, C., & Tarrier, N. (1992). *Families of schizophrenic patients: Cognitive behavioural intervention.* London: Chapman & Hall.

Bateson, G., Jackson, D. D., Haley, J., & Weakland, J. (1956). Toward a theory of schizophrenia. *Behavioral Science, 1,* 251-264.

Bebbington, P., & Kuipers, L. (1992). Life events and social factors. In D. J. Kavanagh (Ed.), *Schizophrenia: An overview and practical handbook* (pp. 126-144). London: Chapman & Hall.

Bellack, A. S., Mueser, K. T., Gingerich, S., & Agresta, J. (2004). *Social skills training for schizophrenia: A step-by-step guide* (2nd ed.). New York: Guilford.

Breslau, N., & Davis, G. (1985). Chronic stress and major depression. *Archives of General Psychiatry, 43,* 309-314.

Bulger, M. W., Wandersman, A., & Goldman, C. R. (1993). Burdens and gratifications of caregiving: Appraisal of parental care of adults with schizophrenia. *American Journal of Orthopsychiatry, 63,* 255-265.

Burland, J. (1998). Family-to-family: A trauma and recovery model of family education. *New Directions in Mental Health Services, 77,* 33-44.

Butzlaff, R. L., & Hooley, J. M. (1998). Expressed emotion and psychiatric relapse. *Archives of General Psychiatry, 55,* 547-552.

Cardin, V. A., McGill, C. W., & Falloon, I. R. H. (1986). An economic analysis: Costs, benefits and effectiveness. In I. R. H. Falloon (Ed.), *Family management of schizophrenia* (pp. 15-123). Baltimore: Johns Hopkins University Press.

Caton, C. L. M., Shrout, P. E., Eagle, P. F., Opler, L. A., & Felix, A. (1994). Correlates of codisorders in homeless and never homeless indigent schizophrenic men. *Psychological Medicine, 24,* 681-688.

Clark, R. (1994). Family costs associated with severe mental illness and substance use: A comparison of families with and without dual disorders. *Hospital and Community Psychiatry, 45,* 808-813.

Clausen, J. A. (1986). A 15- to 20-year follow-up of married adult psychiatric patients. In L. Erlenmeyer-Kimling & N. E. Miller (Eds.), *Life-span research on the prediction of psychopathology* (pp. 175-194). Hillsdale, NJ: Lawrence Erlbaum.

Coldham, E. L., Addington, J., & Addington, D. (2002). Medication adherence of individuals with a first episode of psychosis. *Acta Psychiatrica Scandinavica, 106,* 286-290.

Coyne, J. C., Kessler, R. C., Tal, M., Turnbull, J., Wortman, C. B., & Greden, J. F. (1987). Living with a depressed person. *Journal of Consulting and Clinical Psychology, 55,* 347-352.

Dixon, L., Lucksted, A., Stewart, B., Burland, J., Brown, C. H., Postrado, L., et al. (2004). Outcomes of the peer-taught 12-week family-to-family education program for severe mental illness. *Acta Psychiatrica Scandinavica, 109,* 207-215.

Dixon, L., McFarlane, W., Lefley, H., Lucksted, A., Cohen, C., Falloon, I., et al. (2001). Evidence-based practices for services to family members of people with psychiatric disabilities. *Psychiatric Services, 52,* 903-910.

Dixon, L., Stewart, B., Burland, J., Delahanty, J., Lucksted, A., & Hoffman, M. (2001). Pilot study of the family-to-family education program. *Psychiatric Services, 52,* 965-967.

Edwards, J., & McGorry, P. D. (2002). *Implementing early intervention in psychosis: A guide to establishing early psychosis services.* London: Martin Dunitz.

Falloon, I. R. H., Boyd, J. L., & McGill, C. W. (1984). *Family care of schizophrenia: A problem-solving approach to the treatment of mental illness.* New York: Guilford.

Falloon, I. R. H., Boyd, J. L., McGill, C. W., Williamson, M., Razani, J., Moss, H. B., et al. (1985). Family management in the prevention of morbidity of schizophrenia: Clinical outcome of a two year longitudinal study. *Archives of General Psychiatry, 42,* 887-896.

Falloon, I. R. H., Held, T., Coverdale, J. H., Roncone, R., & Laidlaw, T. M. (1999). Family interventions for schizophrenia: A review of long-term benefits of international studies. *Psychiatric Rehabilitation Skills, 3,* 268-290.

Fromm-Reichman, F. (1948). Notes on the development of treatment of schizophrenics by psychoanalytic psychotherapy. *Psychiatry, 1,* 263-273.

Greenley, J. R. (1986). Social control and expressed emotion. *Journal of Nervous and Mental Disease, 174,* 24-30.

Harris, M. (1998). *Trauma recovery and empowerment: A clinician's guide for working with women in groups.* New York: Free Press.

Hatfield, A. B., & Lefley, H. P. (Eds.). (1987). *Families of the mentally ill: Coping and adaptation.* New York: Guilford.

Institute of Medicine. (2001). *Neurological, psychiatric, and developmental disorders: Meeting the challenges in the developing world.* Washington, DC: National Academy of Sciences.

Kuipers, L., Leff, J., & Lam, D. (2002). *Family work for schizophrenia: A practical guide* (2nd ed.). London: Gaskell.

Leavey, G., Gulamhussein, S., Papadopoulos, C., Johnson-Sabine, E., Blizard, B., & King, M. (2004). A randomized controlled trial of a brief intervention for families of patients with a first episode of psychosis. *Psychological Medicine, 34,* 423-431.

Leff, J., & Vaughn, C. (Eds.). (1985). *Expressed emotion in families.* New York: Guilford.

Lefley, H. P. (1987). Culture and mental illness: The family role. In A. B. Hatfield (Ed.), *Families of the mentally ill* (pp. 30-59). New York: Guilford.

Lefley, H. P. (1996). *Family caregiving in mental illness.* Thousand Oaks, CA: Sage.

Linszen, D., Dingemans, P., Van der Does, A. J. W., Scholte, P., Lenior, R., & Goldstein, M. J. (1996). Treatment, expressed emotion and relapse in recent onset schizophrenic disorders. *Psychological Medicine, 26,* 333-342.

Linszen, D. H., & Dingemans, P. M. (2002). Early psychosis, schizophrenia and the family. In A. Schaub (Ed.), *New family interventions and associated research in psychiatric disorders* (pp. 59-76). Vienna: Springer-Verlag.

Mannion, E., Mueser, K. T., & Solomon, P. (1994). Designing psychoeducational services for spouses of persons with serious mental illness. *Community Mental Health Journal, 30,* 177-189.

McFarlane, W. R. (2002). *Multifamily groups in the treatment of severe psychiatric disorders.* New York: Guilford.

McGoldrick, M., Giordano, J., & Pearce, J. (Eds.). (1996). *Ethnicity and family therapy* (2nd ed.). New York: Guilford.

Miklowitz, D. J., & Goldstein, M. J. (1997). *Bipolar disorder: A family-focused treatment approach*. New York: Guilford.

Miller, R., Dworkin, J., Ward, M., & Barone, D. (1990). A preliminary study of unresolved grief in families of seriously mentally ill patients. *Hospital and Community Psychiatry, 41,* 1321-1325.

Moorman, M. (1992). *My sister's keeper: Learning to cope with a sibling's mental illness*. New York: Norton.

Mueser, K. T., & Fox, L. (2002). A family intervention program for dual disorders. *Community Mental Health Journal, 38,* 253-270.

Mueser, K. T., & Glynn, S. M. (1999). *Behavioral family therapy for psychiatric disorders* (2nd ed.). Oakland, CA: New Harbinger.

Mueser, K. T., Noordsy, D. L., Drake, R. E., & Fox, L. (2003). *Integrated treatment for dual disorders: A guide to effective practice*. New York: Guilford.

Mueser, K. T., Rosenberg, S. D., Goodman, L. A., & Trumbetta, S. L. (2002). Trauma, PTSD, and the course of schizophrenia: An interactive model. *Schizophrenia Research, 53,* 123-143.

Mueser, K. T., Rosenberg, S. D., Jankowski, M. K., Hamblen, J., & Descamps, M. (2004). A cognitive-behavioral treatment program for posttraumatic stress disorder in severe mental illness. *American Journal of Psychiatric Rehabilitation, 7,* 107-146.

Mueser, K. T., Webb, C., Pfeiffer, M., Gladis, M., & Levinson, D. F. (1996). Family burden of schizophrenia and bipolar disorder: Perceptions of relatives and professionals. *Psychiatric Services, 47,* 507-511.

Mueser, K. T., Yarnold, P. R., Rosenberg, S. D., Swett, C., Miles, K. M., & Hill, D. (2000). Substance use disorder in hospitalized severely mentally ill psychiatric patients: Prevalence, correlates, and subgroups. *Schizophrenia Bulletin, 26,* 179-192.

Oldridge, M. L., & Hughes, I. C. T. (1992). Psychological well-being in families with a member suffering from schizophrenia: An investigation into long-standing problems. *British Journal of Psychiatry, 161,* 249-251.

Pilling, S., Bebbington, P., Kuipers, E., Garety, P., Geddes, J. R., Orbach, G., et al. (2002). Psychological treatments in schizophrenia: I. Meta-analysis of family intervention and cognitive behaviour therapy. *Psychological Medicine, 32,* 763-782.

Pitschel-Walz, G., Leucht, S., Bäuml, J., Kissling, W., & Engel, R. R. (2001). The effect of family interventions on relapse and rehospitalization in schizophrenia: A meta-analysis. *Schizophrenia Bulletin, 27,* 73-92.

Randolph, E. T., Eth, S., Glynn, S., Paz, G. B., Leong, G. B., Shaner, A. L., et al. (1994). Behavioural family management in schizophrenia: Outcome from a clinic-based intervention. *British Journal of Psychiatry, 144,* 501-506.

Regier, D. A., Farmer, M. E., Rae, D. S., Locke, B. Z., Keith, S. J., Judd, L. L., et al. (1990). Comorbidity of mental disorders with alcohol and other drug abuse: Results from the Epidemiologic Catchment Area (ECA) study. *Journal of the American Medical Association, 264,* 2511-2518.

Rosenberg, S. D., Mueser, K. T., Jankowski, M. K., Salyers, M. P., & Acker, K. (2004). Cognitive-behavioral treatment of posttraumatic stress disorder in severe mental illness: Results of a pilot study. *American Journal of Psychiatric Rehabilitation, 7,* 171-186.

Solomon, P., Draine, J., Mannion, E., & Meisel, M. (1996). Impact of brief family psychoeducation on self-efficacy. *Schizophrenia Bulletin, 22,* 41-50.

Steadman, H. J., Mulvey, E. P., Monahan, J., Robbins, P. C., Appelbaum, P. S., Grisso, T., et al. (1998). Violence by people discharged from acute psychiatric inpatient facilities and by others in the same neighborhoods. *Archives of General Psychiatry, 55,* 393-401.

Swados, E. (1991). *The four of us: A family memoir.* New York: Farrar, Straus & Giroux.

Tarrier, N., Lowson, K., & Barrowclough, C. (1991). Some aspects of family interventions in schizophrenia: II. Financial considerations. *British Journal of Psychiatry, 167,* 473-479.

Weisman, A. Y., Nuechterlein, K. H., Goldstein, M. J., & Snyder, K. S. (1998). Expressed emotion, attitudes, and schizophrenic symptom dimensions. *Journal of Abnormal Psychology, 107,* 355-359.

CHAPTER 9

Families, Coping Styles, and Health

Arlene L. Vetere and Lynn B. Myers

This chapter describes a series of published studies, designed to explore the relationship between repressive coping style (Weinberger, 1990) and adult romantic attachment style (Simpson, 1990), and the links with self-reported coping and health. We discuss why these links might be important for the practice of family therapists.

We performed a series of small-scale studies on young adults, using self-report psychometric data, to explore the possible relationships between (a) repressive coping style, coping resources, and reported psychological and physical well-being; (b) repressive coping style and adult attachment style; and (c) adult attachment style, coping resources, and reported psychological and physical well-being.

CONCEPTUAL AND OPERATIONAL DEFINITIONS

Before presenting the series of studies and their implications, we describe the main concepts and measures we used in the studies to orient the reader, including repressive coping style (Weinberger, 1990), adult attachment style (Hazan & Shaver, 1987), the Coping Resources Inventory (Hammer & Marting, 1988), the Hazan and Shaver prototypes, the Simpson Questionnaire (Simpson, 1990), the General Health Questionnaire (GHQ-12) (Goldberg, 1992), and the Pennebaker Inventory of Limpid Languidness (Pennebaker, 1982).

Repressive Coping Style

There is increasing research interest in a group of individuals who are said to possess a repressive coping style (i.e., people who avoid negative affect). Repressive coping style is thought to be associated with an avoidant style of information processing (Myers & McKenna, 1996), with restricted access to negative emotional memories (Davis, 1987). Weinberger (1990) concluded that "repressors as a group, seem actively engaged in keeping themselves (rather than just other people) convinced that they are *not* prone to negative affect" (p. 338).

The repressive coping style is operationally defined psychometrically by low scores on a measure of trait anxiety, such as the Bendig version of the Manifest Anxiety Scale (MAS;

Bendig, 1956), and high scores on a measure of defensiveness, such as the Social Desirability Scale (Crowne & Marlowe, 1964). Weinberger (1990) originally proposed a fourfold classification of individuals, using quartile splits, differentiated in terms of their coping styles: repressor (REP; low anxiety and high defensiveness), low anxious (LA; low anxiety and low defensiveness), high anxious (HA; high anxiety and low defensiveness), and defensive high anxious (DHA; high anxiety and high defensiveness).

Most research studies compare the repressor group with the other three extreme scoring "control" groups, often omitting from the comparisons nearly half of the research sample, who do not score within the low and high ranges of the psychometric measures. In our studies, we compared the repressor groups with the traditional control groups and with the total research sample. We justify this on the basis that we are interested in the health behavior of all our participants.

Previous research on the group of people described as having a repressive coping style has produced some robust findings that are crucial to our thinking. First, individuals with a repressive coping style have been defined in a number of studies as comprising between 10% and 20% of research samples (Myers, 1993). Second, in stressful situations, individuals with a repressive coping style report low levels of subjective distress but are physiologically highly reactive (i.e., they seem to exhibit a dissociation between self-report and physiological measures of stress). This finding has been widely replicated (Myers & Vetere, 1997; Vetere & Myers, 2002). Third, there is increasing evidence of an association between repressive coping style and the development and course of disease. For example, studies have reported an association between the repressive coping style and impaired immune function (Jamner, Schwartz, & Leigh, 1988), carcinogenic disease (Jensen, 1987), and

cardiovascular disease risk (Miller, 1991). This possible association between repressive coping and illness is not surprising, considering that dissociations between self-report and physiological measures of arousal may produce adverse health outcomes because somatic signs might be less likely to stimulate health- or help-seeking behaviors designed to relieve distress. Thus, individuals with a repressive coping style comprise a significant minority of people who are of interest to health care practitioners.

Adult Romantic Attachment Style

We were curious about the developmental origins of repressive coping style. There is some indication that it may develop in childhood. For example, in an interview study of women described as having a repressive coping style, Myers and Brewin (1994) found that they had experienced poor relationships with their fathers.

Bowlby (1979) described attachment as the "propensity of human beings to make strong affectional bonds to particular others" (p. 18). The quality of a child's attachment relationship is thought to be rooted in the degree to which the child can rely on his or her caregiver to be a source of security. A basic principle of attachment theory is that attachment relationships continue to be important throughout the life span. Hazan and Shaver (1987) proposed that romantic love between adults is an attachment process. In particular, they proposed that the three primary attachment styles of emotional bonding of a child to an adult caregiver (i.e., secure, avoidant, anxious/ambivalent) also exist in adulthood and influence the ways adults experience romantic love and behave in romantic attachments.

Various studies have found that reported secure adult attachment is related to marital satisfaction and acceptance, and provision of physical and emotional support in anxiety-eliciting situations, whereas insecure attachment styles exhibit the opposite patterns of care. Main and Goldwyn (1984) suggest that early insensitive or rejecting parenting may lead to an adult avoidant attachment style. They describe a group of individuals who devalue the importance of relationships, report extremely positive relationships with their parents (even perfect relationships) that they cannot substantiate with actual memories of empathic or loving episodes, and downplay the influence of childhood experiences. The individuals are said to employ a deactivating strategy for coping. Interestingly, Dozier and Koback (1992) found that individuals who show this pattern of responses exhibit physiological arousal when asked potentially stressful questions concerning their childhood. The research on repressive coping style and on adult romantic attachment styles has been reported in separate literatures. We were interested in whether there was a relationship between them.

MEASURES USED

Coping Resources Inventory

The Coping Resources Inventory (CRI; Hammer & Marting, 1988) is a 60-item questionnaire used to identify resources currently available to individuals for managing stress. It is based on Lazarus's model of stress and coping and measures resources in five domains: cognitive, social, emotional, spiritual/philosophical, and physical. The following are examples of items: "I exercise vigorously 3-4 times per week" (physical), "I actively look for the positive side of people and situations" (cognitive), "I can cry when sad" (emotional), "I enjoy being with people" (social), and "I pray or meditate" (spiritual/philosophical). Each item is rated on a 4-point scale (never/rarely, sometimes, often, and always/almost always).

Hazan and Shaver Prototypes

The Hazan and Shaver prototypes (Hazan & Shaver, 1987) are their original prototypical descriptions of how people feel in close relationships. There are three descriptions that correspond to secure, avoidant, and anxious/ambivalent romantic adult attachment styles. For example, the secure attachment style states, "I find it relatively easy to get close to others and am comfortable depending on them. I don't often worry about being abandoned or about someone getting too close to me." Participants are instructed to read the three descriptions and place a tick in the box beside the statement with which they agree. They are instructed not to tick more than one box.

Romantic Adult Attachment Style Questionnaire

Hazan and Shaver (1987) suggested that a single description may be inadequate for classifying participants into attachment groups because it assumes there are three mutually exclusive styles of attachment. In addition, each description includes statements about both being comfortable with closeness and being able to depend on others. Thus, adults are asked to endorse an entire description that may not reflect their views on all dimensions.

The Romantic Adult Attachment Style questionnaire (Simpson, 1990) responded to this by allowing participants to rate themselves as having more than one style. In addition, being comfortable with closeness and being able to depend on others are presented as separate statements. The Simpson Questionnaire separates the three Hazan and Shaver (1987) descriptions into 13 individual statements, each of which is answered on a 7-point Likert scale ranging from strongly agree to strongly disagree. Five statements correspond to secure attachment (e.g., "I find it relatively easy to get close to others"),

4 statements correspond to avoidant attachment (e.g., "I'm not very comfortable having to depend on others"), and 4 statements correspond to anxious/ambivalent attachment (e.g., "I'm nervous if anyone gets too close to me"). The total score for each attachment style is summed to give each individual three scores: secure, avoidant, and anxious.

General Health Questionnaire

The 12-item version of the General Health Questionnaire (GHQ-12; Goldberg, 1992) is a self-report questionnaire designed to detect nonpsychotic psychiatric disorder and avoid symptoms of physical illness. Each of the 12 items asks respondents if they have recently experienced a particular symptom or item of behavior using a 4-point scale: less than usual, no more than usual, rather more than usual, and much more than usual. A Likert scoring system was used, in which responses score 0, 1, 2, and 3, respectively.

Pennebaker Inventory of Limpid Languidness

The Pennebaker Inventory of Limpid Languidness (PILL; Pennebaker, 1982) is a 54-item measure of reporting common physical symptoms, such as coughing, indigestion, and back pain. Each symptom, which is experienced as occurring at least once a month, scores 1 point.

THE SERIES OF STUDIES

Study 1: Self-Reported Relationship Between Repressive Coping Style and Coping Resources (Myers & Vetere, 1997)

Individuals with a repressive coping style, so described, comprise a significant minority of people of interest to health psychologists. There has been considerable interest in the

way people cope with sources of stress, and many studies have used questionnaire methods. We were interested in the potential relationship between the repressive coping style and self-reported scores on the CRI. We hypothesized that people with a repressive coping style would report more coping resources than the other people in the study.

The participants were 113 adults (age range, 18-38 years; mean age, 22.5 years) studying psychology at Reading University in the United Kingdom. Our four-way classification of extreme scoring groups was selected on the basis of their scores on the MAS and the Marlowe Crowne using quartile splits (REP, LA, HA, and DHA).

We compared the responses of people with a repressive coping style to those of the other three extreme scoring groups, as is traditional in studies of repressive coping style, and to those of all the nonrepressors in our sample. Group differences in the means were tested using one-way analysis of variance. Newman-Keuls tests were used for all post hoc comparisons, with significance levels set at $p < .05$. Regarding the comparison between REP and the other three extreme scoring control groups, there were main effects of group for the total CRI scores and all the individual subscales. When the REP group was compared to all other participants, we found the same pattern of results, namely that the repressive coping group reported significantly more total coping resources than the rest of the sample, and the pattern was repeated for the subscales.

Study 2: Self-Reported Relationship Between Repressive Coping Style and a Measure of Psychological Symptoms and of Physical Symptoms (Myers & Vetere, 1997)

Participants were a different sample of 184 adults between 18 and 54 years old (mean age, 21.3 years) from the University of

Reading. Participants completed the GHQ-12 and the PILL and were separated into the four extreme scoring groups on the basis of their MAS and Marlowe Crowne scores. Similar to Study 1, the repressive coping style group was compared to the three extreme scoring control groups and to the total sample of participants.

As in Study 1, group differences in the means were tested using one-way analysis of variance, and Newman-Keuls tests were used for all post hoc comparisons, with significance levels set at $p < .05$.

First, we compared REP with the other three extreme scoring control groups and found that there was no significant main effect of group for the PILL. There was a main effect of group for the GHQ-12, however, with REP scoring significantly lower than the HA and DHA. Second, when REP was compared to all other participants, there was a main effect of group for the PILL and the GHQ-12, such that REP scored significantly lower on both the PILL and the GHQ-12. When we used the whole sample, REP exhibited a similar pattern to that found in Study 1.

Why is this important? It may be that people defined as having a repressive coping style are simply a group of individuals who are healthy, cope well with sources of stress, and lack psychological and physiological symptoms. The key issue, however, that repressive coping style is linked with physical health problems, would lead us to be curious, if not concerned, by these findings. It seems that people with a repressive coping style are presenting themselves in an overly positive manner on self-report health-related measures. Their low scores on the GHQ-12 are consistent with previous research results that suggest that they are less likely to report negative affect and symptoms of depression than others (Canning, Canning, & Boyce, 1992).

The implications of understanding the repressive coping style, in terms of its contribution to health outcomes and to the prevention of ill health and the promotion of positive well-being, are crucial. These findings led us to want to know more about the developmental origins of the repressive coping style. We examined the adult attachment style research and began to explore a developmental, theoretical basis for these findings.

Study 3: Repressive Coping Style and Adult Attachment Style: Is There a Relationship (Vetere & Myers, 2002)?

A group of people who present themselves in an overly positive light and who are sensitive to the demand characteristics of research situations present a challenge to methodology. If the very nature of the repressive coping style is to protect the self from criticism and cope with a social world that failed somehow to nurture and support the developing person, then research participation may challenge a person's customary mode of coping in an unhelpful way. It was in this study that we found a way to address this difficulty.

We wished to explore whether there was a relationship between adult attachment styles, as defined, and repressive coping style, particularly whether adults who can be described as having a repressive coping style describe themselves as having an avoidant attachment style. It seemed to us that there were similarities between the two groups, based on both our research experience and our clinical experience. The implications of this relationship for subjective well-being, emotional adjustment, and health-related behaviors are important.

Sixty-four adult participants (age range, 18-46 years; mean age, 22.5 years) from an initial pool of 145 undergraduate students were divided into the four classification groups, using quartile splits, based on their MAS and Marlowe Crowne scores (REP,

LA, HA, and DHA). All participants completed the two measures of adult romantic attachment: the Hazan and Shaver prototypes (Hazan & Shaver, 1987) and the Simpson Questionnaire (Simpson, 1990).

We found that the majority of individuals described as having a repressive coping style described themselves as securely attached on the Hazan and Shaver prototypes in this study. It is of interest that two of the other three extreme scoring control groups (i.e., the two high anxious groups, HA and DHA) rated themselves as anxiously/ambivalently attached. The LA group members rated themselves as securely attached.

Given our previous concerns about the wish of the repressive coping style group to present themselves overly positively, we examined their scores on the Simpson Questionnaire, which allowed them to endorse themselves on all three attachment dimensions.

We used one-way analysis of variance to test for group differences in the means and Newman-Keuls tests for post hoc comparisons, and significance levels were set at $p < .05$. There was no main effect of group for secure attachment, but there was a significant main effect of group for avoidant attachment, with REP members rating themselves as significantly more avoidantly attached than LA, HA, and DHA members. Interestingly, there was also a significant main effect of group for anxious attachment, with the HA group members rating themselves as significantly more anxiously attached than the other three groups. There were no significant main effects for gender, nor were there significant attachment style by gender interactions.

We replicated this study using a different sample from Reading University composed of 259 undergraduates between 18 and 54 years old (mean age, 20.7 years). In this replication study, the REP group was compared with the other three extreme scoring control groups and all nonrepressors in the sample group.

We found a similar pattern of results: (a) There were no significant group differences for the mean secure attachment scores, and (b) REP members rated themselves as significantly more avoidantly attached than the other three control groups and the entire sample.

It may be that the reason we found group differences with the Simpson Questionnaire, but not the Hazan and Shaver categorical descriptions, is that the Simpson Questionnaire allows people with a repressive coping style to present themselves positively on the secure attachment items. Thus, a dimensional measure may make it easier to indicate their avoidant tendencies at the same time. Thus, they are not forced to choose a less positive attachment description.

These studies suggest a potential link between the adult attachment literature and the repressive coping style literature. Thus, individuals with an avoidant attachment style may face similar challenges to their emotional and physical well-being as those found in the repressive coping literature.

Study 4: Adult Attachment Style and Health (Myers & Vetere, 2002)

Many studies have explored aspects of romantic adult attachment styles, but very few have examined the implications of different romantic adult attachment styles for health-related attitudes, health-related behaviors, and ways of coping with stress. For example, we are interested to know (a) whether an adult's reported attachment style reflects differences in preferred coping styles, and (b) whether adults who self-report themselves to be insecurely attached in their adult romantic relationships are at higher risk for psychological problems. Such links, if shown, would provide the basis for further exploration of health- and help-seeking behaviors in families.

There were two arms to this study: (a) 113 participants (age range, 18-38 years; mean age, 22.5 years) completed the CRI and the Hazan and Shaver prototypes, and (b) 125 participants (age range, 18-54 years; mean age, 21.3 years) completed the Simpson Questionnaire, the GHQ-12, and the PILL. For the first arm of the study, group differences in the means were tested using one-way analysis of variance, with Bonferroni corrected comparisons for post hoc comparisons ($p < .05$). Individuals with a secure attachment style reported significantly more total coping resources than the avoidant and anxious/ambivalent attachment style groups and also more social and emotional resources on the subscales. The secure attachment group scored higher on the cognitive subscale than the anxious/ambivalent group. There were no group differences for the physical and spiritual/philosophical subscales.

The second arm of the study examining the Simpson Questionnaire, the GHQ-12, and the PILL recorded the following observations: For the GHQ-12 scores, there was a main effect of attachment style, with the secure attachment style group scoring significantly lower than the anxious/ambivalent group. There were no significant group effects for the PILL.

The finding that different coping resources are related to different attachment styles lends support to previous research. For example, Mikulincer and Florian (1998) found that patients with chronic back pain who reported an insecure attachment style relied more on emotion-focused coping strategies, whereas those with a secure attachment style tended to use more problem-focused coping strategies.

We did not find a link between self-reported attachment style and self-reported physical symptoms. We found a tentative link between secure attachment style and low levels of psychological symptoms on the GHQ-12 and between anxious/ambivalent attachment and high levels of psychological symptoms. Kotler, Buzwell, Romeo, and Rowland (1994) suggested that an avoidant romantic attachment style was linked to

symptoms of physical and psychological ill health via high levels of emotional control. The putative relationships between repressive coping style, adult attachment style, and physical and psychological health warrant further investigation.

CONCLUSIONS

We conclude this chapter with a summary of our major findings and a discussion of the implications for the work of couple and family therapists. In our research studies, people described as having a repressive coping style seem to self-report more coping resources both in total scores and on each of the five subscales on the CRI. In addition, they score lower on the PILL and the GHQ-12 compared to all other groups of respondents, both the total sample and the extreme scoring control groups. We have replicated these findings. In addition to these findings, people with a repressive coping style will self-report a secure adult attachment style on a forced-choice measure of adult attachment. On a dimensional self-rating measure of each adult attachment style, however, they will report both a secure and an avoidant attachment style. We have also replicated these findings. This suggests that respondents with a repressive coping style are likely to represent themselves in an overly positive light relative to other respondents. Different self-reported coping resources seem to be related to different self-reported attachment styles. In our studies, we could find no link between self-reported attachment styles and physical symptoms as measured by the PILL. Those who self-report secure attachment styles, however, also score low on the GHQ-12.

We support a biopsychosocial and contextual model that does not divorce our understanding of relationships, beliefs, and narratives from embodied experience and behavioral and health outcomes. Traditionally, health psychologists and cognitive psychologists have not conversed with family systems thinkers, except in the relatively small discipline of family systems medicine. The recent interest in narrative in the family systems field carries the risk that discourse across these discipline and practice boundaries may become even less likely.

We believe that the implications of our small series of studies may be profound for the thinking and practice of relationship therapists. If it is the case that a significant minority of people can be characterized by the current deployment of a repressive coping style, and that there may be a relationship between this group and those who describe themselves as forming adult romantic attachments characterized by avoidance, then many of them are likely to be living in family and relationship systems.

There is increasing evidence of an association between repressive coping, as defined by Weinberger and others, and the development and course of disease. Other studies have suggested that the repressive coping style is associated with an avoidant style of information processing, with restricted access to negative emotional memories, and may well develop during childhood (Myers & Brewin, 1994). Schwartz's (1990) dysregulation theory argues that attention to levels of distress may be needed for a person to maintain health. Thus, failure to pay attention to distress may be important in the development of disease. As Weinberger (1990) concluded, "Repressors as a group, seem actively engaged in keeping themselves (rather than just other people) convinced that they are *not* prone to negative affect" (p. 338). We have shown a tentative link between this group and those with an avoidant romantic attachment style, in which they share the use of deactivating strategies in circumstances of psychological threat. It is no coincidence that the avoidant attachment style has been called "dismissing" (Bartholomew & Horowitz, 1991), which potentially captures its iterative psychological and relationship effects. We know of no

published research that has explored the systemic effects on other family members, such as intimate partners and children, of living with other adults who can be characterized in this way. A connection could be made to the literature on emotional style of relatedness among family group members, with implications for understanding developmental trajectories.

One of the main implications for our practice as systemic therapists would be to question whether this group of people would be likely to seek out the services of relationship therapists. It remains an empirical question, of course, but our experience suggests that they would be more likely to turn to the use of alcohol and other mood-altering substances to avoid negative affect, and that their entry into therapy would be facilitated by family involvement (Vetere & Henley, 2001). Our experience has been that an engagement process with couples and families for family therapy as part of an overall treatment strategy is often very lengthy and probably best characterized as a series of consultations. Such a lengthy engagement process facilitates a thoughtful and less threatening context in which discrepancies between beliefs, emotions, coping behaviors, and physiological arousal can be addressed. Family involvement appears to be key in helping initiate and sustain motivation for change, as has been found in alcohol treatment outcome studies (Edwards & Steinglass, 1995). Our experience supports Schwartz's (1990) observation that clients presenting to a clinical psychologist with psychosomatic problems at a manifest level will disclose a more latent level of broader psychological and relationship difficulties if they are gently coaxed and supported over time. Such an approach relies on the practitioner not being bound by short-term contractual requirements for therapeutic intervention.

If it is the case that people characterized by the use of avoidance and repression are less likely to seek out therapeutic help and are at risk of some adverse health outcomes, but delay medical help-seeking behavior, when they do present for help, the disease process may be more established or have become an acute crisis. It is often in conditions of crisis that a person's constructs are most volatile and available for challenge and modification. Thus, the offer of therapeutic intervention as part of a medical crisis service or immediate referral for therapeutic help or both may have more impact at this time rather than when the crisis has settled or resolved. We do not know of any published research on repressive coping and compliance and adherence with medication, but we suspect this is an area that could be investigated. In the United Kingdom, most acute medical services are not able to offer therapeutic support because of both a physical medicine orientation and a lack of resources. The implications of the previous findings and tentative suggestions, however, are that the resource implications for individuals, family life, and health care providers are potentially greater if we do not engage the particular problems presented by the repressive coping style and the avoidant adult attachment style.

The crucial role that social and intimate relationships can play in buffering individuals against the longer term psychological effects of stress may well be mediated by their attachment styles. Therefore, understanding the development of both an avoidant/dismissing attachment style and a repressive coping style can inform therapeutic interventions. A systemic view of attachment is interested in how the family group provides a network of care and security for all members; for example, a mother-child relationship is influenced by the mother's relationship with her partner, her past and current relationships with her parents, their socioeconomic context, and so on. Attachment is considered to be a construct of importance across the life span. Similarly, we are interested in using retrospective interviews to explore how people described as having a repressive coping style make sense of the development of their style. We previously noted the difficulties of interpretation raised by overly positive self-presentation on questionnaires. Interviews can form part of a triangulated methodology.

Interviews raise some peculiar ethical problems, however. Research is an intervention into people's lives. We are less interested in the certainties of whether childhood memories are true or false and more interested in the beliefs about self, others, and relationships and the perceptions of behavioral options and choices as they develop over time. We are aware of the vulnerabilities of memory and that the process of remembering may be understood in the social context in which it occurs. There is an ethical paradox in trying to research a process some people claim not to remember or that creates ambiguities, threats, and uncertainties for both researcher and research participants. We need to start somewhere, however. We intend to pilot the collection of narrative accounts from a handful of volunteers who can be characterized as possessing a repressive coping style. Initially, we will read the accounts for attachment themes and issues, searching for intergenerational patterning of beliefs about attachment, and the meanings and interconnections of those beliefs, events, and relationships, and any descriptions of change in attachment styles and patterns.

REFERENCES

Bartholomew, K., & Horowitz, L. M. (1991). Attachment styles among young adults: A test of a four-category model. *Journal of Personality and Social Psychology, 61*, 226-244.

Bendig, A. W. (1956). The development of a short form of the Manifest Anxiety Scale. *Journal of Consulting Psychology, 20,* 384.

Bowlby, J. (1979). *The making and breaking of affectional bonds.* London: Tavistock.

Canning, E. M., Canning, R. D., & Boyce, T. (1992). Depressive symptoms and adaptive style in children with cancer. *Journal of American Child and Adolescent Psychiatry, 31,* 1120-1124.

Crowne, D. P., & Marlow, D. A. (1964). *The approval motive: Studies in evaluative dependence.* New York: John Wiley.

Davis, P. J. (1987). Repression and the inaccessibility of affective memories. *Journal of Personality and Social Psychology, 53,* 585-593.

Dozier, M., & Koback, R. (1992). Psychopathology in attachment interviews: Converging evidence of deactivating strategies. *Child Development, 63,* 1473-1480.

Edwards, M., & Steinglass, P. (1995). Family therapy treatment outcomes for alcoholism. *Journal of Marital and Family Therapy, 21,* 475-509.

Goldberg, D. (1992). *General Health Questionnaire (GHQ-12).* London: NFER-Nelson.

Hammer, A. L., & Marting, M. S. (1988). *Manual for the Coping Resources Inventory.* Palo Alto, CA: Consulting Psychologists Press.

Hazan, C., & Shaver, P. R. (1987). Romantic love conceptualised as an attachment process. *Journal of Personality and Social Psychology, 52,* 511-524.

Jamner, L. D., Schwartz, G. E., & Leigh, H. (1988). The relationship between repressive and defensive coping styles and monocyte, eosinophile, and serum glucose levels: Support for the opioid peptide hypothesis of repression. *Psychosomatic Medicine, 50,* 567-575.

Jensen, M. R. (1987). Psychobiological factors predicting the course of breast cancer. *Journal of Personality, 55,* 317-342.

Kotler, T., Buzwell, S., Romeo, Y., & Bowland, J. (1994). Avoidant attachment as a risk factor for health. *British Journal of Medical Psychology, 67,* 237-245.

Main, M., & Goldwyn, R. (1984). Predicting rejection of her infant from mother's representation of her own experience: Implications for the abused-abusing intergenerational cycle. *Child Abuse and Neglect, 8,* 203-217.

Mikulincer, M., & Florian, V. (1998). The relationship between adult attachment styles and emotional and cognitive reactions to stressful events. In J. A. Simpson & W. S. Rholes (Eds.), *Attachment theory and close relationships* (pp. 143-165). New York: Guilford.

Miller, S. B. (1991). Repressive coping style and cardiovascular response to active coping stress. *Psychosomatic Medicine, 53,* 221.

Myers, L. B. (1993). *The origins and nature of the repressive coping style.* Unpublished doctoral dissertation, University of London, London.

Myers, L. B., & Brewin, C. R. (1994). Recall of early experience and the repressive coping style. *Journal of Abnormal Psychology, 103,* 288-292.

Myers, L. B., & McKenna, F. P. (1996). The colour naming of socially threatening words. *Personality and Individual Differences, 6,* 801-803.

Myers, L. B., & Vetere, A. (1997). Repressors' responses to health-related questionnaires. *British Journal of Health Psychology, 2,* 245-257.

Myers, L. B., & Vetere, A. (2002). Adult romantic attachment styles and health-related measures. *Psychology, Health and Medicine, 7,* 175-180.

Pennebaker, J. W. (1982). *The psychology of physical symptoms.* New York: Springer-Verlag.

Schwartz, G. E. (1990). Psychobiology of repression and health: A systems approach. In J. L. Singer (Ed.), *Repression and dissociation* (pp. 405-434). Chicago: University of Chicago Press.

Simpson, J. A. (1990). Influence of attachment styles on romantic attachment. *Journal of Personality and Social Psychology, 59,* 971-980.

Vetere, A., & Henley, M. (2001). Integrating couples and family therapy into a community alcohol service: A pantheoretical approach. *Journal of Family Therapy, 23,* 85-101.

Vetere, A., & Myers, L. B. (2002). Repressive coping style and adult romantic attachment style: Is there a relationship? *Personality and Individual Differences, 32,* 799-807.

Weinberger, D. A. (1990). The construct validity of the repressive coping style. In J. L. Singer (Ed.), *Repression and dissociation* (pp. 337-386). Chicago: University of Chicago Press.

CHAPTER 10

Families, Poverty, and Children's Health

RONALD J. ANGEL AND JACQUELINE L. ANGEL

Although childhood is thought to be a relatively healthy time of life, the health and happiness of childhood are stolen from an increasing number of children by the poverty and social disorganization in which they grow up. Prior to the advent of the U.S. Social Security system, the elderly were at highest risk of poverty; today, children younger than 18 years old are more likely than any other age group to live in poverty (Proctor & Dalaker, 2003). The situation of African American and Hispanic children is particularly serious because a large fraction of these children spend at least some portion of their childhood in poor, single-parent households (Angel & Angel, 1993). The health consequences of poverty are both immediate and long-lasting. Children who grow up in poverty face elevated risks of infectious and chronic diseases associated with poor nutrition, lack of health insurance, and inadequate health care (Angel, Lein, Henrici, & Leventhal, 2001; Newacheck, Hung, Park, & Irwin, 2003; Newacheck & Taylor, 1992). Today, an epidemic of obesity, which has become a disease of the poor, has resulted in the emergence of type 2 diabetes among children, a phenomenon not known in previous decades (Ogden, Flegal, Carroll, & Johnson, 2002). The environmental decay and social instability that poverty brings increase the risk of emotional and behavioral problems that can have long-term negative educational and developmental consequences.

Because of the fact that the United States is unique among developed nations in not providing universal health care coverage to its citizens, unemployment and the lack of employer-based health insurance among poor families create serious problems. The employment-based system of coverage in the United States means that children in middle- and upper-class families in which parents have access to family insurance coverage often get all the preventive and acute care they need. For the unemployed and working poor, health care access depends on a system that is means-tested, often stigmatizing, and difficult to negotiate. Although the State Children's Health Insurance Program (SCHIP) provides coverage to more children in needy families, many eligible children do not take advantage of either Medicaid or SCHIP (Dubay, Kenney, & Haley, 2002). As a consequence, the

United States faces the challenge of providing health care to children in need at a time when health care costs are soaring and public budgets, especially at the state level, are seriously strained. The imperative is great because today's children are tomorrow's adults who will be among the two workers supporting each retired individual. If their productivity is compromised by poor health and its negative developmental and educational consequences, the economic basis of the nation and the well-being of all Americans will be placed in jeopardy.

In this chapter, we summarize a large body of literature and a wide range of data spanning 30 years to document the following: (a) the social factors that affect the physical, emotional, and social health of children; (b) the prevalence of specific physical health conditions among children in different family situations; and (c) the findings of community studies of the prevalence of emotional and behavioral problems among children and adolescents. This literature addresses various aspects of the impact of minority group status and poverty on children's health. We pay close attention to the health consequences of family structure. An exhaustive review of the literature, of course, is impossible in a short chapter. The published literature on the health of children consists of thousands of articles and books. Instead, we focus on studies that provide empirical evidence concerning the overall impact of poverty. This focus includes the complex interactions among factors associated with poverty, such as race and Hispanic ethnicity, on the physical and mental health of children.

We begin with our conclusion: The data clearly show that African American and Hispanic children are at elevated risk of compromised health, and that this increased risk is related to the deleterious consequences of poverty and minority group status. Family disruption and single parenthood greatly increase the risk of poverty and its negative health consequences. On almost every measure of physical and emotional well-being, poor and minority children fare worse than middle-class nonminority children. African American and Hispanic children younger than age 18 years, for example, are less likely than white children to be in excellent health (McCormick, Kass, Elixhauser, Thompson, & Simpson, 2000). Impaired health and vitality are exacerbated by a lack of health insurance and other serious barriers to health care, as well as the general discrimination that minority Americans have traditionally suffered (Newacheck et al., 1998, 2003).

POVERTY AND ILLNESS IN INFANCY, CHILDHOOD, AND ADOLESCENCE

In the United States, the average child who survives the dangers of birth and the neonatal period can look forward to a period of relatively good health. A few children are born with serious congenital problems and birth defects, many of which are the result of incomplete gestation and very low birth weight—problems exacerbated by poverty and teenage pregnancy (March of Dimes, 2002). In the United States, few children die of acute causes (Gwatkin, 2000; Rosenwaike & Bradshaw, 1989). Significant differences between the health of the children of the poor and that of the middle class persist, however (Starfield, Robertson, & Riley, 2002). The health disadvantage faced by poor children begins before birth and persists throughout life. During their first year of life, the children of the poor face an elevated risk of death (Finch, Frank, & Hummer, 2000). African American children are at least twice as likely as white children to die before their first birthday, largely as the result of low birth weight, poverty, and low parental educational levels (Centers for Disease Control and Prevention [CDC], 2002).

Low Birth Weight

Low birth weight is one of the most serious short- and long-term threats to children's health, but it is also an outcome that is relatively easily avoided given current medical knowledge (Sowards, 1999). The risk of prematurity and low birth weight is inequitably distributed in the population. African American infants are more than twice as likely as white and Hispanic infants to be born prematurely (Alexander, Kogan, Himes, Mor, & Goldenberg, 1999). Among African Americans, 13% of infants are born weighing less than 2,500 g as opposed to 6% of non-Hispanic whites (Health Resources and Services Administration [HRSA], 2002). African American infants face a two- or three-fold greater risk of very low birth weight (less than 1,500 g) compared to white children (CDC, 2002). Some of this elevated risk can be accounted for by low educational levels, although even the children of college-educated African American parents face an elevated risk of prematurity, a fact that reflects the independent impact of discrimination and the economic and social disadvantages associated with minority group status (Schoendorf, Hogue, Kleinman, & Rowley, 1992).

A large part of the risk of prematurity is the result of the fact that many African American mothers are young and unmarried (Costa, 2003). One fourth of infants born to mothers 15 years old or younger are premature and experience mortality rates that are twice as high as those of infants born to women who are age 20 to 30 years (Granger, 1982; Menken, 1972). The Apgar scores (a measure of the child's vital status at birth) of the infants of teenage mothers are on average lower than those of the infants of older mothers (Jones & Placek, 1981). The consequences of low birth weight can be tragic. Seriously underweight infants frequently suffer neonatal complications, such as respiratory distress syndrome, hypoglycemia, jaundice, and other metabolic and neurological disorders (Granger, 1982). Low-birth-weight infants experience growth retardation that often results from a mother's poor nutritional status (Balcazar, Aoyama, & Cai, 1991). The reality, then, is that the consequences of poverty and inequality scar children's lives from their very beginning.

Major maternal predictors of adverse birth outcomes include drug abuse, cigarette smoking, prenatal stress, negative attitudes toward pregnancy, and inadequate prenatal care (Zambrana, Dunkel-Schetter, Collins, & Scrimshaw, 1999). Early prenatal care greatly reduces the risk of low birth weight and poor infant health outcomes (Casper & Hogan, 1991). In 1999, however, approximately 17% of pregnant women did not receive care during the first trimester of pregnancy. Some of these women did not receive care until the last trimester of pregnancy, and a significant fraction received no care at all (HRSA, 2002). Again, those most likely to do without adequate prenatal care are disproportionately African American, Native American, Hispanic, and poor. In 2000, approximately one third of pregnant African American and Hispanic women received less than optimal prenatal care. Among these disadvantaged groups, even those who receive care often see the doctor later in their pregnancies and receive less care than is medically recommended (Frisbie, Echevarria, & Hummer, 2001; Hansell, 1991; March of Dimes, 2002).

Lead Poisoning and Other Environmental Pollutants

The magnitude of the problem of lead poisoning is best illustrated by estimates that approximately 1 million young children suffer from lead poisoning (President's Task Force on Environmental Health Risks and Safety Risks to Children, 2000). After the first year, minority children face elevated risks from lead poisoning and other environmental pollutants. Also, poor children are more than twice as likely as middle-class children to suffer lead poisoning (Sherman, 1997). Because they more often live in old, inner-city households that were constructed before modern building codes were adopted, the children of the poor are frequently exposed to lead from lead-based paint and lead plumbing. Exposure to lead from these and other sources can result in damage to the central nervous system and lead to such neurological problems as hearing loss and poor motor coordination. High blood lead levels can also result in impaired blood flow and growth deficits. It is not just old housing that places poor children at risk, however. Congested urban environments are often seriously polluted by automobile exhaust, which until recently contained high levels of lead. Lead, however, is not the only pollutant in poor children's environments. The poor are also exposed to nonphysical pollutants. Children who grow up in disorganized poverty-stricken neighborhoods face an elevated risk of the negative health consequences as the result of noise and a generally stressful environment (Shonkoff & Phillips, 2000).

Growing up in a neighborhood beset by drugs and violence can easily harm children's emotional and mental health as well as their physical health (Jencks & Mayer, 1990; Tienda, 1991). One of the greatest tragedies we face today arises from the fact that the physical decay and social disorganization of many urban neighborhoods place poor children at very high risk of emotional and physical illness (Duncan, Boisjoly, & Harris, 2001; Duncan, Brooks-Gunn, & Aber, 1997; Hewlett, 1991; Schorr, 1990). Numerous observers have noted that today a new type of poverty characterizes our inner cities (Wilson, 1997). It is much harder and more intractable than that characteristic of those same neighborhoods not long ago. The new urban poverty is made particularly harsh by the almost complete absence of good jobs and high youth unemployment in certain blighted zones. The lack of ties to the labor force or school results in a hopelessness and loss of faith in the future that promotes deviant behavior (Wilson, 1987, 1997). In such an environment in which drugs are readily accessible, their use becomes normative.

Again, the risk of damage from such negative social factors disproportionately affects minority Americans. Hispanics are more likely than students from other racial and ethnic groups to report having drugs available to them on school property (National Institute on Drug Abuse, 2003).

Infectious Diseases, Including HIV

Despite a decade of improvements in vaccination, low-income children are still less likely than middle-class children to be fully immunized against diseases such as measles and rubella (Berglas & Lim, 1998). Data from Los Angeles County for the mid-1980s showed that Hispanic preschoolers were at higher risk of contracting measles than non-Hispanic preschoolers (Ewert, Thomas, Chun, Enguidanos, & Waterman, 1991).

Unfortunately, effective vaccines for some diseases are not available. As the AIDS epidemic worsens, it disproportionately victimizes the children of the minority poor. In 2001, African American and Hispanic children comprised approximately one fourth of the population younger than age 15 years but accounted for more than three fourths of pediatric AIDS cases. In cities such as Newark and New York, AIDS is among the leading causes of death for African American and Hispanic children between 1 and 4 years of age (CDC, 2002). The children of the poor are more likely to suffer from hearing and vision disorders than the children of the more affluent (Starfield, 2003). Overall, a large body of data indicates that the children of poor and minority parents are not only at higher risk of illness and impaired development than the children of middle-class parents but also the illnesses they experience are more serious and have more serious long-term effects (Angel & Angel, 1993).

Asthma

Asthma is the most common chronic disease in childhood. Asthma rates in children younger than the age of 5 years increased more than 160% between 1980 and 1994 (CDC, 1998). African American and Hispanic children are at the highest risk (Akinbami & Schoendorf, 2002). Even when they receive Medicaid, asthmatic African American children obtain poorer care than white children (Lieu et al., 2002). The reasons for the increase in childhood asthma are not clear but may include better diagnosis or changing indoor and outdoor environmental exposure to pollutants (Miller, 2000). Although some studies reveal a racial difference in the prevalence of asthma, most of this difference is accounted for by socioeconomic factors and poorer general health care among African Americans (Wissow, Gittelsohn, Szklo, Starfield, & Mussman, 1988).

Higher childhood incidence of asthma among minority populations persists throughout the life course. African Americans and Hispanics have higher lifetime rates of asthma than non-Hispanic whites (Boudreaux, Emond, Clark, & Camargo, 2003). Again, the racial difference is largely a reflection of socioeconomic factors (Wissow et al., 1988). Most poor children have access to some source of asthma treatment, but poor and minority children are less likely than middle-class and nonminority children to receive the best care or the most effective preventive therapy (Boudreaux et al., 2003). Perhaps partially because of language barriers and cultural distance, children in Spanish-speaking families are at particularly high risk of receiving inadequate therapy (Halterman, Aligne, Auinger, Mcbride, & Szilagyi, 2000).

Obesity

As in the case of asthma, the prevalence of childhood obesity is rapidly increasing. The CDC defines overweight as a body mass index (BMI), a ratio of height to weight, of 25 to 29.9 and obesity as a BMI of 30 or higher (National Center for Health Statistics, 2003). Results from the 1999 and 2000 National Health and Nutrition Examination Survey indicate that 15% of children and adolescents between the ages of 6 and 19 years are overweight. More than 10% of children between the ages of 2 and 5 years are overweight, up from 7% in 1994. The rates are even higher for minority school-age children. Twenty-four percent of Mexican American children and 20% of African American children, as opposed to 12% of non-Hispanic white children, between the ages of 6 and 11 years are overweight. The racial disadvantage in obesity persists as children age into their teenage years (National Center for Health Statistics, 2003).

High-fat diets are often identified as a leading cause of the increase in childhood obesity. Because weight gain results from an imbalance between caloric intake and expenditure, exercise is clearly important in avoiding weight gain. Rather than expending energy in outdoor activities, many children spend hours watching television, surfing the Internet, or playing video games. Because of inadequate resources and poor dietary habits, poverty seriously increases the risk of obesity (Himes, 2003). Single-parent households are at particularly high risk of poverty, and many live in dangerous neighborhoods in which a mother is reluctant to allow her children to play outside.

Anemia

Many poor children are seriously under-nourished and, as a consequence, are at elevated risk of anemia (Yip, Binkin, Fleshood, & Trowbridge, 1987). Although the prevalence of childhood anemia in the United States has declined during the past 30 years, iron deficiency remains a nutritional problem among low-income infants and children (Pollitt, 1999). Children in low-income families in certain states face a seriously elevated risk of iron deficiency anemia (Pollitt, 1999). In Orange County, California, for example, approximately one in six children from low-income families suffer from anemia, a ratio much higher than the national average (Orange County Health Care Agency, 2005).

Accidents

Accidents are the leading cause of death among children older than 1 year of age, as well as for adolescents and young adults. Minority children, especially poor African American children, die at higher rates than whites from falls, drowning, gunshot wounds, suffocation, home fires, and car accidents (National Center for Health Statistics, 2002a, 2002b). African Americans younger than age 20 years are twice as likely as whites to die accidentally. In Chicago, between 1992 and 1994, 283 African Americans in this age group suffered fatal accidents compared to 81 Hispanics and 62 non-Hispanic whites (Rogal, 1996). During the same years, accidents claimed the lives of 131 whites, 60 African Americans, and 29 Hispanics in suburban Cook County.

Children from low-income families are twice as likely to die in motor vehicle accidents as children of the middle class; they are four times more likely to drown and five times more likely to die in fires. Children from low-income families live in more hazardous environments that greatly increase their risk of injury. The dangerous aspects of these environments include substandard and overcrowded housing, lack of safe recreational facilities, busy streets, and other physical hazards. Given these dangers, children in poor neighborhoods need even more supervision than children in safer neighborhoods, but they are often poorly supervised (Escarce, 2003; Shonkoff & Phillips, 2000). Also, because of a lack of money, low-income families are less likely to use safety devices that might make their households safer. It is clear, therefore, that a large portion of the racial disparity in injuries can be directly attributed to the risks associated with poverty and the social and environmental disorganization it brings.

Emotional and Behavioral Problems

Childhood and adolescence can be rather traumatic in terms of emotional development. Children and adolescents are engaged in the difficult task of becoming adults at a time of life when they lack the well-defined social statuses and power that those who successfully navigate this part of the life course will later acquire (National Research Council Commission on Behavioral and Social Sciences and Education, 1995). In recent years, major advances have been made in the assessment of emotional and behavioral problems in community samples. Several studies that employ instruments such as the Diagnostic Interview Schedule for Children and the Child Behavior Checklist have shown that emotional and behavioral problems that are serious enough to interfere with normal development or social functioning are common among children and adolescents. In a review of studies, Costello (1986) reported rates of significant psychopathology ranging from nearly 18% to 22%. The data also show that rates of childhood psychopathology are influenced by various vulnerabilities associated with minority group status (Montgomery, Kiely, &

Pappas, 1996). A study of kindergarten children found that 32% live in what are considered high-risk families, including those characterized by low levels of parental education and single or non-English-speaking parents (Zill & West, 2001). A study of Head Start patrons found that over a 10-year period, the proportion of Head Start families facing these multiple demographic risks increased by 22% (Kaiser, Cai, Hancock, & Foster, 2002).

In the past 10 years, the literature on racial and ethnic differences in behavioral and emotional problems has increased. We know much more today about the factors related to such differentials than we did a decade ago. These studies reveal large group differences. For example, African American and Puerto Rican children experience significantly more behavioral problems than non-Hispanic white children (Angel & Angel, 1993, 1996; Canino, Early, & Rogler, 1980; Patterson, Kupersmidt, & Vaden, 1990). This is hardly surprising in light of the socioeconomic disadvantage and discrimination that African Americans and Hispanics experience in U.S. society (McLanahan & Sandefur, 1994).

One major study of racial and ethnic differences in children's mental health in a large sample of children in New York City revealed substantial differences among African American, Hispanic, and non-Hispanic white children in the number and type of mental health symptoms reported by their parents (Langner, Gersten, & Eisenberg, 1974). African American children were more likely than white children to experience delusions and hallucinations, and they were more likely than white children to have problems with memory, concentration, and speech. African American children were also more likely than white children to be delinquent. The study also showed that African American children were more violent than Hispanic children but less violent than white

children. White children were more likely than African American children to feel depressed and to argue with their parents. Hispanic children had more organic developmental problems, including problems with memory and concentration and problems with toilet training, than non-Hispanic white children. Hispanic children were also more likely to suffer from repetitive motor behavior, delayed development, social isolation, dependency, and compulsivity. These data show that many children and adolescents experience significant emotional difficulties, and that the different social situations in which African American, Hispanic, and non-Hispanic white children find themselves influence the type of emotional and behavioral problems they manifest.

Social contextual factors account for much of the difference in rates of emotional and behavioral problems among children from different racial and ethnic groups (Eggebeen & Lichter, 1991; McLeod & Edwards, 1995). Were the negative health effects of poverty and social disorganization only minor or short-lived, there might be less cause for alarm. Unfortunately, emotional problems in childhood appear to have serious long-term effects (Chase-Lansdale, 1997; Guang, 1998; McLanahan, 2000). Studies based on the National Longitudinal Surveys of Youth show that persistent childhood poverty results in high and increasing levels of antisocial behavior (McLeod & Nonnemaker, 2000; McLeod & Shanahan, 1996). These studies show that children in families that are chronically poor display higher rates of antisocial behavior than children in middle-class families or families that are only episodically poor.

Mental Health Service Use

Although there are no good population-based estimates of mental health care use by poor and minority children, data for the general population suggest that most children in need of services never see a mental health professional and, as is the case for adults, most children who receive any care at all for mental health problems are seen exclusively by general practitioners, primarily pediatricians (Angel & Angel, 1993; Boyle et al., 1987; Offord et al., 1987; Wolfe, 1980). Among children with a mental disorder, only one in five receive specialist treatment (Costello, 1986). Again, for poor minority group children, among whom rates of psychopathology related to the stresses of poverty are probably elevated, even this level of contact with mental health care professionals is probably rare. As among younger children, a large fraction of African American adolescents manifest behavioral problems and are much less likely than non-Hispanic white adolescents to have seen a mental health professional (Angel & Angel, 1993). In general, the evidence suggests that there is a great deal of unmet need for mental health care services among children, particularly among poor and minority group children. Providing mental health care to children with serious emotional and behavioral disturbances remains a serious challenge for health care policymakers (Dawson, 1991; Zill & Schoenborn, 1990).

FAMILY AND NEIGHBORHOOD CONTEXTUAL EFFECTS

The research summarized so far makes it clear that social factors are among the most serious threats to children's health. These factors influence every important domain of a child's life, including family, school, and the community. These major social health threats consist of neglect, abuse, drugs and violence, and unsafe neighborhoods. Recent research has examined the impact of these threats on children's health.

Violence Both Outside and Inside the Home

Low family income is associated with higher rates of nearly every form of violence against children. Data from the Third National Incidence Study of Child Abuse and Neglect reveal that children in families with earnings less than $15,000 per year were more than 22 times more likely than those in families with annual incomes higher than $30,000 per year to experience some form of maltreatment (Sedlak & Broadhurst, 1996). School violence mars the academic experiences of many students and challenges parents, teachers, and school officials to respond. Hispanic and African American students are more likely than white students to report the existence of gangs in their schools. According to the National Center for Education Statistics, African American students report high levels of verbal abuse at school (Kaufman et al., 2000).

In addition to poverty, family structure is associated with the risk of violence. The children of single parents are at higher risk of physical abuse and of all types of neglect and are overrepresented among seriously injured, moderately injured, and endangered children. Children in single-parent families are at much higher risk of physical injury or abuse compared to children who live with both parents (Sedlak & Broadhurst, 1996). Although parents are not necessarily, nor even most frequently, the perpetrators of abuse, the increased stresses of single parenthood clearly increase the risk, especially because single-parent families often find themselves in hostile physical environments with inadequate social support. In addition to violence, poor children are at elevated risk of neglect, which can have profound long-term developmental consequences. One study found that abused or neglected children are far more likely to be arrested as adolescents and as adults than are children who have not been abused or neglected (Widom & Maxfield, 2001).

Family Instability and Parental Absence

The evidence clearly shows that the emotional climate of the family has a direct impact on a child's emotional well-being (for reviews, see Angel & Angel, 1993; Garmezy & Rutter, 1983; Rutter, 1985). A harmonious and functioning family can protect a child from the negative effects of poverty, whereas a dysfunctional and strife-ridden family can seriously harm even a middle- or upper-class child's emotional health. Children are particularly sensitive to family discord, and parental conflict often results in serious behavioral and emotional problems (Hetherington, 1989; Rutter, 1985; Wallerstein & Blakeslee, 1989). A weak parent-child bond has been associated with a weak superego and elevated use of cigarettes, alcohol, and marijuana. Such a situation further undermines parental authority and increases mental health problems and substance abuse (Resnick et al., 1997).

It is clear that a large part of the risk associated with single parenthood results from the poverty that such families suffer. A large body of research, however, indicates that the absence of a father or another adult in a child's life can have negative mental health and developmental effects. Children who grow up without a father often experience serious developmental problems, including disturbed sex role identities and antisocial behavior (Angel & Angel, 1993; Angel & Worobey, 1988; Biller, 1971; Dawson, 1991; Garfinkel & McLanahan, 1986; Guidubaldi & Cleminshaw, 1985; Kellam, Ensminger, & Turner, 1977; McLanahan & Sandefur, 1994; Munroe, Boyle, & Offord, 1988). In addition, the data show fairly convincingly that children can suffer major health problems as a consequence of their parent's divorce (Angel & Angel, 1993; Hetherington, Cox, & Cox, 1985a, 1985b; Wallerstein & Blakeslee, 1989; Zill & Schoenborn, 1990).

Most single-parent families are clearly not dysfunctional, nor do all children suffer irreparable damage as the result of divorce (Munroe et al., 1988). Nonetheless, children clearly benefit from a certain degree of family stability, and the economic and social stresses that many female-headed families experience can place a child at increased risk of both mental and physical illness. Physical and emotional health are highly interdependent, and emotional and behavioral problems are part of a package that includes substantial physical comorbidity. Those risk factors that undermine a child's sense of emotional well-being, therefore, can have long-term physical health consequences. As we have documented, given their disadvantaged economic and social situations, African American and Hispanic children are at a disproportionate risk of suboptimal physical and emotional health.

CHILDREN OF IMMIGRANTS

Today, the majority of immigrants to the United States are from Asia and Latin America, and a large number are undocumented and ineligible for government social services, except emergency services. As a result of changes in immigration and welfare laws during the 1990s, even legal immigrants remain ineligible for such services for a period of 5 years (Angel, Angel, & Markides, 2000). These restrictions are intended to discourage the immigration of individuals who might become public charges. The consequence is that the entire burden of caring for a recent immigrant falls on his or her sponsors during that 5-year period. What might well be rational immigration policy represents a potential major health threat to the children of immigrants. Because of a lack of health insurance, both adults and children in immigrant families frequently have no regular source of care. Access to a regular source of health care increases the number of pediatric visits for children and the likelihood that they receive the specialty physical and mental health care services they may need (Newacheck, Hughes, & Stoddard, 1996). Health care coverage represents a tie to the medical care establishment that increases the likelihood of good health. The lack of coverage, then, represents a serious health risk for immigrant children.

The health risks and the health care needs of immigrant adults and children are unique, as are the barriers that often keep them from receiving medical care (Angel & Angel, 2003a, 2003b; Angel et al., 2000, 2001). Although they may be selected for good physical health, immigrants to the United States often endure serious emotional stresses related to difficulties in dealing with a foreign culture, a new language, and new institutions. Such stresses can undermine social and mental adjustment (Hernandez, 1999). Often, the immigrant family is ill equipped to deal with emotional and mental problems or to gain access to the care it needs. Conflicts and strife within the immigrant family that arise as part of the process of cultural change can be the source of emotional problems for both adults and children. Such conflicts can be exacerbated by the isolation that many immigrant families experience. This isolation is revealed by the fact that Puerto Rican women living on the U.S. mainland have significantly less social and emotional support at the time of childbirth than those who remain in Puerto Rico (Landale & Oropesa, 2001).

Immigrant Children in Texas

The situation of immigrants in Texas typifies that of newcomers in the nation as a whole, although Texas fares worse than other states in social services and health insurance

coverage. The immigrant population of Texas is primarily of Mexican origin. On the basis of data from the Urban Institute, more than one third of the children of immigrant parents live in poverty in comparison to less than one fourth of immigrant children nationwide. The study, compiled from data from the 1999 National Survey of American Families, examined several indicators of well-being for children of immigrants in eight states with large immigrant populations: California, Colorado, Florida, Massachusetts, New Jersey, New York, Texas, and Washington. In general, Texas fares far worse in key areas of nutrition, health insurance, housing, and poverty. As Table 10.1 shows, children of immigrants in Texas suffer significantly higher levels of hardship in term of food security (i.e., a condition in which the family has access at all times to nutritionally adequate foods from customary food sources, such as stores, gardens, and restaurants, to maintain an active healthy life), health care, and housing compared to children in other states (Capps, 2001).

In response to welfare reform, legal immigrants' family participation in benefit programs for which they qualify decreased at a much sharper rate than that for low-income citizen families with children (Fix & Passel, 2002). Experts attribute the decline to the erroneous belief among immigrants that the use of social services may jeopardize the immigration status of a family member. Given their ill-defined situation and the fact that the law specifically excludes many forms of assistance for even legal immigrants for 5 years, such a misunderstanding and mistrust is not surprising. The great majority of children affected are U.S. citizens, however, because 78% of the children of immigrants were born in the United States and are citizens. Although these U.S. citizen children are eligible for all benefits, evidence indicates that they are not using these benefits at the same rate as children of native-born parents.

Table 10.1   Social and Economic Well-Being of Children of Immigrants

Indicator	Texas (%)	United States (%)
Poverty rate	36	24
Food concerns	49	37
Uninsured	40	22

SOURCE: Data from the 1999 National Survey of American Families.

HEALTH INSURANCE: MEDICAID AND SCHIP

In the United States, health insurance is an employment benefit. Certain families, especially among the self-employed, purchase private plans, but for the most part, if one does not have a job that is good enough to offer family coverage, it is unlikely to pay enough to allow a family to purchase a private plan. Middle-class families in which one or both parents have access to such plans have immediate access to the best health care in the world. Unfortunately, more than 40 million Americans are either unemployed or work in low-wage service-sector jobs in which health insurance is not offered or offered at a cost that makes full family coverage prohibitively expensive. These, of course, are the types of jobs in which large numbers of minority Americans work. Mexican Americans and African Americans, for example, are far less likely than any other group to be employed in managerial or professional jobs that offer the best health insurance coverage. Minority Americans are disproportionately represented among the working poor, the segment of the population in which even two parents can be employed full-time for the entire year and still be only slightly above the poverty line. This segment of the population, which until recently did not qualify for Medicaid for their children, is at particularly high risk of poor health, a lack of coverage, and inadequate health care.

The poorest families have access to Medicaid, and SCHIP extends coverage to children and some adults up to 200% of the poverty line. Some states offer coverage to children in families that make even more. Even when they are employed, African Americans and Hispanics are at particularly high risk of lacking health insurance (Angel, Angel, & Lein, 2003). Not all eligible children are enrolled in either Medicaid or SCHIP, however. Table 10.2 presents data on the percentage of children with health insurance coverage by race and ethnicity for 2001. This table shows that 26% of Mexican Americans, 18% of Cuban Americans, 14% of African Americans, and 11% of Puerto Ricans lack coverage for health care. At least half of the uninsured Hispanic and African American children in 2002 were eligible for SCHIP or Medicaid (Urban Institute Covering Kids and Families, 2003).

These ethnic disparities in health insurance coverage vary by state and reflect the inequities that are part of our state-based system of insurance for the poor. Table 10.3 presents data from the Three City Study, a large study of the impact of welfare reform in Boston, Chicago, and San Antonio (Winston, 1999). The table presents information on the percentage of children enrolled in Medicaid at various levels of family income expressed in terms of the poverty ratio. The last column presents data from the March 2000 Current Population Survey for the nation as a whole for purposes of comparison. The city differences that the table reveals are striking. In Texas, for example, only 64% of children in families below the poverty line are enrolled in Medicaid, compared to 82% in Boston,

Table 10.2 Selected Types of Health Insurance Coverage for Children Younger Than 18 Years by Race and Hispanic Ethnicity, 2001[a]

	Younger Than 18 Years				
Type of Coverage	*Non-Hispanic White*	*Non-Hispanic Black*	*Mexican American*	*Cuban American*	*Puerto Rican*
Employer (%)	75	51	39	52	45
Medicaid (%)	15	38	35	27	42
None (%)	7	14	26	18	11
Total (in thousands)	44,378	11,227	9,314	270	987

SOURCE: U.S. Census Bureau, *Annual Demographic Supplement* (2002), and unpublished tabulations for Hispanic subgroups.

a. Respondents 15 years or older were asked to indicate all forms of coverage a child living in the household had. Only the most frequently reported are presented here. Categories may overlap.

Table 10.3 Children Covered by Medicaid

Family Income Relative to Federal Poverty (%)	*All Three Cities (%)*	*Boston (%)*	*Chicago (%)*	*San Antonio (%)*	*March 2000 Current Population Survey (%)*
<100	77	82	82	64	60
100-124	58	86	59	30	42
125-149	53	63	61	35	33
150-199	34	64	35	5	23

SOURCE: Welfare, Children, and Families. A Three-City Study.

and coverage decreases precipitously as family income increases in Texas. In families with incomes between 150% and 199% of the poverty line, only 5% of San Antonio children are enrolled in Medicaid compared to 64% in Boston. Massachusetts has taken advantage of all the coverage options allowed by federal law, whereas Texas provides only the minimal coverage required.

The reasons for the low levels of health financing program participation among Mexican-origin children include regional concentration in states such as Texas in which both state policy and labor market difficulties reduce coverage, immigration status, language difficulties, and other access barriers (Feinberg, Swartz, Zaslavsky, Gardner,

& Walker, 2002). Even after controlling for citizenship status, Mexican-origin children in San Antonio are far less likely than children from any other group to have health insurance of any form.

The Marriage Penalty

Since the time of the Elizabethan Poor Laws, poor able-bodied adults have presented a serious dilemma to communities and welfare policymakers. Policy dealing with support of the poor has always been informed by a desire to force adults to support themselves and not become a burden on the State. Welfare policy has always been based on the expectation that nondisabled males should support themselves and their families. In today's world, this creates an often perverse situation in which married couples where the husband or even both parents are employed full-time earn too little to pay for private or employer-based coverage but do not qualify for Medicaid. Families in which there is an unemployed adult male present face particular problems. In poor counties, such as those along the U.S.-Mexico border in which employment opportunities are limited and unemployment rates among heads of household high, intact families are often penalized in terms of health insurance access.

The Personal Responsibility and Work Opportunity Reconciliation Act (PRWORA) requires that states reduce the total cash assistance caseload, but it requires that states decrease the number of couple-headed households on assistance at an even faster rate. The desire is clearly to force fathers to support their dependents. If a male breadwinner cannot do so, the family as a whole suffers. Mexican-origin families are more likely than non-Hispanic families to have both parents present, but they reside in areas with few employment opportunities for the male. In such situations, the family is dependent on the earnings of the mother, or it resorts to other means of support.

In the Three City Study, which consists of a poor, primarily black and Hispanic sample, slightly more than 40% of the study children in families with a single mother and no male in the household received Medicaid. These data suggest that if there is an adult male in the household, whether he and the children's mother are married or not, the household's probability of receiving Medicaid is greatly reduced.

Health Care Access

The fact that minority Americans, and Mexican Americans in particular, have lower levels of health insurance coverage than other groups is a matter of concern. The problem is made far more serious, however, by the fact that the lack of health insurance reduces health care use and thereby potentially undermines educational and work productivity (Agency for Healthcare Research and Quality, 1999). The lack of private health insurance means that the children of the poor often do not receive the same quality of health care as the children of the middle class (Elixhauser et al., 2002). These children often do not have a regular source of care, one of the basic indicators of high-quality care. Neither do poor children have the same access to specialty medical and mental health care as children from more affluent families (Smedley, 2002).

Although all poor children face health care disadvantages, there are significant differences in pediatric health care use among low-income families (Starfield, 2003). In the 1996 Medical Expenditure Panel Survey, approximately 30% of Hispanic and 20% of African American children lacked a usual source of health care compared to less than 16% of non-Hispanic whites (Agency for Healthcare Research and Quality, 2000). The same survey revealed that Hispanic and African American children are more likely than non-Hispanic white children to rely on clinics and emergency rooms for treatment. In addition, poor children often lack continuity of care, one of the major indicators of high-quality care (Edwards, Bronstein, & Rein, 2002).

SUMMARY AND POLICY RECOMMENDATIONS

We return to our original observation that the health care vulnerabilities suffered by children are not equally distributed. Poor and minority children are at the highest risk of illness, injury, and death, as well as of inadequate health care coverage. They are at highest risk of growing up in single-parent households that are economically unable to escape disorganized neighborhoods. Adequate adult supervision is even more important in such dangerous neighborhoods, but the families who are trapped there are exactly the ones who lack the capacity to provide it. This situation represents a crisis because the number of children involved is large and increasing. These children are tomorrow's workers on whose shoulders the support of the elderly and of younger age groups will fall. If poor physical and mental health in childhood interferes with the social development and education of a large fraction of these children, the productivity of the United States will be undermined.

Given their higher fertility rates, the future labor force will consist heavily of African Americans and Hispanics, groups that today are at elevated risk of poor health and inadequate health insurance coverage. Such a situation threatens to give an increasing racial and ethnic dimension to conflicts between age groups as a politically powerful and predominantly non-Hispanic white retired population draws on the earnings of a working-age population that is heavily Hispanic and black. Inequality is not simply an injustice; it is a threat to everyone's well-being. The situation clearly demands serious attention to the health of children of all groups. Their health represents our most valuable social resource every bit as important as oil or any precious mineral. For most children, good health can be purchased rather cheaply. They do not need the expensive interventions that the chronic illnesses of the elderly demand. Clearly, covering the needs of all children will be expensive, but the return on the investment justifies the expense. We offer a few suggestions for beginning a dialog directed toward improving the health of children and ensuring that their health care safety net does not contain holes through which some might fall.

Full Use of Existing Programs

Even as cash assistance rolls have been drastically reduced as part of welfare reform,

legislation that preserves and even expands the health care safety net for children has been introduced. As part of PRWOA, eligibility for Medicaid was uncoupled from cash assistance. Transitional Medicaid ensures that even after leaving the cash assistance rolls, families can receive Medicaid for up to 1 year. Medicaid is an important program for poor children and, along with other health-related programs, should be adequately funded (O'Brien & Mann, 2003). One strong motivation for states to maintain Medicaid enrollment, in addition to the fact that it benefits poor children, is that reductions in state Medicaid enrollment and spending result in losses in federal funding (Wachino, 2003). Nationally, 57% of Medicaid funds and 70% of SCHIP spending are financed with federal funds (Institute of Medicine, 2000).

The fact that states have substantial discretion in setting eligibility criteria and payment amounts means that health insurance coverage for children varies widely. In Rhode Island, Massachusetts, Vermont, and Wisconsin, less than 5% of children are not covered by any health insurance plan. In contrast, southern states and states with large Hispanic populations fare worse. In Arizona, New Mexico, California, Nevada, Oklahoma, and Texas, approximately 20% of children lack health insurance (Bhandan & Gifford, 2003). Between 2000 and 2003, Texas led the nation in the number of uninsured children, with approximately 1.5 million children lacking coverage. The state has had extreme difficulty reaching out to uninsured children with their nonprofit organization, TexCare, and has only recently experienced significant declines in the number of children without insurance. Consequently, Texas has not been able to use the vast majority of its SCHIP allocation. In Illinois, KidCare provides health insurance to children and pregnant women and also plays an important role in insuring the children of working, lower-income immigrants. One estimate suggests that 16% of children younger than age 18 years received KidCare benefits compared with 24% of undocumented immigrants living in Illinois (Mehta, Theodore, Mora, & Wade, 2002).

Build on the State Children's Health Insurance Program

SCHIP is an ambitious and useful program for providing health care coverage to children and adolescents from working-class families. Medicaid serves the needs of the poorest families, but those with incomes close to 200% of the poverty line, a level of family income that makes the purchase of even employer-based family coverage difficult, have traditionally had to rely on charity or go into debt. SCHIP addresses the needs of many more children in working poor families. Unfortunately, tight state budgets and an increasing federal deficit threaten its full implementation in many states. The potential losses to state economies and the negative consequences for children's health of the failure to fully implement SCHIP are major and should be emphasized.

Massachusetts is one of six states that have obtained approval to use both Medicaid and SCHIP funds to subsidize insurance premiums of low-income employees and their families. The implementation of two premium assistance programs has led to considerable increases in coverage among children, two thirds of whom were uninsured prior to enrollment (Mitchell & Osber, 2002). Of course, the states that take advantage of opportunities to expand coverage are the same ones that had high rates of coverage to begin with. The expansion of SCHIP and other programs in states such as Texas has been far more modest and only to the level required by federal law. Unfortunately, barriers to expanding enrollment in health insurance premium payment programs abound.

Universal Health Care Coverage: The Single Payer Model

Ultimately, universal health care coverage for all Americans or the transformation of Medicaid into a universal program will be necessary to address all the health care needs of all poor families. Despite our best efforts at piecemeal reform, many poor children will remain uncovered or will not participate in programs such as SCHIP. Programs that are means-tested are inevitably stigmatizing and difficult to administer. Many observers have noted what has been called "churning" in health care coverage among the poor as families move from private sources of coverage to public sources to no coverage at all. Such churning has negative consequences for a family's access to needed care. Even with SCHIP, it is still common that in some families certain children are covered and others are not.

The only comprehensive solution for the U.S.'s health care coverage crisis is governmentally sponsored financing as in Canada. Ever since the Progressive Party and its call for national health insurance were defeated in 1912, no attempt to introduce universal health care has come even close to success. There are reasons to suspect that the situation may change in the not too distant future, however. Certainly, the plight of the poor by itself will not lead to significant reform. What is changing rapidly, though, is health care coverage for the middle class. As medical care inflation skyrockets, employers are forced to pass a larger fraction of the cost of health plans on to employees. At the same time, plans cover less and require higher deductibles. Retirees who were promised lifetime supplemental coverage find that they are not receiving it. Meanwhile, more than 40 million Americans remain uninsured as an ever-growing fraction of the gross national product goes to health care. With the aging of the population, the situation will only worsen, and the need to coordinate services and bring economic rationality to the system will require basic changes in the way health care is paid for. The needs of the middle class, rather than the needs of the poor, may result in a system that is more equitable and that covers everyone. Barring such a comprehensive approach, the only solutions are partial and entail efforts to facilitate the enrollment of eligible individuals in existing programs.

We conclude by reiterating the observation with which we began, which is that the data we have reviewed clearly show that African American and Hispanic children are at elevated risk of compromised health, and that this increased risk is related to the deleterious consequences of poverty and minority group status. It is also clear that family disruption and single parenthood greatly increase the risk of poverty and its negative health consequences. On almost every measure of physical and emotional well-being that we have examined, poor and minority children fare worse than middle-class nonminority children. This poverty and its long-term health consequences bode ill for the economic security of the United States as a whole. Given the relative youth of the African American and Hispanic populations and the general aging of the population, in the future the working-age population will be increasingly minority. These young minority workers will be responsible for supporting a growing older, non-Hispanic white population and for maintaining the economic productivity of the country as a whole. If the productivity of tomorrow's workers is compromised by poor health and low educational levels, the United States' position as a global economic superpower may be undermined. Health care inequalities and disadvantages, therefore, represent more than individual or group tragedies; they represent a serious social problem that affects us all.

REFERENCES

Agency for Healthcare Research and Quality. (1999). *Annual report on access to and utilization of health care for children and youth in the United States* (Publication No. 00-R014). Silver Spring, MD: Government Printing Office.

Agency for Healthcare Research and Quality. (2000). *Fact sheet identifying racial and ethnic disparities in health care* (Publication No. 00-PO41). Silver Spring, MD: Government Printing Office.

Akinbami, L. J., & Schoendorf, K. C. (2002). Trends in childhood asthma: Prevalence, health care utilization, and mortality. *Pediatrics, 110,* 315-322.

Alexander, G. R., Kogan, M. D., Himes, J. H., Mor, J. M., & Goldenberg, R. (1999). Racial differences in birth weight for gestational age and infant mortality in extremely low-risk U.S. populations. *Paediatric and Perinatal Epidemiology, 13,* 205-217.

Angel, J. L., Angel, R. J., & Markides, K. S. (2000). Late-life immigration, changes in living arrangements, and headship status among older Mexican-origin individuals. *Social Science Quarterly, 81,* 389-403.

Angel, R., Lein, L., Henrici, J., & Leventhal, E. (2001). Health insurance coverage for children and their caregiver in low-income neighborhoods. *Welfare, children, and families* (Policy Brief No. 01-2). Baltimore: Johns Hopkins University Press.

Angel, R. J., & Angel, J. L. (1993). *Painful inheritance: Health and the new generation of fatherless families*. Madison: University of Wisconsin Press.

Angel, R. J., & Angel, J. L. (1996). Physical co-morbidity and medical care use in children with emotional problems, *Public Health Reports, 3*, 8-14.

Angel, R. J., & Angel, J. L. (2003). Family, the State, and health care: Changing roles in the new century. In J. Treas (Ed.), *Sociology of the family* (pp. 233-252). Oxford, UK: Blackwell.

Angel, R J., & Angel, J. L. (2003). Hispanic diversity and health care coverage. *Public Policy and Aging Report, 13*, 8-12.

Angel, R. J., Angel, J. L., & Lein, L. (2003). *The health care safety net for Mexican Americans* (Center for Health and Social Policy Working Paper Series, No. 03-1). Austin, TX: LBJ School of Public Affairs. Retrieved February 9, 2004, from http://www.utexas.edu/lbj/research/chasp/wp_0503.pdf

Angel, R. J., & Worobey, J. L. (1988). Single motherhood and children's health. *Journal of Health Social Behavior, 29*, 38-52.

Balcazar, H., Aoyama, C., & Cai, X. (1991). Interpretative views on Hispanics' perinatal problems of low birth weight and prenatal care. *Public Health Reports, 106*, 420-426.

Berglas, N., & Lim, J. J. (1998, November). *Racial and ethnic disparities in maternal child health* (Policy Brief No. 3). Arlington, VA: National Center for Education in Maternal and Child Health Policy.

Bhandan, S., & Gifford, E. (2003). Children without health insurance: 2003. *Current population reports* (Publication No. P60–224). Washington, DC: U.S. Bureau of the Census.

Biller, H. B. (1971). The mother-child relationship and the father-absent boy's personality development. *Merrill Palmer Quarterly, 17*, 227-241.

Boudreaux, E. D., Emond, S. D., Clark, S., & Camargo, C. A. (2003). Race/ethnicity and asthma among children presenting to the emergency department: Differences in disease severity and management. *Pediatrics, 111*, 615-621.

Boyle, M. H., Offord, D. R., Hoffman, H. G., Catlin, G. P., Byles, J. A., Cadman, D. T., et al. (1987). Ontario child health study I: Methodology. *Archives of General Psychiatry, 44*, 826-831.

Canino, I. A., Earley, B. F., & Rogler, L. H. (1980). *The Puerto Rican child in New York City: Stress and mental health* (Monograph No. 4). Bronx, NY: Fordham University, Hispanic Research Center.

Capps, R. (2001). *Hardship among children of immigrants: Findings from the 1999 National Survey of American Families* (Policy Brief No. B-29 in the series New Federalism: National Survey of America's Families). Washington, DC.: Urban Institute.

Casper, L. M., & Hogan, D. P. (1991). Family networks in prenatal and postnatal health. *Social Biology, 37*, 84-101.

Centers for Disease Control and Prevention. (1998). Surveillance for asthma: United States, 1960-1995. *Morbidity and Mortality Weekly Report, 47*, 1-28.

Centers for Disease Control and Prevention. (2002). *U.S. HIV and AIDS cases reported through December 2001* (Vol. 13, No. 2, Table 15). Atlanta, GA: Author. Retrieved March 8, 2003, from http://www.cdc.gov/hiv/stats/hasr1302/table15.htm

Chase-Lansdale, L. P. (1997). *Escape from poverty: What makes a difference for children?* New York: Cambridge University Press.

Costa, D. L. (2003). *Race and pregnancy outcomes in the twentieth century: A long-term comparison* (Working Paper No. 9593). Cambridge, MA: National Bureau of Economic Research.

Costello, E. J. (1986). Primary care pediatrics and child psychopathology: A review of diagnostic, treatment, and referral practices. *Pediatrics, 78*, 1044-1051.

Dawson, D. A. (1991). Family structure and children's health and well-being: Data from the 1988 National Health Interview Survey on Child Health. *Journal of Marriage and the Family, 53*, 573-584.

Dubay, L., Kenney, G., & Haley, J. (2002). Children's participation in Medicaid and SCHIP: Early in the SCHIP era. *New Federalism National Survey of America's Families* (Series B, No. B-40). Washington, DC: Urban Institute.

Duncan, G., Brooks-Gunn, J., & Aber, J. L. (Eds.). (1997). *Neighborhood poverty: Context and consequences for children*. New York: Russell Sage Foundation.

Duncan, G. J., Boisjoly, J., & Harris, K. M. (2001). Sibling, peer, neighbor and schoolmate correlations as indicators of the importance of context for adolescent development. *Demography, 38*, 437-447.

Edwards, J. N., Bronstein, J., & Rein, D. B. (2002). Do enrollees in "look-alike" Medicaid and SCHIP programs really look alike? *Health Affairs, 21*, 240-248.

Eggebeen, D., & Lichter, D. (1991). Race, family structure, and changing poverty among children. *American Sociological Review, 56*, 801-817.

Elixhauser, A., Machlin, S. R., Zodet, M. W., Chevarley, F. M., Patel, N., McCormick, M. C., et al. (2002). Health care for children and youth in the United States: 2001 annual report on access, utilization, quality, and expenditures. *Ambulatory Pediatrics 2*, 419-437.

Escarce, J. J. (2003). Editorial column: Socioeconomic status and the fates of adolescents. *Health Services Research, 38*, 12-29.

Ewert, D. P., Thomas, J. C., Chun, L. Y., Enguidanos, R. C., & Waterman, S. H. (1991). Measles vaccination coverage among Latino children aged 12 to 59 months in Los Angeles County: A household survey. *American Journal of Public Health, 81*, 1057-1059.

Feinberg, E., Swartz, K., Zaslavsky, A., Gardner, J., & Walker, D. K. (2002). Language proficiency and the enrollment of Medicaid-eligible children in publicly funded health insurance programs. *Maternal and Child Health Journal, 6*, 5-18.

Finch, B. K., Frank, R., & Hummer, R. A. (2000). Race/ethnic disparities in infant mortality: The role of behavioral factors. *Social Biology, 47*, 244-263.

Fix, M. E., & Passel, J. S. (2002). *Scope and impact of welfare reform's immigrant provisions. Assessing the new federalism* (Discussion Paper No. 02-03). Washington, DC: Urban Institute.

Frisbie, W. P., Echevarria, S., & Hummer, R. A. (2001). Prenatal care utilization among non-Hispanic whites, African Americans, and Mexican Americans. *Journal of Maternal and Child Health, 5*, 21-33.

Garfinkel, I., & McLanahan, S. (1986). *Single mothers and their children: A new American dilemma*. Washington, DC: Urban Institute.

Garmezy, N., & Rutter, M. (Eds.). (1983). *Stress, coping and development in children*. New York: McGraw Hill.

Granger, C. (1982). Maternal and infant deficits related to early pregnancy and parenthood. In N. J. Anastasiow (Ed.), *The adolescent parent* (pp. 33-45). Baltimore: Brookes.

Guang, G. (1998). The timing of the influences of cumulative poverty on children's cognitive outcomes in childhood and early adolescence. *Social Forces, 77,* 257-287.

Guidubaldi, J., & Cleminshaw, H. (1985). Divorce, family health, and child adjustment. *Family Relations, 34,* 35-41.

Gwatkin, D. R. (2000). Health inequalities and the health of the poor: What do we know? What can we do? *Bulletin of the World Health Organization, 78*(1), 3-18.

Halterman, J. S., Aligne, C. A., Auinger, P., Mcbride, J. T., & Szilagyi, P. G. (2000). Health and health care for high-risk children and adolescents: Inadequate therapy for asthma among children in the United States. *Pediatrics, 105*(Suppl.), 272-276.

Hansell, M. J. (1991). Sociodemographic factors and the quality of prenatal care. *American Journal of Public Health, 81,* 1023-1028.

Health Resources and Services Administration. (2002). *Child health USA 2002.* Washington, DC: U.S. Department of Health and Human Services, Maternal and Child Health Bureau.

Hernandez, D. J. (1999). *Children of immigrants: Health, adjustment, and public assistance.* Washington, DC: National Research Council Committee on the Health and Adjustment of Immigrant Children and Families.

Hetherington, E. M. (1989). Coping with family transitions: Winners, losers, and survivors. *Child Development, 60,* 1-14.

Hetherington, E. M., Cox, E. M., & Cox, R. (1985a). Long-term effects of divorce and remarriage on the adjustment of children. *Journal of the American Academy of Psychiatry, 24,* 518-530.

Hetherington, E. M., Cox, E. M., & Cox, R. (1985b). Play and social interaction in children following divorce. *Journal of Social Issues, 35,* 26-49.

Hewlett, S. A. (1991). *When the bough breaks: The cost of neglecting our children.* New York: Basic Books.

Himes, C. (2003, May). *Family structure and adolescent obesity.* Paper presented at the meeting of the Population Association of America, Minneapolis, MN.

Institute of Medicine. (2000). *From neurons to neighborhoods: The science of early childhood development.* Washington, DC: National Academy Press.

Jencks, C., & Mayer, S. E. (1990). The social consequences of growing up in a poor neighborhood. In L. Lynn & M. McGeary (Ed.), *Inner city poverty in the United States* (pp. 111-186). Washington, DC: National Academy Press.

Jones, A. E., & Placek, P. J. (1981). Teenage women in the United States: Sex, contraception, pregnancy, fertility and maternal health. In T. Ooms (Ed.), *Teenage pregnancy in a family context* (pp. 49-72). Philadelphia: Temple University Press.

Kaiser, A. P., Cai, X., Hancock, T. B., & Foster, E. M. (2002). Teacher-reported behavior problems and language delays in boys and girls enrolled in Head Start. *Behavioral Disorders, 28,* 23-39.

Kaufman, P., Chen, X., Choy, S. P., Ruddy, S. A., Miller, A. K., Fleury, J. K., et al. (2000). *Indicators of school crime and safety, 2000* (NCES 2001-017/NCJ-184176). Washington, DC: U.S. Departments of Education and Justice.

Kellam, S. G., Ensminger, M. E., & Turner, F. J. (1977). Family structure and the mental health of children. *Archives of General Psychiatry, 34,* 1012-1022.

Landale, N. S., & Oropesa, R. S. (2001). Migration, social support and perinatal health: An origin-destination analysis of Puerto Rican women. *Journal of Health and Social Behavior, 42,* 166-183.

Langner, T. S., Gersten, J. C., & Eisenberg, J. G. (1974). Approaches to measurement and definition in the epidemiology of behavior disorders: Ethnic background and child behavior. *International Journal of Health Services, 4,* 483-501.

Lieu, T. A., Lozana, P., Finkelstein, J. A., Chi, F. W., Jensvold, N. G., Capra, A. M., et al. (2002). Racial/ethnic variation in asthma status and management practices among children in managed Medicaid. *Pediatrics, 109,* 857-865.

March of Dimes. (2002). *Ten leading causes of infant mortality, 1999.* Retrieved January 3, 2003, from www.marchofdimes.com/aboutus/1529.asp

McCormick, M. C., Kass, B., Elixhauser, A., Thompson, J., & Simpson, L. (2000). Annual report on access to and utilization of health care for children and youth in the United States—1999. *Pediatrics, 105,* 219-230.

McLanahan, S. (2000). Family, state, and child well-being. *Annual Review of Sociology, 26,* 703-706.

McLanahan, S., & Sandefur, G. (1994). *Owing up with a single parent.* Cambridge, MA: Harvard University Press.

McLeod, J. D., & Edwards, K. (1995). Contextual determinants of children's responses to poverty. *Social Forces, 73,* 1487-1516.

McLeod, J. D., & Nonnemaker, J. M. (2000). Poverty and child emotional and behavioral problems: Racial/ethnic differences in processes and effects. *Journal of Health and Social Behavior, 41,* 137-161.

McLeod, J. D., & Shanahan, M. J. (1996). Trajectories of poverty and children's mental health. *Journal of Health and Social Behavior, 37,* 207-220.

Mehta, C., Theodore, N., Mora, L., & Wade, J. (2002). *Chicago's undocumented immigrants: An analysis of wages, working conditions, and economic contributions.* Washington, DC: Center for Urban Economic Development.

Menken, J. (1972). The health and social consequences of teenage childbearing. *Family Planning Perspectives, 4,* 54-63.

Miller, J. (2000). The effects of race/ethnicity and income on early childhood asthma prevalence and health care use. *American Journal of Public Health, 90,* 428-32.

Mitchell, J. B., & Osber, D. S. (2002). Medicaid/SCHIP to insure working families: The Massachusetts experience. *Health Care Financing Review, 23,* 35-45.

Montgomery, L. E., Kiely, J. L., & Pappas, G. (1996). The effects of poverty, race, and family structure on U.S. children's health: Data from the NHIS, 1978 through 1980 and 1989 through 1991. *American Journal of Public Health, 86,* 1401-1405.

Munroe, H. B., Boyle, M. H., & Offord, D. R. (1988). Single-parent families: Child psychiatric disorder and school performance. *Journal of Child and Adolescent Psychiatry, 27,* 214-219.

National Center for Health Statistics. (2002a). Deaths: Final data for 2001, Table 1. *National Vital Statistics Report, 50*(16), 13.

National Center for Health Statistics. (2002b). Deaths: Final data for 2001, Table 2. *National Vital Statistics Report, 50*(16), 49.

National Center for Health Statistics. (2003). *Prevalence of overweight among children and adolescents: United States, 1999-2000.* Retrieved February 9, 2004, from http://www.cdc.gov/nchs/products/pubs/pubd/hestats/overwght99.htm

National Institute on Drug Abuse. (2003). *Drug use among racial/ethnic minorities* (NIH Publication No. 03-3888). Bethesda, MD: National Institutes of Health.

National Research Council Commission on Behavioral and Social Sciences and Education. (1995). *Losing generations: Adolescents in high-risk settings.* Washington, DC: National Academy Press.

Newacheck, P. W., Hughes, D. C., & Stoddard, J. J. (1996). Children's access to primary care: Differences by race, income, and insurance status. *Pediatrics, 97,* 26-32.

Newacheck, P. W., Hung, Y. Y., Park, M. J., & Irwin, C. E. (2003). Disparities in the adolescent health and health care: Does socioeconomic status matter? *Health Services Research, 38,* 1235-1252.

Newacheck, P. W., Strickland, B., Shonkoff, J. P., Perrin, J. M., McPherson, M., McManus, M., et al. (1998). An epidemiologic profile of children with special health care needs. *Pediatrics, 102,* 117-123.

Newacheck, P. W., & Taylor, W. R. (1992). Childhood chronic illness: Prevalence, severity, and impact. *American Journal of Public Health, 82*(3), 364-371.

O'Brien, E., & Mann, C. (2003). *Maintaining the gains: The importance of preserving coverage in Medicaid and SCHIP.* Washington, DC: Georgetown University Press. Retrieved February 18, 2005, from http://coveringkidsandfamilies.org/ckf/files/maintaining_the_gains.pdf

Offord, D. R., Boyle, M. H., Szatmari, P., Rae-Grant, N. I., Links, P. S., Cadman, D. T., et al. (1987). Ontario Child Health Study II: Six-month prevalence of disorder and rates of service utilization. *Archives of General Psychiatry, 44,* 832-836.

Ogden, C. L., Flegal, K. M., Carroll, M. D., & Johnson, C. L. (2002). Prevalence and trends in overweight among U.S. children and adolescents, 1999-2000. *Journal of the American Medical Association, 288,* 1728-1732.

Orange County Health Care Agency. (2005). *Anemia prevention.* Santa Ana, CA: Nutrition Services.

Patterson, C. J., Kupersmidt, J. B., & Vaden, N. A. (1990). Income level, gender, ethnicity, and household composition as predictors of children's school-based competence. *Child Development, 61,* 485-494.

Pollitt, E. (1999). Early iron deficiency anemia and later mental retardation. *American Journal of Clinical Nutrition, 69,* 4-5.

President's Task Force on Environmental Health Risks and Safety Risks to Children. (2000). *Eliminating childhood lead poisoning: A Federal strategy targeting lead paint hazards.* Washington, DC: Environmental Protection Agency.

Proctor, B., & Dalaker, J. (2003). Poverty in the United States: 2002. *Current population reports* (P60-222). Washington, DC: U.S. Census Bureau.

Resnick, M. D., Bearman, P. S., Blum, R. W., Bauman, K. I., Harris, K. M., Jones, J., et al. (1997). Protecting adolescents from harm. Findings from the National Longitudinal Study on Adolescent Health. *Journal of the American Medical Association, 278,* 823-832.

Rogal, B. J. (1996). Death comes by accident in poor, black neighborhoods. *The Chicago reporter.* Retrieved September 26, 2003, from http://www.chicagoreporter.com/1996/07-96/0796accident.htm

Rosenwaike, I., & Bradshaw, B. S. (1989). Mortality of the Spanish surname population of the Southwest: 1980. *Social Science Quarterly, 70,* 631-641.

Rutter, M. (1985). Resilience in the face of adversity: Protective factors and resistance to psychiatric disorder. *British Journal of Psychiatry, 147,* 598-611.

Schoendorf, K. C., Hogue, C. J., Kleinman, J. C., & Rowley, D. (1992). Mortality among infants of black as compared with white college educated parents. *New England Journal of Medicine, 326,* 1522-1526.

Schorr, L. (1990). *Within our reach: Breaking the cycle of disadvantage.* Garden City, NY: Doubleday.

Sedlak, A. J., & Broadhurst, D. D. (1996). *Executive summary of the third National Incidence Study of Child Abuse and Neglect.* Washington, DC: U.S. Department of Health and Human Services, National Center on Child Abuse and Neglect, Administration for Children, Youth, and Families.

Sherman, A. (1997). *Poverty matters: The cost of child poverty in America.* Washington, DC: Children's Defense Fund.

Shonkoff, J. P., & Phillips, D. A. (Eds.). (2000). *From neurons to neighborhoods: The science of early childhood development.* Washington, DC: National Research

Council Committee on Integrating the Science of Early Childhood Development, Board on Children, Youth, and Families.

Smedley, B. (2002). *Unequal treatment: Confronting racial and ethnic disparities in health care*. Washington, DC: Institute of Medicine.

Sowards, K. A. (1999). What is the leading cause of infant mortality? A note on the interpretation of official statistics. *American Journal of Public Health, 89,* 1752-1754.

Starfield, B. (2003). Public health and primary care: Challenges and opportunities for partnerships. *Ethnicity and Disease, 13,* S3-12-S3-13.

Starfield, B., Robertson, J., & Riley, A. W. (2002). Social class gradients and health in childhood. *Ambulatory Pediatrics, 2,* 238-246.

Tienda, M. (1991). Poor people and poor places: Deciphering neighborhood effects on poverty outcomes. In J. Huber (Ed.), *Macro-micro linkages in sociology* (pp. 244-262). Newbury Park, CA: Sage.

Urban Institute Covering Kids and Families. (2003). *Number of uninsured children declines, but millions remain without coverage: Report by Covering Kids and Families program office*. Princeton, NJ: Robert Wood Johnson Foundation.

Wachino, V. (2003, September). *Medicaid and the state fiscal crisis: A national perspective*. Presentation to the Foundation for a Healthy Kentucky's Medicaid Forum: Building our common health: Kentucky at a crossroads—Crisis I: Medicaid, Frankfort, KY. Retrieved December 15, 2003, from http://www.healthyky .org/PDFs/Victoria%20Wachino.pdf

Wallerstein, J. S., & Blakeslee, S. (1989). *Second chances: Men, women, and children a decade after divorce*. New York: Ticknor & Fields.

Widom, C. S., & Maxfield, M. G. (2001). *An update on the "cycle of violence"* (National Institute of Justice Research in Brief). Washington, DC: U.S. Department of Justice.

Wilson, W. J. (1987). *The truly disadvantaged: The inner city, the underclass and public policy*. Chicago: Chicago University Press.

Wilson, W. J. (1997). *When work disappears: The world of the new urban poor*. New York: Vintage.

Winston, P. (1999). *Welfare, Children, and Families. A Three-City Study: Overview and design*. Baltimore: Johns Hopkins University Press.

Wissow, L. S., Gittelsohn, A. M., Szklo, M., Starfield, B., & Mussman, M. (1988). Poverty, race, and hospitalization for childhood asthma. *American Journal of Public Health, 78,* 777-782.

Wolfe, B. L. (1980). Children's utilization of medical care. *Medical Care, 18,* 1196-1207.

Yip, R., Binkin, N. J., Fleshood, L., & Trowbridge, F. L. (1987). Declining prevalence of anemia among low-income children in the United States. *Journal of the American Medical Association, 258,* 1619-1623.

Zambrana, R. E., Dunkel-Schetter, C., Collins, N., & Scrimshaw, S. C. (1999). Mediators of ethnic-associated differences in infant birth weight. *Journal of Urban Health, 76,* 102-116.

Zill, N., & Schoenborn, C. A. (1990). Developmental, learning, and emotional problems: Health of our nation's children, United States, 1988. *Advanced data from the vital and health statistics* (No. 190). Hyattsville, MD: National Center for Health Statistics.

Zill, N., & West, J. (2001). *Entering kindergarten: Findings from the condition of education: 2000*. Washington, DC: U.S. Department of Education, Office of Educational Research and Improvement.

CHAPTER 11

Parental HIV/AIDS

An Empirical Model of the Impact on Children in the United States

Debra A. Murphy, William D. Marelich,
Dannie Hoffman, and Mark A. Schuster

This chapter addresses the impact of parental HIV/AIDS on children in the United States. Since the first published case reports of five gay men in Los Angeles with *Pneumocystis carinii* pneumonia (Centers for Disease Control and Prevention [CDC], 1981), HIV/AIDS has reached pandemic proportions, with 650,000 to 900,000 people living with HIV/AIDS in the United States (Fleming et al., 2002) and 40 million estimated to be infected worldwide (United Nations Programme on HIV/AIDS, 2003). Although in the beginning of the pandemic most infections were diagnosed among gay men and intravenous drug users, the epidemiology dramatically changed in the late 1980s and the following decade.

The 1990s brought changes to how the epidemic was perceived. Researchers began to note an increase in heterosexually transmitted HIV (CDC, 1997). At that time, HIV started to clearly bridge into the previously perceived "safe harbor" of families. Previously, there was little research on HIV-affected families,

and government funding, action, and resources were slow to be applied (Epstein, 1996). The number of HIV-positive women, especially women of childbearing age (Gwinn et al., 1991), increased dramatically, however. Given the high mortality rate of those with AIDS, researchers began estimating the number of youth who would be orphaned by AIDS-related deaths (Michaels & Levine, 1992). Studies published in the mid-1990s revealed that the majority of women with HIV were of childbearing age (Schable et al., 1995), and approximately 75% of them had children (Forsyth, 1995), with an average of 2.6 children (Smith, 1996). A survey of medical records of HIV-positive women in 11 U.S. cities found that 16% were pregnant, and an additional 9.9% became pregnant within 2 years (Chu, Hanson, & Jones, 1995). Moreover, the development of highly active antiretroviral treatments in the 1990s prolonged survival (Palella et al., 1998), thus lengthening the time that HIV-infected women might have children.

CURRENT PROJECTION ESTIMATES OF FAMILIES IN THE UNITED STATES AFFECTED BY HIV/AIDS

Using a representative U.S. sample collected in 1996 and 1997 for the HIV Cost and Services Utilization Study (HCSUS), Schuster et al. (2000) estimated that 62,800 (28%) of adults receiving care for HIV/AIDS had at least one child younger than 18 years of age. Furthermore, across the entire sample, 45% of women and 6% of men reported living with at least one of their children. Thus, the total number of families directly affected by parental HIV/AIDS was at least 33,000 (our estimate) in 1996 and 1997. Applying the HCSUS figures to CDC's (1998) estimate of 650,000 to 900,000 living with HIV, and adjusting for gender distributions of those living with HIV/AIDS and children younger than 13 years of age (CDC, 2002), we can extrapolate that the number of affected families exceeds 100,000. That is approximately 1 in every 346 families, assuming 34.6 million families with children younger than 18 years of age (Fields & Casper, 2001). Given the estimated figure of 2.6 children per mother described previously, the calculations translate to a conservative estimate of at least 200,000 children living with an HIV/AIDS-infected parent. These numbers are expected to increase with the anticipated continuing increase in HIV-infection among women. HIV/AIDS is the leading cause of death for African American women in the United States between the ages of 25 and 34 years, and it is the sixth leading cause of death for Hispanic women in the same age category (Anderson & Smith, 2003). Our estimates of families affected by HIV/ AIDS underscore the importance of understanding and predicting the effect that parental HIV/AIDS has on children and adolescents. In this chapter, we discuss an empirical model of child and adolescent outcomes for those affected by parental HIV/AIDS that addresses the many facets that influence family functioning.

AN EMPIRICAL MODEL OF FAMILIES AFFECTED BY HIV/AIDS

The advent of new antiretroviral medication regimens has shifted HIV from a terminal illness to a chronic disease (Valdiserri, Holtgrave, & West, 1999), meaning that HIV-infected patients are living longer. With this shift, children are living long term with chronically ill parents who have a highly stigmatized disease. Research has shown that chronic illness is a major stressor for family members. Illness severity has been linked to higher levels of psychological distress in chronically ill adults (Derogatis et al., 1983; Woods, Haberman, & Packard, 1993) and their children (Armistead, Klein, & Forehand, 1995; Worsham, Compas, & Ey, 1997). Only recently have the effects of parental HIV on children and adolescents begun to be examined.

PARENTS AND CHILDREN COPING TOGETHER MODEL

The literature predicts that both parent and child background and situational factors will affect long-term child outcomes (i.e., behavioral adjustment, mental health status, and social adjustment) in response to chronic parental illness. Figure 11.1 outlines the model of the effects of maternal HIV on child outcomes developed by Murphy for her study of mothers living with HIV/AIDS and their well children (Murphy, Marelich, Dello Stritto, Swendeman, & Witkin, 2002; Murphy, Steers, & Dello Stritto, 2001) titled Parents and Children Coping Together (PACT). PACT was an adaptation of

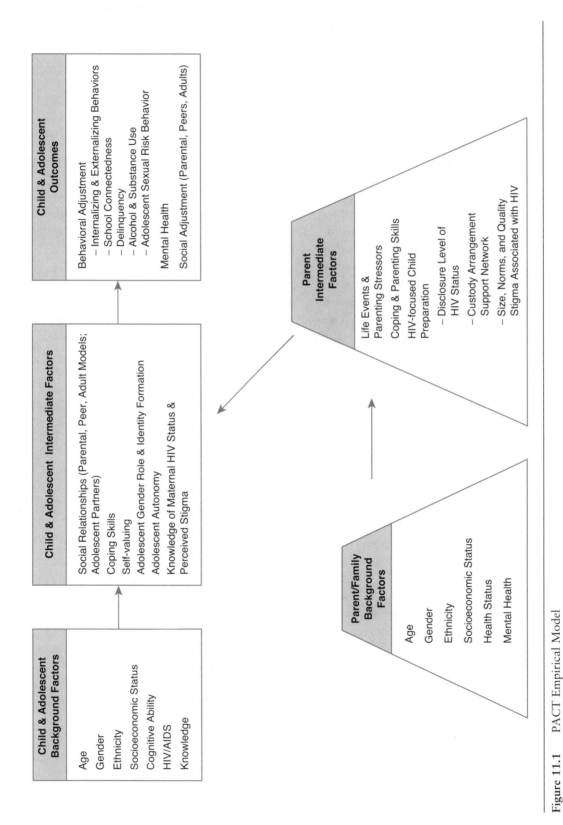

Figure 11.1 PACT Empirical Model

SOURCE: Adapted from Murphy, D. A., Marelich, W. D., Dello Stritto, M. E., et al. (2002).

Sandler's work (Sandler, Tein, & West, 1994; Sandler et al., 1992; West, Sandler, Baca, Pillow, & Gersten, 1991) describing child and maternal situational and background factors anticipated to affect child adjustment in response to disruptive events (e.g., divorce and parental death). Although PACT was a study of the impact on children of maternal HIV, and much of the literature cited is derived from maternal HIV research, we suggest that the model can be applied effectively to paternal HIV. The emphasis on maternal HIV throughout this chapter is justified by the higher percentage of HIV-infected women than HIV-infected men living with their children (Schuster et al., 2000). In the PACT model, background and intermediate outcomes of parents and children are anticipated to impact child adjustment and long-term child outcomes. In the following sections, we review the components of the model.

CHILD AND PARENTAL BACKGROUND FACTORS

Age, Gender, and Ethnicity

Age, gender, and ethnicity are powerful variables in family responses to HIV. They shape perceptions of illness, health care use, and attitudes toward providers (Chavez, Hubbell, McMullin, Martinez, & Mishra, 1995; Clark, 1998; Sargent & Brettell, 1996). In addition, children's age can affect both how they use resources to cope and what information adults give them. For example, child age is often a determinant of mothers' disclosure decisions (Murphy et al., 2001). Among children coping with parental HIV, younger children are especially dependent on caregivers for protection and thus are vulnerable to declines in the quality of parenting (Garmezy, 1991; Masten, Best, & Garmezy, 1990). Older

children and adolescents, although also dependent, are able to make use of psychological buffering systems, seeking protective relationships outside their family or environment when needed. Gender and ethnicity can also influence individuals' experience of sickness and their relationship with health care providers, and ethnicity influences the way individuals experience pain, label symptoms, and communicate about illness (Clark, 1998; McGoldrick, Pearce, & Giordano, 1982; Rapp, 1998). Among HIV-positive adults, ethnicity was found to be a factor in treatment status, with ethnic minorities, primarily African Americans, more likely to be untreated (Kalichman, Graham, Luke, & Austin, 2002). Among HIV-infected adults, rates of disclosure to family and friends are significantly lower for African Americans and Asians than for whites (Petrak, Doyle, Smith, Skinner, & Hedge, 2001). Furthermore, HIV-positive African American women report significantly more depression than Caucasian men or women (Lichtenstein, Laska, & Clair, 2002), and HIV-positive women report significantly lower positive well-being and social support than men, despite having less advanced disease (Cederfjaell, Langius-Ekloef, Lidman, & Wredling, 2001).

Socioeconomic Level

Socioeconomic status (SES) is one of the most widely studied constructs in the social sciences, and the effect of SES on morbidity and mortality is well-known (Frank, Elon, & Hogue, 2003). Health increases as SES increases (Adler & Snibbe, 2003) from childhood through adulthood, and SES operates to affect health similarly for different ethnic and racial groups (Ostrove, Feldman, & Adler, 1999). It has been proposed that low SES environments are stressful and reduce an individual's capacity to manage stress, thus increasing vulnerability (Gallo & Matthews,

2003). SES is a better predictor of knowledge of AIDS than race or ethnicity (Sweat & Levin, 1995), and among HIV-positive individuals, SES has been associated with quality of life (Flannelly & Inouye, 2001).

PARENT BACKGROUND FACTORS

Health

As illness progresses among parents with HIV, the parent is likely to exhibit a number of maladaptive behaviors that disrupt relationships with their children (Cates, Graham, Boeglin, & Tiekler, 1990; Lamping et al., 1991). When HIV-infected mothers remain healthy, the children are less likely to exhibit depressive symptoms (Murphy, Marelich, & Hoffman, 2002). Dorsey et al. (1999) found a linear increase in children's report of externalizing and internalizing difficulties as their mothers progressed through stages of HIV infection and then AIDS. HIV-positive mothers with late-stage HIV/AIDS exhibit extraordinarily high levels of psychological disturbance related to spending time in bed, non-HIV-related medical conditions, and having difficulty caring for their children due to ill health (Silver, Bauman, Camacho, & Hudis, 2003). Finally, health affects psychological distress, with illness severity associated with higher levels of psychological distress (Derogatis et al., 1983; Woods et al., 1993).

Mental Health

Research has found that a parent's mental health status affects parenting behaviors and child resiliency, parental monitoring, family support, and family problem solving and coping. Rates of depression among HIV-positive individuals have been found to be twice as high as those in the general population (Lyketsos et al., 1996), with rates of diagnosable depressive disorders estimated at

4 to 14% (Lyketsos et al., 1996). Among HIV-positive women, studies have shown rates of clinically significant anxiety and depression of approximately 30% to 40% (Kaplan, Marks, & Mertens, 1997; Miles, Burchinal, Holditch-Davis, & Wasilewski, 1997; Swartz, Markowitz, & Sewell, 1998). Tompkins, Henker, Whalen, Axelrod, and Comer (1999) found that HIV-positive women had elevated rates of depression compared to uninfected women, and in particular women who were mothers were more depressed than women without children. Depressed parents may be limited in their interactions with their children (Webster-Stratton & Hammond, 1988). In PACT families in which the mother was depressed, family functioning was also poorer; specifically, family cohesion and sociability were worse (Murphy, Marelich, Dello Stritto, et al., 2002). Depression among the PACT mothers was also associated with increased child responsibilities for household tasks.

PARENT INTERMEDIATE FACTORS

Life Events and Parenting Stressors

Life stress is a predictor of early disease progression (Kimerling et al., 1999). Higher levels of maternal HIV-associated stressors are associated with more child adjustment problems reported by both mothers and children (Hough, Brumitt, Templin, Saltz, & Mood, 2003).

Coping

The use of maladaptive coping strategies has been associated with lower levels of energy and social functioning among people living with HIV/AIDS (Vosvick et al., 2003). It has also been associated with significantly lower psychological quality of life, as defined by cognitive functioning, mental health, and health distress (Vosvick et al., 2002). For example, Kotchick, Forehand, Wierson, Armistead, and Klein (1996) found that in families with fathers with hemophilia (45% of whom were also HIV infected), avoidant coping was associated with poorer adjustment for all family members. Avoidant coping by either parent was related to greater child adjustment problems.

Parenting Skills

HIV-infected mothers report less monitoring of children's activities than do non-infected mothers (Kotchick et al., 1997), suggesting that HIV infection may disrupt effective parenting. Parental monitoring of adolescents has been significantly associated with such outcomes as academic achievement, less drug use (Brown, Mounts, Lamborn, & Steinberg, 1993), and greater self-reliance (Linver & Silverberg, 1995). Parental monitoring is associated with girls' risky sexual behavior (Wilson, 2001) and middle adolescent-onset delinquency (Steinberg, 1987).

Disclosure

Parental disclosure of HIV can affect child adjustment, parent-child relationships, and the ability of parents to access resources to effectively cope with the family's situation. In a sample of 135 mothers and their young children, Murphy et al. (2001) found that only 30% of mothers had disclosed their serostatus. The majority did not disclose because they thought the child might be too young to understand. Many mothers also expressed concern that the child would disclose to others, or that the child would be angry, fear the parent, or withdraw from the parent. Mothers who did disclose reported having a stronger social support network in terms of having people with whom they could share personal and private feelings.

Decision making about disclosure may cause high levels of tension and stress (Marks et al., 1992); in focus groups held with HIV-infected women, a major concern of participants was disclosure to their children (Moneyham et al., 1996).

Social Support

Perceived low social support among HIV-infected women has been found to be predictive of loneliness, stress, and the presence of depressive symptoms (Serovich, Kimberly, Mosack, & Lewis, 2001). Social support among HIV-infected mothers has been found to have a direct influence on their level of emotional distress, even after accounting for coping behavior (Hough et al., 2003). In some studies, HIV-infected mothers and children have been found to report less social support compared to non-HIV-affected families (Reyland, McMahon, Higgins-Delessandro, & Luthar, 2002). This may be due in part to fear of reaching out for social support for HIV-related stressors because of perceived stigma. In one study, 27% of HIV-positive women reported changes in their social networks, and approximately two thirds experienced severe disruption of their personal relationships following their diagnosis (Pergami et al., 1993). Therefore, it is difficult to determine the relationship of HIV to social support systems because some social isolation is likely to result from stigma associated with HIV.

Stigma

HIV-related stigma is associated with psychological distress and can interfere with coping, adjustment, and management of disease (Chesney & Smith, 1999). Maternal concerns include fear, anger, blame, and stigmatization from family and friends (e.g., being perceived as an irresponsible or "bad" mother), as well as from their children, and further disclosure to others through the children (Faithful, 1997; Murphy, Roberts, & Hoffman, 2002; Murphy et al., 2001). The relationship between social support, disclosure, and stigma illustrates the interplay among factors represented in the PACT model. Women with good social support are more likely to disclose their serostatus to their children (Murphy et al., 2001). Disclosure can facilitate utilization of existing social support and identification and access of additional social resources. Fear of negative outcomes of disclosure, resulting from the stigma associated with HIV/AIDS, can inhibit such utilization.

CHILD AND ADOLESCENT BACKGROUND FACTORS

Cognitive Ability and Knowledge of HIV/AIDS

Understanding of illness and health varies with age (Lansdown & Benjamin, 1985; Perrin & Gerrity, 1981). Children of kindergarten age view illness as stemming from a concrete action that was or was not done, and they identify illness only when told (e.g., "You have to stay in bed") or when they view external signs. Children, however, can discuss illness concepts such as death even though they do not fully understand its meaning and finality. By approximately age 9 years, a developmental shift occurs and children can differentiate internal and external phenomena; they can also understand the finality of death at this age. Children can then typically define illness as a set of symptoms; they believe it to be caused by germs that have predetermined effects on their bodies, and they think of it as preventable (e.g., "Don't be around sick people"). They expect that ill people will recover by taking medication and following the doctor's orders. Finally, by age 12 or 13 years, children can comprehend that there are multiple causes of illness, and that bodies respond variably to it. Understanding of AIDS follows a similar developmental progression across age (Osborne, Kistner, & Helgemo, 1993). By age 10 years, the majority of children are aware of its existence (Sly, Eberstein, Quadagno, & Kistner, 1992).

CHILD AND ADOLESCENT INTERMEDIATE FACTORS

Social Relationships

Social support is an important part of child and adolescent functioning. Social support has been found to assist children who are living with a depressed parent to maintain positive psychosocial functioning over time (Garber & Little, 1999). Similarly, more socioemotional support from HIV-infected mothers has been associated with less depressed mood and disruptive behavior among their children (Klein et al., 2000). Compared to early and middle adolescents in families not affected by HIV, however, those with HIV-infected mothers report lower perceived social support available from parents, friends, and teachers and perceptions of more indifference and hostility in the mother-child relationship (Reyland et al., 2002). These findings are of concern, given the important role social support plays in the promotion of adaptive adjustment during adolescence (Taylor, 1996; Wills & Cleary, 1996) and the relationship between social support and resiliency in children (Murphy, Marelich, & Hoffman, 2004).

Resiliency refers to the process of, capacity for, or outcome of successful adaptation despite challenging or threatening circumstances (Masten et al., 1990). Resiliency is usually assessed as good outcomes among children living in high-risk situations over time, sustained competence under stress, and recovery from traumatic events. Resilient children who experience chronic adversity have often had an ongoing relationship with a supportive adult (Brown, Harris, & Bifulco, 1986; Garmezy, 1985; Garmezy & Rutter, 1985; Masten et al., 1990). Among families affected by maternal HIV, resiliency has been associated with parent-child relationship, parental monitoring, and parental structure (Dutra et al., 2000). Murphy et al. (2004) found that children of mothers with AIDS who were classified as resilient reported significantly higher levels of handling their problems well, higher satisfaction with handling their problems, higher confidence that they handled their problems better than other children, and higher confidence they can handle things in the future. The resilient children also had lower levels of negative self-esteem, lower levels of depression, and reported greater happiness compared to nonresilient children.

Coping

Interpersonal problem-solving and coping skills play a crucial role in adjustment (Shure, 1988; Shure & Spivack, 1987). Lack of coping skills and limited competence (affective, social, or achievement) increase the risk of adjustment problems among children and adolescents (Wills, Blechman, & McNamara, 1996). Maladaptive coping has been associated with psychological problems and, among older children, with drug use.

As children mature, more complex coping strategies emerge. Young children often rely on parental support as a primary means of coping, whereas adolescents may rely more on peer support. Therefore, coping among younger children may be affected greatly if HIV-positive mothers become too ill to be a primary resource. The type of coping strategy that children use may also influence behavioral or mental health outcomes:

Compas, Worsham, Ey, and Howell (1996) found that children's avoidance of thoughts about parental cancer was related to greater symptoms of anxiety and depression.

Gender Role and Identity Formation and Self-Valuing

Research indicates that identity develops through processes of individuation and connectedness within the family (Hamilton, 1996). Identity development is related to both self-valuing and gender roles, both of which can influence a number of factors, including decisions regarding risk behavior (Rosenthal & Smith, 1997). Having an HIV-infected mother is likely to affect developmental processes related to identity formation occurring in early and middle adolescence. To our knowledge, however, there have been no HIV-specific studies of child and adolescent gender role and identity formation and how maternal HIV/AIDS may interact with these processes and affect child outcomes.

Autonomy

Another important factor in normative child and adolescent social development is that of positive autonomy (Allen, Hauser, Bell, & O'Connor, 1994). Adolescents who demonstrate positive autonomous behaviors are more likely to have positive relationships with peers and have better social competence. A press for early autonomy, or in Udry's (1990) words a "strain toward maturity," may be associated with a too early detachment from parental guidance and supervision. Having a mother with HIV/AIDS is likely to influence whether children and adolescents develop autonomy within normal developmental parameters. For example, HIV-positive mothers have concerns about their children assuming adult roles too early due to parental illness (Brackis-Cott, Mellins, & Block, 2003). Adult role-taking among adolescents of HIV-infected parents has been associated with their mother having AIDS, being female, and greater parental drug use (Stein, Riedel, & Rotheram-Borus, 1999). Such adult role-taking predicted more internalized emotional distress among the adolescents. Expectation of early autonomy has been associated with greater use of illicit drugs (Rosenthal, Smith, & de Visser, 1999) and misconduct and lack of restraint (Feldman & Quatman, 1988).

Disclosure and Stigma

Despite the fact that many HIV-positive mothers chose not to disclose their HIV status, previous research indicates that even for children who are not told, psychological distress may be apparent due to guilt they feel for a disordered family environment whose source they cannot identify (Weiner & Septimus, 1990). Children of HIV-infected mothers who found out their mothers' status frequently report that they knew something was wrong but felt unable to ask about the cause (Nagler, Adnopoz, & Forsyth, 1995). For example, regardless of whether mothers living with HIV have disclosed, children are often aware that their mothers are taking medications, and they ask about their mothers' health (Murphy et al., 2001).

For those children whose mothers have disclosed to them, the most prevalent child response is anxiety, primarily focused on the mother's health and fear of her death (Murphy, Roberts, & Hoffman, 2003b). For most children, the anxiety decreased over time, although for a small number it sustained and became maladaptive. Most mothers (68%), however, report they do not regret having disclosed (Murphy, Roberts, & Hoffman, 2003a), although many recommend follow-up support for the children. Murphy et al. (2001) found that children informed by their mothers exhibited lower levels of aggressiveness and were somewhat more likely to report lower levels of negative self-esteem compared to uninformed children.

Stigma associated with HIV complicates the process of disclosure, affecting not only the HIV-infected mothers but also their families (Madru, 2003). Young children whose mothers have disclosed their serostatus are very protective of their mothers, but the children also express concern about their friends finding out and ostracizing them or assuming they are infected (Murphy, Roberts, et al., 2002). Similarly, early adolescents of HIV-positive mothers have reported concern about stigma and ostracism (Brackis-Cott et al., 2003). Reactions related to stigma may be exacerbated among young adolescents, who are often learning about HIV/AIDS transmission, treatment, and potential outcomes as they transition to early and middle adolescence.

Some investigators suggest healthy children in families affected by HIV may be at risk for poor developmental outcomes as a consequence of stigma (Fair, Spencer, Weiner, & Riekert, 1995), and that stigma and secrecy associated with HIV often lead families into seclusion, resulting in abnormal grief reactions (Gossart-Walker & Moss, 1998). Rehm and Franck (2000) reported that the need for stigma management prevents families from defining their lives as normal, and they deliberately use normalization strategies to enhance family well-being. Bauman, Camacho, Silver, Hudis, and Draimin (2002), however, reported that child behavior problems among HIV-affected children were not related to stigma.

CHILD MENTAL HEALTH, BEHAVIORAL, AND SOCIAL OUTCOMES

As can been seen by the previous review of background factors and intermediate factors that may affect child outcomes, children affected by parental HIV/AIDS are at risk for poorer mental health, behavioral, and social outcomes. Children of HIV-positive mothers have been found to have more difficulties in all domains of psychosocial adjustment (Forehand et al., 1998; Hough et al., 2003). In one study, children living with a seropositive mother showed greater disturbance in the parent-child relationship and greater disturbance in psychological functioning than other children attending public school in the same community (Reyland et al., 2002). Children living with mothers who have HIV symptoms or are diagnosed with AIDS have also been found to have poorer grades than children living with noninfected mothers (Biggar et al., 2000). Among adolescents of parents with HIV, somatic symptoms were found to persist during adolescence (Lester, Stein, & Bursch, 2003).

SUMMARY

Given the relatively poor outcomes of children affected by parental HIV/AIDS, there is a crucial need for service and intervention for this population. We now have some understanding from studies reviewed here of the variables that need to be targeted in such service provision. For example, we know that when parents disclose their status, children may need short-term support to deal with the disclosure. They may also need assistance with their anxiety about "catching" HIV and their fear of losing their parent. We also know that children are aware of the stigma related to HIV/AIDS and have concerns about their parents being stigmatized as well as concerns about being stigmatized themselves (Murphy, Roberts, et al., 2002). We know very little about how to provide services effectively, however: It may be best to work on improving parental intermediate factors affecting child outcomes, it may be best to work on improving child intermediate factors affecting child outcomes, or it may be best to adopt a multipronged approach to improve child outcomes. As can be seen from this review, the state of research in this area has only progressed to the stage of identifying factors associated with child outcomes. Investigators need to use this information to identify successful methods of improving the outcomes of children affected by parental HIV/AIDS.

REFERENCES

Adler, N. E., & Snibbe, A. C. (2003). The role of psychosocial processes in explaining the gradient between socioeconomic status and health. *Current Directions in Psychological Science, 12,* 119-123.

Allen, J. P., Hauser, S. T., Bell, K. L., & O'Connor, T. G. (1994). Longitudinal assessment of autonomy and relatedness in adolescent-family interactions as predictors of adolescent ego development and self-esteem. *Child Development, 65,* 179-194.

Anderson, R. N., & Smith, B. L. (2003). Deaths: Leading causes for 2001. *National Vital Statistics Reports, 52*(9), 1-86.

Armistead, L., Klein, K., & Forehand, R. (1995). Parental physical illness and child functioning. Special Issue: The impact of the family on child adjustment and psychopathology. *Clinical Psychology Review, 15,* 409-422.

Bauman, L. J., Camacho, S., Silver, E. J., Hudis, J., & Draimin, B. (2002). Behavioral problems in school-aged children of mothers with HIV/AIDS. *Clinical Child Psychology & Psychiatry, 7,* 39-54.

Biggar, H., Forehand, R., Chance, M. W., Morse, E., Morse, P., & Stock, M. (2000). The relationship of maternal HIV status and home variables to academic performance of African American children. *AIDS & Behavior, 4,* 241-252.

Brackis-Cott, E., Mellins, C. A., & Block, M. (2003). Current life concerns of early adolescents and their mothers: Influence of maternal HIV. *Journal of Early Adolescence, 23,* 51-77.

Brown, B. B., Mounts, N., Lamborn, S. D., & Steinberg, L. (1993). Parenting practices and peer group affiliation in adolescence. *Child Development, 64,* 467-482.

Brown, G. W., Harris, T. O., & Bifulco, A. (1986). Long-term effects of early loss of parent. In M. Rutter, C. E. Izard, & P. B. Read (Eds.), *Depression in young people: Developmental and clinical perspectives* (pp. 251-296). New York: Guilford.

Cates, J. A., Graham, L. L., Boeglin, D., & Tiekler, S. (1990). The effect of AIDS on the family system. *Families in Society, 71,* 195-201.

Cederfjaell, C., Langius-Ekloef, A., Lidman, K., & Wredling, R. (2001). Gender differences in perceived health-related quality of life among patients with HIV infection. *AIDS Patient Care and STDs, 15,* 31-39.

Centers for Disease Control and Prevention. (1981). Pneumocystis pneumonia–Los Angeles. *Morbidity and Mortality Weekly Report, 30,* 250-252.

Centers for Disease Control and Prevention. (1997). Update: Trends in AIDS incidence–United States, 1996. *Morbidity and Mortality Weekly Report, 46,* 861-867.

Centers for Disease Control and Prevention. (1998). *Trends in the HIV and AIDS epidemic.* Retrieved September 12, 2003, from http://www.cdc.gov/nchstp/od/trends.htm

Centers for Disease Control and Prevention. (2002). *HIV/AIDS surveillance report.* Atlanta, GA: Author.

Chavez, L. R., Hubbell, F. A., McMullin, J. M., Martinez, R. G., & Mishra, S. I. (1995). Structure and meaning in models of breast and cervical cancer risk factors: A comparison of perceptions among Latinas, Anglo women, and physicians. *Medical Anthropology Quarterly, 9,* 40-74.

Chesney, M. A., & Smith, A. W. (1999). Critical delays in HIV testing and care: The potential role of stigma. *American Behavioral Scientist, 42,* 1162-1174.

Chu, S. Y., Hanson, D., Jones, J., & the Adult/Adolescent Spectrum of HIV Disease (ASD) Project Group, Centers for Disease Control and Prevention. (1995, October). *Pregnancy rates among HIV-infected women.* Paper presented at the annual meeting of the American Public Health Association, San Diego, CA.

Clark, L. (1998). Gender and generation in poor women's household health production experiences. In P. J. Brown (Ed.), *Understanding and applying medical anthropology* (pp. 158-168). Mountain View, CA: Mayfield.

Compas, B. E., Worsham, N. L., Ey, S., & Howell, D. C. (1996). When mom or dad has cancer: II. Coping, cognitive appraisals, and psychological distress in children of cancer patients. *Health Psychology, 15,* 167-175.

Derogatis, L. R., Morrow, G. R., Fetting, J., Penman, D., Piasetski, S., Schmale, A. M., et al. (1983). The prevalence of psychiatric disorders among cancer patients. *Journal of the American Medical Association, 249,* 751-757.

Dorsey, S., Forehand, R., Armistead, L. P., Morse, E., Morse, P., & Stock, M. (1999). Mother knows best? Mother and child report of behavioral difficulties of children of HIV-infected mothers. *Journal of Psychopathology & Behavioral Assessment, 21,* 191-206.

Dutra, R., Forehand, R., Armistead, L., Brody, G., Morse, E., Morse, P. S., et al. (2000). Child resiliency in inner-city families affected by HIV: The role of family variables. *Behaviour Research & Therapy, 38,* 471-478.

Epstein, S. (1996). *Impure science: AIDS, activism, and the politics of knowledge.* Berkeley: University of California Press.

Fair, C. D., Spencer, E. D., Weiner, L., & Riekert, K. (1995). Healthy children in families affected by AIDS: Epidemiological and psychosocial considerations. *Child & Adolescent Social Work Journal, 12,* 165-181.

Faithful, J. (1997). HIV-positive and AIDS-infected women: Challenges to mothering. *American Journal of Orthopsychiatry, 67,* 144-151.

Feldman, S. S., & Quatman, T. (1988). Factors influencing age expectations for adolescent autonomy: A study of early adolescents and parents. *Journal of Early Adolescence, 8,* 325-342.

Fields, J., & Casper, L. M. (2001). America's families and living arrangements: March 2000. In *Current population reports* (pp. 20-537). Washington, DC: U.S. Census Bureau.

Flannelly, L. T., & Inouye, J. (2001). Relationships of religion, health status and socioeconomic status to the quality of life of individuals who are HIV positive. *Issues in Mental Health Nursing, 22,* 253-272.

Fleming, P. L., Byers, R. H., Sweeney, P. A., Daniels, D., Karon, J. M., & Janssen, R. S. (2002, February). *HIV prevalence in the United States, 2000.* Paper presented at the ninth Conference on Retroviruses and Opportunistic Infections, Seattle, WA.

Forehand, R., Steele, R., Armistead, L., Morse, E., Simon, P., & Clark, L. (1998). The Family Health Project: Psychosocial adjustment of children whose mothers are HIV infected. *Journal of Consulting and Clinical Psychology, 66,* 513-520.

Forsyth, B. W. C. (1995). A pandemic out of control: The epidemiology of AIDS. In S. Geballe, J. Gruendel, & W. Andiman (Eds.), *Forgotten children and the AIDS epidemic* (pp. 19-31). New Haven, CT: Yale University Press.

Frank, E., Elon, L., & Hogue, C. (2003). Transgenerational persistence of education as a health risk: Findings from the women physicians' health study. *Journal of Women's Health, 12,* 505-512.

Gallo, L. C., & Matthews, K. A. (2003). Understanding the association between socioeconomic status and physical health: Do negative emotions play a role? *Psychological Bulletin, 129,* 10-51.

Garber, J., & Little, S. (1999). Predictors of competence among offspring of depressed mothers. *Journal of Adolescent Research, 14,* 44-71.

Garmezy, N. (1985). Stress-resistant children: The search for protective factors. In J. E. Stevenson (Ed.), *Recent research in developmental psychopathology* (pp. 213-233). New York: Pergamon.

Garmezy, N. (1991). Resiliency and vulnerability to adverse developmental outcomes associated with poverty. *American Behavioral Scientist, 34,* 416-430.

Garmezy, N., & Rutter, M. (1985). Acute reactions to stress. In M. Rutter & L. Hersov (Eds.), *Child psychiatry: Modern approaches* (2nd ed., pp. 152-176). Oxford, UK: Blackwell Scientific.

Gossart-Walker, S., & Moss, N. E. (1998). Support groups for HIV-affected children. *Journal of Child & Adolescent Group Therapy, 8,* 55-69.

Gwinn, M., Pappaioanou, M., George, J. R., Hannon, W. H., Wasser, S. C., Redus, M. A., et al. (1991). Prevalence of HIV infection in childbearing women in the United States. *Journal of the American Medical Association, 265,* 1704-1708.

Hamilton, L. A. (1996). Dyadic family relationships and gender in adolescent identity formation: A social relations analysis. *Dissertation Abstracts International, 57,* 4056. (UMI No. AAM96–33181)

Hough, E. S., Brumitt, G., Templin, T., Saltz, E., & Mood, D. (2003). A model of mother-child coping and adjustment to HIV. *Social Science & Medicine, 56,* 643-655.

Kalichman, S. C., Graham, J., Luke, W., & Austin, J. (2002). Perceptions of health care among persons living with HIV/AIDS who are not receiving antiretroviral medications. *AIDS Patient Care and STDs, 16,* 233-240.

Kaplan, M. S., Marks, G., & Mertens, S. B. (1997). Distress and coping among women with HIV infection: Preliminary findings from a multiethnic sample. *American Journal of Orthopsychiatry, 67,* 80-91.

Kimerling, R., Calhoun, K. S., Forehand, R., Armistead, L., Morse, E., Morse, P., et al. (1999). Traumatic stress in HIV-infected women. *AIDS Education & Prevention, 11,* 321-330.

Klein, K., Armistead, L., Devine, D., Kotchick, B., Forehand, R., Morse, E., et al. (2000). Socioemotional support in African American families coping with maternal HIV: An examination of mothers' and children's psychosocial adjustment. *Behavior Therapy, 31,* 1-26.

Kotchick, B. A., Forehand, R., Brody, G., Armistead, L., Simon, P., Morse, E., et al. (1997). The impact of maternal HIV-infection on parenting in inner-city African American families. *Journal of Family Psychology, 11,* 447-461.

Kotchick, B. A., Forehand, R., Wierson, M., Armistead, L., & Klein, K. (1996). Coping with illness: Interrelationships across family members and predictors of psychological adjustment. *Journal of Family Psychology, 10,* 358-370.

Lamping, D. L., Sewitch, M., Clark, E., Ryan, B., Gilmore, N., Grover, S. A., et al. (1991, June). *HIV-related mental health distress in persons with HIV infection, caregivers, and family members/significant others: Results of a cross-Canada survey.* Paper presented at the International Conference on AIDS, Florence, Italy.

Lansdown, R., & Benjamin, G. (1985). The development of the concept of death in children aged 5-9 years. *Child: Care, Health, and Development, 11,* 13-20.

Lester, P., Stein, J. A., & Bursch, B. (2003). Developmental predictors of somatic symptoms in adolescents of parents with HIV: A 12-month follow-up. *Journal of Developmental & Behavioral Pediatrics, 24,* 242-250.

Lichtenstein, B., Laska, M. K., & Clair, J. M. (2002). Chronic sorrow in the HIV-positive patient: Issues of race, gender, and social support. *AIDS Patient Care and STDs, 16,* 27-38.

Linver, M. R., & Silverberg, S. B. (1995). Parenting as a multidimensional construct: Differential prediction of adolescents' sense of self and engagement in problem behavior. *International Journal of Adolescent Medicine & Health, 8,* 29-40.

Lyketsos, C. G., Hoover, D. R., Guccione, M., Dew, M. A., Wesch, J. E., Bing, E. G., et al. (1996). Changes in depressive symptoms as AIDS develops. The Multicenter AIDS Cohort Study. *American Journal of Psychiatry, 153,* 1430-1437.

Madru, N. (2003). Stigma and HIV: Does the social response affect the natural course of the epidemic? *Journal of the Association of Nurses in AIDS Care, 14,* 39-48.

Marks, G., Bundek, N. I., Richardson, J. L., Ruiz, M. S., Moldonado, N., & Mason, H. R. C. (1992). Self-disclosure of HIV infection: Preliminary results from a sample of Hispanic men. *Health Psychology, 11,* 300-306.

Masten, A. S., Best, K. M., & Garmezy, N. (1990). Resilience and development: Contributions from the study of children who overcome adversity. *Development and Psychopathology, 2*, 425-444.

McGoldrick, M., Pearce, J., & Giordano, J. (Eds.). (1982). *Ethnicity and family therapy.* New York: Guilford.

Michaels, D., & Levine, C. (1992). Estimates of the number of motherless youth orphaned by AIDS in the United States. *Journal of the American Medical Association, 268*, 3456-3461.

Miles, M. S., Burchinal, P., Holditch-Davis, D., & Wasilewski, Y. (1997). Personal, family, and health-related correlates of depressive symptoms in mothers with HIV. *Journal of Family Psychology, 11*, 23-34.

Moneyham, L., Seals, B., Demi, A., Sowell, R., Cohen, L., & Guillory, J. (1996). Experiences of disclosure in women infected with HIV. *Health Care for Women International, 17*, 209-220.

Murphy, D. A., Marelich, W. D., Dello Stritto, M. E., Swendeman, D., & Witkin, A. (2002). Mothers living with HIV/AIDS: Mental, physical, and family functioning. *AIDS Care, 14*, 633-644.

Murphy, D. A., Marelich, W. D., & Hoffman, D. (2002). A longitudinal study of the impact on young children of maternal HIV serostatus disclosure. *Clinical Child Psychology and Psychiatry, 7*, 55-70.

Murphy, D. A., Marelich, W. D., & Hoffman, D. (2004). *Resiliency in young children whose mothers are living with HIV/AIDS.* Manuscript submitted for publication.

Murphy, D. A., Roberts, K. J., & Hoffman, D. (2002). Stigma and ostracism associated with HIV/AIDS: Children carrying the secret of their mothers' HIV+ serostatus. *Journal of Child and Family Studies, 11*, 191-202.

Murphy, D. A., Roberts, K. J., & Hoffman, D. (2003a). Regrets and advice from mothers who have disclosed their HIV+ serostatus to their young children. *Journal of Child and Family Studies, 12*, 307-318.

Murphy, D. A., Roberts, K. J., & Hoffman, D. (2003b). *Young children's reactions to mothers' disclosure of maternal HIV+ sersostatus.* Manuscript submitted for publication.

Murphy, D. A., Steers, W. N., & Dello Stritto, M. E. (2001). Maternal disclosure of mother's HIV serostatus to their young children. *Journal of Family Psychology, 15*, 441-450.

Nagler, S., Adnopoz, J., & Forsyth, W. (1995). Uncertainty, stigma, and secrecy: Psychological aspects of AIDS for children and adolescents. In S. Geballe, J. Gruendel, & W. Andemann (Eds.), *Forgotten children of the AIDS epidemic* (pp. 71-82). New Haven, CT: Yale University Press.

Osborne, M. L., Kistner, J. A., & Helgemo, B. (1993). Developmental progression in children's knowledge of AIDS: Implications for education and attitudinal change. *Journal of Pediatric Psychology, 18*, 177-192.

Ostrove, J. M., Feldman, P., & Adler, N. E. (1999). Relations among socioeconomic status indicators and health for African-Americans and whites. *Journal of Health Psychology, 4*, 451-463.

Palella, F. J., Jr., Delaney, K. M., Moorman, A. C., Loveless, M. O., Fuhrer, J., Satten, G. A., et al. (1998). Declining morbidity and mortality among patients with advanced human immunodeficiency virus infection. *New England Journal of Medicine, 338*, 853-860.

Pergami, A., Gala, C., Burgess, A., Durbano, F., Zanello, D., Riccio, M., et al. (1993). The psychosocial impact of HIV infection in women. *Journal of Psychosomatic Research, 37,* 687-696.

Perrin, E. C., & Gerrity, P. S. (1981). There's a demon in your belly: Children's understanding of illness. *Pediatrics, 67,* 841-849.

Petrak, J. A., Doyle, A.-M., Smith, A., Skinner, C., & Hedge, B. (2001). Factors associated with self-disclosure of HIV serostatus to significant others. *British Journal of Health Psychology, 6,* 69-79.

Rapp, R. (1998). Accounting for amniocentesis. In P. J. Brown (Ed.), *Understanding and applying medical anthropology* (pp. 366-374). Mountain View, CA: Mayfield.

Rehm, R. S., & Franck, L. S. (2000). Long-term goals and normalization strategies of children and families affected by HIV/AIDS. *Advances in Nursing Science, 23,* 69-82.

Reyland, S. A., McMahon, T. J., Higgins-Delessandro, A., & Luthar, S. S. (2002). Inner-city children living with an HIV-seropositive mother: Parent-child relationships, perception of social support, and psychological disturbance. *Journal of Child & Family Studies, 11,* 313-329.

Rosenthal, D. A., & Smith, A. M. (1997). Adolescent sexual timetable. *Journal of Youth & Adolescence, 26,* 619-636.

Rosenthal, D. A., Smith, A. M., & de Visser, R. (1999). Personal and social factors influencing age at first sexual intercourse. *Archives of Sexual Behavior, 28,* 319-333.

Sandler, I. N., Tein, J., & West, S. G. (1994). Coping, stress, and the psychological symptoms of children of divorce: A cross-sectional and longitudinal study. *Child Development, 65,* 1744-1763.

Sandler, I. N., West, S. G., Baca, L., Pillow, D. R., Gersten, J. C., Rogosch, F., et al. (1992). Linking empirically based theory and evaluation: The Family Bereavement Program. *American Journal of Community Psychology, 20,* 491-521.

Sargent, C., & Brettell, C. (1996). Introduction: Gender, medicine, and health. In C. Sargent & C. Brettell (Eds.), *Gender and health: An international perspective* (pp. 1-21). Englewood Cliffs, NJ: Prentice Hall.

Schable, B., Diaz, T., Chu, S. Y., Caldwell, M. B., Conti, L., Alston, O. M., et al. (1995). Who are the primary caretakers of children born to HIV-infected mothers? Results from a multistate surveillance project. *Pediatrics, 95,* 511-515.

Schuster, M. A., Kanouse, D. E., Morton, S. C., Bozzette, S. A., Miu, A., Scott, G. B., et al. (2000). HIV-infected parents and their children in the United States. *American Journal of Public Health, 90,* 1074-1081.

Serovich, J. M., Kimberly, J. A., Mosack, K. E., & Lewis, T. L. (2001). The role of family and friend social support in reducing emotional distress among HIV-positive women. *AIDS Care, 13,* 335-341.

Shure, M. B. (1988). How to think, not what to think: A cognitive approach to prevention. In L. A. Bond & B. M. Wagner (Eds.), *Families in transition: Primary prevention programs that work* (pp. 170-199). Newbury Park, CA: Sage.

Shure, M. B., & Spivack, G. (1987). Competence-building as an approach to prevention of dysfunction: The ICPS model. In J. A. Steinberg & M. Silverman (Eds.), *Preventing mental disorders: A research perspective* (pp. 124-139). Rockville, MD: National Institute of Mental Health.

Silver, E. J., Bauman, L. J., Camacho, S., & Hudis, J. (2003). Factors associated with psychological distress in urban mothers with late-stage HIV/AIDS. *AIDS & Behavior, 7*, 421-431.

Sly, D. F., Eberstein, I. W., Quadagno, D., & Kistner, J. A. (1992). Young children's awareness, knowledge, and beliefs about AIDS: Observations from a pretest. *AIDS Education and Prevention, 4*, 227-239.

Smith, J. M. (1996). *AIDS and society.* Upper Saddle River, NJ: Prentice Hall.

Stein, J. A., Riedel, M., & Rotheram-Borus, M. J. (1999). Parentification and its impact on adolescent children of parents with AIDS. *Family Process, 38*, 193-208.

Steinberg, L. (1987). Familial factors in delinquency: A developmental perspective. *Journal of Adolescent Research, 2*, 255-268.

Swartz, H. A., Markowitz, J. C., & Sewell, M. C. (1998). Psychosocial characteristics of pregnant and nonpregnant HIV-seropositive women. *Psychiatric Services, 49*, 1612-1614.

Sweat, M. D., & Levin, M. (1995). HIV/AIDS knowledge among the U.S. population. *AIDS Education & Prevention, 7*, 355-375.

Taylor, R. D. (1996). Adolescents' perceptions of kinship support and family management practices: Association with adolescent adjustment in African American families. *Developmental Psychology, 32*, 687-695.

Tompkins, T. L., Henker, B., Whalen, C. K., Axelrod, J., & Comer, L. K. (1999). Motherhood in the context of HIV infection: Reading between the numbers. *Cultural Diversity & Ethnic Minority Psychology, 5*, 197-208.

Udry, J. R. (1990). Hormonal and social determinants of adolescent sexual initiation. In J. Bancroft & J. M. Reinisch (Eds.), *Adolescence and puberty* (Vol. 3, pp. 841-855). New York: Oxford University Press.

United Nations Programme on HIV/AIDS. (2003). *AIDS epidemic update: 2003.* Geneva: United Nations Programme on HIV/AIDS/World Health Organization.

Valdiserri, R. O., Holtgrave, D. R., & West, G. R. (1999). Promoting early HIV diagnosis and entry into care. *AIDS, 13*, 2317-2330.

Vosvick, M., Gore-Felton, C., Koopman, C., Thoresen, C., Krumboltz, J., & Spiegel, D. (2002). Maladaptive coping strategies in relation to quality of life among HIV+ adults. *AIDS & Behavior, 6*, 97-106.

Vosvick, M., Koopman, C., Gore-Felton, C., Thoresen, C., Krumboltz, J., & Spiegel, D. (2003). Relationship of functional quality of life to strategies for coping with the stress of living with HIV/AIDS. *Psychosomatics: Journal of Consultation Liaison Psychiatry, 44*, 51-58.

Webster-Stratton, C., & Hammond, M. (1988). Maternal depression and its relationship to life stress, perceptions of child behavior problems, parenting behaviors, and child conduct problems. *Journal of Abnormal Child Psychology, 16*, 299-315.

Weiner, L., & Septimus, A. (1990). Psychological consideration and support for the child and family. In P. Pizzo (Ed.), *Pediatric AIDS: The challenge of HIV infection in infants, children and adolescents* (pp. 577-594). New York: Williams & Wilkins.

West, S. G., Sandler, I., Baca, L., Pillow, D. R., & Gersten, J. C. (1991). The use of structural equation modeling in generative research: Toward the design of a preventive intervention for bereaved children. *American Journal of Community Psychology, 19*, 459-480.

Wills, T. A., Blechman, E. A., & McNamara, G. (1996). Family support, coping, and competence. In E. M. Hetherington & E. A. Blechman (Eds.), *Stress, coping, and resiliency in children and families. Family research consortium: Advances in family research* (pp. 107-133). Hillsdale, NJ: Lawrence Erlbaum.

Wills, T. A., & Cleary, S. D. (1996). How are social support effects mediated? A test with parental support and adolescent substance use. *Journal of Personality & Social Psychology, 71,* 937-952.

Wilson, H. W. (2001, July). *Risky behaviors in clinically disturbed girls: Which relationships matter—Parents, peers, or partners?* Paper presented at the NIMH Annual International Research Conference on the Role of Families in Preventing and Adapting to HIV/AIDS, Los Angeles.

Woods, N. F., Haberman, M. R., & Packard, N. J. (1993). Demands of illness and individual, dyadic, and family adaptation in chronic illness. *Western Journal of Nursing Research, 15,* 10-25.

Worsham, N. L., Compas, B. E., & Ey, S. (1997). Children's coping with parental illness. In S. A. Wolchik & I. N. Sandler (Eds.), *Handbook of children's coping: Linking theory and intervention* (pp. 195-213). New York: Plenum.

CHAPTER 12

Families, Health, and Genomics

MARCIA VAN RIPER AND AGATHA M. GALLO

In April 2003, 50 years after Watson and Crick discovered the double helix structure of deoxyribonucleic acid (DNA), researchers working on an international effort known as the Human Genome Project (HGP) completed a high-quality, comprehensive sequence of the human genome (Collins, Green, Guttmacher, & Guyer, 2003). The sequencing of the human genome is a major accomplishment that promises to have a profound impact on our understanding of the role of genetic factors in human health and disease. It provides unparalleled opportunities to study the complex interplay between genetic and environmental factors that trigger, accelerate, or exacerbate the disease process (Desiere, 2004; Greco, 2003).

Professionals in the family and health sciences need to understand how individuals and families are affected by advances in genomics because an increasing number of genomic advances are already being applied to the prevention, diagnosis, and treatment of disease (Guttmacher & Collins, 2003): Preimplantation genetic diagnosis is being used to help families affected by devastating genetic conditions have unaffected children (Jones, 2004; Sermon, Van Steirteghem, &

Liebaers, 2004), genetic testing for BRCA1/2 mutations is becoming an integral component of the care of individuals whose family history indicates an increased risk for hereditary breast and ovarian cancer (Lerman & Shields, 2004; Mincey, 2003), new approaches to gene therapy are being used to deter the progression of disease to end-organ failure and transplantation (Cashion, 2002), and genomic mapping tools are being used to develop safer and more effective drugs (Roses, 2004). Although advances such as these have the potential to benefit many families, there is also the potential that these and other advances in genomics will be distributed unequally, resulting in a society of genetic haves and have-nots (Mehlman & Botkin, 1998).

One of our challenges as professionals in the family and health sciences is to provide every family with a chance to obtain access to advances in genomics. Another challenge is to identify effective ways of addressing the ethical, legal, and social implications of genomic advances (Clayton, 2003). For example, we need to determine the best way to approach the "duty to warn" issue in families with an increased risk of hereditary conditions

(Offit, Groeger, Turner, Wadsworth, & Weiser, 2004). Because of our genetic makeup, we are linked with each other, not only within our families but also in larger communities and the world. Therefore, decisions about the disclosure of genetic information cannot be merely considered as, and reduced to, a matter of individual choice; in decisions about whether, when, or how genetic information should be shared, one must always be aware of both the interests of the individual and the interests of those who they are linked to genetically (de Wert, ter Meulen, Mordacci, & Tallacchini, 2003). In our work with families in which one or more individuals undergo genetic testing, we will need to find a way to respect and protect the individual's right to privacy while simultaneously preventing harm and promoting the welfare of other family members (Doukas & Berg, 2001; Jacobs & Deatrick, 1999).

The purpose of this chapter is to provide an overview of the existing literature on how families make sense of, respond to, and use advances in genomics. It is hoped that this effort will stimulate the development of additional family research in this area—research that will ultimately lead to the testing and implementation of tailored, culturally sensitive interventions for individuals and families who are being tested for and living with genetic conditions.

A SHIFT FROM GENETICS TO GENOMICS

As genetic knowledge has increased, there has been a gradual shift from genetics to genomics in health care (Khoury, 2003). According to Guttmacher and Collins (2002), genetics is the "study of single genes and their effects" (p. 1512), whereas genomics is the "study not just of single genes, but the functions and interactions of all the genes in the genome" (p. 1512). Khoury (2003) described the shift from genetics to genomics as a

continuum ranging from the concept of disease in genetics to the concept of genetic information in genomics. Medical genetics has traditionally focused on hereditary conditions resulting from either a mutation in a single gene (e.g., cystic fibrosis, sickle cell disease, and Huntington disease) or an abnormal number of chromosomes (e.g., trisomy 21 and Turner's syndrome). For these conditions, which affect a relatively small number of individuals in the population, genetic services usually include genetic counseling, education, and support. Geneticists, genetic counselors, and nurses or other health care professionals with genetics expertise typically provide these genetic services.

Genomics is a broader term. It reflects complex interactions involving multiple genes and interactions between genes and environmental factors, such as nutrition, drugs, infectious agents, chemicals, behavioral factors, and physical agents that trigger, accelerate, or exacerbate the disease process (Desiere, 2004; Greco, 2003). Gene-gene and gene-environment interactions are thought to play a critical role in the development of many common diseases, such as heart disease, cancer, diabetes, and Alzheimer's disease (Collins et al., 2003; Greco, 2003; Guttmacher & Collins, 2002; Khoury, 2003; Newell, 2004; Wung, 2002). In the future, it is likely that some type of genetic screening will be offered to populations or subgroups of high-risk individuals and families in an effort to prevent, diagnose, and treat these and other common diseases (Collins & McKusick, 2001; Khoury, McCabe, & McCabe, 2003).

INCREASED DEMAND FOR PROFESSIONALS WITH EXPERTISE IN GENOMICS

The shift from genetics to genomics has created an increased demand for health care professionals who understand the contribution of genetic and environmental factors to health and disease, as well as the impact of genomic advances on disease management (Collins & Guttmacher, 2001; Greco, 2003). Recent advances in genomics have quelled the nature versus nurture debate (de Waal, 1999; Greco, 2003). It is no longer a question of if genes or environment determine human behavior but a question of how genes and environment influence human behavior. According to de Waal (1999),

> Trying to determine how much of a trait is produced by genes and how much by the environment is as useless as asking whether the drumming that we hear in the distance is made by the percussionist or by his instrument. (p. 947)

Many health care professionals lack the knowledge base necessary to integrate genome-based knowledge into their practice (Burke & Emery, 2002; Collins & Guttmacher, 2001; Doukas & Berg, 2001; Khoury, 2003; Olsen et al., 2003). This is due, in part, to the fact that most health care professionals have had little or no formal education in genomics (Burke & Emery, 2002; Greendale & Reed, 2001; Hetteberg, Prows, Deets, Monsen, & Kenner, 1999). In addition, advances in genomics have been occurring so rapidly that it may be difficult for health care professionals to keep abreast of new discoveries. Moreover, for some health care professionals, the relevance of genomics may not be obvious (Wulfsburg, 2000); therefore, they may have minimal interest in becoming better educated about genomics (Greendale & Reed, 2001).

Fortunately, interest in genomics appears to be growing among health care professionals, and there has been a significant increase in the number and type of educational offerings in genomics for health care professionals. In addition to workshops and annual conferences for organizations such as the International Society of Nurses in Genetics, the American Society of Human Genetics,

and the American College of Medical Genetics, there have been special issues devoted to genomics in a wide variety of professional journals (e.g., *New England Journal of Medicine, Biological Research for Nursing,* and *Seminar in Oncology Nursing*). Furthermore, the number of online resources in genomics has expanded dramatically. Because many of these educational offerings were developed with funding from the National Human Genome Research Institute (NHGRI), they are available free of charge (see http://www.genome.gov/Education/).

TRANSLATION OF HUMAN GENOME PROJECT PROMISES INTO BENEFITS

Efforts by NHGRI and Researchers Funded by the Ethical, Legal, and Social Implications Research Program of NHGRI

NHGRI has taken a lead role in translating the promises of the HGP into benefits for individuals and families (Collins et al., 2003). In addition to providing funding for genomic research, NHGRI provides funding for professional and public education in genomics. Much of NHGRI's funding for genomic education is provided through the Ethical, Legal, and Social Implications Research Program (ELSI) of NHGRI.

Ethical, Legal, and Social Implications Research Program

The ELSI program was started in 1990 at the same time the HGP began. Five percent of the HGP's funds are designated to the ELSI program. In 2002, this amounted to approximately $16.5 million (Olsen et al., 2003). Of high priority for the ELSI program are issues surrounding the completion of the human DNA sequence and the study of human genetic variation; issues raised by the integration of genetic technologies and information into health care and public health activities; issues raised by the integration of knowledge about genomics and gene-environment interactions into nonclinical settings; ways in which new genetic knowledge may interact with a variety of philosophical, theological, and ethical perspectives; and how socioeconomic factors and concepts of race and ethnicity influence the use and interpretation of genetic information, the utilization of genetic services, and the development of policy. All these issues are relevant to families and may be examined using a family perspective.

Only a minority of the studies funded by the ELSI program have used the family as the unit of analysis: Culture and Family Interpretation of Genetic Disorders (Grant R01 HG02164) by Skinner and colleagues; Family Disclosure of Cancer Risk: An Ethnographic Study (Grant R01 HG001885) by Press and colleagues; and Parents' Interpretation and Use of Genetic Information (Grant R01 HG002036) by Gallo and colleagues. Other studies funded by the ELSI program have examined how individuals respond to genetic testing within the context of the family: Use of Amniocentesis by Mexicans and Mexican-Americans and also Genetic Counseling Strategies With Mexican-Origin Women (Grant R01 HG01384) by Browner and colleagues; Hemophilia "A" Carrier Testing—Acceptance and Reactions (Grant R01 HG01445) by Sorenson and colleagues; and Parent Communication of BRCA1/2 Test Results to Children (Grant R01 HG002686) by Tercyak and colleagues.

National Coalition for Health Professional Education in Genetics

In the late 1990s, NHGRI, the American Medical Association, and the American Nurses Association initiated the National Coalition for Health Professional Education in Genetics (NCHPEG), a national effort to promote health professional education and access to information about advances in human genetics. NCHPEG is an interdisciplinary group composed of leaders from approximately 120 diverse health professional organizations, consumer and voluntary groups, government agencies, private industries, managed-care organizations, and genetics professional societies. A list of core competences in genetics essential for all health professionals (http://www.nchpeg.org) has been endorsed by NCHPEG members. These core competencies represent the minimum knowledge, skills, and attitudes necessary for health care professionals from all disciplines to provide patient care that involves awareness of genetic issues and concerns. By including consumer and voluntary groups, NCHPEG makes it possible for the voices of families affected by genetic conditions to be heard.

Integration of Genome-Based Knowledge Into Health Care

Despite notable examples of how advances in genomics are being applied in health care, it could take years, possibly generations, before much of the genome-based knowledge from the HGP and other genomic research is translated into health benefits for individuals and families (Bell, 2003; Collins et al., 2003). One example of where genome-based knowledge is being routinely applied in health care is in the area of genetic testing. According to the GeneTests Web site (http://www.genetests .org), a publicly funded medical genetics information resource developed for physicians, other health care providers, and researchers, there are more than 1,000 genetic tests being used commercially, and many of these are being marketed directly to consumers (Burke, 2004; Gray, 2003; Hull & Prasad, 2001; McCabe & McCabe, 2004).

Although most genetic tests are being used to diagnose genetic disease, other uses of genetic tests include the identification of future health risk, the prediction of drug responses, and the assessment of risks for future children (Burke, 2002).

Unfortunately, effective treatment is available for only a minority of the genetic conditions being tested for, such as phenylketonuria and hereditary hemochromatosis. Thus, although it is possible for health care professionals to use genetic tests to determine whether an individual has or is likely to develop more than 1,000 conditions, it is not possible for health care professionals to offer effective treatment for most of these. The delay that exists between the ability to test and the ability to treat creates ethical, legal, and social consequences for families (Green, 1999; Johnson, Wilkinson, & Taylor-Brown, 1999; Juengst, 1997, 1999).

According to Thomson (1997), the major risk associated with genetic testing is that of gaining information: information that may result in increased anxiety, altered family relationships, discrimination, or stigmatization; information that may be difficult to keep confidential; and information about which little can be done, in most cases. Thomson also noted that informed consent is very difficult to ensure when some of the outcomes, benefits, and risks of genetic testing remain unknown. In addition, many of the tests being used are imperfect. That is, they do not have a 100% detection rate. Individuals and families who receive false-positive results may terminate an unaffected pregnancy or undergo unnecessary risk-reducing surgery. Also, individuals and families who receive false-negative results may fail to follow surveillance strategies designed to improve their health outcomes because they have been falsely reassured that they are not at increased risk for a genetic condition.

BRCA1/2 Testing for Women Newly Diagnosed With Breast Cancer: Exemplar of the Integration of Genetic Information Into Individual and Family Responses to Illness.

As knowledge of the genetic basis of disease and behavior continues to increase, increasingly more individuals and families will be called on to integrate genetic information into their responses to illness challenges. For example, women newly diagnosed with breast cancer are increasingly being asked to consider undergoing BRCA1/2 testing before they make decisions about treatment options (Daly, 2004; Meijers-Heijboer et al., 2003; Schwartz et al., 2004; Weitzel et al., 2003). This is occurring largely because a number of studies have shown that a woman's short-term risk of developing a second breast cancer is substantially affected by whether she carries a BRCA1/2 mutation, and prophylactic surgery has been found to decrease the risk of breast and ovarian cancer by more than 90% (Hartmann, Degnim, & Schaid, 2004; McDonnell et al., 2001; Meijers-Heijboer et al., 2003; Rebbeck et al., 2004). It is estimated that 5% to 10% of all breast cancers result from the inheritance of a mutation in a gene, such as the BRCA gene.

The main advantage to offering BRCA1/2 testing prior to the onset of treatment is that it gives women who are found to carry a deleterious mutation the option of choosing risk-reduction surgery concurrent with therapeutic surgical treatment. That is, women with newly diagnosed breast cancer are given the option of choosing to undergo a bilateral mastectomy or a bilateral mastectomy and bilateral oophorectomy rather than breast conserving surgery, the treatment option chosen by many women with breast cancer. Carriers of a BRCA1/2 mutation who opt for a bilateral mastectomy can prevent future breast cancers and avoid unnecessary radiation treatment and possibly a second surgery should they later decide to or need to have their other breast removed (Schwartz et al., 2004; Weitzel et al., 2003).

The main disadvantages to offering BRCA1/2 testing prior to the onset of treatment are that women who are already dealing with the stress of a new cancer diagnosis have to deal with the added stress of genetic testing; the cost of the BRCA1/2 testing is high—$2975 for a comprehensive BRCA analysis or $350 if a mutation has already been identified in the family; and the results may be uninformative (negative result with a high residual risk that it is a false negative or a variant of unknown significance. Another disadvantage is that there may be a delay in definitive surgical treatment because of the need to wait for the results of genetic testing (Daley, 2004).

Although some women newly diagnosed with breast cancer may welcome the opportunity to incorporate information about their mutation status into their decision making about treatment options, others may find this overwhelming. Moreover, some may be too distraught over the diagnosis of breast cancer to make well-informed decisions about genetic testing and subsequent treatment, and they may make decisions that have negative consequences for their psychological well-being.

Little is known about the experiences of women who are offered BRCA1/2 testing soon after they are diagnosed with breast cancer, and even less is known about how other members of their family respond. Because BRCA1/2 mutations are inherited in an autosomal dominant manner, each offspring of a woman who carries a BRCA mutation has a 50% chance of carrying the same mutation. Therefore, the results of BRCA1/2 testing have profound implications not only for the women who are being offered genetic testing for BRCA mutations but also for members of their immediate and extended family.

Women who choose to undergo BRCA testing need to decide whether, when, and how they want to share this information with other family members. If and when this information is shared with other family members, some family members may respond positively, whereas others may not. For example, some may view this as helpful information; they may use this information to help make their own decisions about BRCA1/2 testing, or they may use this information to guide their decision making about the use of available management options. In contrast, other family members may strongly disagree with genetic testing; they may believe it will create too much distress, or they may believe it is "fooling with God's plan." Differences in opinion about the need for and value of genetic testing may result in an increase in family conflict and a decrease in family functioning. Ultimately, this may result in the woman who is newly diagnosed with breast cancer receiving less support from her family at a time when family support could play a critical role in both her physical and her psychological well-being.

Genetic Testing for Huntington's Disease: Exemplar of Delay Between Ability to Test and Ability to Treat. The story of genetic testing for Huntington's disease (HD) exemplifies the delay that often exists between advances in genomics and the availability of effective treatment. It has been more than 20 years since researchers discovered the location of the mutation that causes this progressive, neurodegenerative disorder (Gusella et al., 1983), and mutation analysis for HD has been available since 1993 (Huntington's Disease Collaborative Research Group, 1993). Nonetheless, a treatment that will alter the natural history of HD has yet to be found, and the onset of HD continues to be somewhat difficult to predict (Smith, Michie, Stephenson, & Quarrell, 2002). Findings suggest that given the lack of effective treatment for HD, only a minority of at-risk individuals (5-25%) choose to undergo genetic testing for HD (Harper, Lim, & Craufurd, 2000; Hayden, 2000).

Individuals who choose to undergo testing for HD may experience both positive and negative consequences. Potential positive consequences are relief from uncertainty, the chance to avoid passing on a gene mutation to future generations, and prudent future planning (Chapman, 2002; Codori & Brandt, 1994; Codori, Slavney, Young, Miglioretti, & Brandt, 1997; Williams, Schutte, Evers, & Forcucci, 1999). Potential negative consequences are sadness, depression, anxiety, anger, stigmatization, discrimination, survivor guilt, uncertainty, suicide, increased family conflicts, and decreased family functioning (Harper, 1996; Lawson et al., 1996; Sobel & Cowan, 2000b; Williams, Schutte, Evers, & Holkup, 2000; Tibben, Timman, Bannink, & Duivenvoorden, 1997). Negative consequences have been reported in both those who test positive and those who test negative. The most common ethical issues associated with genetic testing for HD are concerns about autonomous decision making, anonymity, confidentiality, disclosure to others, stigmatization, insurance discrimination, the testing of children for an adult disorder, and discrimination in the workplace (Binedell & Soldan, 1997; Chapman, 2002; Hakimian, 2000; Harper, 1993; Post, 1992; Sobel & Cowan, 2000a; Stone & Miles, 1999).

FAMILIES AND GENOMICS

Genomic research has resulted in burgeoning information and outcomes that have direct consequences for families and their members. Although researchers and clinicians acknowledge that genetic information and genetic testing decisions may affect family relationships, most family genetic studies are epidemiological studies that focus on molecular biology and the collection of biological data; they typically do not focus on the family as a social unit affected by recent genomic discoveries. The findings from these studies are valuable and add to existing knowledge about the genetic basis of disease and behavior, but they do not address how families make sense of, respond to, and use recent advances in genetics.

The Family Experience of Genetic Testing

Despite increasing awareness that genetic testing is inherently a family experience (Doukas & Berg, 2001; Feetham, 1999; Juengst, 1999; McDaniel & Campbell, 1999; Richards, 1998; Sorenson & Botkin, 2003; Street & Soldan, 1998), relatively few researchers have used a family perspective in their studies of the genetic testing experience. Most researchers interested in the genetic testing experience have explored the following topics: (a) factors that influence the choices individuals make regarding genetic testing, (b) psychological consequences for individuals who undergo genetic testing, and (c) use of management options following genetic testing (surveillance, risk-reducing surgery, chemoprevention, and lifestyle changes).

In a special issue of *Families Systems & Health* that focused on genetic testing and the family, McDaniel and Campbell (1999) wrote, "Families and genetic testing is an area yet to be studied, one that cries out for clinical innovation and scientific inquiry" (p. 2). In the same issue, Feetham (1999) noted, "The paucity of attention to family systems and family relationships in the collection and dissemination of genetic information places family members and families at increased risk" (p. 27).

In a special issue on genetic testing and the family in the *American Journal of Medical Genetics*, Sorenson and Botkin (2003) reported that there has been an increase in research on genetic testing and the family, and much of this research has focused on the disclosure of genetic information within the family in the context of genetic testing.

Sorenson and Botkin went on to argue that "an increased understanding of the role of the family is critical to fostering better clinical care and more humane and ethically acceptable genetic testing policies" (p. 2).

Prenatal Testing and the Family

Much of the existing research on prenatal testing and the family has focused on the genetic testing experiences of pregnant women. There have been a few researchers, however, such as Browner and colleagues, who have explored how women respond to prenatal testing within the context of the family. Findings from the studies by Browner and colleagues have made a significant contribution to the literature on how individuals and families are affected by recent advances in prenatal testing (Browner & Preloran, 1999a, 1999b, 2000a, 2000b, 2000c, 2000d; Browner, Preloran, Casado, Bass, & Walker, 2003; Browner, Preloran, & Cox, 1999; Browner, Preloran, & Press, 1996; Markens, Browner, & Press, 1999: Press & Browner, 1993, 1997, 1998; Root & Browner, 2001). By focusing on maternal serum screening and amniocentesis, two types of prenatal testing that were widely adopted into mainstream health care within a relatively short time, Browner and colleagues have been able to bring to the foreground some of the complex ethical, legal, and social issues raised by the integration of advances in genomics into health care activities.

To fully understand the importance of the research by Browner and colleagues, one needs to have a basic understanding of how the development of prenatal screening tests, such as the various forms of maternal serum screening, dramatically changed the landscape of prenatal testing for Down syndrome and other genetic disorders (Cuckle, 2000; Holding, 2002). Initially, the primary approach used to make a prenatal diagnosis of Down syndrome was to offer a diagnostic test, such as an amniocentesis, to pregnant

women who were considered to be at high risk for having a child with Down syndrome (women older than 34 years of age and women who had already given birth to a child with Down syndrome). Then, in the early 1980s, it was discovered that maternal serum screening or alpha-feta protein screening during the second trimester of pregnancy (a test used to screen for neural tube defects since the 1970s) could be used to screen for Down syndrome and other chromosomal disorders. Subsequently, additional markers (human chorionic gonadotrophin, unconjugated estriol, and inhibin) were added to improve the sensitivity and specificity of the screening test. By the late 1990s, maternal serum screening was a routine part of prenatal care. It was often described to pregnant women and their families as "just a simple blood test" or "a way to see if your baby is healthy." Pressure for earlier screening eventually led to the discovery that markers, such as PAPP-A and free beta-hCG, could be used to screen for Down syndrome in the first trimester. It was also discovered that nuchal translucency and other morphological markers visualized by ultrasound could be added to the screening protocol to provide a better risk assessment (Ferguson-Smith, 2004).

According to Ferguson-Smith (2004), there are three main options for prenatal screening: (a) a combination of maternal serum markers and nuchal translucency during the first trimester (detection rate, 85%; false-positive rate, 2-6%), (b) a four-marker screening test during the second trimester (detection rate, 85%; false-positive rate, 6-10%), and (c) an integrated test in which the first two options are combined and families are given the results after the completion of the second option (detection rate, 85%; false-positive rate, 1-2%). Unfortunately, access to these options varies depending on factors such as where the expectant family lives (certain services are not available in some geographic areas), from whom they receive care, and whether they have the insurance coverage or personal resources necessary to cover the cost of the services.

When prenatal screening first became available, most of the women who underwent screening were white, well-educated, middle- to upper-income women. Then, as maternal serum screening became more widely used, it was introduced to a much more diverse group of pregnant women and their families (Browner et al., 1999). An increasing number of women being offered screening had no prior knowledge of or experience with genetic services. In addition, many had limited formal education and inadequate financial resources. Moreover, many were from cultures that did not share mainstream U.S. views about the role of medicine and prenatal care or the meaning of disability (Browner & Preloran, 2000c).

Browner and colleagues used a variety of approaches to examine the decisions that pregnant women and their families make about the use of prenatal testing: They reviewed the medical charts of more than 500 pregnant women, conducted semistructured interviews with hundreds of pregnant Mexican immigrant and Mexican American women and their partners, and observed interactions between health care professionals and pregnant women. One of their key findings was that by including maternal serum screening under the rubric of routine prenatal care, health care professionals not only encouraged pregnant women to undergo this type of prenatal screening but also simultaneously discouraged the women and their families from giving much thought to their decision (Browner et al., 1996; Markens et al., 1999; Press & Browner, 1993, 1997). Another key finding was that the information given to minority women and their partners about prenatal screening may not be adequate, clearly understandable, or culturally sensitive (Browner et al., 2003). Common sources of miscommunication were medical jargon, the nondirective nature of genetic counseling, inhibitions of genetic counselors related to misplaced cultural sensitivity, problems of translation, and problems of trust.

Findings from the research by Browner and colleagues suggest that the routine use of prenatal tests, such as maternal serum screening and amniocentesis, places a considerable decision-making burden on the pregnant women and families to whom they are offered: The genetic issues involved are complex, and the appropriate course of action is often ambiguous (Browner et al., 2003). To illustrate this, Browner and Preloran (2000c) offered a narrative account of one woman's decision to undergo an amniocentesis, despite the fact that she had experienced considerable confusion and turmoil after learning that her test results were positive. According to Browner and Preloran, this woman found herself caught between the promise of reassurance that a negative, or normal, amniocentesis would offer and the criticism she expected she would endure within her own family, church, and neighborhood should she subject her fetus to the test's known risks. The way she managed this difficult dilemma was to represent herself as a "victim of circumstances," one who had "no choice" but to agree to the amniocentesis. By rationalizing that the decision was out of her control, she was able to follow clinical recommendations, gain information, and leave open the option of abortion. At the same time, she was able to act according to what she regarded as maternally appropriate behavior.

Santalahti and colleagues have also explored how women respond to prenatal testing within the context of the family (Santalahti, Aro, Hemminki, Helenius, & Ryynanen, 1998; Santalahti, Hemminki, Aro, Helenius, & Ryynanen, 1999; Santalahti, Hemminki, Latikka, & Ryynanen, 1998; Santalahti, Latikka, Ryynanen, & Hemminki, 1996). Findings from their interviews with

45 pregnant women who had received positive screening results and 46 control women illustrate possible negative consequences of prenatal screening. One of the 33 women who chose to undergo an amniocentesis reported that while she was waiting for the results she had fights with her partner, smoked constantly, and drank beer. She indicated that she did not know if she drank because of the prenatal test or because of the fights, or whether the fights arose as a result of the stress caused by having to wait for the test results. Another woman reported that she had not planned to tell the positive screening result to others but had to do so because she started to cry whenever anyone asked how she felt or how her pregnancy was proceeding. A third woman described the 4 weeks that she spent waiting for the results of the amniocentesis as the most difficult time in her life. She reported that during the time she had to wait for her results, she was nervous, tearful, and hypersensitive. Even after the results came back negative, she did not feel better. She felt that something had happened to her: "Serum screening had struck her down" (p. 106).

Helm, Miranda, and Chedd (1998) interviewed 10 women who decided to continue their pregnancy after an amniocentesis revealed that the fetus had Down syndrome. According to their findings, decisions to continue the pregnancy were based on a number of interrelated themes, including broad moral values, past religious experiences, personal experiences with other people with disabilities, "seeing" the fetus on the monitor after experiencing years of infertility, and the responses of friends and relatives. One mother noted that both her parents and her in-laws were uninformed and unrealistic, with one side believing that the baby would be a "comatose vegetable" and the other side expecting that the baby would have "only a mild case of Down syndrome." In one family, the expectant parents had almost decided to terminate the pregnancy, but

they changed their mind when they heard that there was a waiting list for families interested in adopting children with Down syndrome.

Findings from a cross-sectional study of 999 socioeconomically and racially and ethnically diverse pregnant women (Learman et al., 2003) suggest that there are racial and ethnic differences in pregnant women's views on motherhood; attitudes about giving birth to an infant with Down syndrome; and the degree of influence on prenatal genetic testing decisions accepted from partners, family, faith and religion, and health care providers. For example, African Americans and Latinas were more likely than Caucasians and Asians to agree with the statement, "A child with Down syndrome would be accepted in my community." They were also more likely to state that their faith or religion would influence the prenatal testing decision and that "accepting what is given" is a part of their cultural belief system. Asian women were more likely than women in the other ethnic and racial groups to state that their family's feelings about having a child with Down syndrome would influence their decision. The authors noted that although racial and ethnic differences did exist in social and familial attitudes and influences on decision making, these differences were dwarfed by the substantial variation that remained unexplained within each racial and ethnic group.

Carrier Screening and the Family

Carrier screening is available for a number of genetic conditions that are inherited in an autosomal recessive manner, such as cystic fibrosis, sickle cell disease, and Tay-Sachs disease (de Wert et al., 2003): Cystic fibrosis is a genetic disorder characterized by severe respiratory problems and inadequate pancreatic functioning; sickle cell disease is a group of disorders in which the affected individual has heightened susceptibility to infections, variable degrees of hemolysis, and intermittent episodes of vascular occlusion resulting in tissue ischemia and acute and chronic organ dysfunction; and Tay-Sachs is a devastating neurological disorder that is usually fatal within the first few years of life. Individuals with autosomal recessive conditions have inherited two defective genes for the condition, one from each parent. In contrast, carriers of autosomal recessive conditions have inherited only one defective gene. Carriers typically show no signs or symptoms of the genetic condition, but they do have an increased risk of being the parent of an affected child.

Initially, carrier screening was offered primarily to adults with family members who had autosomal recessive conditions. Then, carrier screening programs were developed for individuals from ethnic or racial groups known to be at increased risk for specific autosomal recessive conditions. For example, in the 1970s, there was a screening program for sickle cell disease that focused on African Americans. Screening programs have also been conducted for Tay-Sachs disease in Ashkenazi Jewish communities. Although these programs may help to decrease the incidence of the specific condition, they may also increase the risk of discrimination for the individual and his or her family, especially if they are not conducted in a culturally sensitive manner that takes into account the ethical, legal, and social implications of carrier screening.

For example, in the early years of sickle cell disease screening, many people thought that carriers for sickle cell disease actually had sickle cell disease. Thus, individuals found to be carriers for sickle cell disease were discriminated against in health and life insurance, employment, school athletics, and the Armed Services (Beeson & Duster, 2002; Bowman, 1998). Reports of poor quality care, inadequate information, and professional insensitivity permeated parental accounts of screening and counseling for sickle cell disease in a study by Atkin, Waquar, and Anionwu (1998).

Carrier screening is becoming a routine part of preconceptual and prenatal care. Couples interested in undergoing preconceptual or prenatal carrier screening may choose to undergo stepwise or sequential screening or couple-based screening (Tinkle, 2002). In stepwise or sequential screening, one partner (usually the woman) is tested, and if she is found to be a carrier, then the other partner is tested. If both partners are determined to be carriers, they have a 25% chance of having an affected child with each pregnancy. They also have a 50% chance of having a child who is a carrier with each pregnancy. In couple-based screening, both partners are tested at the same time. Stepwise or sequential screening can minimize health costs, but it can also limit available reproductive options if it is done late in pregnancy. Couple-based screening is most advantageous in situations in which gestational age and reproductive choices are a concern.

To date, research concerning the carrier screening experience has focused almost exclusively on the decision to be tested. That is, researchers have examined factors that influence the decision to be tested (Cheuvront, Sorenson, Callanan, Stearns, & DeVellis, 1998; Levenkron, Loader, & Rowley, 1997; Poppelaars et al., 2004; Sorenson et al., 1997; Wertz, Janes, Rosenfield, & Erbe, 1992) and barriers to testing (Fanos & Johnson, 1995). Few researchers have examined how individuals and families choose a course of action in response to the results of carrier screening.

Wertz and colleagues (1992) used anonymous survey questionnaires, supplemented by interviews, to explore psychosocial factors underlying decisions about the use of prenatal screening for cystic fibrosis (CF) in 227 families of affected children. Of these families, 118 (51%) included one spouse who had been sterilized; 39 (18%) had a spouse, partner, or both who were older than age 45 years, widowed, or divorced or had adopted the affected child; and 70 (31%) were still considered to be at risk for having an affected child (both partners were still fertile, and they each carried a defective gene). Forty-four percent of the 70 at-risk families intended to have more children, and 77% of these had or were considering prenatal testing for CF. Among those who intended to use prenatal diagnosis for CF, 44% indicated they would carry a fetus with CF to term, 28% would abort an affected fetus, and 28% were undecided. According to Wertz and colleagues, these findings suggest that many families affected by CF would rather curtail childbearing than use selective abortion for CF.

Williams and Schutte (1997) used a qualitative approach to examine the experiences of 34 adults requesting carrier screening for four genetic disorders (i.e., cystic fibrosis, Tay-Sachs disease, Duchenne muscular dystrophy, and fragile-X syndrome). Interviews were done 1 month after receipt of test results. According to Williams and Schutte, noncarriers experienced benefits of emotional relief and freedom to move ahead with reproductive planning. In contrast, carriers experienced burdens of sadness and loss of reproductive expectations. Some individuals in both groups experienced difficulty disclosing results to selected family members. Concerns about disclosure of test results to insurance providers were also expressed.

Findings from a study by Ormond, Mills, Lester, and Ross (2003) suggest that the frequency and reasons for disclosing CF carrier status differ between individuals with and without a family history of CF. The 30 CF carriers with a family history of CF told 100% of their living parents, siblings, and half-siblings, whereas the 18 CF carriers without a family history of CF told 84% of their living parents and 56% of their siblings. The most common reason for disclosing

information was a close social relationship with a relative as well as the need for social support in a time of crisis.

In a study of communication patterns about carrier screening within families affected by hemophilia A, Sorenson, Jennings-Grant, and Newman (2003) focused on three aspects of the family context of genetic testing among women at risk to be carriers: (a) the extent to which there was discussion of carrier screening for hemophilia within these families before it was offered to the at-risk women; (b) with which family members these women communicated the results of their carrier screening; and (c) concerns these women had about communicating their results to relatives, including their children. Findings from this study suggest that these women discussed carrier screening with other family members prior to it being offered to them. Communication about carrier screening within these families was selective, not universal, largely following gender lines for this X-linked disorder (X-linked disorders are carried in genes on the X chromosome, and they affect males more often than females because males have only one X chromosome). Family members had limited concern about communicating carrier information to children and other relatives.

Ambivalence about confidentiality was evident in the cross-sectional interview study by Plantinga et al. (2003). Findings from this study of approximately 600 participants comparing the experiences, attitudes, and beliefs of individuals with a single-gene condition (e.g., CF and sickle cell disease) to those of individuals with multifactoral conditions (diabetes, HIV, breast cancer, and colon cancer) suggest that participants did not think family members should be able to get information about them without their knowledge. They did believe, however, that it was their responsibility to disclose information about hereditary conditions to other family members. In general, the views did not differ by the participant's type of condition (genetic vs. multifactoral). The majority of participants believed that health care professionals should be punished for releasing information without the patient's permission.

In one of the only studies focusing on the genetic testing experiences of minor siblings of individuals with X-linked and autosomal recessive conditions, James, Holtzman, and Hadley (2003) explored adolescent sisters' perceptions of their reproductive risks, attitudes toward carrier screening, and resources for information and support by interviewing 14 parents and 9 adolescent sisters of males with chronic granulomatous disease (CGD). CGD is a primary immunodeficiency disorder inherited in both an X-linked and an autosomal recessive manner. All of the adolescents knew that CGD is an inherited condition, and they each had thought about the possibility of having a child with CGD. They all considered their parents to be their best source of information and support, but a number of them had difficulty initiating discussions about CGD with their parents because they were afraid it would upset them. All of the adolescents and the parents considered carrier screening vital for relationship building and reproductive decision making. The adolescents favored testing at a later age than did their parents, however, and they expressed more concerns about the psychological consequences associated with testing.

Predictive Testing and the Family

There are two types of predictive testing: presymptomatic and predispositional. Mutation analysis for HD is an example of presymptomatic testing. If the gene mutation for HD is present, symptoms of HD are certain to appear if the individual lives long enough. Genetic testing for breast and ovarian cancer susceptibility is an example of predispositional testing. Predispositional testing differs from presymptomatic testing in that a positive result (indicating that either a BRCA1 or BRCA2 mutation is present) does not indicate a 100% risk of developing the condition (breast cancer).

Research on Disclosure of Genetic Information Within the Family

Since 2000, there have been at least 10 published studies concerning the disclosure of genetic information within the family in the context of predictive genetic testing (Burgess & d'Aincourt-Canning, 2001; Claes et al., 2003, 2004; Costalas et al., 2003; d'Agincourt-Canning, 2001; Daly et al., 2001; Forrest et al., 2003; Foster, Eeles, Ardern-Jones, Moynihan, & Watson, 2004; Foster, Watson, Moynihan, Ardern-Jones, & Eeles, 2002; Hallowell et al., 2002; Hallowell, Foster, Eeles, Ardern-Jones, & Watson, 2003; Hughes et al., 2002; Kenen, Ardern-Jones, & Eeles, 2004; Peterson et al., 2003; Sermijn et al., 2004). Eight of the 10 studies were about genetic testing for hereditary breast and ovarian cancer susceptibility (1 also included families in which one or more family members were tested for HD), and 1 was about genetic testing for hereditary nonpolyposis colon cancer. Most of the studies used a qualitative approach. Study participants were primarily white, well-educated, middle- to upper-income women who were offered testing through a specialty clinic or a research program. Sample size ranged from 15 women in the grounded theory study by Foster and colleagues (2004) to 162 women for the survey by Costalas and colleagues (2003). None of the studies used a family approach to data collection. In the qualitative studies, individual rather than family interviews were conducted.

Findings from these 10 studies suggest that the disclosure of genetic information within the family in the context of predictive genetic testing for adult-onset disorders is a complex issue that is influenced by both preexisting and cultural factors and individuals' responses to risk information. According to d'Agnincourt-Canning (2001), most of the individuals who underwent testing believed their relatives had a right to know this information, and they believed that it was their responsibility to inform family members of their genetic risk. Most of the participants in these studies had intended to disclose their results to other family members. For many, however, disclosure was more difficult than anticipated. Many experienced what Forrest and colleagues (2003) have described as a "disclosure dilemma": They were torn between a desire to disclose at the right time and a need to protect family members from what they perceived as problematic information, especially if they had been told they carried a gene mutation.

In these 10 studies, women were typically the ones who disclosed the information about genetic testing to other family members, and they usually focused on disclosing the information to first-degree relatives, especially their sisters and other first-degree female relatives. Communication with distant relatives about genetic testing tended to be more problematic than communication with first-degree relatives. Individuals found to carry a gene mutation were more likely to experience difficulty and distress disclosing their results than were individuals who were told that their results were negative. Some of the women who had intended to disclose their results ultimately decided that it was too difficult. Others decided to disclose their results to a limited number of individuals. Some disclosed their results but shared incorrect information. In the study by Sermijn and colleagues (2004), women who underwent BRCA1/2 testing had a good understanding of various aspects of testing, but the information they transferred to other family members was less than adequate and at times inaccurate. Less than half of their 107 first-degree relatives knew about the existence of hereditary breast and ovarian cancer, the availability of BRCA1/2 testing, and the cancer risk incurred by mutation carriers. Only one third of their family members knew about risk-reducing surgeries and other management strategies.

Research on Duty to Warn At-Risk Family Members

When an individual with a known gene mutation refuses to disclose this information to other relatives, health care professionals are faced with an ethical dilemma (Dugan et al., 2003). On one side of the dilemma is the obligation to respect and protect the individual's right to privacy. On the other side is the obligation to prevent harm and promote the welfare of the family members. Health care professionals who warn the at-risk relatives without the patient's consent may have to face a malpractice suit. According to Offit and colleagues (2004), failure to warn family members about hereditary diseases has resulted in at least three lawsuits against physicians in the United States.

There has been limited research on the duty to warn at-risk family members. The studies that do exist have been from the perspective of the genetic professional, not the perspective of the patient or the at-risk family member. In a survey of 259 genetic counselors (Dugan et al., 2003), almost half of the respondents (119) indicated that they had had at least one patient who had refused to notify an at-risk relative. Of these 119 genetic counselors, 24 (21%) had seriously considered warning the family member without the patient's consent, but only 1 genetic counselor actually did disclose without the patient's consent. The most commonly cited reasons for patient refusal to notify at-risk relatives were estranged family relationships, insurance discrimination, fear of altering family relationships, and employment discrimination. These findings suggest that although genetic counselors often encounter conflict about informing at-risk relatives, the situation seldom remains unresolved to the extent that genetic counselors actually warn at-risk relatives without the patient's consent.

Findings from a survey of 206 medical geneticists (Falk, Dugan, O'Riordan, & Matthews, 2003) indicated that 143 (69%) of the geneticists believed they did bear responsibility to warn their patient's relatives about hereditary disease risks. Thirty-one of the 143 who had faced this issue seriously considered disclosing the information to at-risk relatives without the patient's consent, but only 4 of the study participants actually proceeded to warn at-risk relatives of their status.

Research on the Family Response to Genetic Testing

There are few published studies on the family response to genetic testing. There are four notable exceptions, however, and all are about how families respond to genetic testing for HD. In the first study (Cox & McKellin, 1999), in-depth individual interviews were conducted with 41 family members from 21 families. Findings from this study suggest that Mendelian theories of inheritance patterns seldom provide an adequate framework for families to understand the risk of HD as it emerges within everyday life. Theories of Mendelian genetics provide a framework for calculating the odds of inheriting a disorder, but they do not take into account the social, biographical, and temporal factors that families consider when discussing risk and its modification through genetic testing. Families develop their own lay constructions of risk. These differ from the Mendelian theories in a number of ways: They are fluid and contingent rather than static; they are intersubjective rather objective; and they are creative yet coherent.

In the second study (Sobel & Cowan, 2000a, 2000b, 2003), in-depth family interviews were conducted with 18 families (55 family members participated in the interviews). Areas of affected family functioning noted by the respondents included family membership, family patterns of communication, and future caregiving concerns as they influenced current relationships. Eighty-one percent of families reported experiencing changes in family membership (e.g., changes due to marriage, divorce, and birth). Members in 50% of families experienced changes in patterns of communication, and 56% of those interviewed reported changes in current relationships in response to test results and their implications for future caregiving. According to Sobel and Cohen (2000b), key findings from their research are that families need to

(a) address "unfinished business" associated with the decision for testing; (b) bring family members, peripheral in the decision for testing, into the loop; (c) reorganize patterns of communication and roles altered by the testing and heal ruptures in family membership; and (d) revise family stories about illness to provide a meaning for HD and explain the test results in a way that leaves them with a sense of mastery. (p. 237)

The final two studies are a quantitative, longitudinal study by Richards and Williams (2004) and a qualitative study by Richards (2004) based on family systems theory. In the quantitative study, no significant difference in the level of marital adjustment over time was found between couples in which the at-risk partner had undergone predictive testing (testing group) and couples in which the at-risk partner had not undergone testing (nontesting group). Within the testing group, however, couples who received a noncarrier result experienced an adverse effect on their relationship, whereas the couples who received a carrier result did not.

The qualitative study (Richards, 2004) was designed to complement the quantitative longitudinal study by using semistructured interviews to investigate the experiences of 14 couples in more depth. All the interviews were individual interviews, not couple interviews. In 6 of the 14 couples, the at-risk partner had undergone testing: 3 were carriers, and 3 were not carriers. Five of the couples included at-risk partners who had not undergone testing. In the final 3 couples, the at-risk partner was symptomatic for HD. Three of the couples from the testing group were separated at the time of the interviews and another subsequently separated. The reason for the separation was not the test result, however. Most of the couples reported that receiving a predictive test result had little or no adverse effect on their relationship. For the 2 couples who separated after the at-risk partner received a noncarrier result, emotional factors associated with living with the risk of HD had caused irreparable damage to their relationship, not the test results. In the other 2 couples, the at-risk partner was symptomatic, and the separations were attributed to emotional distancing and the obsessive behavior of the affected individual. According to Richards, findings from this study highlight both the individuality and the complexity of psychological effects on the intimate relationships of couples who live with the risk or reality of HD.

CONCLUSION

Findings from the literature on genetic testing and the family suggest that the genetic testing experience is both an individual and a family experience. The genetic testing experience can have a profound impact on individual and family well-being. One factor that seems to play a critical role in how individuals and families respond to the genetic testing experience is family communication. As professionals in the family and health sciences, we need to use our expertise in family communication in particular, and family theory in general, to help design and implement tailored, culturally sensitive interventions for individuals and families who are being tested for and living with genetic conditions. These interventions need to take into account the fact that certain groups of individuals and families may be particularly vulnerable to the ethical, legal, and social implications of recent advances in genomics because of factors such as age, ethnicity, race, education level, socioeconomic status, role in the family, and mutation status. More research is needed to determine the best way to address these unique vulnerabilities.

REFERENCES

Atkin, K., Waquar, I. U., & Anionwu., E. (1998). Screening and counseling for sickle cell disorders and thalassaemia: The experience of parents and health care professionals. *Social Science and Medicine, 11,* 1639-1651.

Beeson, D., & Duster, T. (2002). African American perspectives on genetic testing. In J. Alper, C. Ard, A. Asch, J. Backwith, P. Conrad, & L. Geller (Eds.), *The double-edged helix* (pp. 151-174). Baltimore: Johns Hopkins University Press.

Bell, J. I. (2003). The double helix in clinical practice. *Nature, 421,* 414-416.

Binedell, J., & Soldan, J. R. (1997). Nonparticipation in Huntington's disease predictive testing: Reasons for caution in interpreting findings. *Journal of Genetic Counseling, 6,* 419-431.

Bowman, J. E. (1998). Minority health issues and genetics. *Community Genetics, 1,* 142-144.

Browner, C. H., & Preloran, H. M. (1999a). Male partners' role in Latinas' amniocentesis decisions. *Journal of Genetic Counseling, 8,* 85-108.

Browner, C. H., & Preloran, H. M. (1999b). Why women say yes to prenatal diagnosis. *Social Science Medicine, 45,* 979-989.

Browner, C. H., & Preloran, H. M. (2000a). Characteristics of women who refuse an offer of prenatal diagnosis: Data from the California maternal serum alpha feto-protein blood test experience. *American Journal of Medical Genetics, 8,* 433-445.

Browner, C. H., & Preloran, H. M. (2000b). Interpreting low-income Latinas' amniocentesis refusals. *Hispanic Journal of Behavioral Sciences, 22*(3), 346-368.

Browner, C. H., & Preloran, H. M. (2000c). Latinas, amniocentesis and the discourse of choice. *Culture, Medicine, & Psychiatry, 3,* 353-375.

Browner, C. H., & Preloran, H. M. (2000d). Para sacarse la espina (To get rid of the doubt): Mexican immigrant women's amniocentesis decisions. In A. R. Saetnan, N. Oudshoorn, & M. Kirejczyk (Eds.), *Bodies of technology: Women's involvement with reproductive medicine* (pp. 368-383). Columbus: Ohio State University Press.

Browner, C. H., Preloran, H. M., Casado, M. C., Bass, H. N., & Walker, A. P. (2003). Genetic counseling gone awry: Miscommunication between prenatal genetic service providers and Mexican-origin clients. *Social Science & Medicine, 56,* 1933-1946.

Browner, C. H., Preloran, H. M., & Cox, S. J. (1999). Ethnicity, bioethics, and prenatal diagnosis: The amniocentesis decisions of Mexican-origin women and their partners. *American Journal of Public Health, 89,* 1658-1666.

Browner, C. H., Preloran, H. M., & Press, N. (1996). The effects of ethnicity, education and an informational video on pregnant women's knowledge and decisions about a prenatal diagnostic screening test. *Patient Education & Counseling, 27,* 135-146.

Burgess, M. M., & d'Aincourt-Canning, L. (2001). Genetic testing for hereditary disease: Attending to relational responsibility. *Journal of Clinical Ethics, 12,* 361-372.

Burke, W. (2002). Genetic testing. *New England Journal of Medicine, 5,* 1867-1875.

Burke, W. (2004). Genetic testing in primary care. *Annual Review of Genomics and Human Genetics, 5,* 1-14.

Burke, W., & Emery, J. (2002). Genetics education for primary-care providers. *Nature Reviews: Genetics, 3,* 561-566.

Cashion, A. (2002). Genetics in transplantation. *MEDSURG Nursing, 11,* 91-94.

Chapman, E. (2002). Ethical dilemmas in testing for late onset conditions: Reactions to testing and perceived impact on other family members. *Journal of Genetic Counseling, 11,* 351-367.

Cheuvront, B., Sorenson, J. R., Callanan, N. P., Stearns, S. C., & DeVellis, B. M. (1998). Psychosocial and educational outcomes associated with home- and clinic-based pretest education and cystic fibrosis carrier testing among a population of at-risk relatives. *American Journal of Medical Genetics, 75,* 461-468.

Claes, E., Evers-Kiebooms, G., Boogaerts, A., Decruyenaere, M., Denayer, L., & Legius, E. (2003). Communication with close and distant relatives in the context of genetic testing for hereditary breast and ovarian cancer in cancer patients. *American Journal of Medical Genetics, 116A,* 11-19.

Claes, E., Evers-Kiebooms, G., Boogaerts, A., Decruyenaere, M., Denayer, L., & Legius, E. (2004). Diagnostic genetic testing for hereditary breast and ovarian cancer in cancer patients: Women's looking back on the pre-test period and a psychological evaluation. *Genetic Testing, 8,* 13-21.

Clayton, E. W. (2003). Ethical, legal, and social implications of genomic medicine. *New England Journal of Medicine, 349,* 562-569.

Codori, A., & Brandt, J. (1994). Psychological costs and benefits of predictive testing for Huntington's disease. *American Journal of Medical Genetics, 54,* 174-184.

Codori, A., Slavney, P. R., Young, C., Miglioretti, D. L., & Brandt, J. (1997). Predictors of psychological adjustment to genetic testing for Huntington's disease. *Health Psychology, 16,* 36-50.

Collins, F. S., Green, E. D., Guttmacher, A. E., & Guyer, M. S. (2003). A vision for the future of genomics research. A blueprint for the genomic era. *Nature, 422,* 835-847.

Collins, F. S., & Guttmacher, A. E. (2001). Genetics moves into the medical mainstream. *Journal of the American Medical Association, 286,* 2322-2324.

Collins, F. S., & McKusick, V. (2001). Implications of the Human Genome Project for medical science. *Journal of the American Medical Association, 285,* 2447-2448.

Costalas, J. W., Itzen, M., Malick, J., Babb, J. S., Bove, B., Godwin, A. K., et al. (2003). Communication of BRCA1 and BRCA2 results to at-risk relatives: A cancer risk assessment program's experience. *American Journal of Medical Genetics, 119C,* 11-18.

Cox, S. M., & McKellin, W. (1999). "There is this thing in our family": Predictive testing and the construction of risk for Huntington disease. *Sociology of Health & Illness, 21 ,*622-646.

Cuckle, H. (2000). Biochemical screening for Down syndrome. *European Journal of Obstetrics & Gynecology and Reproductive Biology, 92,* 97-101.

d'Agincourt-Canning, L. (2001). Experiences of genetic risk disclosure and the gendering of responsibility. *Bioethics, 15,* 231-246.

Daly, M. B. (2004). Tailoring breast cancer treatment to genetic status: The challenges ahead. *Journal of Clinical Oncology, 22,* 1-2.

Daly, M. B., Barsevick, A., Miller, S. M., Buckman, R., Costalas, J., Montgomery, S., et al. (2001). Communicating genetic test results to the family: A six-step skills-building strategy. *Family and Community Health, 24*(3), 13-26.

Desiere, F. (2004). Towards a systems biology understanding of human health: Interplay between genotype, environment, and nutrition. *Biotechnological Annual Review, 10,* 51-84.

de Waal, F. B. M. (1999). The end of nature versus nurture. *Scientific American, 281,* 94-99.

de Wert, G., ter Meulen, R., Mordacci, R., & Tallacchini, M. (2003). *Ethics and genetics: A workbook for practitioners and students.* New York: Berghahn.

Doukas, D., & Berg, J. W. (2001). The family covenant and genetic testing. *American Journal of Bioethics, 1,* 2-7.

Dugan, R. B., Wiesner, G. L., Juengst, E. T., O'Riordan, M., Matthews, A. L., & Robin, N. H. (2003). Duty to warn at-risk relatives for genetic disease: Genetic counselors' clinical experience. *American Journal of Medical Genetics, 119C,* 27-34.

Falk, M. J., Dugan, R. B., O'Riordan, M. A., & Matthews, A. (2003). Medical geneticists' duty to warn at-risk relatives for genetic disease. *American Journal of Medical Genetics, 120A,* 374-380.

Fanos, J. H., & Johnson, J. P. (1995). Barriers to carrier testing for adult cystic fibrosis sibs: The importance of not knowing. *American Journal of Medical Genetics, 23,* 85-91.

Feetham, S. L. (1999). Families and the genetic revolution: Implications for primary healthcare, education, and research. *Families, Systems, and Health, 17,* 27-43.

Ferguson-Smith, M. A. (2004). Which prenatal screening protocol? *Prenatal Diagnosis, 24,* 761.

Forrest, K., Simpson, S. A., Wilson, B. J., van Teijlingen, E. R., McKee, L., Haites, N., et al. (2003). To tell or not to tell: Barriers and facilitators in family communication about genetic risk. *Clinical Genetics, 64,* 317-326.

Foster, C., Eeles, R., Ardern-Jones, A., Moynihan, C., & Watson, M. (2004). Juggling roles and expectations: Dilemmas faced by women talking to relatives about cancer and genetic testing. *Psychology and Health, 19,* 439-455.

Foster, C., Watson, M., Moynihan, C., Ardern-Jones, A., & Eeles, R. (2002). Genetic testing for breast/ovarian cancer predisposition: Cancer burden and responsibility. *Journal of Health Psychology, 7,* 469-484.

Gray, S. (2003). Direct-to-consumer marketing of genetic tests for cancer: Buyer beware. *Journal of Clinical Oncology, 21,* 3191-3193.

Greco, K. E. (2003). Nursing in the genomic era: Nurturing our genetic selves. *Medical Surgical Nursing, 12,* 307-312.

Green, R. (1999). Genetic medicine and the conflict of moral principles. *Families, Systems and Health, 17,* 63-74.

Greendale, K., & Reed, P. (2001). Empowering primary care health professionals in medical genetics: How soon? How fast? How far? *American Journal of Medical Genetics, 106,* 223-232.

Gusella, J. F., Wexler, N. S., Conneally, P. M., Naylor, S. L., Anderson, M. A., Tanzi, R. E., et al. (1983). A polymorphic DNA marker genetically linked to Huntington's disease. *Nature, 306,* 234-238.

Guttmacher, A. E., & Collins, F. S. (2002). Genomic medicine. *New England Journal of Medicine, 347,* 1512-1520.

Guttmacher, A. E., & Collins, F. S. (2003). Welcome to the genomic era. *New England Journal of Medicine, 349,* 996-998.

Hakimian, R. (2000). Disclosure of Huntington's disease to family members: The dilemma of known but unknowing parties. *Genetic Testing, 4,* 359-364.

Hallowell, N., Foster, C., Eeles, R., Ardern-Jones, A., Murday, V., & Watson, M. (2002). Balancing autonomy and responsibility: The ethics of generating and disclosing genetic information. *Journal of Medical Ethics, 29,* 74-83.

Hallowell, N., Foster, C., Eeles, R., Ardern-Jones, A., & Watson, M. (2003). Accommodating risk: Responses to BRCA1/2 genetic testing of women who have had cancer. *Social Science & Medicine, 59,* 553-565.

Harper, P. S. (1993). Insurance and genetic testing. *Lancet, 341,* 184.

Harper, P. S. (1996). *Huntington's disease* (2nd ed.). London: W. B. Saunders.

Harper, P. S., Lim, C., & Craufurd, D. (2000). Ten years of presymptomatic testing for Huntington's disease (HD): The experience of the UK Huntington's Disease Prediction Consortium. *Journal of Medical Genetics, 37,* 567-571.

Hartmann, L. C., Degnim, A., & Schaid, D. J. (2004). Prophylactic mastectomy for BRCA 1/2 carriers: Progress and more questions. *Journal of Clinical Oncology, 22,* 981-983.

Hayden, M. R. (2000). Predictive testing for Huntington's disease: The calm after the storm. *Lancet, 356,* 1944-1945.

Helm, D. T., Miranda, S., & Chedd, N. A. (1998). Prenatal diagnosis of Down syndrome: Mothers' reflections on supports needed from diagnosis to birth. *Mental Retardation, 36,* 55-61.

Hetteberg, C., Prows, C. A., Deets, C., Monsen, R., & Kenner, C. (1999). National survey of genetics content in basic nursing preparatory programs in the United States. *Nursing Outlook, 47,* 168-174.

Holding, S. (2002). Current state of screening for Down syndrome. *Annals of Clinical Biochemistry, 39,* 1-11.

Hughes, C., Lerman, C., Schwartz, M., Peshkin, B. N., Wenzel, L., Narod, S., et al. (2002). All in the family: Evaluation of the process and content of sisters' communication about BRCA1 and BRCA2 genetic test results. *American Journal of Medical Genetics, 107,* 143-150.

Hull, S., & Prasad, K. (2001). Reading between the lines: Direct-to-consumer advertising of genetic testing in the U.S. *Reproductive Health Matters, 9,* 44-48.

Huntington's Disease Collaborative Research Group. (1993). A novel gene containing a trinucleotide repeat that is expanded and unstable on Huntington's disease chromosomes. *Cell, 72,* 971-983.

Jacobs, L. A., & Deatrick, J. A. (1999). The individual, the family, and genetic testing. *Journal of Professional Nursing, 15,* 313-324.

James, C. A., Holtzman, N. A., & Hadley, D. W. (2003). Perceptions of reproductive risk and carrier testing among adolescent sisters of males with chronic granulomatous disease. *American Journal of Medical Genetics, 119C,* 60-69.

Johnson, A. M., Wilkinson, D. S., & Taylor-Brown, S. (1999). Genetic testing: Policy implications for individuals and families. *Families, Systems, and Health, 17,* 49-61.

Jones, S. (2004). The confluence of two clinical specialties: Genetics and assisted reproductive technologies. *MEDSURG Nursing, 13,* 114-121.

Juengst, E. (1997). Caught in the middle again: Professional ethical considerations in genetic testing for health risks. *Genetic Testing, 1,* 189-200.

Juengst, E. (1999). Genetic testing and the moral dynamics of family life. *Public Understanding of Science, 8,* 1-13.

Kenen, R., Arden-Jones, A., & Eeles, R. (2004). We are talking, but are they listening? Communication patterns in families with a history of breast/ovarian cancer (HBOC). *Psycho-oncology, 13,* 335-345.

Khoury, M. J. (2003). Genetics and genomics in practice: The continuum from genetic disease to genetic information in health and disease. *Genetics in Medicine, 5,* 261-268.

Khoury, M. J., McCabe, L. L., & McCabe, E. R. B. (2003). Population screening in the age of genomic medicine. *New England Journal of Medicine, 348,* 50-58.

Lawson, K., Wiggins, S., Green, T., Adam, S., Bloch, M., Hayden, M. B., & the Canadian Collaborative Study of Predictive Testing. (1996). Adverse psychological events occurring in the first year after predictive testing for Huntington's disease. *Journal of Medical Genetics, 33,* 856-862.

Learman, L. A., Kupperman, M., Gates, E., Nease, R. F., Gildengorin, V., & Washington, A. E. (2003). Social and familial context of prenatal genetic testing decisions: Are there racial and ethnic differences? *American Journal of Medical Genetics, 15*(119C), 19-26.

Lerman, C., & Shields, A. E. (2004). Genetic testing for cancer susceptibility: The promise and the pitfalls. *Nature Reviews, 4,* 234-241.

Levenkron, J. C., Loader, S., & Rowley, P. T. (1997). Carrier screening for cystic fibrosis: Test acceptance and one year follow-up. *American Journal of Medical Genetics, 73,* 378-386.

Markens, S., Browner, C. H., & Press, N. (1999). "Because of the risks": How U.S. pregnant women account for refusing prenatal screening. *Social Science Medicine, 49,* 359-369.

McCabe, L. L., & McCabe, E. R. B. (2004). Direct-to-consumer genetic testing: Access and marketing. *Genetics in Medicine, 6,* 56-59.

McDaniel, S. H., & Campbell, T. L. (1999). Genetic testing and families. *Families, Systems, and Health, 17,* 1-3.

McDonnell, S. K., Schaid, D. J., Myers, J. L., Grant, C. S., Donohue, J. H., Woods, J. E., et al. (2001). Efficacy of contralateral prophylactic mastectomy in women with a personal and family history of breast cancer. *Journal of Clinical Oncology, 19,* 3938-3943.

Mehlman, M., & Botkin, J. R. (1998). *Access to the genome: The challenge of equality.* Washington, DC: Georgetown University Press.

Meijers-Heijboer, H., Brekelmans, C. T., Menke-Pluymers, M., Seynaeve, C., Baalbergen, A., Burger, C., et al. (2003). Use of genetic testing and prophylactic mastectomy and oophorectomy in women with breast or ovarian cancer from families with a BRCA1 and BRCA2 mutation. *Journal of Clinical Oncology, 21,* 1675-1681.

Mincey, B. A. (2003). Genetics and the management of women at high risk for breast cancer. *The Oncologist, 8,* 466-473.

Newell, A. M. (2004). Genetics for targeting disease prevention: diabetes. *Primary Care, 31,* 743-766.

Offit, K., Groeger, E., Turner, S., Wadsworth, E. A., & Weiser, M. A. (2004). The "duty to warn" a patient's family members about hereditary disease risk. *Journal of the American Medical Association, 292,* 1469-1478.

Olsen, S. J., Feetham, S. L., Jenkins, J., Lewis, J. A., Nissly, T., Sigmon, H. D., et al. (2003). Creating a nursing vision for leadership in genetics. *MEDSURG Nursing, 12,* 177-184.

Ormond, K. E., Mills, P. L., Lester, L. A., & Ross, L. F. (2003). Effect of family history on disclosure patterns of cystic fibrosis carrier status. *American Journal of Medical Genetics, 119C,* 70-77.

Peterson, S. K., Watts, B. G., Koehly, L. M., Vernon, S. W., Baile, W. F., Kohlmann, W. K., et al. (2003). How families communicate about HNPCC genetic testing: Findings from a qualitative study. *American Journal of Medical Genetics, 119C,* 78-86.

Plantinga, L., Natowicz, M. R., Kass, N. E., Hull, S. C., Gostin, L. O., & Faden, R. (2003). Disclosure, confidentiality, and families: Experiences and attitudes of those with genetic versus nongenetic medical conditions. *American Journal of Medical Genetics, 119C,* 51-59.

Poppelaars, F., Henneman, L., Ader, H., Cornel, M., Hermens, R., Van Der Wal, G., et al. (2004). Preconceptual cystic fibrosis carrier screening: Attitudes and intentions of the target population. *Genetic Testing, 8,* 80-89.

Post, S. G. (1992). Huntington's disease: Prenatal screening for late onset disease. *Journal of Medical Ethics, 18,* 75-78.

Press, N., & Browner, C. H. (1993). Collective fictions: Similarities in reasons for accepting maternal serum alpha-fetoprotein screening among women of diverse ethnic and social class backgrounds. *Fetal Diagnosis and Therapy, 8,* 97-106.

Press, N., & Browner, C. H. (1997). Why women say yes to prenatal diagnosis. *Social Science Medicine, 45,* 979-989.

Press, N., & Browner, C. H. (1998). Characteristics of women who refuse an offer of prenatal diagnosis: Data from the California maternal serum alpha fetoprotein blood test experience. *American Journal of Medical Genetics, 78,* 433-445.

Rebbeck, T. R., Friebel, T., Lynch, H. T., Neuhausen, S. L., van 't Veer, L., Garber, J. E., et al. (2004). Bilateral prophylactic mastectomy reduces breast cancer risk in BRCA1 and BRCA2 mutation carriers: The PROSE study group. *Journal of Clinical Oncology, 22,* 1055-1062.

Richards, F. (2004). Couples' experiences of predictive testing and living with the risk or reality of Huntington disease: A qualitative study. *American Journal of Medical Genetics, 126A,* 170-182.

Richards, F., & Williams, K. (2004). The impact on couple relationships of predictive testing for Huntington disease: A longitudinal study. *American Journal of Medical Genetics, 15,* 161-169.

Richards, M. (1998). Annotation: Genetic research, family life, and clinical practice. *Journal of Child Psychology and Psychiatry, 39,* 291-305.

Root, R., & Browner, C. H. (2001). Practices of the pregnant self: Compliance with and resistance to prenatal norms. *Culture, Medicine, and Psychiatry, 25,* 195-223.

Roses, A. D. (2004). Pharmacogenetics and drug development: The path to safer and more effective drugs. *Nature Reviews: Genetics, 5,* 645-656.

Santalahti, P., Aro, A. R., Hemminki, E., Helenius, H., & Ryynanen, M. (1998). On what grounds do women participate in prenatal screening? *Prenatal Diagnosis, 18,* 153-165.

Santalahti, P., Hemminki, E., Aro, A. R., Helenius, H., & Ryynanen, M. (1999). Participation in prenatal screening tests and intentions concerning selective termination in Finnish maternity care. *Fetal Diagnosis and Therapy, 14,* 71-79.

Santalahti, P., Hemminki, E., Latikka, A. M., & Ryynanen, M. (1998). Women's decision-making in prenatal screening. *Social Science Medicine, 46,* 1067-1076.

Santalahti, P., Latikka, A., Ryynanen, M., & Hemminki, E. (1996). Women's experiences of prenatal serum screening. *Birth, 23,* 101-107.

Schwartz, M. D., Lerman, C., Brogan, B., Peshkin, B. N., Halbert, C. H., DeMarco, T., et al. (2004). Impact of BRCA1/BRCA2 counseling and testing on newly diagnosed breast cancer patients. *Journal of Clinical Oncology, 15,* 1823-1829.

Sermijn, E., Goelen, G., Teugels, E., Kaufman, L., Bonduelle, M., Neyns, B., et al. (2004). The impact of proband mediated information dissemination in families with a BRCA1/2 gene mutation. *Journal of Medical Genetics, 41,* 1-7.

Sermon, K., Van Steirteghem, A., & Liebaers, I. (2004). Preimplantation genetic diagnosis. *Lancet, 3363,* 1633-1641.

Smith, J. A., Michie, S., Stephenson, M., & Quarrell, O. (2002). Risk perception and decision-making in candidates for genetic testing for Huntington's disease: An interpretative phenomenological analysis. *Journal of Health Psychology, 7,* 131-144.

Sobel, S. K., & Cowan, D. B. (2000a). Impact of genetic testing for Huntington disease on the family system. *American Journal of Medical Genetics, 90,* 49-59.

Sobel, S. K., & Cowan, D. B. (2000b). The process of family reconstruction after DNA testing for Huntington disease. *Journal of Genetic Counseling, 9,* 237-251.

Sobel, S. K., & Cowan, D. B. (2003). Ambiguous loss and disenfranchised grief: The impact of DNA predictive testing on the family as a system. *Family Process, 42,* 47-57.

Sorenson, J. R., & Botkin, J. R. (2003). Genetic testing and the family. *American Journal of Medical Genetics, 119C,* 1-2.

Sorenson, J. R., Cheuvront, B., DeVellis, B., Callanan, N., Silverman, L., Koch, G., et al. (1997). Acceptance of home and clinic-based cystic fibrosis carrier education and testing for first, second, and third degree relatives of cystic fibrosis patients. *American Journal of Medical Genetics, 70,* 121-129.

Sorenson, J. R., Jennings-Grant, T., & Newman, J. (2003). Communication about carrier testing within hemophilia A families. *American Journal of Medical Genetics, 119C,* 3-10.

Street, E., & Soldan, J. (1998). A conceptual framework for the psychosocial issues faced by families with genetic conditions. *Families, Systems, and Health, 16,* 217-232.

Stone, H. W., & Miles, R. (1999). Moral direction in genetic counseling: Prenatal testing and Huntington's disease. *Families, Systems and Health, 17,* 75-86.

Thomson, E. (1997). Ethical, legal, social, and policy issues in genetics. In F. R. Lashley (Ed.), *The genetics revolution: Implications for nursing* (pp. 15-26). Washington, DC: American Academy of Nursing.

Tibben, A., Timman, R., Bannink, E., & Duivenvoorden, H. (1997). Three-year follow-up after presymptomatic testing for Huntington's disease in tested individuals and partners. *Health Psychology, 16,* 20-35.

Tinkle, M. B. (2002, April/May). Carrier screening: Are nurses ready to be on the front line? *AWHONN Lifelines,* 135-139.

Weitzel, J. N., McCaffrey, S. M., Nedelcu, R., MacDonald, D. J., Blazer, K. R., & Cullinane, C. A. (2003). Effect of genetic cancer risk assessment on surgical decisions at breast cancer diagnosis. *Archives in Surgery, 138,* 1323-1328.

Wertz, D. C., Janes, S. R., Rosenfield, J. M., & Erbe, R. W. (1992). Attitudes toward the prenatal diagnosis of cystic fibrosis: Factors in decision making among affected families. *American Journal of Human Genetics, 50,* 1077-1085.

Williams, J., & Schutte, D. (1997). Benefits and burdens of genetic carrier identification. *Western Journal of Nursing Research, 19,* 71-81.

Williams, J. K., Schutte, D. L., Evers, C. A., & Forcucci, C. (1999). Adults seeking presymptomatic gene testing for Huntington disease. *Journal of Nursing Scholarship, 31,* 109-114.

Williams, J. K., Schutte, D. L., Evers, C., & Holkup, P. A. (2000). Redefinition: Coping with normal results from predictive gene testing for neurodegenerative disorders. *Research in Nursing and Health, 23,* 260-269.

Wulfsberg, E. A. (2000). The impact of genetic testing on primary care: Where's the beef? *American Family Physician, 61,* 971-972, 974, 977-978.

Wung, S. (2002). Genetic advances in coronary artery disease. *MEDSURG Nursing, 11,* 296-301.

Part II

ISSUES OF AGING
AND CAREGIVING

CHAPTER 13

Treatment Decisions When Death Is Near

The Family's Role

THOMAS E. FINUCANE

Gravely ill patients who are near death, and their families, often face a tragic choice. Treatment may be available for the illness, but it may be only partially effective and in many cases will cause intensified suffering. The alternative to active treatment is to elect a more palliative approach in which comfort and dignity are the primary focus of care. A familiar example is a patient with advanced lung disease who develops acute pneumonia. In many cases, the patient could survive for an uncertain time if put on a ventilator and would very likely die quickly if mechanical ventilator support were withheld. On the one hand, mechanical ventilation in an intensive care unit may be a hectic and frightening experience. On the other hand, there is a widespread and deeply held desire not to be dead, even if the death were promised to be comfortable and dignified.

Four boundary conditions ensure that decisions such as these will continue to be difficult. First, life is good. This is the North Star of medical ethics. Second, death is certain. Immortality is specifically confined to single-cell organisms such as amoebae, which do not age and die (although many die traumatic deaths). Third, suffering is bad, although various cultures view suffering differently. Some view suffering as redemptive, for example, but in general suffering may be defined as a situation that one would like to avoid. Fourth, most people can imagine situations that are worse than death. How to define when someone would be "better off dead" is an extremely difficult subject.

Decisions at the end of life have only recently become common. This is largely because of the development of effective, often invasive, technology. Until fairly recently, truly life-sustaining treatments were the exception. Because of advances in technology, many patients now must choose between a longer life with more suffering and a shorter life with comfort and dignity. Because deaths from infectious disease and trauma have been greatly reduced in the United States, fewer patients are dying at a young or middle age.

Accordingly, most patients who face difficult and critical decisions regarding death are elderly. Because of the increasing prevalence of cognitive impairment among the very old, and because sickness can cause delirium, especially among the elderly, acutely ill patients often have a diminished ability to make these life and death decisions about their own illness and treatment.

Making these decisions is not easy. For the elderly patient with advanced lung disease who must decide about mechanical ventilation, the choices can be described in very negative ways. If the patient and his or her family choose mechanical ventilation, it is possible to think that we are torturing a vulnerable elderly person in what are almost certainly the last few days of life. If the decision is not to put the patient on a ventilator but, rather, to offer palliative care, it could be said that we are withholding potentially life-sustaining treatment from a vulnerable human being. Unfortunately, strident activists have taken extreme positions on the simple-minded edges of what is most often a complex, intensely personal, and deeply tragic situation.

One additional factor serves to sharpen the challenge here. Autonomy has become the overwhelmingly dominant principle of medical ethics in the United States. On the basis of a particular conception of how to show respect for people, with roots in the consumer movement and the rise of lawyers, the right to self-determination has out-stripped all other important ethical rights. In the United States, it is thought that if you wish to know what is best to do for a person, you should ask that person. With the developing preeminence of autonomy, and the advance of effective technology, many gravely ill patients are being asked to make tragic life-and-death decisions about their own care. In even more cases, they have become so ill that they are unable to make these decisions, and someone else must do so.

STANDARD PARADIGM FOR END-OF-LIFE DECISION MAKING

In most states, a stereotyped pathway has developed in health care for trying to make these life-and-death decisions. Step 1 is to try to get a decision from the patient himself or herself. Although this step seems straight-forward, at least three problems are well recognized. The first is determination of competence. Questions of competence or capacity frequently arise: Does this elderly, acutely ill person have the ability to make a reasoned decision? In general, such determinations are extremely difficult and almost always subjective. If a person has the capacity to make decisions, the general rule is that the patient's wishes should be honored. The second serious problem that arises is the futility exception. When is treatment so unlikely to benefit the patient that, even if the patient requests the treatment, it should not be given? In general, the claim of futility and the attendant decision to forgo treatment despite a patient's request can be valid only in extremely circumscribed circumstances. The converse of this situation, when a competent patient declines treatment but is forced to take it, is the third problematic area within Step 1. In general, the right to say "Keep your hands off of me" is the cornerstone principle of modern medical ethics, and few exceptions are recognized. Step 1, do what the patient asks, encounters these three problems. Capacity, futility, and forced treatment are areas of significance and are beyond the scope of this chapter.

Step 2 involves advance directives. Advance directives are intended to honor the autonomy of a person who has lost the ability to make decisions. Theoretically, while still competent, the patient makes and communicates decisions about medical decision making for a hypothetical and contingent future. If the person then becomes incapacitated, his or her previously expressed wishes provide guidance about how decisions are to be made. A person who wishes to establish an advance directive must imagine two hypothetical situations. The person must imagine first that he or she is so ill that decisions about life-sustaining treatment must be made and second that the person has become incapacitated and thus unable to make those decisions. This is a complex matter.

A patient can leave guidance for personal wishes in one of two ways. First, the person can attempt to envision specific treatment decisions that might arise, such as attempted cardiopulmonary resuscitation, tube feeding, or mechanical ventilation, and state in advance directives to provide or withhold such specific treatments. The second way to leave guidance is to designate a person who will have the authority to make decisions. The former is frequently called a living will. The latter is often known as a health care agent or durable power of attorney for health care, although both have many other names in various states.

Most studies show that the large majority of elderly people have not completed advance directives (Hanson, Tulsky, & Danis, 1997; Hofmann et al., 1997; Pendergast & Luce, 1997), and that many will not do so even if every effort is made to assist them (Carresse & Rhodes, 1995; Costantini-Ferrando, Foley, & Rapkin, 1998; Fadiman, 1997; Finucane, 2002; Hanson et al., 1997; Hines et al., 1999; Hofmann et al., 1997). Thus, many gravely ill patients will become incapacitated and will lack advance directives at a time when critical decisions must be made about treatment. Step 3 of the standard paradigm simply states that someone will act by default when these decisions must be made.

An explanation of nomenclature is important. A substitute decision maker, usually a close family member, may act on behalf of a patient because he or she has been designated by the patient in an advance directive or by default because the family member is the logical choice. In some states, the designated decision maker is called a proxy, and the default decision maker is called a surrogate. In other states, the nomenclature is reversed, and the designated decision maker is called surrogate, whereas the default decision maker is called proxy. As noted previously, the terms *durable power of attorney* and *health care agent* are also frequently used for the designated family member making the decision. Several additional terms are used in various jurisdictions, also ambiguously and variously. It is extremely important, both in reading the literature on medical ethics and in taking care of gravely ill patients, to be clear about the facts and the nomenclature of substitute decision making.

In some situations, this default decision maker must be established by judicial proceedings. Here, too, there is some inconsistency in nomenclature. Most commonly, a person who is named by a judge to make health care decisions and other personal decisions for an incapacitated person is known as a *guardian*, although the term *conservator* is used in some jurisdictions. Most commonly, a person who is appointed to be responsible for a patient's financial assets is known as a conservator, but this is also variable.

PROBLEMS WITH THE PARADIGM FOR END-OF-LIFE DECISIONS

Although this step-by-step approach to decision making seems coherent, there are major problems with it at every step. Step 1 assumes that frail, vulnerable elderly people who are acutely ill and retain capacity will be willing to participate in informed consent discussions about life-and-death matters. In other societies, this assumption would be considered barbaric. For such a person to make a truly informed decision, he or she would have to be carefully educated about the severity of the physical condition, how burdensome the treatment would be, and how likely was death with or without treatment. Evidence shows that many, and perhaps most, patients do not wish to take the reins in the course of their own serious illness and manage their own downward spiral to death (Costantini-Ferrando et al., 1998; Finucane, 2002).

Step 2 is extremely problematic. Living wills are so circumscribed as to be almost useless. In most states, for example, a living will is only effective by statute if the patient is terminally ill or in a persistent vegetative state. Very few states have special descriptions of clinical situations, such as severe advanced dementia, for which a living will may be effective. In general, however, they are not broadly applicable. States are reluctant to allow patients wide latitude in making decisions to forgo treatment. The reasons for this are fascinating but are beyond the scope of this chapter. The basis for this limitation on living wills can be seen, however, in a situation that arises frequently during the care of patients with lung disease. It is not uncommon for a patient who has recently been on a mechanical ventilator to state that he or she would never want to be placed on the ventilator again. In many cases, however, when such a patient again becomes critically ill, and the choice is between mechanical ventilation and death, the patient will elect to repeat mechanical ventilation. Several related lines of clinical evidence argue that healthy patients often make glib remarks about refusing treatment and then change their minds when they are actually facing death.

SUBSTITUTE DECISION MAKING

In many cases, acutely ill elderly patients are incapable of making treatment decisions for themselves, and the state limits the situations in which advance directives can be used to direct the decision making. Thus, a substitute decision maker will be necessary, either a previously designated person or someone who is acting by default. State-to-state variability in the rules about substitute decision making is enormous.

In some states, there is a strong presumption that family members are the optimal people to be substitute decision makers. They are most likely to be well intentioned and most likely to be aware of the patient's wishes. If the patient has not specifically expressed wishes about these often unimaginable choices that must be made, the family is considered well situated to make inferences based on the patient's known goals, fears, and previously stated desires. These states may make little distinction between designated family members and those acting by default.

Other states take the position that family members cannot be trusted to make decisions to withhold potentially life-sustaining treatment. The state's interest in preserving life outweighs the family's interest to act on behalf of the patient, particularly because the family may be uninformed or unfortunately motivated.

Still other states make a major distinction between substitutes who are acting because they were designated and those who are acting by default. These states give a great deal of authority to a substitute decision maker who has been specifically named by the patient for the purpose, whereas they are much more restrictive in the authority granted to substitutes who are making decisions only because there is no one better positioned to do so.

Several trends promise to exacerbate the tensions in this arena. Families are smaller and more geographically dispersed. Nontraditional families and families with divorce are common. The cost of life-sustaining treatment is increasing. Respect for values of cultural subgroups is more widely honored. Mistrust of conventional medicine is on the rise. Managed care organizations have powerful, purely financial motives to limit life-sustaining treatment when death is near. (Woody Allen reportedly said, "Death is a great way to cut expenses.") Cross-cultural understandings are nearly inevitable as the various parties attempt to assign the values of life, suffering, cognitive impairment, and death.

Simple resolution of these difficult problems is impossible and may not be desirable. In many cases, there is no single "correct" course of action. There are several decisions that are entirely morally plausible. What is needed is an open, fair, and consensual process for choosing among the morally acceptable options. It is often in the negotiation and interview that trust develops, communication is enriched, mutual confidence is established, and good decisions are made.

Four suggestions are made here. The first is that young and healthy people should not belittle, discourage, discount, or disrespect the very deep-seated desire of seriously ill people not to die. When people, and their families, facing certain death ask for burdensome treatment with little chance of benefit, health care providers and others should never express impatience or contempt. This desire not to be dead should be expected and accepted, never disparaged.

Second, professionals, especially those from a Western European intellectual tradition, who place a high value on the life of the mind, should be very clear that in many cultural traditions a living body loses little or no worth when cognitive impairment develops. In *The Spirit Catches You and You Fall Down*, Fadiman (1997) described a young girl in a persistent vegetative state. Her family took her home from the hospital because hospital personnel were so insistent that little was to be gained by further treatment. One year later, the girl was still alive, still in a persistent vegetative state, and a fully loved and valued member of the family.

Third, because of the United States' pluralism, patients are probably well advised to discuss their wishes about care near the end of life with trusted companions. Patients and their care providers should be aware of state laws, and if certain formalities would increase the likelihood that patients can get the kind of care they want, then those formalities should be completed. In many states, it is very important to name a health care agent (also known as durable power of attorney). In some states, it is advisable to put into writing specific wishes about limiting artificial nutrition and hydration. In almost all situations, it helps to have had some kind of conversation that considers the choice between painful survival and comfortable death, when death is near in either case.

Finally, tolerance is essential. The case of Nancy Cruzan is exemplary. She was a young woman in a persistent vegetative state. After several years, when her prognosis was certain, her family unanimously requested that tube feeding be withdrawn, stating they were sure she would not have wanted to be kept alive in those circumstances. The case eventually went to the Supreme Court, with several mentions that the motives of the family were clearly and entirely altruistic. The Supreme Court refused the family's request, however, and the feeding tube was continued. After new evidence developed, a lower court allowed the family to have the tube removed. People associated with activist groups demonstrated outside the nursing home, calling the patient's parents murderers and at one point attempting to use force against the nursing home. In the end, the patient died comfortably and quietly in the presence of her loving family. The advocacy group's disregard for the parents' wishes, especially when there was never even the smallest question of the parents' good intentions, is unlikely to improve the morality of the decision-making process. We are all going to die. Many of us will suffer before death. Many will develop severe cognitive impairment. Tragic decisions will be necessary. We are working here in a great mystery.

CONCLUSION

Family decision making on behalf of incapacitated elderly patients is a common occurrence and is likely to become more so. Different states have different rules about what is permissible. In all cases, the state is trying to balance reverence for life with the critical right to say, "Keep your hands off of me." Allowing vulnerable people to die of neglect is intolerable. Causing meaningless suffering in vulnerable people in the days before their deaths is also intolerable. Wishes expressed previously by an incapacitated person should be considered carefully. Respectful dialogue and respect for the rights of the patient's loved ones are essential to good decision making. There is usually more than one morally acceptable decision; the key problem is to find a fair way to make the decision and to be able to respect the decisions of others if the decisions are made in good faith and within legal guidelines. These are critical issues for families.

REFERENCES

Carresse, J. A., & Rhodes, L. A. (1995). Western bioethics on the Navajo reservation: Benefit or harm? *Journal of the American Medical Association, 274*(10), 826-829.

Costantini-Ferrando, M. J., Foley, K. M., & Rapkin, B. D. (1998). Communicating with patients about advanced cancer. *Journal of the American Medical Association, 280*(16), 1403 [Author reply, 1404].

Fadiman, A. (1997). *The spirit catches you and you fall down.* New York: Farrar, Straus, & Giroux.

Finucane, T. E. (2002). Care of patients nearing death: Another view. *Journal of the American Geriatric Society, 50*(3), 551-553.

Hanson, L. C., Tulsky, J. A., & Danis, M. (1997). Can clinical interventions change care at the end of life? *Annals of Internal Medicine, 126*(5), 383-388.

Hines, S. C., Glover, J. J., Holley, J. L., Babrow, A. S., Badzek, L. A., & Moss, A. H. (1999). Dialysis patients' preferences for family-based advance care planning. *Annals of Internal Medicine, 130*(10), 825-828.

Hofmann, J. C., Wenger, N. S., Davis, R. B., Teno, J., Connors, A. F., Jr., Desbiens, N., et al. (1997). Patient preferences for communication with physicians about end-of-life decisions. SUPPORT investigators. Study to understand prognoses and preference for outcomes and risks of treatment. *Annals of Internal Medicine, 127*(1), 1-12.

Prendergast, T. J., & Luce, J. M. (1997). Increasing incidence of withholding and withdrawal of life support from the critically ill. *American Journal of Respiratory Critical Care Medicine, 155*(1), 15-20.

CHAPTER 14

Assessing Eldercare Needs

An Application of Marketing
Orientation Within the Nonprofit Sector

ROBERT J. PARSONS

There is a reality that humanity has either actively resisted or stoically accepted since the dawn of human history. That reality is aging—the passage of time and the inevitable toll it takes on the human body and mind. No one knows better what that toll is than those professionals and families who provide long-term care for the elderly, unless it is the elderly themselves. Community leaders, most of whom are in the prime of life, are even farther removed from the personally disquieting truth of just what it means to be old, and yet they must form policies and allocate limited community resources to provide care for this growing segment of U.S. society. Families along with community leaders must be aware of the needs of the elderly before they are able to meet them. This can best be done by a needs assessment study. Conduct of regular needs assessment studies directed specifically toward a community's senior citizens is an important channel of communication between the elderly and those who take care of them, such as their families. A needs assessment eliminates the two greatest pitfalls for caregivers: assuming knowledge of the needs of the elderly without accurate information and making decisions based on inadequate information.

BACKGROUND

The aging of America and changing patterns of family life are greatly increasing the demands on family and other informal caregivers who provide long-term care for older relatives and friends. Not only are there now more older adults but also they are living longer. As they age beyond 75 years, many begin to experience some type of physical or mental limitation. Nearly half the older population will report being limited in the amount or kind of activity they perform at some point, and eventually they will need some form of assistance. Approximately 80% of caregiving is provided by a family member who often helps by finding, managing, and offering appropriate assistance (Clark & Weber, 1997). This is why this particular study is so relevant. At every age, people are likely to have more elderly people in their families today than in the past. These profound changes will affect nearly every U.S. family in the future.

The U.S. Census Bureau (1986) estimates that by 2030, approximately 64 million people, or 20% of the population, will be age 65 years or older. In response to the challenges an older population will pose to the human resources of the United States, the Older Americans Act was created at the federal, state, and local levels to administer and to plan the service programs that will assist the nation's elderly (National Association of Area Agencies on Aging, 1992). Federal funds were allocated among states on the basis of the size of the elderly population within each state. The states in turn develop local geographic areas on aging to address the needs and concerns of all senior citizens at the local level. This chapter describes one example of how a local community can use marketing as an efficient way to obtain data from significant segments in the community. These data can then be used to help plan and organize programs and policy to assist the elderly in their respectful communities. In this chapter, we describe how Utah's Provo City formed an Eldercare Coalition to address the elderly population's needs and concerns within the community.

Provo City has a total population of more than 110,000 and an elderly population, 62 years of age or older, of 7,000. Provo is located in the central part of the state of Utah. The city has experienced a 5% increase in its elderly population during the past 10 years. The objectives of the Provo City Eldercare Coalition are to promote the welfare of the senior citizens in Provo, to help them maintain an independent lifestyle, to promote quality of life for the senior citizen, and to ease the burdens of caregivers. An initial mission statement adopted by the Provo City Eldercare Coalition included a needs assessment study of the Provo population. The study evaluated the current environment for senior citizens in Provo City, the senior citizens' basic needs, current programs available to assist seniors, barriers that senior citizens encounter to access certain programs, and how these needs could be better communicated to senior citizens and these caregivers.

METHODS

A multiple input model termed the *convergence model* was used for the Provo City senior citizens needs assessment study. The convergence model provides for appropriate benchmarking of perceptions and attitudes, which will enable the Coalition to replicate the needs assessment over time with the benefit of longitudinal analysis. In addition, the convergence model provides for multiple data points in the planning process for the Coalition.

The major research tasks of the research design included the approval to interview human subjects and the use of focus groups of both frail (elderly who need assistance with daily living activities) and nonfrail senior citizens and their caregivers as a way to assess the needs and concerns of the senior citizen population. The results of the focus groups were used to develop (a) a communitywide survey of 400 households, (b) 100 telephone interviews with the nonfrail elderly, and (c) 50 personal interviews with frail elderly. Twelve individual case studies were conducted as a way to validate the earlier findings of the study and to provide a qualitative analysis of the needs and concerns of senior citizens. A special subsample was used to address the needs and concerns of the elderly Latino population in Provo City.

FINDINGS

General Perceptions

A series of three questions dealing with general community perceptions was asked each respondent from the four populations surveyed in the needs assessment study. Each of the surveys asked for length of residence in Provo City, the rating of Provo as a place to live, and the perceived percentage of the Provo population that is 60 years of age or older. First, the length of residence in Provo from the community survey coincided with actual data provided by the Provo City Economic Development office (Table 14.1). Second, Provo was viewed as a good to excellent place to live by all individuals involved in the different surveys (Table 14.2). Third, the latest census data indicate that less than 10% of Provo's population is 60 years of age or older, whereas the perceptions

among those interviewed were that there are more senior citizens in Provo than actually exist (Table 14.3).

Needs Assessment

Each of the survey populations was asked to give perceptions and overall assessment concerning the current and future needs and concerns of those 60 years of age or older. To assess current needs, all respondents were asked to respond to the following statement: "Please tell us if any of your family, friends, or acquaintances who are 60 years of age or older have needs in any of the following areas." Respondents were then given a list of 11 to 17 different needs to consider. The weighted averages of these responses are summarized for each group in Table 14.4. The weighted sum is calculated by multiplying the frequency of response by the appropriate

Table 14.1   Length of Residence in Provo City

Category	Community, n = 400 (%)	Nonfrail, n = 100 (%)	Frail, n = 50 (%)	Latino, n = 24 (%)
Five or fewer years	53	5	16	57
Six or more years	47	95	84	44

Table 14.2   Ranking of Provo as a Place to Live

Category	Community, n = 400 (%)	Nonfrail, n = 100 (%)	Frail, n = 50 (%)	Latino, n = 24 (%)
Excellent	35	53	58	20
Good	56	40	34	50
Excellent or good	91	93	92	70

Table 14.3   Perceived Percentage of the Provo Population Who Are 60 Years of Age or Older

Category	Community, n = 400 (%)	Nonfrail, n = 100 (%)	Frail, n = 50 (%)	Latino, n = 24 (%)
Average percentage	35	28	42	34
Less than 10%	5	12	0	23

Table 14.4 Perception Ranking of Needs

Rank	Community (n = 400)		Nonfrail (n = 100)		Frail (n = 50)		Latino (n = 24)	
	Area of Need	Weighted Sum	Area of Need	Weighted Sum	Area of Need	Weighted Sum	Area of Need	Weighted Sum
1	Affordable health care	1,035	Coping with rising costs	157	Convenient transportation	104	Socialization with others	198
2	Adequate health care	967	Low-income adequate housing	146	Coping with rising costs	83	Transportation by bus	168
3	Coping with rising costs	936	Affordable health care	144	Socializing with others	72	Transportation by car	162
4	Loneliness	929	Adequate health care	132	Affordable health care	72	Participating in sports	154
5	Convenient transportation	929	Middle-income adequate housing	132	Assistance in daily living	70	Participating in hobbies	134
6	Physicians' acceptance of Medicare patients	854	Socializing with others	107	Loneliness	62	Coping with rising costs	134
7	Low-income adequate housing	821	Protection from scams	106	Leisure activities	55	Help in processing claims	133
8	Socializing with others	812	Leisure activities	105	Adequate health care	50	Taking medications at prescribed times	124
9	Relief for families	810	Taking medications at prescribed times	90	Low-income adequate housing	46	Protection from scams	117

	Community (n = 400)		Nonfrail (n = 100)		Frail (n = 50)		Latino (n = 24)	
Rank	Area of Need	Weighted Sum	Area of Need	Weighted Sum	Area of Need	Weighted Sum	Area of Need	Weighted Sum
10	Personal safety	807	Convenient transportation	86	Help in processing claims	40	Relief for family	105
11	Taking medications at prescribed times	772	Personal safety	85	Protection from scams	37	Assistance in daily living	72
12	Leisure activities	747	Physicians' acceptance of Medicare patients	82	Middle-income adequate housing	31		
13	Assistance in daily living	727	Loneliness	76	Relief for family	30		
14	Help in processing claims	726	Relief for family	67	Taking medications at prescribed times	28		
15	Middle-income adequate housing	689	Help in processing claims	64	Physicians' acceptance of Medicare patients	27		
16			Assistance in daily living	56	Personal safety	24		
17			Exploitation by family	55	Exploitation by family	11		

weight and then adding all the weighted sums. For the community, the weights were as follows: 3, major need; 2, moderate need; and 1, minor need. For the nonfrail and frail, the weights were as follows: 3, major need; 2, moderate need; 1, minor need; and 0, no need. The weights for the Latino sample were calculated on a scale of 1 to 10, with 1 representing no need and 10 representing a major need. Because the number of respondents and weights were different for each population, the weighted sums vary from group to group.

The major needs of the senior citizens of Provo deal with the difficult task of living on fixed incomes and coping with rising costs and adequate medical insurance to cover medical and dental costs. In addition, the lack of adequate transportation, especially for the frail elderly, and the need to socialize with others were cited by many in the needs assessment study. The other concerns expressed dealt with housing issues, primarily for the low- and middle-income senior citizens, and how to perform several household chores that are beyond the senior citizen's physical capacity. The senior citizens want the opportunity to pursue their interests and hobbies, and to feel that they are contributing to society, so as to sense that they have a quality life. Families and friends of senior citizens also need a network that will provide them with some respite from the daily and weekly demands of caring for a loved one.

To assess future concerns, respondents were asked the following open-ended question: "Are there any future concerns, in the next 3 to 5 years, that you think will be more urgent than they are now?" The major future concern expressed in response to the open-ended question was for adequate care for elderly, including both health care and daily living. The second most frequently mentioned concern was adequate housing, followed closely by financial security. All populations were generally in agreement on these issues. Table 14.5 outlines these future concerns.

Latino Population

Because the area of need section in the Latino survey instrument was administered slightly differently than that for the other three populations, a separate discussion regarding these findings is presented. As Table 14.4 shows, socializing with others and some form of leisure activity are ranked very high. In addition, transportation, either by bus or by car, was viewed as a major need. Only 10 of the needs were ranked on a 10-point scale of need; the other need categories were asked as "yes" or "no" questions, with some of the categories broken down further into two or three questions (e.g., regarding access and cost of health care). Table 14.6 summarizes these "yes" and "no" questions.

In summary, the majority of Latin Americans reported that they do not have a problem accessing health care, do not feel lonely, feel relatively safe in their homes and neighborhoods, and do not feel they are taken advantage of.

Overall Perception Ranking

Using a weighted sum again, an overall ranking of the current needs summarized in Table 14.4 was obtained for the community, nonfrail, and frail populations. (The Latino population ranking was not included in this overall ranking because of the different structure used with the survey instrument.) Table 14.7 summarizes this overall ranking.

From the previous discussion, as well as the focus groups and case studies conducted, the following conclusions can be drawn regarding the current and future areas of need:

Coping with rising costs: Senior citizens with fixed income will always have difficulty with budgetary concerns as prices rise over time.

Health care: Acquiring adequate medical insurance is an increasing concern for the elderly population, especially the frail elderly. In addition, the cost of medications is a worry.

Table 14.5   Future Concerns Facing the Elderly Population

Category	Community (n = 400)	Nonfrail (n = 100)	Frail (n = 50)	Latino (n = 24)
First concern	Adequate health care (50%)	Adequate care (29%)	Adequate care (36%)	Adequate health care (20%)
Second concern	Adequate housing (20%)	Transportation (9%)	Finances (20%)	Adequate housing (15%)
Third concern	Increasing number of elderly to provide services to (10%)	Taxes (8%) Personal health 6%	Finances (4%) Personal health (4%)	Financial security(24%)

Table 14.6   Area of Need: Responses to "Yes" and "No" Questions, Latino Population (n = 24)

Question	Yes (%)	No (%)
Do you feel lonely?	15.0	85.0
Do you know what Medicare is?	66.7	33.3
Do physicians accept you as a Medicare patient?	87.5	12.5
Do you have access to a doctor?	77.8	22.2
Do you have access to a clinic?	58.9	41.1
Do you have access to a hospital?	66.7	33.3
Do you have access to a nurse?	53.8	46.2
Do you have access to mobile health care?	41.7	58.3
Do you feel safe in your neighborhood?	85.7	14.3
Do you feel safe in your home?	90.0	10.0
Do you feel you are taken advantage of?	21.1	78.9
Are you given too many responsibilities for you to handle at home?	50.0	50.0

Access to health care does not appear to be a major problem, but the elderly have difficulty over time seeing a physician as more doctors refuse to accept patients covered by Medicare.

Transportation: The lack of adequate transportation, especially for the frail elderly, surfaced as a major need. Running errands, going to doctor appointments, attending church, visiting family or friends, and getting to and from recreational opportunities are very difficult for the frail. In addition, those in assisted living facilities lack the opportunity to participate in recreational activities outside their care center because no organizations provide this service.

Loneliness/socializing with others: The issue that surfaced repeatedly was the need for someone to visit. Those older than 60 years of age, both frail and nonfrail, crave the opportunity to interact with others.

Housing: Housing is a concern for those in the low- and middle-income categories. Although the majority of senior citizens prefer to stay in their own homes as their health deteriorates, housing will be an increasing need for individuals who need assistance with their daily living.

Household chores: Deep cleaning, such as defrosting a refrigerator and washing windows,

Table 14.7   Overall Perception Ranking of Needs: Community, Nonfrail, and Frail ($n = 550$)

Rank	Area of Need	Weighted Sum
1	Coping with rising costs	42
2	Affordable health care	40
3	Adequate health care	34
4	Convenient transportation	33
5	Socializing with others	31
6	Low-income adequate housing	30
7	Loneliness	26
8	Leisure activities	22
9	Physicians' acceptance of Medicare patients	17
10	Middle-income adequate housing	17
11	Taking medications at prescribed times	16
12	Assistance in daily life	15
13	Relief for family	14
14	Personal safety	13
15	Help in processing claims	10

is a challenge to some of the nonfrail as they progress in years, as is maintenance, both inside and outside, and yard work. Snow removal in the winter is a similar need.

Some of the other needs not as apparent from the telephone interviews but surfacing as major needs during the focus groups and case studies were the following:

Quality of life: Quality of life is defined as being able to pursue one's interests and hobbies (e.g., swimming, computer use, and arts and crafts). This need to create, contribute, and participate is perceived as a crucial need by the senior citizens as a means to feel like they are still an important part of society.

Caretaker relief: Assistance is needed for the family and others who provide the support network for frail senior citizens.

Current Service Programs

All the various populations were asked in an open-ended question where they would

turn for help with particular problems the elderly might face in the process of daily living. There were nearly a dozen specific problems mentioned in the survey. Both those problems and the responses are summarized in Table 14.8.

Medical Emergencies

When asked where they would go for help in a medical emergency, a very high percentage (more than 70%) of the nonfrail and frail populations said they would call 911, an ambulance, the hospital, or the emergency room. A surprisingly large percentage of the community at large and the Latino population (28% and 17%, respectively) said they did not know where to go. It was evident that the frail population (who had probably had this need on occasion) knew who to call for help because none of them responded that they did not know. The case is similar for the nonfrail; only 3% responded that they did not know.

Table 14.8   Where Elderly Would Go for Help With Specific Daily Living Situations[a]

Help With	Program	Community, n = 400 (%)	Non-frail, n = 100 (%)	Frail, n = 50 (%)	Latino, n = 24 (%)
Medical emergencies	Hospital, emergency room, ambulance	42	74	82[b]	56[b]
	Didn't know	28	3	0	17
	Other sources	5	23	18	27
	Subtotal	75	100	100	100
Personal care	Didn't know	36	28	0	0
	Family/friends	13	38	14	50
	Home health programs	12	34	50	8
	Subtotal	61	100	64	58
Transportation	Didn't know	25	19	0	17
	United Way	23	5	15	0
	UTA	18	8	0	25
	Family/friends	15	53[c]	55	25
	Subtotal	81	85	70	67
Paying for appropriate medical care	Didn't know	36	31	38	36
	Medicare/Medicaid	18	11	14	36
	Family	7	11	12	14
	Hospital	7	2	4	7
	Subtotal	68	55	68	93
Household chores	Family/friends	31	29	20	27
	Didn't know	28	13	12	47
	Church	17	8	2	0
	Hire someone	0	23	20	7
	Home health agency	0	0	22	0
	Subtotal	76	73	76	81
Nourishing meals	Meals on Wheels	47	43	56	0
	Didn't know	19	14	14	9
	Family/friends	13	25[d]	8	64
	Church	6	2	2	0
	Senior citizens center	0	0	0	18
	Subtotal	85	80	80	91
Preventing physical, mental, and emotional abuse	Didn't know	41	48	56	40
	Family/friends	9	14	6	7
	Police	7	6	4	7
	Social services	7	2	4	0
	Subtotal	64	70	70	54
When abuse has occurred	Didn't know	—[e]	36	40	33
	Police	—	16	10	27
	Family/friends	—	14	18	7
	Church	—	10	6	0
	Subtotal	—	76	74	67
Social/recreational opportunities	Didn't know	27	10	28	42
	Senior citizens center	23	17	42	5
	Eldred Center	18	14	0	21
	Church/BYU	11	26	8	5
	Subtotal	79	67	78	73

(Continued)

Table 14.8 (Continued)

Help With	Program	Community, n = 400 (%)	Non-frail, n = 100 (%)	Frail, n = 50 (%)	Latino, n = 24 (%)
Legal problems	Didn't know	40	14	14	71
	Lawyer	17	40	24	7
	Legal aid society	8	6	20	7
	Family/Friends	6	17	40	0
	State legal services	5	1	0	0
	Subtotal	76	78	98	85
Processing claims and monthly bills	Didn't know	47	21	18	38
	Family/friends	20	29	56	19
	Self/no need	0	21	0	0
	Senior citizens center	4	2	0	0
	Mountainland Association	0	0	0	6
	Subtotal	71	73	74	63

a. In every case, only those sources that were mentioned by 5% or more of the respondents were included in the summary. When there is a source with less than 5%, one or more of the four populations mentioned it.

b. A variety of "other sources" were mentioned, but no single source was mentioned by more than 4% of the respondents. "Dial 911" was included as a response for both the frail and Latino populations, along with hospital, ambulance, and emergency room.

c. Also included in this category for the nonfrail population was the comment "drive ourselves."

d. Also included in this category for the nonfrail population was the response "rely on ourselves."

e. This question was not asked in the survey to the community at large.

Personal Care

In response to help with personal care (e.g., bathing, dressing, and taking medication), again it was evident that the frail population had identified some sources because none of them indicated they did not know where to turn for help, and only 14% said they relied on family or friends. Most of the frail relied on some type of a home health program. The individual case studies among the frail show that home health nursing provides much care, supplemented where possible by the family. The response of the Latino population reflected its family solidarity; the majority responded that they would turn to their family and friends for help.

Transportation

The issue of where people would turn for help with their transportation needs showed a real contrast between what the community expected seniors to do and what the seniors said they would do. Only 15% of the community believed that family or friends should provide the transportation for the elderly. More than 40% said the elderly could rely on United Way or the Utah Transit Authority state bus service. In reality, more than half of the frail and nonfrail said they relied on family and friends. A large portion of the nonfrail, however, responded that they "drove themselves."

Medical Care Payment

Being able to pay for appropriate medical care is a concern of many people, but it can be a major issue for elderly who may be on a fixed income. Slightly more than one third of all four populations did not know where they would go for help or what they would do if they needed medical care that they could not afford. Obviously, Medicare or Medicaid were mentioned, but surprisingly they were mentioned by less than 20% of the respondents in three of the four populations, whereas they were mentioned by 36% of the Latino population. Seven to 14% of all four populations said they would rely on family. Another 2% to 7% of each population said they would hope the hospital would absorb the cost of what they could not afford.

The individual case studies indicated that the elderly were concerned that in the future they would not have the money to buy needed medications and supplemental health insurance. In these cases, they would have to rely on their family to help when that time came.

Household Chores

For many of the elderly who stay in their own homes or apartments, it is a struggle to do simple household chores, such as vacuuming, dusting, and cleaning appliances. The heavier chores, such as laundry, cleaning walls and window blinds, and defrosting refrigerators and freezers, are almost impossible. Minor repairs, both inside and outside, and yard work and snow removal become virtually impossible, especially for the frail elderly.

In the community at large and the Latino population, 28% and 47%, respectively, said they did not know where the elderly would go for help with household chores. From 20% to 31% of all four populations said they turned to family and friends for help. Only the community mentioned the church to any extent. Twenty-three percent of the nonfrail said they would hire someone; 20% of the frail said they had hired someone, and 22% said they used the services provided by the Home Health Agency. All the frail case study individuals who still lived in apartments or their own home said they had someone coming into their home for at least

2 hours each week (some individuals were receiving more help) to do cleaning and other miscellaneous chores.

Nourishing Meals

Another concern of the elderly living in their own home was for nourishing meals when they could not cook for themselves. In response to where one would go for help in this regard, 43% to 56% of three of the four populations indicated they would turn to Meals on Wheels for help. None of the Latino population responded with Meals on Wheels, however, but nearly two thirds of them (64%) said they would turn to family or friends. An additional one fifth of the Latino population said they would go to the senior citizens center (which was not mentioned by any of the other three populations). Sometimes, as discovered in the case studies, people's preference for food is so restrictive that they will not eat any meals prepared and delivered by the Meals on Wheels organization. In these cases, the only help available is close family members.

Abuse

In regard to where the elderly would go for help to prevent physical, mental, and emotional abuse, 40% to 56% of all four populations said they did not know—the highest "did not know" percentage of all the particular problems studied relating to daily living activities. Very few sources were suggested outside of family or friends, the police, and social services.

An interview with a daughter of a frail person identified subtle ways that abuse of elderly occurs. The daughter had been a practicing attorney in Provo for approximately the past 12 years. She indicated in an interview that a few months ago, an 82-year-old woman asked for her professional help to develop an estate plan. The elderly woman wanted to give all her property to a man and a woman who were not married to each other and who were not related to the elderly woman. The attorney probed for reasons why they, rather than her children, should receive her property. The attorney found out that both the man and the woman lived in the general neighborhood where this elderly woman lived. They had convinced her that they were the only people who cared enough about her to visit her regularly. They had also convinced her that for their effort they expected some remuneration. The elderly woman had been paying the man $50 each month for a 1-hour visit. She had also been paying the woman $15 each week for a 1-hour visit.

The attorney believed this situation happened because the elderly woman was desperate for company. Loneliness can be a major issue among the elderly, and both the frail and nonfrail older than 60 years of age crave an opportunity to interact regularly with others. This natural tendency makes the elderly (especially those who try to stay in their own homes) vulnerable to schemes perpetrated by people in their community. These schemes are not hatched only by outsiders. The attorney knew of elderly people who had been taken advantage of by their own family members.

A prime example is the response received when people were asked where they would go for help when physical, mental, and emotional abuse had already occurred. One third and two fifths of the nonfrail, frail, and Latino populations responded that they did not know. The only other suggested sources of help were family, friends, police, and the church. (The community at large was not asked this particular question.) As mentioned previously, both abuse issues had larger percentages of "did not know" responses than any of the other daily living activities asked of the four different populations. It is disturbing that the response of family and friends was almost as large as the response

for police. Those elderly who are being abused by family members or friends simply may not be aware of any other source of help and may be reluctant to report abuse by their family members to the police.

Social and Recreational Opportunities

Social and recreational opportunities enhance the quality of life. When the elderly were asked where they would go for social and recreational opportunities, the community at large, the nonfrail, and even the frail populations frequently mentioned a particular or generic "senior citizens center." For all three populations, between 31% and 42% responded in that vein. Slightly more than one fourth of the Latino population mentioned a senior citizens center, but 42% said they did not know. Approximately one fourth of the nonfrail population responded that the local university or church met most of their social and recreational needs. No other population had a higher rate for that particular response.

Legal Aid

Forty percent of the community and 71% of the Latino population responded that they did not know where to go for legal help. Most of the responses from both the nonfrail and frail populations included lawyers, the legal aid society, and family or friends.

Processing Medical Claims and Monthly Bills

All four populations were asked where they would go for help with processing medical claims and monthly bills. Forty-seven percent of the community and 38% of the Latino population said they did not know where to turn for help. Fifty-six percent of the frail and 29% of the nonfrail populations indicated that they received help from their family or friends. Another 21% of the nonfrail said they did not need any help.

CONCLUSIONS REGARDING CURRENT SERVICE PROGRAMS

Communication

The most alarming factor that emerges from the results is the large percentage of all four populations who said they did not know where to go for help when they needed it. On average, 29% of all the populations across all 11 of the daily living activities said they did not know where to turn for help. This represents nearly one third of everyone surveyed who were frustrated by not having a central source for referrals to agencies or programs that can provide support for regularly needed activities for the elderly.

All the needs previously identified are compounded by the fact that people do not know were to turn for help if help is needed. Communication issues are reiterated by the findings.

Transportation

The lack of adequate transportation, especially for the frail, is a crucial need. As indicated previously, however, more than 40% of the three elderly populations could rely on local bus service or the United Way. In addition, the nonfrail are still able to drive themselves. People are at least somewhat aware of avenues to pursue in fulfilling this need, but more resources need to be made available to the elderly.

Health Care

The problem of obtaining adequate supplemental medical insurance was identified as a major need by the elderly. This need is compounded by the finding that approximately one third of the respondents did not know where they could obtain additional help for covering medical costs.

Household Chores

To some extent, depending on the activity level, both the nonfrail and the frail populations have needs in this area. The frail population had a lower percentage of "did not know" responses than the other populations who indicated their use of household services. The other three populations, however, need to be educated on the options available to them as their need for this service becomes greater. The Meals on Wheels organization has done a good job of educating the public in regard to its service; perhaps other organizations providing assistance with household duties should do the same.

Quality of Life

Another aspect of this need comes into play with regard to the prevention of physical, mental, and emotional abuse of seniors. As discussed previously, abuse occurs more often by people familiar to the senior (i.e., family and friends) than by people unknown to the senior. Again, alarmingly high percentages of "did not know" responses were given. Also, combating loneliness could improve the quality of life for many of the elderly.

Loneliness/Socializing With Others

Because seniors have a great need to socialize and interact with others, every effort should be made to communicate social and recreational opportunities. More than one third are informed enough to know that the senior citizens center can provide this experience. For the frail, it may be difficult to take advantage of this facility due to lack of transportation. More effort needs to be made to create social outlets for the elderly. It was obvious from many of the

Table 14.9   Overall Ranking of Barriers: Community, Nonfrail, Frail, and Latino (N = 574)

Rank	Barrier	Weighted Sum
1	Poor health	37
2	The weather	30
3	Limited money to pay for services or activities	29
4	Dislike going to activities alone	28
5	Lack of information	24
6	Lack of transportation	23
7	Problem remembering things	18
8	Language or cultural differences	13
9	Afraid to try "new" things	10
10	Wanting to be "left alone"	8

personal interviews that seniors want only the opportunity to talk to at least one other person regularly because many of them are profoundly lonely.

In summary, all the populations in the needs assessment were asked where they would turn for assistance with particular problems the senior citizen might encounter in the process of daily living: medical emergencies, personal care, transportation, payment for medical care, household chores, nourishing meals, prevention of several types of elderly abuse, social and recreational opportunities, legal problems, and the task of processing monthly bills. There is an important and crucial need to better communicate information about the availability of current services and programs that provide assistance to senior citizens in the areas previously defined. The level of awareness of these programs, knowing who to contact for assistance if a need exists, and the apparent fragmented system imply the need for a central source for such information.

The issues of transportation, health care, and household chores, along with quality of life issues and loneliness factors, were also prevalent from the assessment of current programs regarding assistance in daily living activities.

BARRIERS TO ACCESSING SENIOR CITIZEN PROGRAMS

A concern of the Eldercare Coalition was to identify the major obstacles or barriers that keep senior citizens from enjoying a better quality of life and access to services, programs, and social activities. To address this issue, each respondent was asked to respond to the following statement: "Please rate each of the following barriers that might prevent you from using existing services or attending scheduled activities." Table 14.9 summarizes the overall ranking of barriers when all four populations were analyzed together using a weighted sum. The major obstacles identified are poor health, the weather, limited resources, and the dislike of going to activities alone. The lack of information and transportation are cited as additional barriers that prohibit senior citizens from participating in some activities and programs. Language and cultural differences are major barriers for the Latino population.

COMMUNICATION ISSUES

An important concern of the Eldercare Coalition was to assess how well existing services and activities were being communicated to the citizens, both elderly and the community at large. To address this issue, an open-ended question was asked: "Do you know of a centralized source to which you can turn to find out what services and activities are available to the elderly?"

Senior citizens and the community at large identified with a particular community senior center, the Eldred Center, as a primary source of information for needs, concerns, and programs for the elderly in Provo. Second, the public believed that the burden rested on their local government. This level of awareness and loyalty, however, needs to be expanded and strengthened as a means to provide a central source where senior citizens, the community, and caregivers can access information and outreach programs to meet the needs and concerns identified in the needs assessment study.

PERCEPTIONS OF SENIOR CITIZEN SERVICES

To help identify possible services that should be provided to citizens older than 60 years of age, six statements regarding potential services were read to the respondents in each population. After each statement, the respondent was asked whether he or she strongly agreed, agreed, disagreed, or strongly disagreed with each statement.

Potential services that were identified that may be of interest to senior citizens and the community included taxi service, in-home services, adult day care centers, a fully staffed senior citizens center, and opportunities for volunteer service for the senior citizen. These perceptions reinforce the need for addressing the lack of transportation for many frail senior citizens, the difficulty they may have with certain physically strenuous household chores, the need to socialize with others, and the relief caregivers would experience from the existence of an adult day care center in Provo.

SUMMARY OF ISSUES

A major advantage of the convergence model is the quality and quantity of the data that are generated relative to the needs of the elderly population in a given community. All the perception data gathered from the surveys and focus groups completed by the Eldercare Coalition provided an excellent summary regarding the services, programs, and needs of the elderly living in Provo. The following is a summary of the findings:

Communication: The majority of people we interviewed, both by telephone and in person, are not aware of services and opportunities available to citizens 60 years of age or older. Approximately 17% to 20% of the respondents did not even know whom they would call for assistance with an important need or concern. Communication channels need to be improved.

Loneliness: The issue that surfaced repeatedly was the need for someone to visit. Those older than 60 years of age, both frail and non-frail, crave the opportunity to interact with others.

Household chores: Deep cleaning, such as defrosting a refrigerator and washing windows, is a challenge to some of the nonfrail as they progress in years. Snow removal in the winter is a similar need.

Quality of life: Quality of life is defined as being able to pursue one's interests and hobbies (e.g., swimming, computer usage, and arts and crafts). This need to contribute and participate is perceived as crucial by the senior citizens as a way to feel they are still an important part of society.

Latino population: The language and cultural differences serve as a major barrier for this population. Special programs need to be developed that are sensitive to the cultural requirements of the Latino population.

Transportation: The lack of adequate transportation, especially for the frail elderly, surfaced as a major need. Running errands, going

Table 14.10 Groups Especially Affected by Issues

Issue	Nonfrail			Frail			
	Independent and Active	Semiindependent, Family Support	Health Deteriorating, No Family Support	Homebound, Poor Health, Family Support	Homebound, Poor Health, No Support	Assisted Living Facility	Latino
Communication	X	X	X	X	X	X	X
Transportation				X	X	X	X
Loneliness			X	X	X	X	X
Health care			X	X	X	X	
Household chores		X	X	X	X		
Rising costs	X	X	X	X	X	X	X
Housing					X	X	X
Quality of life			X	X	X	X	
Caretaker relief				X	X		X

to doctor's appointments, attending church, and getting to and from recreational opportunities are very difficult for the frail. In addition, those in assisted living facilities lack the opportunity to participate in recreational activities outside their care center because no organizations provide this service.

Health care: Acquiring adequate medical insurance is an increasing concern for this segment, especially the frail elderly. The cost of medications is also a worry. Access to health care does not appear to be a major problem, but the elderly have difficulty over time seeing a physician as more doctors refuse to accept Medicare patients.

Caretaker relief: Assistance is needed for the family and others who provide the support network for frail senior citizens.

Coping with rising costs: Senior citizens with fixed incomes will always face budget challenges as prices rise over time.

Housing: Housing is a concern for those in the low- and middle-income categories. Although most senior citizens prefer to stay in their own homes as their health deteriorates, housing will be an increasing need for individuals who need assistance with their daily living.

The senior citizen population segments that were evident from the needs assessment study are presented in Table 14.10. The important implication of these different groups is that implementation of strategies and programs will need to vary depending on which group is affected by the specific issue. This is also essential when the Eldercare Coalition envisions ways to reduce the barriers that affect different senior citizen groups.

To help the Eldercare Coalition, with its significant responsibilities, implement the needs assessment findings, each of the senior citizen issues is presented systematically with suggested implementation ideas. These suggestions provide an initial beginning position for the Coalition and prioritize the issues.

CONCLUSION

Caregiving will remain an intrinsic part of the experience of U.S. families well into the 21st century. Therefore, it is vital to conduct needs assessment surveys to help caregivers and communities identify high-priority areas of need for the elderly population. Implementation of senior citizens' requests, stratified to meet their various circumstances and concerns, is an enormous task, but it is also an exciting one. The successful implementation of a needs assessment study such as the one described in this article can be a first and major step in that task. Such an assessment provides the caregiver for the elderly with a sense of mission and direction by identifying those programs and services that the elderly give highest priority.

In Provo City, doing a needs assessment study of its senior citizens was much like taking the vital signs of its seniors. Investing the time and effort to focus on them—to listen to the "pulse" of their needs, their fears, their hopes, and their suggestions—revealed a segment of the city's population who are in spirit and desire very much alive, willing and eager to be active participants in their community. The reality is that when senior citizens' needs are met, the whole community benefits. Moreover, the convergence model is an excellent method to obtain needs assessment data regarding the elderly population in other communities. The quality of the data reported here relate to the broad range of issues, needs, and policies that attest to the model's strength to obtain and portray such data.

REFERENCES

Clark, J. A., & Weber, K. A. (1997). *Challenges and choices: Family relationships—Elderly caregiving.* Columbia: University of Missouri, Department of Human Development and Family Studies.

National Association of Area Agencies on Aging for the Administration on Aging. (1992, April). *The National Network on Aging and the role of the Area Agencies on Aging.* Washington, DC: Emprise Designs.

U.S. Census Bureau, Congressional Research Service. (1986). *Current population survey.* Washington, DC: Government Printing Office.

CHAPTER 15

Death, Grief, and Bereavement in Families

BETH VAUGHAN-COLE

A nurse talks with a mother holding a final vigil over a daughter with cystic fibrosis with complications. During the past 5 months, mother and daughter have been at the hospital more than they have been at home. There are three other children at home 300 miles away in a small rural town. The mother reports that her teenage son is causing trouble at home and that her 3 year-old would not sit in her lap when she returned home because she was angry with her for leaving.

Billy, almost 8 years old, was referred to the Child Guidance Center for unusual behavior—running in front of moving cars and jumping off high perches. Intake interviews with the parents revealed that Billy was 6 when his 8 year old brother died of leukemia. Because Billy was so young, and his parents' grief so profound, his parents did not talk about the death, and tried to protect Billy from their sadness. Without correct information, Billy believed that boys in his family died at the age of 8. As he now approached his next birthday, he was profoundly anxious yet drawn to questioning how people die.

What happens in families when death occurs? In the first vignette, a mother is estranged from her family as she invests time and attention in her dying daughter. After the death, she will need to integrate back into a family that has attempted to continue its daily activities without her. In the second vignette, the parents' silence led a young boy to misperceive the cause of his brother's death. The boy lived in terror as he approached his eighth birthday, believing it would precipitate his death.

There are volumes of literature about death, dying, and bereavement. Novels, movies, artwork, television, newspapers, magazines, Internet Web sites, and one's lived experience bring death and the associated grief into our awareness. Yet academics suggest that we have only scratched the surface in our understanding. Sorrow and suffering in response to the death of a loved one forcefully impact the lives of the living, and most of our living is conducted in close proximity to others, usually family groups.

The focus of this chapter is on an event, the death of a family member, and how that death impacts families. Although Weiss (2001) makes a case for studying "affiliation relationships," it is the "attachment relationships" of the immediate and closely extended family that are examined. Usually, these refer to parent-child, spouse-spouse or couple, sibling, and relationships of all the family members together. The nuclear family of parents and children living together no longer represents the majority of households. Single, divorced, or never married parents living with children, or grandparents raising grandchildren, are more common than in past decades. Households may include nuclear families plus additional relatives. Also, with the aging population, couples often live in households for many years without children.

This chapter presents an overview of the significance and relevance of a death of a family member to individuals and their families. Individual variables of the deceased (age at time of the death, cause of death, and family roles and relationships) interact with individual variables of the survivors (age at time of the death of the family member, relationship with deceased, emotional and physical responses to grief, mental health, and coping responses) in the human crucible of the family.

DEFINITIONS OF TERMS

Several authors (DeSpelder & Strickland, 2005; Rando, 1993; Weiss, 2001) have suggested a need for clarification of terms related to the experience of death. The term *bereavement* is a noun and generally refers to the loss of a loved one by death or to the bereaved condition. The verb *to bereave* is defined as to be deprived or robbed of a relationship, to be left desolate and alone. *Grief* is a noun defined as sorrow, anguish, or deep sadness. *Mourning* is a noun and has

a number of definitions that include the acts of a person who mourns, such as sorrowing and lamentation, or the period during which black or other displays of sorrow are worn. *To mourn* is to feel or express deep sorrow or grief (Random House Webster's College Dictionary, 1996). Thus, there is some attempt to separate the event of the death of a loved one from the feelings and responses of a person to the death and from the outward acts that a person demonstrates in response to a significant death.

HOW DEATH OCCURS IN THE UNITED STATES

In 2001, there were 2,416,425 deaths in the United States (National Center for Health Statistics [NCHS], 2003). This represented 854.5 deaths per 100,000 of the U.S. population. Very few people live in total isolation, and most live in family groups of some kind. It is reasonable to suggest that on average the deceased would have three to five significant relationships. Therefore, 7 to 12 million people are affected annually by the death of a loved one. This number, and the fact that every person is mortal, emphasizes the hunger to understand how death affects the living.

Table 15.1 shows the top 13 causes of death in the United States in 2001 according to the NCHS (2003). These represent 80% of all deaths. A major variable influencing the grieving process of individuals and their families is how the death occurred. Acute and chronic illnesses represent the most frequent causes of death, with the rest being sudden and unexpected deaths. Although the cause of death has implications for individual and family responses to the loss, the implications extend further. Deaths due to accidents, homicide, or suicide may involve long legal and criminal investigations, media attention, or stigma, which influence the

Table 15.1   The Top 13 Causes of Death in the United States in 2001

1. Heart disease	8. Alzheimer's disease
2. Cancer	9. Nephritis, nephritic syndrome, and nephrosis
3. Stroke	10. Septicemia
4. Chronic lower respiratory diseases	11. Suicide
5. Accidents (unintentional injuries)	12. Chronic liver disease
6. Diabetes	13. Homicide
7. Influenza/pneumonia	

SOURCE: NCHS (2003).

grieving process. Acute and chronic illnesses generally include contact with health care professionals and institutions that can also influence the grieving process.

Age and Causes of Death

The following rankings are from the 2001 vital statistics (NCHS, 2003). The major causes of infant mortality are congenital malformations, deformations, and chromosomal abnormalities. Accidents represent the most common cause of death of people 1 to 45 years of age. After age 45 years, accidents are the third most common cause until age 65, when they decline to the ninth most common cause.

The second and third most frequent causes of death of children, ages 1 to 14 years, are congenital malformations and malignant neoplasms. The second and third most frequent causes of death of people aged 15 to 24 years are assault (homicide) and intentional self harm (suicide). Malignant neoplasms and diseases of the heart are the second and third most frequent causes of death for people 25 to 44 years of age, respectively. From ages 45 to 65 years, the first and second most frequent causes of death are malignant neoplasms and diseases of the heart, respectively. For ages 65 years and older, the three main causes of death are diseases of the heart, malignant neoplasms, and cerebrovascular diseases.

Age is a significant factor for families who experience a loss. The age of the deceased, as well as the age of each family member, draws relevant associations for family structure, dynamics, relationships, and the meaning that death has to the remaining family members over a lifetime. The death of an infant has different implications for a family than the death of the breadwinner of a family. Family roles, responsibilities, and relationships are associated with family members' ages.

It is impossible in a brief chapter to present all the relevant theories that have developed throughout the years to explain individual and family grieving. The scholarly literature on grief emerges from a variety of disciplines, such as sociology, psychology, medicine, nursing, social work, epidemiology, and anthropology. Although each contributes a view that enhances our understanding of grief, many, including Shaver and Tancredy (2001), bemoan the lack of a single unifying theory or framework

The next section addresses individual grief responses to bereavement in the following areas: attachment theory, grief and psychopathology, bereavement and physiology, grief and resilience, age and grief responses, and cause of death and grieving. The section on grief from a family perspective addresses young parents and the loss of a child, parents and the death of an adult child, parenting children when a spouse dies, parent-to-parent behaviors after loss, sibling-to-sibling relationships after a death, and extended family responses. The section on families grieving together addresses three major theories useful in understanding grieving families: family systems theory and a typology of grieving families, the resiliency model of family stress, and family development theory. The chapter ends with a final conclusion.

INDIVIDUAL GRIEF RESPONSES

Most of the theoretical and research literature has approached the phenomenon from how grief affects individuals. As with all social and behavioral research, there is variation in how grief affects individuals. Summarizing across groups has been helpful. It is by noting the commonalities, trends, and outcomes that a body of literature increases our understanding about the human experience of grieving. Individual differences are often important to note, however, especially as clinicians develop interventions to decrease suffering and long-term negative influences of the death of a loved one.

Attachment Theory

According to Weiss (2001), "Relationships are formed of all the events occurring between people. Interpersonal bonds are the emotional linkages that underlie these events" (pp. 54-55). Grieving is the predictable consequence of the loss of a relationship or attachment. Other consequences of the loss of a relationship of attachment depend on the constellation of bonds and feelings carried by that relationship.

Attachment theory has a fairly long history. Although Freud was most interested in the intrapsychic world, he clearly recognized the role that people had in influencing the personality of another. He approached the phenomenon of grief in his paper titled

Mourning and Melancholia (1919). Freud called the psychological processing in response to loss "grief work" and projected that the curative process for grieving was to "let go" of the strong emotional bond with the deceased.

Amid the bombing of London during World War II, Spitz (1945) engaged in a unique research study created by natural circumstances. His interest was in normal and pathological infant development. He carefully observed infants and very young children who were separated from their parents and placed in a rural foundling home, a safe haven from the explosions occurring in the city. The high incidence of mortality was surprising because the institution worked diligently to maintain a clean environment and to provide good food and compassionate care, though infrequent and inconsistent. Spitz compared the growth and development of infants in the foundling home to those of infants with their mothers in a prison and infants and mothers in a rural, seaside community. Movies taken at the foundling home of the infants underscored the unfolding tragedy Spitz attributed to infants being deprived of their mothers with no replacement. He identified a cluster of behaviors as "protest" and "despair" and coined the term *anaclitic depression* as the response of infants to the loss of a consistent nurturing mothering figure (Spitz, 1946).

Grief and Psychopathology

Other researchers were in search of the origins of psychopathology and depression. In the early 1950s, Robertson and Bowlby (1952) studied the responses of children separated from their parents. In Bowlby's three-volume treatise, he catalogued related studies and their contribution to his theory of attachment, separation, and loss. His focus was on children and identifying the origins and evolutionary necessity of psychological relationships. Bowlby (1969, 1973, and 1980) described children's responses to the death of one or both parents.

Robertson (1953a) augmented reports with videotapes of toddlers separated from their mothers, who were hospitalized with the deliveries of their newborns. Again, the visual data offered evocative images of toddlers' psychological distress to separation over time. Robertson, however, identified some of the mediating environmental variables that seemed to prevent the most extreme suffering from separation (Robertson, 1953a, 1953b, 1956; Robertson & Bowlby, 1952).

In 1942, a fire broke out in a nightclub in Boston. The Coconut Grove fire killed 492 people. Lindemann (1944) followed up with families of the victims. More than 100 family members sought mental health support after the fire. He chronicled adult acute grief responses that he suggested were "normal" grief responses. Common symptoms noted were anger, apathy, loneliness, emptiness, disbelief, yearning, and searching.

Anderson (1949), later validated by Parkes (1965), wrote about the increased incidence of recent death of a family member and other significant people in the histories of hospitalized patients with mental illness. Piper, Ogrodniczuk, Azim, and Weideman (2001) reported that more than half of a large group of outpatients in a mental health clinic had experienced significant losses, and one third of these patients met the criteria for moderate or severe long-term complicated grief.

The relationship of grief to mental illness has been a major focus of research and clinical studies since Freud. There was clear evidence, however, that most people who had a significant loss did not develop severe mental illness. Thus, there had to be some differentiation between those who developed mental illness and those who did not. Parkes and Weiss (1983) identified three risk factors that predicted later adjustment: unanticipated grief, conflicted grief, and chronic grief.

The most common psychopathologies, associated with grief and mourning, are depression and anxiety. Rando (1993) noted that the association between loss and depression has been studied extensively and listed many of the studies. After a decade of research, Kim and Jacobs (1993) suggested that between 17% and 27% of bereaved people had "unremitting depression" at the end of the first year of the loss. Obviously, the strong relationship is serious, but it does not represent the majority of the population.

Klerman, Weissman, Rounsaville, and Chevron (1984) described event-triggered depression versus constitutional depression. The fourth edition, text revision of the *Diagnostic and Statistical Manual of Mental Disorders* (*DSM-IV-TR*; American Psychiatric Association [APA], 2000) describes bereavement separately from major depression, although the symptoms are similar. If major depressive symptoms occur as a reaction to the death of a loved one and resolve within 2 months, they do not fall into the category of major depression. Many symptoms of major depression, however, are elaborated symptoms and responses associated with grief.

Similar to the association between grief and depression, there is a strong relationship between grief and anxiety. Bryne and Raphael (1997) found a closer relationship between grief and anxiety than between grief and depression, and they found a strong overlap of depression and anxiety in their research populations. Anxiety and its associated symptoms are particularly troublesome to individuals and to family dynamics and functioning. In the *DSM-IV-TR* (APA, 2000), 13 subtypes of anxiety disorders were identified. Acute stress disorder is the most common cluster of symptoms in response to a death of a loved one.

Studies of traumatic grief and its relationship to posttraumatic stress disorder (PTSD) have been conducted by Prigerson and Jacobs (2001). They identified two symptom categories associated with traumatic grief: symptoms of separation distress and symptoms of traumatic distress. These clusters of symptoms were previously referred to as complicated mourning or pathological mourning. The authors note that traumatic grief (TG) is similar to PTSD, except that in PTSD there is an avoidance of something, whereas in TG there is an active searching for reminders of the deceased (p. 619).

A third mental health problem often related to people grieving is substance abuse. Often described as an attempt to numb the pain of sorrow, mourners will seek alcohol or other prescription and nonprescription drugs. The relationship between bereavement and alcohol and substance abuse is discussed by several scholars (Atchley & Barusch, 2004; Hudak, Krestan, & Repko, 1999; Rando, 1993), who have described a pattern in which individuals who face many losses choose escape behaviors, including alcohol and drug abuse. They call it an inability in self-regulation. The strong relationships between alcohol and substance abuse and domestic violence, automobile accidents, homicide, missed work days, and homelessness suggest the seriousness of these mental health problems and family functioning.

Bereavement and Physiology

In recent decades, more light has been shed on the genetic and biochemical factors that are associated with grief reactions. The brains of those who are grieving, like the brains of individuals who have traumatic physical injuries, show significant increases in a variety of stress hormones. The brain secretes more adrenocorticotropic hormones, which leads to the adrenal glands secreting more glucocorticoids. These hormones can lead to increased blood pressure, decreased tissue healing, and suppression of immune system function through lower T cell and natural killer cell activity. With the body

physically compromised, grieving people have an increased rate of infectious illnesses, heart disease, and malignancy (Chrousos & Elenkov, 2001).

Neurotransmitters especially play important roles in the physiology of grief and depression. Neurotransmitters interact with a variety of receptors on neuron systems that regulate such global states as sleep, concentration, appetite, and mood. There are prominent changes in the monoamine neurotransmitter systems, which include the dopamine, norepinephrine, and serotonin pathways. Depression is strongly linked with low serotonin levels and raised norepinephrine levels. Many medications, including the selective serotonin receptor inhibitor family of drugs and tricyclic antidepressants, used to treat depression associated with chronic stress will alter the effective levels of neurotransmitters to more normal levels. Effective antidepressant therapy results in renormalization of not only the neurotransmitter balance in the brain but also the stress hormone levels secreted by other organs and tissue (Chrousos & Elenkov, 2001).

Understanding the brain's neurophysiology has given rise to new and effective medications for depression and anxiety. Future studies on brain functioning and sleep, appetite, and mood in the bereaved will increase our understanding of the mechanisms and will probably give rise to new medications to address some of the debilitating symptoms of grief.

Grief and Resilience

Rando (1993) identified seven high-risk factors in adapting to a significant loss. The first grouping addressed specific death factors: "(a) sudden, unexpected death (especially when traumatic, violent, mutilating, or random); (b) death from an overly lengthy illness; (c) loss of a child; and (d) the mourner's perception of the death as preventable" (p. 5). The second grouping addressed aspects of the mourner: "(a) a premorbid relationship with the deceased that was markedly angry or ambivalent, or markedly dependent; (b) prior or concurrent mourner liabilities, specifically, unaccommodated losses and/or stresses and mental health problems; and the (c) mourner's perceived lack of social support" (p. 5).

Kubler-Ross (1969) worked with dying patients and identified a pattern of adjusting to a life-threatening diagnosis, which she called stages of grief: (a) shock and denial, (b) anger, (c) bargaining for time, (d) depression, and (e) acceptance. There is a strong attraction to the idea of her stages. Grieving people, and the clinicians who work with them, want to feel that the griever is moving toward some resolution of the consuming pain and sorrow. Subsequent studies, however, have demonstrated that these were not really stages. The concepts were significant, often common, grief experiences for dying patients and those who loved them, but they were not progressive stages.

Rando (1993) clearly recognized that although there are no clearly marked stages, there are probably three phases. Rando calls the three phases avoidance, confrontation, and accommodation. In the avoidance phase, the mourner must recognize the loss and acknowledge the death.

The confrontation phase requires the mourner to react to the separation by experiencing the pain and identify and mourn the secondary losses, such as lost hopes, roles, and expectations that were associated with the person who died. In addition, the mourner must be able to recollect and reexperience the deceased and their relationship, to "review and remember realistically the person and their relationship," and "revive and reexperience the feelings" of "thousands of attachment bonds" (Rando, 1993, pp. 45-50).

In the accommodation phase, the mourner readjusts and adapts to the new world without forgetting the old. The mourner reframes his or her assumptive world. Both Rando (1993) and Janoff-Bulman (1992) described the importance of personal world views and how individuals see themselves in that world in response to trauma or loss. Rando suggested that the mourner must develop a new relationship with the deceased, adopt new ways of being in the world, and form a new identity. The last task requires the mourner to reinvest time, energy, and being into new activities and efforts.

It seemed important to describe the elements of healthy adaptation to the death of a loved one, after describing the more dysfunctional characteristics that mourners may exhibit, and how healthy adaptation may go awry. Although many of the older explanatory theories of grief were posed to foster understanding of grief as a dysfunctional process, several of the newer theories postulate that death of a loved one is a stressful, often traumatic, life event, but that there can be healthy adaptation (Horowitz, 2001; Rando, 1993). Shaefer and Moos (2001) have gone even further and developed a model that includes not only adjustment and nonadjustment but also actual growth from the adversity of the mourning experience.

Age and Grief Responses

Rando (1993) listed many common responses to loss. She categorized them as psychological (affects, cognitions, perceptions, and defenses or attempts at coping or both), behavioral, social, and physical. For the purposes of this discussion, 13 common grief responses routinely identified in the literature are addressed. Although not every bereaved person experiences each one, nearly everyone experiences some. As evidenced in the qualitative and longitudinal research, people who grieve experience a wide variety of psychological and physiological responses as well as an erratic and rocky fluctuation in their physical and emotional lives.

Other authors (Cole, 1998; Cole, Harvey, & Miles, 2003) have identified the common grief responses shown in Table 15.2. This list is important in understanding individual adjustment to grief. It is understanding these individual behaviors and recognizing how the responses influence family dynamics and relationships that is central to this discussion, however.

Grief and the Elderly

The bereaved elderly (older than age 65 years) constitute a special group of adults. Researchers have studied bereaved elderly spouses' adjustment for several decades (Barusch, Rogers, & Abu-Bader, 1999; Barusch & Spaid, 1989; Caserta & Lund, 1992; Caserta, Lund, & Dimond, 1989; Moss, Moss, & Hansson, 2001). They have noted the following age-specific issues. As the normal view of death at an older age looms in the face of the elderly, their grief is often ignored and brushed aside as expected and part of the aging process. Each year, as a person ages, more siblings, spouses, friends, and associates die. The compounding of losses (one risk factor for complicated mourning) increases with age.

Marriages that spanned from high school or early adulthood to the aging years encounter the death of one spouse. The intertwined lives of a couple make grieving painful, and shortened life expectancy impacts their view of the future. Physical health is often compromised in the elderly, which adds another factor to the burden of coping with grief and bereavement. Caserta and Lund (1992), however, discussed the resiliency of the elderly due to improved coping skills developed through life experience.

Children and Grief

Children's responses to loss will be influenced by their age, developmental level, cognitive ability, relationship to the deceased, and support system. The most significant deaths for children are parent losses, followed by the death of a sibling. The impact of death of grandparents and extended family members is often very important to children as well as the death of close friends.

The research on children's grief has generally focused on loss of a parent. Fathers are the most frequent losses for children in childhood. Because most fathers raising children are in the 24- to 44-year-old age group, accidents, homicide, suicide, and cancer are the most common causes of death. Spitz (1945, 1946) and Bowlby (1969, 1973, 1980) identified the loss of security as having the most dramatic impact on children when they lose a parent. Unable to care for themselves, even young children are acutely aware of their vulnerability. Cole et al. (2003) and Shapiro (1994) described the cognitive, affective, and physical responses of infants, children, and adolescents by age groups.

Ainsworth, Blehar, Waters, and Wall (1978) studied the time during infant development when children are able to distinguish their mothers (or primary caretakers) from others with stranger anxiety. Very young children can sense changes in routines and caretakers. Kaplan (1978) and Sullivan (1953) stated that it is through frequent breast- or bottle-feeding experiences with the mother (or primary caretaker) that infants organize information about the world around them. The primary feeder or nurturer becomes the most significant person to the child. Through these feeding experiences, children begin to differentiate one person from another.

Understanding changes in routines cannot be mediated by explanation or logic because infants' and toddlers' cognitive and verbal worlds are just beginning to develop.

Table 15.2   Common Grief Responses of Adults

Grief Response	Description of Terms
Shock, numbness, and denial	First responses to the death Asking if information is true Seeking additional confirmation of death Feeling of watching oneself Feeling like one is in a dream
Sadness	Crying frequently and for long periods Showing sad face (furrowed brow, down-turned mouth, puffy eyes from crying, bloodshot eyes)
Guilt	Blaming oneself for the death Anger toward self Perceived view that something could have been done to prevent the death Guilt by association with deceased Survivor guilt
Depression	More than just sadness Irritability, agitation Loss of interest or pleasure in most activities Alterations in sleep or eating (can be an increase or decrease) Somatic symptoms (headaches, stomach aches, diffuse pain, fatigue) Hopelessness
Anxiety	Feelings or thoughts of excessive worry Fear about the future Exaggerated sense of vulnerability to death or injury Somatic sensations of difficulty breathing or choking
Anger	Intense negative emotion associated with the loss Directed at family, friends, health care providers, police, etc. Directed at God Increased aggressiveness Decreased impulse control
Relief	Usually experienced when death occurs after a long illness or when the deceased has suffered a great deal of pain Experienced when caregiving has been long term and burdensome, physically and mentally Often combined with guilt
Loneliness	Feel lost, alone, and isolated Change in a large portion of daily activities
Confusion and disorientation	Disorganized thoughts Difficulty concentrating Difficulty sequencing events Difficulty remembering appointments, recently learned information, or skills
After death experiences	Occurs in approximately 50% of bereaved Dreams Auditory or sensory perception Occasional visual perceptions Fear of discussion due to perceived sacred or aberrant experience
Spirituality	May increase or decrease after the death of a loved one Shattered assumptions about self or the world
Other grieving behaviors	Frequent visits to cemetery Making a place into a shrine for the deceased Remove all material related to the deceased Set out photographs, other items, in memory of deceased

Affective development is primitive and unorganized. Infants' and toddlers' distress in response to the loss of their caretakers is evidenced by crankiness, crying, altered sleep patterns, changes in eating habits, and other patterns of behavior.

Preschool children, ages 3 to 5 years, generally believe that death is reversible. Although they can understand that death can be permanent for other living creatures, they believe that the parent or deceased could return if he or she wanted to do so. Their limited language to describe emotions or explore the world verbally may create confusion and misunderstanding. Because they are often egocentric in their thinking, they may believe that their thoughts or behavior may have caused the death of their family members. Preschool children often misunderstand euphemisms, such as "has gone to sleep" or "gone to their home in the sky/heaven." These misperceptions can cause serious consequences, for example, if they refuse to fall asleep for fear of dying or want to be with the deceased. Not only does the loss of their loved one affect their functioning but also it changes many other aspects and routines of their daily lives. Thus, as devastating as the loss may be, the changes in other relationships, surroundings, and expected routines can equally devastate young children's worlds.

Physical activity often becomes a medium for managing the emotional distress of grief for young children. Increased irritability, aggressiveness, and demanding behaviors are often seen in this age griever, but the opposite may also be observed. Young children may withdraw from their usual activities, choose to play alone, or cry frequently or in response to very simple frustrations. Other physical responses to death may be difficulty sleeping, lack of appetite, regression of toileting behavior, thumb sucking, and clinging behavior.

Children at the elementary school age can be characterized by their burgeoning intellectual development. They have learned that death is permanent, and that dead people do not eat, sleep, walk, or talk. Death, however, may still be perceived as a person or creature that comes and takes away the life of a person. They can formulate questions and hypothesize cause-and-effect relationships. Their cognitive abilities can help them understand death's permanence and the implications of a death on their lives and the lives of their family.

Similar to younger children, school-age children may become more physically aggressive, irritable, impulsive, and argumentative. In addition, they may choose to withdraw and be alone, cry frequently, or select themes of death and dying in their play.

Family members comprise the small number of significant relationships of school-age children. Thus, when school-age children experience the death of a parent or sibling, their world of significant relationships is greatly diminished. By comparison, adults generally have more relationships that can offer support, and they have increased cognitive acumen to negotiate the world after the loss. Adults have previous life experiences that may assist them in keeping their world balanced. The vulnerability of school-age children is often heightened by adult misconceptions that children understand too little or too much.

Adolescents exhibit increased maturity in thinking and self-perception. They are able to more accurately perceive the circumstances around death, and they are more capable of initiating and participating in their own daily care. They are unable to protect themselves from their own emotional distress, however, and use a great deal of psychic energy to ward off the feelings or manage the psychological distress. Adolescents are acutely aware of how the death of a family member changes the family organization and patterns. It also makes them different from their peers, which is often an issue of importance to teenagers (Balk & Corr, 2001).

Although they are more like adults in their distress behavior, bereaved adolescents have an increased incidence of sexual activity, substance abuse, confrontations with law enforcement, and other acting out behaviors after the death of a family member. Adolescents may exhibit pronounced withdrawal behaviors, such as staying in their rooms for long hours at a time.

Rando (1993), Kaplan (1995), and Oltjenbruns (2001) discussed a "re-grief" phenomenon. Usually, the authors refer to this process in which children periodically review their loss in relation to their current experience. Others talk about children's and adults' conscious review of a loss, allowing integration of the loss in a new way. With greater cognitive ability of increased age and maturity, children and adults are able to rework the loss experience and make new sense of who they are or new meaning of what it is to lose a loved one.

Cause of Death and Grieving

As mentioned previously, if the mourner perceives that the death was preventable, it increases the risk of more complicated mourning (Rando, 1993). Deaths by suicide, homicide, and accidents or other sudden and unexpected deaths have unique contributions to the grieving process. Often, it is not only the perception of preventability but also the social stigma associated with some deaths that increase the distress of grieving.

Suicide

Suicide is most common in young adults ages 15 to 24 years and in the elderly. The reasons for suicide are somewhat different for each age group, depending on the stage in the life cycle. Although the most common precursor for suicide is severe depression, there is strong social stigma associated with death due to suicide. Chronic physical pain and life-threatening illness are also precursors for suicide. Family members often endure serious personal social criticism or ostracism in response to a family member's suicide.

In 2001, there were 29,423 suicide deaths in the United States (NCHS, 2003). Most scholars believe that suicide is underreported due to social stigma, and that many accidents may be acts of self-injury. Shniedman (1980) and colleagues have spent decades studying suicide and its causes. DeSpelder and Strickland (2005) discussed suicide in its social context. Firestone (1997) wrote a scholarly approach to understanding suicide by identifying the disruptive and demeaning inner voice (inner thoughts) described by suicidal people. Although they may understand the reasons for suicide, family members are often left pondering unanswered questions that inevitably arise. Guilt is often pronounced in survivors of sudden and unexpected deaths. The internal conflict of anger and love toward the deceased further complicates adjustment for survivors.

Homicide

Homicide, like suicide, occurs more frequently in certain age groups. Males age 15 to 24 years are the most frequent victims of homicide by a margin of two to one. Homicide involves law enforcement and the criminal justice system. Interactions with people from law enforcement and the criminal justice system can be extremely difficult for family survivors of homicide. Already impacted by the death of their loved ones, interactions with a slow-moving justice system may prolong the grieving process. In addition, many homicides are caused by a family or former family member, thus compounding the traumatic loss and individual and family adjustments.

Media professionals and nonprofessionals often intrude on the bereaved, who are at the mercy of insensitive questions and personal confrontations. Occasionally, media personnel can be helpful to the bereaved by keeping the story of the homicide in the news until the perpetrator is apprehended. Most survivors of homicide, however, are novices to the media world and are vulnerable to its frequent exploitation of tragedy.

GRIEVING FROM A FAMILY PERSPECTIVE

Understanding grief from an individual perspective lays the foundation for understanding how grief affects families. Generalizations about the "typical" family can be extrapolated to particular family situations. Obviously, the death of a family member alters the family structure and who is in the family. The death may alter family dynamics, family decisions, family roles, and family use of space. There are changes in economic conditions and access to psychological and physical resources. Whether parental responsibilities are designated by gender or by task, these usually include purchasing or gathering and preparing food on a daily basis; housekeeping; nurturing and disciplining young children; employment for economic support and gain; task delegation; decision making; religious education; and planning for family activities, leisure, and goals.

Children also have roles and responsibilities in a family, which may include dependency on their parents, accepting discipline, following directions and routines, learning their parents' beliefs about family and social responsibility, and mastering developmental tasks.

There are dramatic differences if a single mother dies versus one parent in a two-parent family. Also, in many automobile accidents, there may be multiple deaths, which place unique demands on grievers.

Young Parents and the Loss of a Child

Which family member died becomes differentially significant. The age of the deceased is important, as is the age of the bereaved parent, sibling, or grandparent. Rando (1986) wrote one of the seminal works on parental bereavement of a child. Loss of a child is often interpreted as the loss of the future. Children represent hopes and dreams for what might be. Historically, children participated in contributing to families' economic welfare. In modern America, children play an important psychological and social role in families.

The loss of a young child or teenager can be a life-shattering experience for parents. Several authors speak to the overwhelming sense of persistent guilt that engulfs many young parents who lose a child (Rando, 1986; Rubin & Malkinson, 2001; Shapiro, 1994). Their role as protector was unfulfilled, and they report intense feelings of failure. If the child who died was an only child, there is an additional sense of failure because the role of parent is taken away. DeSpelder and Strickland (2005) described mothers of perinatal losses who reported feeling a sense of failure in not being able to produce a viable child.

Obviously, parenting after the death of a child can be difficult. Common grieving responses can compromise energy and thinking processes, including judgment. Affective responses overwhelm psychological and physical systems. Bereaved parents experiencing confusion and disorientation have difficulty attending to the immediate demands and concerns of their children. Other grieving responses can interfere with attending and performing the parenting role. Some parents express concern that they are preoccupied with the deceased child to the detriment of their other children. The opposite of less functional parenting can be increased attention and investment in parenting. Rubin and Malkinson (2001) reported a greater investment in parent relationships with the remaining children.

Parents and the Death of an Adult Child

Rubin and Malkinson (2001) noted that middle-age and older parents who lose a child report fewer problems in functioning than do younger parents. Older parents, however, report that the mourning process continued for many years. The parenting role generally changes as children reach adulthood and move into their own parenting and work roles. Adult children who commit suicide often have long-standing mental illnesses, and their bereaved parents often believe the health care system has failed. Adolescent and young adults who are members of gangs participate in violent and risky activities. Death due to violence may not be unexpected, but parents experience the same sorrow and shattered confidence in the world around them. Where countries are engaged in military conflict, young adults are generally killed in greater numbers than older members of the military. Death of young adults can devastate a country as well as the families.

Parenting Children When a Spouse Dies

According to Holmes and Masuda (1974), the death of a child or a spouse is the most stressful life event. Parents of young children often face multiple losses along with the loss of their spouses. Young fathers are more likely than mothers to die in their youth, although thousands of young mothers die each year as well. The death of either parent dramatically affects subsequent family and individual development.

Along with the obvious immediate and long-term changes in family dynamics are the changes in numerous other aspects of family life. For example, if it is the father-breadwinner who dies, there may be economic challenges to the spouse. The spouse may have to return to work, or the family may have to change residences. With more limited resources, family activities, social status, and social relationships outside the family may change for parents and children.

If a mother dies and she is the housekeeper and child caretaker, these important activities need to be taken on by the spouse or someone else. Depending on the ages of the children, this may require changes in employment, economic expenses, or moving closer to or in with relatives who can assist with these tasks. Again, the enormity of these changes can increase the burden associated with family grieving.

Researchers of maternal depression and parenting (Jameson, Gelfand, Kulcsar, & Teti, 1997) have noted that low energy, irritability and anger, and withdrawal behaviors associated with grief interfere with parenting. Modulating the erratic emotions of grief is exhausting work. Grieving parents may not attend to their children's needs in the same way they did prior to their loss. Children may escalate their negative behaviors to get attention. Due to increased irritability and anger, parents may overrespond to disciplining their children. If they recognize this excessive response, they may experience increased guilt.

Children experience their parents' grief in many ways. Although they may recognize the cause of their parents' negative behavior or lack of interaction, they want their parents back, with familiar rules and patterns. Even very young children recognize their parents' sorrow and try to engage their parents in positive interactions. A pattern of concern is when children work hard to protect their parents. They may avoid making loud noises or asking for their own needs, never bringing up the subject of the loss, or even taking on adult responsibilities, such as housework or caring for siblings.

Grieving adolescents often take out their anger on their peers, which interferes with keeping good peer relationships. Acting-out behaviors, such as alcohol abuse, drug abuse, sexual activity, gang behavior, and oppositional behavior, can increase negative parent-child interactions and lead to long-term problems.

Parent-to-Parent Behavior After a Loss

There is a wide variety of grieving behaviors. In a small group such as a family, there may be little tolerance for these differences. Many of the common grieving behaviors interfere with maintaining close personal relationships. Anger, withdrawal, and bouts of crying focus attention inward rather than engaging others (DeSpelder & Strickland, 2005).

Many people describe grieving as a roller coaster ride. This fluctuation in emotion makes close personal relationships between spouses difficult. The usual intimate and supportive behaviors that are expressed between couples may decrease in frequency. One spouse may want and expect support and comfort from the other, but a grieving spouse may be unavailable for comfort. Due to differences in grieving patterns and timing of grief responses, couples may experience increased couple tension or conflict.

Comfort behaviors that were exchanged prior to the loss, such as talking together, leisure activities, sexual intimacy, and sharing meals, may decrease. Due to depression, fatigue, and poor sleeping, sexual activity may decrease, and the lack of this intimate behavior can become a source of couple irritation. Because grief is self-absorbing, the bereaved may pay less attention to others and the world around them. In contrast, other grieving behaviors may include hypervigilance. Either extreme can be problematic in interpersonal relationships.

DeSpelder and Strickland (2005) recognized that "each couple has to come to terms with spouse's grieving behavior" (p. 385).

Normalizing, a term used by Knafl, Deatrick, and Kirby (2001), or *reframing*, a term used by many family therapists (Haley, 1971; Minuchin, 1974; Satir, 1967; Satir & Bitter, 1982), is the process of understanding a behavior in a new context or perspective. McCubbin and McCubbin (1996) identified normalizing as a variable in their resilience model of family stress, adjustment, and adaptation. Reframing a spouse's behavior in the context of recent loss allows a spouse to accept behavior he or she would otherwise find unacceptable.

Sibling-to-Sibling Relationships After a Death

Although it is socially expected that adults refrain from destructive behaviors, children may not have learned how to control themselves. As noted previously, children may respond to their own grief with more aggressive behavior. Sibling rivalry and normal conflicts of growing up often make children vulnerable to guilt. If the death in the family is a sibling or an adult, children may exacerbate their normal behaviors. The sex, role, and age of the deceased interact with the sex, role, and age of the child and influence identity formation.

Remarriages after the death of a parent are common. If there are children from previous marriages, there are usually profound adjustments for the parents and the children. Joining two families is usually the choice of the parents. The new stepbrothers and stepsisters have to struggle to establish a new living environment. These relationships are often fraught with conflict, tension, and loyalty issues.

Extended Family Responses

Grandparents, aunts, uncles, cousins, and others can be as touched by a loss as the immediate family members. Some extended families are intimately involved in the day-to-day activities of their relatives, and their grief may be as profound. Friends and other family members may overlook their sorrow, however. Moss et al. (2001) noted that grieving grandparents have the same responses as other adults, but that grandparents "yield to the priority of their adult child's grief" (p. 249). In addition, grandparents revive their own protective parenting roles related to their children.

FAMILIES GRIEVING TOGETHER

Vaughan-Cole (1998) noted the difficulties of gathering data that reflect family characteristics versus individual characteristics of family members. Family research is often conducted from one family member's view (usually the mother's). A few resolute scholars have attempted to examine grief from a family perspective, but the struggle to measure and interpret grieving families from a family perspective is still in its infancy.

Family systems theory dominated the intellectual curiosity of sociology and psychology during the second half of the 20th century. Understanding families became the goal for unanswered questions of mental health and social functioning. Three of these are discussed in more detail as they relate to grieving families: family focused grief therapy, the family resiliency model, and the family life cycle.

Family Systems Theory

First, a brief introduction of some of the salient concepts in family systems theory is presented. In this chapter, the more formal differentiations of model, framework, and theory are cast as theories. In its broadest and most general usage, *theory* refers to a coherent explanation for understanding phenomena.

Early family systems theorists drew liberally on von Bertalanffy's (1968) general systems theory. Von Bertalanffy's concept of *wholeness* or *holism* assumes that the family unit cannot be subdivided and still remain the same, it is a goal-directed unit, and the whole is more than the sum of its parts. The family and its parts exist in time and space (Friedman, Bowden, & Jones, 2003; Vaughan-Cole, 1998). The family and its parts as well as the family and society are in dynamic interaction. Family structure and organization are essential to family systems. Family structure refers to roles, power, and status. Family organization refers to the delegation of responsibilities, the family boundaries, and rules that are essential to homeostasis. These rules may be invisible or real lines and processes that define family members, relationships, and behavior (Friedman et al., 2003; Vaughan-Cole, 1998).

Systems theory recognizes that systems do not function in isolation. The individual human system is embedded in a family system, which is embedded in a larger social system composed of many family systems. This concept of embedded systems is significant because many discussions of family theory explicate the relationship of individual to family and family to society. Family adaptation is the process by which families and their members modify their behavior to each other and to their outer world as the situation demands. Through its feedback loop, the family adapts by accepting or rejecting incoming elements in an attempt to balance or achieve homeostasis or equilibrium. The obvious subsystems of a nuclear family are parent, parent-child, and sibling.

Kissane and Bloch (2002) studied grieving families. Their research addressed families with a member dying from cancer, bereaved families after the death of a family member due to cancer, and a control group of families. Their research included the Family Relationships Index and also the Family Adaptability and Cohesion Evaluation Scales

(FACES III) (Olsen, Russell, & Sprenkle, 1986). These tools are grounded in family systems theory.

In their first study (which they call their palliative care sample), Kissane and Bloch (1994) studied 102 families, which included 79 patients, 84 spouses, and 179 offspring for a sample size of 362 subjects. Kissane, Bloch, Dowe, McKenzie, and Posterino (1996a, 1996b) conducted a longitudinal study of 115 families for 13 months after one of the spouses died. In this sample, there were 100 spouses and 101 offspring who completed the study. Through a rigorous analytic review, they developed a typology of families and their adjustments to the death of a family member.

The researchers identified three essential dimensions of family functioning that differentiated five family types. Family cohesion was identified by the cohesion subscales of the FACES III and FES. They defined family cohesion as a family's ability to function together as a team. It is the central characteristic of well-functioning families. High cohesiveness acts as a buffer in the other dimensions. The second dimension was family conflict, a subscale of the FES. High conflict is indicative of family dysfunction, whereas the ability to resolve conflict demonstrates family adaptability. The third dimension is family expressiveness, another subscale from the FES. Family expressiveness includes the communication of both thoughts and feelings. Again, families who score low on this subscale tend to be dysfunctional. Within a framework of grieving families, reciprocal expressions of deep feelings would be both expected and respected (Kissane & Bloch, 2002).

The five family types are supportive, conflict resolving, hostile, sullen, and intermediate. High cohesiveness, good expressiveness, and the absence of conflict define the supportive family. This group of highly functioning families is characterized by family intimacy, the ability to share distress, and mutual comfort. Conflict is absent in these families. In conflict resolving families, family variables include moderate conflict with high cohesiveness and above average expressiveness. Closeness and open communication with an ability to resolve differences characterize these families (Kissane & Bloch, 2002). Hostile families are considered the most dysfunctional. They are high on conflict and low on cohesion and expressiveness. These families are defined by high conflict and what they do not do together. Described as chaotic and highly conflicted, they are not organized and rarely do things together. The sullen family is a second type of dysfunctional family. They have reduced cohesiveness, mild to moderate conflict, and poor expressiveness. Although they demonstrate high levels of control in their family life, they are rigid and require family conformity while blocking family feelings. The last family type, the intermediate family, is characterized by moderate cohesiveness, moderate conflict, and moderate expressiveness. The families are inflexible and exert great control over family life (Kissane & Boch, 2002).

As psychiatrists, Kissane and Bloch's research purpose was to identify families at high risk for poor outcomes to the death of a spouse. A typology of grieving families would support a strategy for developing therapeutic interventions for the most dysfunctional adjustments to bereavement. For each family type, they described a pattern of adaptation to bereavement. The supportive families adjusted well to the death of a family member. Supportive families were able to use mature coping strategies. Conflict resolving families experienced low levels of psychological morbidity and grief post-bereavement. Hostile families post-bereavement were the most distressed and yet the most difficult to engage in treatment. Sullen families demonstrated the most intense levels of grief and although very needy, they were amenable to help. The last family group, intermediate families, exhibited a great deal of depression and anxiety, needed a great deal of help, but were easily engaged in therapy (Kissane & Bloch, 2002).

Building on their research, Kissane and Bloch developed family-focused grief therapy. Their aim was to improve family functioning by enhancing cohesiveness, communication, and conflict resolution and to promote the expression of grief, and their approach is an important contribution to the literature.

Resiliency Model of Family Stress, Adjustment, and Adaptation

In 1949, Hill proposed the ABCX model of family stress theory. The basis of this theory focused on the separation and reunion of armed service personnel after World War II. In this model, he identified a set of variables, with A being the event and related hardships, B the family's crisis in meeting resources, and C the definition of meaning that the family makes of the event. These variables interact to produce X, the crisis. He then identified three adjustment variables the family faces: a time of disorganization, the angle of recovery, and reorganization and new level of family functioning (Friedman et al., 2003).

McCubbin and Patterson (1983) revised the model by including a pileup of stressors along with the initial stressor in factor A. They added the concept of coping to the model, which explained the differential postcrisis adjustment. Over time, the model developed into the resiliency model of family stress, adjustment, and adaptation (McCubbin & McCubbin, 1996). According to Friedman et al. (2003), the current resiliency model emphasizes the strengths and resiliencies of families, and it now includes established patterns of functioning and family types and family's schema or worldview. In

addition, problem solving has been added to the coping variable.

Originally, the family resiliency model was adapted for studying families coping with illnesses (usually the illness of a child). The concepts are adaptable for use in studying and understanding families who experience the death of a family member, however. Instead of an illness stressor, the death of a family member becomes the family stressor.

The initial stressor (A) influences a family, which has vulnerabilities (V) due to life changes and pileup of stresses. The family, with its family vulnerabilities, enters the adjustment phase, in which the family addresses four variables: family types and established patterns of functioning (T), appraisal of the stressor and its severity (C), problem solving and coping (PSC), and family resistance resources (B). The outcome of the adjustment phase is either adjustment or maladjustment of the crisis situation (X).

For those who experience maladjustment due to the crisis situation, the family progressed to family crisis situation (X), with pileup stressors, strains, and transitions. The family moves to the adaptation phase, within which there are six interacting variables: family types and newly instituted patterns of functioning (R); family appraisal: schema and meaning (CCC); situational appraisal of family capability (CC); problem solving and coping (PSC); family resources (BB); and social support (BBB). From these interacting elements, the family moves again to adaptation or maladaptation, a crisis situation (XX).

For each of the variables, the McCubbins have clear definitions. In addition, they developed instruments for measuring the variables. The recognition of short-term adjustment and long-term adaptation to the death of a family member is consistent with most descriptions of grief responses. Much of the literature on grief responses describes a short initial adjustment phase followed by a longer period of integrating and adapting to the loss in everyday life. Malone (1998) discussed the family resiliency model as useful in clinical practice. Using the concepts and variables in this model, Malone discussed families' responses to acute illness in children; adults in ambulatory care, acute care, and home care settings; and elderly in ambulatory care, acute care, and rural home settings. Thus, this model is useful in clinical work and as an explanatory research model.

The family resiliency model is well organized and conceptualized. Research using this model in the area of grief is lacking. Because the model manages family stressful events, this model may be adapted for the family stress of a family member's death. The research would be valuable in addressing family resiliency as well as family dysfunction.

Family Development Theory

Family development theory is also called family life cycle theory. Most family development theories describe family life over time as families progress through identifiable stages. Both structure and characteristic relationship interactions are common across families and are specific to a stage. Each stage covers a set time, with transitional times assisting families to move from one stage to another (Friedman et al., 2003).

Duvall (1977) identified eight stages in families' life cycles based on three elements: major changes in family size, the oldest child's developmental stage, and the breadwinner's work status. Carter and McGoldrick (1980, 1999) revised Duval's stages and others into what they call the expanded family life cycle. They call it a "multicontextual framework." In this framework, the individual is nested in an "immediate household," which is nested in an extended family, which is nested in a community with social connections, which is nested in a larger society. Their focus is not so much on explaining the family as a social system but on assisting clinicians in assessing

and diagnosing families along a continuum of common or normative characteristics that influence adjustment. This assessment then allows family therapists to develop plans for assisting families in their adjustment. They describe the family as a system moving through time (Carter & McGoldrick, 1999, p. 1).

Unique to their extended family life cycle framework, Carter and McGoldrick (1999) began their family cycle with "leaving home: Single young adults." In this stage of young adulthood, members accept "emotional and financial responsibility for [them]selves" (p. 2), which requires additional changes in their families of origin. The additional changes require single adults to differentiate themselves from their family, develop intimate peer relationships, and establish themselves in work and financial independence.

The second stage of the family life cycle is "joining of families through marriage: The new couple" (Carter & McGoldrick, 1999). The emotional task is the commitment to a new system with the "formation of the marital system and a realignment of relationships with extended families and friends to include the spouse" (p. 2).

The third stage of the family life cycle is "families with young children," during which couples accept new members into their system (Carter & McGoldrick, 1999). They must "adjust their marital system to make room for children, join together in child rearing, financial and household tasks, and realign relationships to include parenting and grandparenting roles" (p. 2).

The fourth stage is "families with adolescents" (Carter & McGoldrick, 1999). Families are required to "increase flexibility of family boundaries to permit children's independence and grandparent's frailties." Parent-child relationships have to adjust to "permit adolescents to move into and out of the system." The couple "refocuses on marital and career issues." Also, there is a "beginning shift toward caring for older generations" (p. 2).

The fifth stage is "launching children and moving on." According to Carter and McGoldrick (1999), this stage requires families to accept "a multitude of exits from and entries into the family system." The couple has to renegotiate the "marital system as a dyad." The family must develop "adult-adult relationships between grown children and their parents," and "there is a new realignment of relationships to include in-laws and grandchildren." Also, the family must deal with "disabilities and death of parents (grandparents)" (p. 2).

The last stage in their system is "families in later life" (Carter & McGoldrick, 1999). The focus of this family stage is "accepting the shifting generational roles." Second-order family changes in this stage include individual and couple "functioning and interest in the face of physiological decline"; "supporting the central role of middle generation"; "making room in the system for the wisdom and experience of the elderly, supporting the older generation without overfunctioning for them'" and "dealing with loss of spouse, siblings, and other peers and preparation for death" (p. 2).

McGoldrick and associates (Carter & McGoldrick, 1999; McGoldrick & Walsh, 1999) fostered and enhanced the development and use of genograms for identifying significant recurring family patterns and identifying structure, family demographics, functioning, and relationships in the family life cycle stages. Although the genogram can stand alone and inform significant family characteristics, it is through the development of family genograms over time (also called a family map) and the discussion of the elements that reveal important family structure, interactions, roles, and functions. Conducting a family genogram for each family life stage can be very informative. McGoldrick's genogram notes family members; family roles and relationships; and dates of births, marriages, and deaths of extended family members. She notes family members' employment and health data.

McGoldrick and Walsh (1999) discussed death and the family life cycle. With their emphasis on family structure or membership, family stages, roles, and relationships, the death of a family member is placed in the context of these elements. They described the processes needed to negotiate this family life transition. Essential to accomplishing this family transition is family adaptation. Family adaptation to a family member's death requires family members to reorganize family roles, relationships, identity, and purpose. They stated that adaptation does not require families to completely resolve their relationships with the deceased, but these are reviewed and integrated throughout the life cycle. Two family tasks facilitate short- and long-term positive adaptation to a death, however. The first is the "shared acknowledgment of the reality of death and shared experience with the loss" (p. 186). Clear information and open communication are essential for families' acceptance of a death. Funeral rituals and memorial rituals assist mourning families in putting the death in a meaningful perspective, which includes managing the negative aspects of the loss into ongoing family life. The second family task requires that family systems reorganize and reinvest in other relationships and life pursuits (p. 186). Part of the adjustment of families experiencing the death of a family member requires realignment of relationships and redistribution of role functions. This single sentence understates the effort and painful struggle necessary to reestablish family equilibrium.

Although death of a family member is expected in later years, early or untimely death may place the family at higher risk for dysfunction. Other high-risk factors include the concurrence of the death with other major life cycle changes, a family history of traumatic loss and unresolved mourning, the way the death occurred, and the roles and functions that the deceased exercised within the family.

With adaptation the necessary element, McGoldrick and Walsh (1999) discussed family death in the context of each family life stage. Their discussion is greatly abbreviated here. The death of a young adult requires the launching family to integrate the death just as the child was reaching maturity, with all the hopes and dreams for the next generation about to come to fruition. The loss of a parent to a young adult can also have dramatic effects. Initiative and independence are contemplated with greater reassurance when there is family support in the wings. New family responsibilities may be forced on the young adult, which may interfere with educational or career goals. The death of a grandparent may affect young adults differently according to their relationship with the person. The grandparent may have been a central caregiver or a distant relative.

Young couples may face infertility, miscarriage, or perinatal losses. Each loss has its own influence on the adjustment of a couple. Combined with the transitioning of the relationship, any of these losses can challenge a couple's adjustment. Young couples who lose a parent at this time must incorporate this loss as they are adjusting to their new relationship. One member of the couple may be grieving more profoundly, and that grief influences many aspects of the relationship, including sexuality, initiative, energy, and joy.

Families with young children or adolescents who experience a death incur many adjustments. The loss of a child profoundly affects parents, siblings, and extended family members. The death of a child is out of the expected sequence of the family life cycle. Children who lose a parent during this stage recognize their vulnerability and must adapt to the loss in a culture that expects two parents.

Death of young adults often occurs during the family launching stage. Loss of a spouse may occur in this midlife stage for adults. Widows and widowers experience different societal expectations. One spouse may have to learn new skills that the other spouse had accomplished on a routine basis. Death of a breadwinner can jeopardize family financial stability and many other aspects of family functioning.

Families in later life were discussed previously. Death of aging parents is not unexpected, but the loss can be painful for the remaining spouse, siblings, and children. One spouse generally dies before the other, leaving one person to adjust to a new life alone. In general, children are engaged in newly launched adulthood or invested in their own families.

The expanded family life cycle framework organizes information about the death of a family member around the concepts of a family as a system through time, adaptation in response to death, and common differential adaptations depending on the stage of family life cycle when the death occurs.

Shapiro (2001) developed a developmental approach or framework that she considered useful for clinical practice. She elaborated on the family life cycle approach and gave clinical descriptions of the dynamics and stages, which would be useful to clinicians treating people with grief-related disorder.

A great deal of research on grieving families remains to be done. Little research has been performed on what happens within families when there is a death of a family member. Hypotheses-driven research should be implemented to diffuse myths and lead to substantive theory.

CONCLUSION

In 2001, there were approximately 2.5 million deaths in the United States, and these deaths impacted millions more. Acute and chronic illnesses are the most frequent causes of death after 1 year of age. Sudden and unexpected deaths, such as those caused by accidents, suicide, or homicide, rank in the top 13 most frequent causes of death.

Death of a family member is considered one of the most stressful and traumatic events of human experience. Although most individuals and families manage to adjust or adapt to the death of a loved one, a significant proportion do not. This chapter addressed common individual grieving responses, grieving family member-to-member interaction patterns, and total family patterns of adjustment to grief. It addressed the variables of age, role, and cause of death and how these influence adjustment to grief.

The individual's perspective has received the lion's share of attention in research and theory. Most individuals live in family groups, however. Taking what we know about individual grief and casting it in the larger view of family member-to-member interaction improves our understanding of families and grief, somewhat. The impact of death on the whole family needs more focus and understanding, however. Sorrow and suffering may be individual experiences, but families experience grief together. Understanding these family dynamics should help to preserve and enhance family functioning during the extreme stress of bereavement.

REFERENCES

Ainsworth, M. D. S., Blehar, M. C., Waters, E., & Wall, S. (1978). *Patterns of attachment: A psychological study of the strange situation.* Hillsdale, NJ: Lawrence Erlbaum.

American Psychiatric Association. (2000). *Diagnostic and statistical manual of mental disorders* (4th ed.). Washington, DC: Author.

Anderson, C. (1949). Aspects of pathological grief and mourning. *International Journal of Psychoanalysis, 30,* 48-55.

Atchley, R. C., & Barusch, A. S. (2004). *Social forces & aging: An introduction to social gerontology* (10th ed.). Belmont, CA: Wadsworth/Thomson Learning.

Balk, D. E., & Corr, C. A. (2001). Bereavement during adolescence: A review of research. In M. S. Stroebe, R. O. Hansson, W. Stroebe, & H. Schut (Eds.), *Handbook of bereavement research* (pp. 199-218). Washington, DC: American Psychological Association.

Barusch, A. S., Rogers, A., & Abu-Bader, S. (1999). Depressive symptoms among the frail elderly: Physical and psycho-social correlates. *International Journal of Aging and Human Development, 49,* 107-125.

Barusch, A. S., & Spaid, W. M. (1989). Gender differences in caregiving: Why do wives report greater burden? *The Gerontologist, 29,* 667-676.

Bowlby, J. (1969). *Attachment and loss: Vol. 1. Attachment.* New York: Basic Books.

Bowlby, J. (1973). *Attachment and loss: Vol. 2. Separation: Anxiety and anger.* New York: Basic Books.

Bowlby, J. (1980). *Attachment and loss: Vol. 3. Loss: Sadness and depression.* New York: Basic Books.

Bryne, G., & Raphael, B. (1997). The psychological symptoms of conjugal bereavement in elder men over the first 13 months. *International Journal of Geriatric Psychiatry, 12,* 241-251.

Carter, E., & McGoldrick, M. (1980). *The family life cycle.* New York: John Wiley.

Carter, E., & McGoldrick, M. (1999). *The expanded family life cycle: Individual, family and social perspectives* (3rd ed.). Boston: Allyn & Bacon.

Caserta, M. S., & Lund, D. A. (1992). Bereavement stress and coping among older adults: Expectations versus the actual experience. *Omega, 25,* 33-45.

Caserta, M. S., Lund, D. A., & Dimond, M. F. (1989). Older widow's early bereavement adjustments. *Journal of Women and Aging, 1,* 5-27.

Chrousos, G. P., & Elenkov, I. J. (2001). Interactions of the endocrine and immune systems. In L. J. Degroot & J. L. Jameson (Eds.), *Endocrinology* (4th ed., Vol. 1, pp. 571-586). Philadelphia: W. B. Saunders.

Cole, B. V. (1998). *What are common responses to the loss of a loved one? Grief support group manual.* Salt Lake City, UT: Caring Connections.

Cole, B. V., Harvey, J., & Miles, L. (2003). *Dealing with sudden and unexpected death: A handbook for survivors.* Salt Lake City, UT: Caring Connections.

DeSpelder, L. A., & Strickland, A. L. (2005). *The last dance: Encountering death and dying* (7th ed.). Boston: McGraw-Hill.

Duval, E. (1977). *Marriage and family development* (5th ed.). Philadelphia: J. B. Lippincott.

Firestone, R. W. (1997). *The inner voice.* Thousand Oaks, CA: Sage.

Freud, S. (1919). Mourning and melancholia. In J. Strachey (Ed. & Trans.), *The standard edition of the complete psychological works of Sigmund Freud.* London: Hogarth.

Friedman, M. M., Bowden, V. R., & Jones, E. G. (2003). *Family nursing: Research, theory, and practice* (5th ed.). Upper Saddle River, NJ: Prentice Hall.

Haley, J. (1971). *Changing families.* New York: Grune & Stratton.

Holmes, T. H., & Masuda, M. (1974). Life change and illness susceptibility. In B. S. Dohrenwend & B. P. Dohrenwend (Eds.), *Stressful life events: Their nature and effects* (pp. 45-72). New York: John Wiley.

Horowitz, M. J. (2001). *Stress response syndromes: Personality styles and interventions* (4th ed.). Northvale, NJ: Jason Aronson.

Hudak, J., Krestan, J. A., & Repko, C. (1999). Alcohol problems and the family life cycle. In B. Carter & M. McGoldrick (Eds.), *The expanded family life cycle: Individual, family and social perspectives* (3rd ed., pp. 455-469). Boston: Allyn & Bacon.

Jameson, P. B., Gelfand, D. M., Kulcsar, E., & Teti, D. M. (1997). Mother-toddler interaction patterns associated with maternal depression. *Developmental Psychopathology, 9*(3), 637-650.

Janoff-Bulman, R. (1992). *Shattered assumptions: Towards a new psychology of trauma.* New York: Free Press.

Kaplan, L. J. (1978). *Oneness and separateness: From infant to individual.* New York: Simon & Schuster.

Kaplan, L. J. (1995). *No voice is ever wholly lost.* New York: Touchstone.

Kim, K., & Jacobs, S. (1993). Neuroendocrine changes following bereavement. In M. S. Stroebe, W. Stroebe, & R. O. Hansson (Eds.), *Handbook of bereavement: Theory, research and intervention* (pp. 143-159). New York: Cambridge University Press.

Kissane, D. W., & Bloch, S. (1994). Family grief. *British Journal of Psychiatry, 164,* 728-740.

Kissane, D. W., & Bloch, S. (2002). *Family focused grief therapy.* Philadelphia: Open University Press.

Kissane, D. W., Bloch, S., Dowe, D. L., McKenzie, D., & Posterino, M. (1996a). The Melbourne family grief study: I. Perceptions of family functioning in bereavement. *American Journal of Psychiatry, 153,* 650-658.

Kissane, D. W., Bloch, S., Dowe, D. L., McKenzie, D., & Posterino, M. (1996b). The Melbourne family grief study: II. Psychosocial morbidity and grief in bereaved families. *American Journal of Psychiatry, 153,* 659-666.

Klerman, G. L., Weissman, M. M., Rounsaville, B. J., & Chevron, E. S. (1984). *Interpersonal psychotherapy of depression.* New York: Basic Books.

Knafl, K. A., Deatrick, J. A., & Kirby, A. (2001). Normalization promotion. In M. Craft-Rosenberg & J. Denehy (Eds.), *Nursing interventions for infants, children and families* (pp. 373-388). Thousand Oaks, CA: Sage.

Kubler-Ross, E. (1969). *On death and dying.* New York: Macmillan.

Lindemann, E. (1944). Symptomatology and management of acute grief. *American Journal of Psychiatry, 101,* 141-148.

Malone, J. A. (1998). The resiliency model of family stress, adjustment, and adaptation; Implications for family nursing practice. In B. Vaughan-Cole, M. A. Johnson, J. A. Malone, & B. L. Walker (Eds.), *Family nursing practice.* Philadelphia: W. B. Saunders.

McCubbin, H. I., & McCubbin, M. A. (1996). Resiliency in families: A conceptual model of family adjustment and adaptation in responses to stress and crises. In H. I. McCubbin, A. Thompson, & M. McCubbin (Eds.), *Family assessment: Resiliency, coping, and adaptation—Inventories for research and practice* (pp. 1-64). Madison: University of Wisconsin System.

McCubbin, H. I., & Patterson, J. M. (1983). Family transitions: Adaptation to stress. In H. I. McCubbin & C. R. Figley (Eds.), *Stress and the family: Coping with normative transitions* (pp. 5-25). New York: Brunner/Mazel.

McGoldrick, M., & Walsh, F. (1999). Death and the family life cycle. In B. Carter, R. H. Moos, & B. S. Moos (Eds.), *Family environment scale manual.* Stanford, CA: Consulting Psychologists Press.

Minuchin, S. (1974). *Families and family therapy.* Cambridge, MA: Harvard University Press.

Moss, M. S., Moss, S. Z., & Hansson, R. O. (2001). Bereavement and old age. In M. S. Stroebe, R. O. Hansson, W. Stroebe, & H. Schut (Eds.), *Handbook of bereavement research* (pp. 241-260). Washington, DC: American Psychological Association.

National Center for Health Statistics. (2003). *HHS study finds life expectancy in the U.S. rose to 77.2 years in 2001.* Retrieved March 29, 2003, from http://www .cdc.gov/nchs/releases/03news/lifeex.htm

Olson, D. H., Russell, C. S., & Sprenkle, D. H. (Eds.). (1986). *Circumplex model: Systemic assessment and treatment of families.* New York: Springer.

Oltjenbruns, K. A. (2001). Developmental context of childhood: Grief and re-grief phenomena. In M. S. Stroebe, R. O. Hansson, W. Stroebe, & H. Schut (Eds.), *Handbook of bereavement research* (pp. 169-198). Washington, DC: American Psychological Association.

Parkes, C. M. (1965). Bereavement and mental illness: Part I. A clinical study of the grief of bereaved psychiatric patients. Part II. A classification of bereavement reactions. *British Journal Medical Psychology, 38,* 1-26.

Parkes, C. M., & Weiss, R. S. (1983). *Recovery from bereavement.* New York: Basic Books.

Piper, W. E., Ogrodniczuk, J. S., Azim, H. F., & Weideman, R. (2001). Prevalence of loss and complicated grief among psychiatric outpatients. *Psychiatric Services, 52,* 1069-1074.

Prigerson, H. G., & Jacobs, S. C. (2001). Traumatic grief as a distinct disorder: A rationale, consensus criteria, and a preliminary empirical test. In M. S. Stroebe, R. O. Hansson, W. Stroebe, & H. Schut (Eds.), *Handbook of bereavement research* (pp. 613-646). Washington, DC: American Psychological Association.

Rando, T. A. (Ed.). (1986). *Parental loss of a child.* Champaign, IL: Research Press.

Rando, T. A. (1993). *Treatment of complicated mourning.* Champaign, IL: Research Press.

Random House Webster's college dictionary. (1996). New York: Random House.

Robertson, J. (1953a). *A two-year-old goes to hospital* [Film], Tavistock Child Development Research Unit. New York: New York University Film Library.

Robertson, J. (1953b). Some responses of young children to loss of maternal care. *Nursing Times, 49,* 382-386.

Robertson, J. (1956). A mother's observation on the tonsillectomy of her four-year-old daughter with comments by Anna Freud. In *The psychoanalytic study of the child: 11* (pp. 410-433). New York: International Universities Press.

Robertson, J., & Bowlby, J. (1952). Responses of young children to separation from their mothers. *Courier of the International Children's Centre,* 131-140.

Rubin, S. S., & Malkinson, R. (2001). Parental response to child loss across the life cycle: Clinical and research perspectives. In M. S. Stroebe, R. O. Hansson, W. Stroebe, & H. Schut (Eds.), *Handbook of bereavement research.* Washington, DC: American Psychological Association.

Satir, V. (1967). *Conjoint family therapy.* Palo Alto, CA: Science & Behaviour Books.

Satir, V., & Bitter, J. R. (1982). The therapist and family therapy: Satir's human validation process model. In A. M. Horne & J. L. Passmore (Eds.), *Family counseling and therapy.* Itasca, IL: F. E. Peacock.

Schaefer, J. A., & Moos, R. H. (2001). Bereavement experiences and personal growth. In M. S. Stroebe, R. O. Hansson, W. Stroebe, & H. Schut (Eds.), *Handbook of bereavement research* (pp. 145-168). Washington, DC: American Psychological Association.

Shapiro, E. R. (1994). *Grief as a family process: A developmental approach to clinical practice.* New York: Guilford.

Shapiro, E. R. (2001). Grief in interpersonal perspective: Theories and their implications. In M. S. Stroebe, R. O. Hansson, W. Stroebe, & H. Schut (Eds.), *Handbook of bereavement research* (pp. 301-328). Washington, DC: American Psychological Association.

Shaver, P. R., &Tancredy, C. M. (2001). Emotion, attachment, & bereavement. In M. S. Stroebe, R. O. Hansson, W. Stroebe, & H. Schut (Eds.), *Handbook of bereavement research* (pp. 63-88). Washington, DC: American Psychological Association.

Shniedman, E. S. (Ed.). (1980). *Suicide: Current perspectives* (2nd ed.). Mountain View, CA: Mayfield.

Spitz, R. (1945). Hospitalism. *Psychoanalytic Study of the Child, 1,* 53-74.

Spitz, R. (1946). Hospitalism: A follow up report. *Psychoanalytic Study of the Child, 2,* 113-117.

Sullivan, H. S. (1953). *Interpersonal theory of interpersonal relationships.* New York: Norton.

Vaughan-Cole, B. (1998). Family nursing research. In B. Vaughan-Cole, M. A. Johnson, J. A. Malone, & B. L. Walker (Eds.), *Family nursing practice* (pp. 347-364). Philadelphia: W. B. Saunders.

von Bertalanffy, L. (1968). *General system theory.* New York: George Braziller.

Weiss, R. S. (2001). Grief, bonds and relationships. In M. S. Stroebe, R. O. Hansson, W. Stroebe, & H. Schut (Eds.), *Handbook of bereavement research* (pp. 25-45). Washington, DC: American Psychological Association.

Part III

ISSUES FOR POLICY AND RESEARCH

CHAPTER 16

Family-Centered Health Policy Analysis

Sven E. Wilson

A common feature of much public policy analysis is methodological individualism, meaning that individuals are the primary unit of analysis. Health policy analysis, in particular, focuses on individuals because so many health variables—blood pressure, life expectancy, disease status, body mass, smoking history, and so on—are intrinsically characteristics of individuals.

However, even though we cannot (and would not want to) purge the individual from our analyses, the premise of this chapter is that public policies related to health are best analyzed within a family context, since families both shape and are shaped by the health of individuals within the family.

Although the centrality of the family seems obvious, the concept of family is virtually nonexistent in the scientific literature used to support health policy analysis. Family scholars often study health, but other social science literature on health, the biomedical literature, and the health policy literature have largely ignored families. For example, the American Psychological Association recently published an important handbook titled *Integrating Behavioral and Social Sciences With Public Health* (Schneiderman, 2001). This volume contains no articles on families, nor does it contain even a single reference to marriage or family in the cumulative index. A search of texts on health policy reveals a similar neglect of the family (see Litman & Robins, 1997; Longest, 2002; Patel & Rushefsky, 1999).

What might family-centered health policy look like and how will family-centered proposals fare in the policy arena? What follows is a first step in crafting an analytical framework for policy analysis that integrates family into the standard techniques of policy analysis, including the fundamental role of normative criteria and attention to the politics of policy making. The nascent nature of this inquiry will, it is hoped, spur scholars from a wide variety of disciplines to incorporate the health-family nexus into future analyses.

AUTHOR'S NOTE: I acknowledge the financial support of the National Institute on Aging (Grant No. AG10120). I thank Jonathan Wunderlich for research assistance and Elaine Marshall, Gary Bryner, and members of the Political Science faculty seminar (Winter, 2004) at Brigham Young University for insightful comments.

ANALYTICAL FRAMEWORK

Public policy analysis is a multidisciplinary and comprehensive approach to understanding and addressing a variety of social problems. Policy analysis begins with the definition of a social problem, proceeds to the specification of possible policy alternatives to address the problem, and then compares each policy alternative in light of normative criteria that encompass the goals of the alternatives. Health policy analysis relies on empirical research from many different disciplines, such as medicine, epidemiology, sociology, social work, economics, politics, and demography.

Preliminaries

Defining the term "family" is a highly controversial endeavor, particularly given the politics of our time. Cherlin (1999) argued that no single definition is satisfactory for all purposes, and many of the analytical issues presented here are equally applicable to alternative definitions and theoretical constructs. This chapter will use the term in the following two ways.

First, a family is a social unit composed of individuals sharing the same household and linked together by blood relation or marriage. The second, more important usage treats family not as a noun but as an adjective: family relationships are pieces of a larger social network. The concept of a family network emphasizes that individual families (and individuals within families) are connected to each other in far-reaching ways. Family networks are usually distinguished from other social networks (consisting of friends, co-workers, neighbors, schoolmates, etc.) by the intimacy and permanence of the connecting bonds. These connections are reinforced by genetic ties, public and private commitments such as marriage, and by family history.

Rather than focusing on what a family is, or how families differ from one another, the purpose here is to concentrate on how families function. Three roles are prominent. These roles could be used to discuss families in other domains, but the focus here will be on health. First, the protective role of families is to provide for children or adults who cannot live independently, and an important part of this protective role is to preserve and promote the health of dependent family members. The family's protective role can be supported, replaced, or diminished by public policy, such as when family income is supplemented by Title XVI Supplemental Security Income Disability (SSID) payments or when Medicaid pays for nursing home care, allowing an elderly adult to live independently from his or her family.

Second, family networks play a mediating role. Policies to promote health must recognize that families influence all aspects of individuals' health: what they eat, where they live, the type of insurance coverage they have, how much they exercise, how hard they work, how much disposable income they have, which physicians they choose, how well they follow doctors' orders, the medical options they choose during a health crisis, who cares for them when they are disabled, and so forth. The mediating role differs from the protective role because individuals are not dependent on other family members, but the choices they make are shaped fundamentally by family networks. For example, use of Medicare services by independent seniors may interact in important ways with the family networks the seniors participate in.

Third, families create, preserve, and transmit values—the instrumental-normative role of the family. Families are a storehouse of values, norms, and customs that are transmitted across space and time by family networks. How family members treat one another and what they view as obligations to one another changes over time within a family network. Public policy can alter the ability of the families to fulfill their obligations to dependent members; shape the values taught to children; and influence the flow of information and values across family networks.

Public policy analysis that is effective in the long run must look at how the policies of today will shape the structure and function of families in the future. When policy has long-term effects on the concept of the family, it changes, for instance, the way that families fulfill their protective and mediating roles as discussed above.

The recent decade has seen an explosion in scholarly attention to social capital (e.g., Baron, Field, & Schuller, 2001; Fukuyama, 1995; Putnam, 2000), which is the idea that social networks embody a productive capacity that is greater than the sum of the capacities of individual members of the network. Similarly, family networks embody a similar capacity, what I call "family capital," which is a prominent aspect of the instrumental-normative function of families. A well-functioning marriage, for instance, can (possibly) generate happiness, good health, and material well-being for the spouses involved that goes far beyond what they could create for themselves living alone. Knowledge about maintaining and exploiting family capital (economists might call such knowledge family technology) is also a value transmitted across family networks.

Given these preliminaries, a useful question is, "What is a pro-family public policy?" Three answers seem possible. First, pro-family policies directly promote the welfare of dependent family members. Second, pro-family policies create a social environment (legal, institutional, cultural) that raises the incentives for family units to form and persist. Third, pro-family policies strengthen the connections within family networks—both within a family unit and across extended family pathways. In other words, they augment family capital.

Health-Related Characteristics of Families

Kamerman and Kahn (1978) made a distinction between explicit and implicit family policies. Explicit policies have a stated goal of being pro-family while implicit policies affect families in important ways but have another stated intention, such as promoting health. Most implicit family policy in the health area addresses the protective role of the family. Relevant policy variables may include the availability of insurance; access to medical care; and specific federal programs such as Medicaid or CHIP, welfare reform, pharmaceutical testing, or accident prevention programs. A common emphasis for study in this area is the health of children.

Policy variables related to children include such things as divorce and single parenthood, low birth weight, secondhand smoke, nutrition, immunizations, and access to pediatric care. It is logical, therefore, to think of health policy as implicit family policy (and vice versa).

An immediate objective, therefore, is to identify key characteristics of the health-family nexus that will generate a new, family-centered analysis of health policy. To this end, seven prominent and policy-relevant characteristics of families are enumerated and discussed below.

Genetic Ties. Genetic risk factors play an increasingly important role in identifying the causes of disease. Research designs in genetic epidemiology incorporate this fact, but it is often neglected when it comes to policy. For instance, disease screening programs should be explicitly designed to reach related family members when positive test results are obtained. Similarly, treatment programs (such as changes in diet recommended to diabetics) may be more effective if implemented on the family level, since family members may face high risks for the same disease.

Common Environmental Risks. To the extent that environmental factors affect health, family members will face many of the same types of health problems. For instance, recent research has shown the effects of neighborhood on health (Chandola, 2001; Kawachi & Berkman, 2003; Pickett & Pearl, 2001; Robert, 1999; Ross & Mirowsky, 2001). Since family members who live together share a common neighborhood, the problems associated with unhealthy neighborhoods will be highly concentrated among the families who live in those neighborhoods, rather than randomly distributed through the population.

Behavioral Coordination. Family members often pursue a set of common objectives and face common constraints, which leads to coordinated behavior. In the area of family finances, coordination is readily apparent in the way families purchase health insurance and medical care.

In the area of health behavior, many behavioral risk factors, such as diet, exercise, or smoking, are best thought of as behaviors of the family group, not just behaviors of individuals. Although research indicates the dangers of secondhand smoke (Asbridge, 2004; Green, Courage, & Rushton, 2003; Kmietowicz, 2003; Li et al., 2003), a quantitatively more important effect is the strong positive association in smoking behavior among members of families. For instance, people are much more likely to smoke if they have a spouse who smokes (Lau, Lee, Lynn, Sham, & Woo, 2003; Monden, de Graaf, & Kraaykamp, 2003). The same pattern holds for physical exercise and diet (Wilson, 2002). In general, health promotion programs will be much more likely to succeed if they are focused on family behaviors, rather than behaviors of individuals.

Hierarchical Structures. Internal family networks are often hierarchical, which can cause resources to be allocated in ways not intended by the policymaker. For instance, when health coverage is extended to children, the decision makers can divert the funds previously allocated to children's health to other ends that may not benefit children at all, thereby mitigating the total effect of the subsidized coverage (Blumberg, Dubay, & Norton, 2000).

Common Pool of Information. Social networks shape the flow of information, and families are a critical part of any extended social network. Communities with stronger extended families are likely to have a faster and more extensive flow of health information (and misinformation) than families where extended kin networks are weaker, holding other factors constant. The success of health education programs, therefore, will depend on the strength of family networks.

Shared History. The health of an individual depends not only upon current contextual variables, but on a variety of historical behaviors and events. Genetics are not the only rationale for paying attention to family health histories because a shared history may lead to the same types of diseases among family members. Even spouses, who are typically not closely related, share a history that can shape their health. Recent research has even shown that spouses tend to get the same types of chronic illnesses as their partners (Hippisley-Cox, Coupland, Pringle, Crown, & Hammersley, 2002), and the overall level of general health and disability is strongly correlated between spouses (Wilson, 2001). The ill health of an individual may be an important warning sign of undetected health problems in his or her spouse, which implies a need for health care providers to treat couples and families, not just individuals. It may turn out that the treatment of women's health issues (a very popular topic in the past decade) is less important than the treatment of *couple's* health.

Commitment. Hardship for one individual in a family is likely to be shared voluntarily by other members of the family. Even in wealthy countries with very extensive health care systems, family members provide informally much of the most important health care. This can include something as small as reminding a spouse to take a medication or as large as providing round-the-clock nursing care, as happens in numerous families with a disabled person. The delivery of this care depends fundamentally on commitment. Social policies that weaken commitment between family members will, in turn, weaken the delivery of informal care. The legacy of high divorce rates and low fertility rates is certain to be a weaker informal health care sector in the coming years, since committed family members provide the bulk of informal care.

Families and Epidemiology

A critical component of health policy analysis is the epidemiological model that is used to understand and explain health processes in the population. The standard public health approach uses the traditional epidemiologic triangle, which is the idea that risk factors can be categorized in three ways: factors that affect (1) the host, (2) the disease agent, and (3) the environment.

> Host factors represent intrinsic characteristics that influence an individual's susceptibility to disease. These include immune status, general health status, genetic makeup, lifestyle practices, age, sex, and socioeconomic status. Agents consist of biological, chemical, and physical hazards that can induce disease. . . . Environmental factors are extrinsic characteristics that can affect exposure to the agent, effectiveness or virulence of the agent, or susceptibility of the host. Examples include weather conditions, adequacy of living conditions, general levels of sanitation, population density, and access to health care. (Oleckno, 2002, p. 24)

The reader should note the individualistic formulation inherent in this description. A large literature has blossomed in recent years on what is often called "social epidemiology," which has been conducted both by sociologists and demographers interested in health and epidemiologists interested in the social aspects of disease. The concept of family has played an important role in this literature, giving rise to numerous studies exploring the health benefits of marriage for both adults and children. Cassell (1976) and Cobb (1976) were important early proponents of the idea that social support had important influences on health, and marriage and family were seen as the primary components of an individual's social support network. Waite and Gallagher (2000) and Ribar (2004) provide extensive reviews of this literature. In the past decade, however, social inequalities have dominated the field of social epidemiology and have displaced the emphasis on the family. Controversial work by Wilkinson (1996) and others point to population-level inequality measures as determinants of individual-level health outcomes. They argue that low social status leads to poor health, even after controlling for the individual level characteristics (education, income, smoking behavior, etc.) that affect health.

The economic critique (or economic epidemiology) of the public health approach is that many risk factors are determined by choices made by individuals. To a large extent people choose their environment, including their sexual partners, spouses, number of children, education, employment, and place of residence. The public health approach assumes that extrinsic risk factors (using Oleckno's terminology from above) can be altered by policy, whereas the economic model assumes that people will respond to changes in their behavior, so effective policy must anticipate the behavioral responses. For instance, the economic model predicts that the spread of diseases such as HIV/AIDS are self-limiting as individuals adapt their behavior in response to changes in the costs and benefits of risky sexual behaviors (Philipson & Posner, 1993). The economic critique demands that policy analysis incorporate a model of individual health behavior when examining public health programs that seek to alter environmental variables because environmental risk factors are determined in part by individual choice.

The family-relevant characteristics of the economic model are many, though economists have done very little work in bringing the family into the study of health behavior (Bolin, Jacobson, & Lindgren, 2001, 2002 and Wilson, 2002 are recent exceptions). Family and social networks constrain the flow of disease and influence the expected costs and benefits of a variety of behaviors, with HIV/AIDS and other STDs being an important case in point. Other examples are smoking and other unhealthy behaviors that are more common among single people than married people. Moreover, for a variety of reasons, marriage and family formation shape behavior by changing incentives. Family commitments can fundamentally alter the expected costs and benefits of a variety of behaviors and account for the stark behavioral changes (particularly among young men) that often occur at marriage (Miller-Tutzauer, Leonard, & Windle, 1991; Waite & Gallagher, 2000).

Although family variables are part of social and economic epidemiology, a family-centric epidemiology is yet to be fully developed. In such an approach the host's membership in a family network would be central. Lifestyle practices and socioeconomic status would be seen as family characteristics, and the fundamental environmental conditions, such as the sanitation of the home and choice of residence, would be determined by the family. Family members would also share environmental risk factors such as population density and air quality. Likewise, many disease agents interact with the family structure. Family members often come into more direct and intimate contact than individuals in the larger environment, which may facilitate the spread of disease (with sexually transmitted diseases being a salient example).

Stages of Policy Analysis

The result of policy analysis is a recommendation for some kind of action (or, if the analysis warrants, inaction). To arrive at such a recommendation, the analyst needs to carefully work through a process that melds the positive and normative dimensions of policy choice into a coherent whole. A suitable descriptive model has the following four stages: (1) problem definition, (2) specification of policy alternatives, (3) identification of policy effects, and (4) policy choice. Several excellent texts describe this analytical model in considerable detail (Bardach, 2000; Patton & Sawicki, 1993). This section illustrates briefly how family affects the nature of the analysis at every stage.

Problem Definition. The first stage of analysis is the identification of the problem: what is wrong, who is being hurt, and what are the likely causes? For the task of problem definition, a family-centered approach can significantly alter the scope of the analysis. Family-centered analysis will bring the problems associated with families—divorce, single parenthood, child poverty, domestic abuse, and so on—into the forefront. For example, poor health may raise the likelihood of divorce, and divorce may lead to poor health. At a fundamental level, it is impossible to separate family problems from health problems.

Specification of Policy Alternatives. Families are not only an integral part of health problems;

they also may be an integral part of policy solutions. For example, recently family therapy has been shown to improve not only the effectiveness of therapy for an individual with mental illness but the physical health of family members, and to lower the use of medical services by the family (Law, Crane, & Mohlman-Berge, 2003). Furthermore, if strong families promote health, as the previously cited literature suggests, then mechanisms to strengthen the family should be part of the policy alternatives considered by a policy analysis.

Identification of Policy Effects. This step usually constitutes the largest part of an analysis. It includes a specification of who has "standing," meaning who gets counted in the analysis. The process also includes mapping out the complex pathways by which each policy alternative may affect the lives of individuals and the vitality of institutions and communities. In some cases, the effects are easily quantifiable, such as dollars spent on hospitalization, but they are often difficult to measure, such as the pain from medical treatment or the grief suffered with the loss of a loved one. Many other outcomes can be measured, such as number of deaths from cancer, but cannot easily be assigned a monetary value.

Family-centered analysis starts with the assumption that anything that affects an individual is likely to affect members of the individual's family. Because the family is the first line of defense against the burdens of poor health, the magnitude of those burdens is in direct proportion to the ability of the family to cope with them. Also, when two or more people in the same family are facing severe health problems, the total cost of disease may be called super-additive, meaning that the sum is greater than what the two individuals would bear if they were sick within otherwise healthy families. When,

for instance, a husband and wife are both disabled, both individuals must cope with their own disability and do it without a healthy partner to provide assistance. This is a serious public health concern because the occurrence of multiple health problems is much more likely in families of low socio-economic status (Wilson, 2001).

The family may also play an important role in the way public programs actually function. The family may augment the effectiveness of those programs by, for example, providing informal health care or providing useful information to family members. Or the family may mitigate its effectiveness, such as when parents respond to health insurance subsidies by diverting funds to other uses not anticipated by the policy (another way of saying this is the public support of health care can "crowd out" private support).

A complete policy analysis addresses the instrumental-normative role of the family, as discussed earlier. Whenever the state steps in to address a role previously undertaken by families, there is the potential that the family will be weakened in the process. On the other hand, the state may provide knowledge and assistance to families that relieve stressors and add to the family's ability to cope with health issues—in other words, increase family capital. Some would argue government policies such as child care credits, Medicaid, and children's health insurance lower the financial risks associated with having children, which may make couples more willing to become parents and provide future generations to perform the work of society. Others would point out that these same assistance programs may reduce the need for fathers to be in the home, leading to increases in single motherhood, which is a strong correlate of a host of negative indicators for child well-being. (Biblarz & Raftery, 1999; Haveman & Wolfe, 1995; Jonsson & Gahler, 1997; Wallerstein, Lewis, & Blakesee, 2000). While passions run high on these types of issues, very little is known about how public policies affect the long-term status and function of families in society.

Policy Choice. There are three important subparts to this stage of the analysis. The first is an identification of criteria used to evaluate each policy alternative. While there are several commonsense criteria that analysts may apply (fairness to different groups, efficiency, etc.), ultimately the criteria are derived from normative theories discussed in the next section. The second subpart is an evaluation and ranking of the alternatives based on the normative criteria. The third subpart is an analysis of the prospects of each alternative given the political landscape. Some alternatives make great sense from the position of an "objective" observer but may be entirely infeasible from a political perspective. These issues are discussed in more detail in the section on politics of families and health.

NORMATIVE CRITERIA
IN POLICY ANALYSIS

The normative component of policy analysis addresses the fundamental question of what governments should (and should not) do. In modern life, social policy is pulled by a variety of normative claims that often come into conflict in both the academic and political spheres. This conflict can be characterized as the tension between four fundamental social values: individual liberty, equality, utility, and community. The general polity tends to believe in all four of these values, but it is useful to characterize different normative traditions in terms of the weight they give to each value in defining the role of the state.

The libertarian school of thought places paramount value on individual liberty and argues for minimal government intrusion in both economic and social life. For example,

Nozick (1974) and Barnett (1998) are modern articulations of libertarian or "classical liberal" thought.

Unfortunately, libertarian scholars have seldom paid attention to the family as a fundamental social institution that produces adults who are (according to the libertarian tradition) both entitled to their freedom and responsible for their actions. Although libertarians view family affairs as largely outside the appropriate scope of government, they have not developed a theoretical apparatus to determine the way in which the state should treat children differently from adults.

Children require support from adults and, sometimes, protection from adults—even from adults in their own family. Indeed, promoting the health and welfare of children is an area of government involvement that many libertarians would accept as necessary in a free society, though it is very difficult in practice to draw the line between the right of children to be protected by the state and the right of parents to raise children as they see fit.

The nature and role of marriage also poses challenges to theories about individual rights. Currently, American society is embroiled in a debate about the definition of marriage, particularly as it relates to same-sex relationships. While almost all libertarians would allow consenting adults the right to form whatever type of intimate relationships they see fit, it is unclear whether the state should sanction such relationships (or any relationships, for that matter).

Currently married persons have rights under the law not afforded to non-married partners. These include the right to be the "next of kin," which can be important in making critical health care decisions in times of crisis. Non-married partners also have no claim to custody of dependent children when their partner dies, which can have consequences for the health of these children.

The second political value is equality. From a political perspective, egalitarians believe the fundamental role of the state is to remove, or at least diminish, the inequalities between people that are caused by an unequal position at birth, differences in native abilities, fortune, and the self-interest of others. In recent decades, theories of policy analysis have been enriched by the influential work of John Rawls (1971). His analysis argues for strong forms of egalitarianism that are derived (in part) from notions of individual liberty, thus encroaching to a degree on the territory claimed by libertarians.

As is the case with any political ideology, egalitarianism takes many forms and is mingled, in practice, with other political values. Many egalitarians, for instance, hold a belief in individual liberty and even limited property rights, but they would still allow the state to confiscate significant resources from citizens in order to promote economic equality.

Egalitarianism in its most extreme form abandons economic and even political liberties altogether and allows the state to collect and redistribute virtually all of the material resources of the society. A practical middle ground between libertarian and egalitarian views is occupied by those who hold that while the state must do more than just protect basic liberties—à la libertarianism—it need not go so far as to ensure more equitable socioeconomic outcomes. Rather, it is an "equality of opportunity" that is favored. How one separates providing opportunities from ensuring outcomes is not always clear, but the debate here is vigorous.

In the case of health policy, egalitarianism has been enormously successful over the past several decades, though less so in the United States than in other industrialized countries. The great majority of public health advocacy groups have policy agendas firmly rooted in egalitarian ground. Examples include probably the two most prominent goals of the modern public health profession: (1) to provide universal health care and (2) to eliminate inequalities in health that exist between different racial, ethnic, and economic groups. Furthermore, egalitarians have recast the drive for health equity in the language of civil rights. For many, this "right" to health care extends not only to life-preserving care, but to care that only promotes the quality of life.

As is the case with libertarianism, the concept of family plays no central role in egalitarian thought. Because children are relatively powerless, some egalitarians are vocal advocates for child welfare, though a concern for families, per se, is only of indirect concern.

Similarly, egalitarianism is a foundation for the feminist assault on gender inequalities within social institutions, including families. Radical egalitarians are willing to attack any institution seen as limiting the equality of individuals. For instance, under a strict egalitarian norm, parents have no special claim to authority over children. In sum, the value of family to egalitarians is essentially an empirical question—it has value only if, in practice, it tends to diminish inequalities.

While liberty and equality remain important political values for the general public, the most prominent normative foundation of policy analysis today is utilitarianism. The utilitarian objective of "the greatest good for the greatest number" is reached by undertaking policies that maximize total utility (well-being or happiness) in society. In policy analysis, utilitarianism takes the form of cost-benefit analysis (CBA), which consists of assigning monetary values to the costs and benefits associated with different policy alternatives and then comparing alternatives based on their net benefits (benefits minus costs).

The goal of CBA is to assign values for social costs and benefits that are a direct function of valuations made by the people affected by policy (rather than values held by, say, the policy analyst). In practice, however, CBA has numerous problems that hinder the reliability of the enterprise, including difficulty in identifying those who are affected by policy and measuring those effects. The family is implicitly included in the calculations to the extent that individuals value families, but a typical CBA study would not consider the potential long-term effects when policies strengthen or weaken the institution of the family (though it is a false critique to say that CBA cannot be used to value future generations).

A fundamental characteristic of CBA is that the willingness-to-pay estimates that CBA relies upon are a function of ability to pay. CBA estimates are based on individuals' demand for goods and services, and demand usually increases with income and wealth. CBA, therefore, automatically assigns greater weight to the rich than to the poor. This tendency is mitigated, however, by the fact that CBA also accounts for the number of people affected, meaning that narrow elites typically do not do well under CBA because of their small numbers.

Applying CBA on a routine basis, therefore, can have serious distributional consequences. Because marriage typically improves the economic standing of individuals, choosing policies based on CBA will tend to favor the married over the unmarried. Similarly, children in single-parent families (who are often among the poorest parts of society) come out very poorly under CBA. CBA would also tend to favor the interests of the elderly over the interests of children since the elderly, as a group, are much wealthier than children. Whether or not families are routinely better off under CBA depends to a large extent on what type of families we are talking about. Any group that has both low income and low numbers of people will fare very poorly.

The final political value to be discussed here is community—a very popular word in modern discourse, but very difficult to define. Most challenges to the dominant economic/ CBA mode of thinking in policy analysis undertake an appeal to communitarian values. In particular, they argue that communities embody values that are distinct from those derived from the preferences or values of individuals within the community—in other words, the whole is greater than the sum of its parts. Scholars such as Barry (1990, p. 192) argue that there are "nonassignable interests" that people share in common that are distinct from their individual interests and that it is the role of government to promote these interests. Similarly, Deborah Stone (1997, p. 18) has argued that public policy is about "communities trying to achieve something as communities," not about satisfying individual interests. Indeed, many contentious political debates in a highly pluralistic society such as the United States are not as much about the interests of individuals as they are about who gets to set community goals and standards.

From a communitarian perspective, the family is a problematic concept. To a degree, a family is the smallest communitarian structure, and the same arguments that apply to promoting communities can be applied to promoting families and extended families. For instance, family members are able to pool resources, thereby lowering risks faced by individual members, and pass on education and other valuable resources between family members.

However, families tend to care much more about the welfare of individuals within the family than about those outside it, which may obstruct more general communitarian aims. Family networks create and preserve family capital and other resources, but they also keep resources from flowing to community members outside of the family network.

Although CBA can be extremely flexible, as a practical concern most cost-benefit studies ignore communitarian concerns. In particular, CBA seldom addresses the impact of policy on social institutions. Because the family is a fundamental social institution, a natural starting point for bringing in communitarian values is to address the instrumental-normative role of family networks.

For instance, as social insurance programs are introduced, the incentives for extended family to support dependent members are weakened. This may, in turn, weaken family bonds between generations, resulting in additional consequences, such as lessening of the emotional support useful to maintaining strong emotional and physical health.

THE POLITICS OF FAMILIES AND HEALTH

Assessing the political prospects of each policy alternative under consideration is an essential component of policy analysis. The political process will influence the likelihood of the recommendation being turned into policy, the chance that policymakers will change the recommendation in important ways (and thereby possibly undermine the rationale for the recommendation), and the tendency of administrative agencies to implement the policy in a fashion that might not be consistent with either the recommendation of the analyst or the aim of the policymaker. This section discusses the politics of families and health as they relate to electoral politics. (Space does not allow an analysis of judicial and bureaucratic politics.)

The Electoral Connection

Before they can pursue any policy agenda, politicians must get elected. Even though politicians will lose very few votes by claiming to be pro-family, election slogans do not necessarily translate into policy. The success of a policy proposal depends on the interaction between voter preferences and institutional features of the political system. Winner-take-all electoral systems with single-member districts are predominant in the United States. Given this institutional context, voters tend to elect candidates with policy positions at the center of the distribution of voter preferences,

a powerful result known as the median voter theorem (Black, 1958). Although the rhetoric in political primaries may be more extreme (as candidates try to appeal to the median position of party members), positions tend to moderate in the general election (as candidates must appeal to the median position in the general electorate). Because the United States is a federal system, policies can differ quite sharply across states because the median voter's political preferences differ from state to state. However, state variation in policy is tempered by policies instituted at the national level, and many of the funds to run state-level programs come from the federal government. While significant distinctions between party positions persist (for reasons that cannot be explained here), policy change in America will almost always be incremental, regardless of the party in power.

The ideological allegiances of the electorate ebb and flow, but one fact remains paramount: the median American voter is getting older. The demographer Sam Preston noted in 1984 that during the 1960s and 1970s, even though the number of children fell and the number of elderly rose, the well-being of children deteriorated while the well-being of the elderly improved dramatically. This suggests an impact on health and welfare as a result of the dramatic increases in public support to the elderly relative to children. More recent evidence also points to large income transfers to the elderly and relatively few to children (Lee, 1994; Stecklov, 1997) even though the elderly are, as a group, much wealthier than children. And as the median voter ages, politicians will be more and more likely to pay attention to the political demands of seniors. The elderly have distinct political advantages over children and younger adults. The elderly vote at higher rates than younger adults (Leighley & Nagler, 1992); they are more likely to be single-issue voters (Bernstein, 1995); and their numbers are growing rapidly.

Elderly people, of course, are part of family networks; thus this demographic shift is not necessarily anti-family. Indeed, one could argue that assisting the elderly to live independently is a pro-family policy because it protects families from the burden of having to support and care for aged relatives. Three arguments speak against the claim, however. First, if transfers from the state crowd out transfers from extended family members, then the independence of the elderly may come at the expense of weakening family and other social networks that have traditionally provided elder care. Second, the elderly are likely to have fewer people dependent upon them for support than younger adults, who often have children. Third, and most important, a large portion of government transfers to the elderly are going to provide benefits to the wealthy (wealthy individuals pay the same Medicare premiums as do the poor, for instance). Even though a relatively large percentage of the elderly are wealthy, means testing (tying benefits to financial need) of Medicare or Social Security is not on the agenda of either dominant political party in the United States. Conservative Republicans generally favor means testing, but it is strongly opposed by most Democrats, who view means testing as a slippery-slope threat to the universality of social insurance. For instance, in the passage of the recent Medicare bill in 2003, most Democrats and a significant number of moderate Republicans killed an effort to means-test Medicare benefits in spite of (1) support for means testing by traditionally left-leaning groups such as the Urban Institute and the Center on Budget and Policy priorities (Pear, 2003) and (2) the increase in dollars that means testing would make available for benefits to the non-wealthy.

The Power of Concentrated Interests

Traditional, pluralistic models of politics predict success for those policies that are supported by large interests (the number of people weighted by the intensity of their preferences). If this were true, pro-family policy would be central, given that families are ubiquitous. Tax deductions for interest on home mortgages, federally funded child health insurance (CHIP), and large percentage increases in child tax credits in recent years provide some evidence for this view. Policies to promote child health generally have strong bipartisan support (Longest, 2002), though many would say U.S. child welfare policies, in general, lag far behind other industrialized nations (for example, the U.S. is the only economically advanced nation not to mandate paid maternity leave, which is arguably a child health issue).

The influence of the American Association of Retired Persons (AARP) is an example of a case in which a large group of individuals is represented by a highly effective association. But this case is relatively anomalous, and is due to the relatively narrow, intense interests of the elderly and their willingness to go to the polls. More often than not, successful associations represent small, narrow interests, not the diverse interests of large groups such as, say, women, Hispanics, or employed persons. For instance, producers of mohair and honey are able to maintain large federal subsidies year after year even though their numbers are small and they are far outside public consciousness. Small groups (beekeepers) can have a much larger influence than do large groups (honey eaters), holding other variables constant. Narrow interests have lobbying power that often runs directly in contrast to the electoral power of the median voter. Many social policy issues generate intense lobbying but lack enough salience at the ballot box to sufficiently counter the efforts of narrow interests.

Public choice theorists argue that the advantages faced by small groups are twofold. First, small groups can solve the internal collective action problem of getting members of the group to participate actively in the cause (Olson, 1971). Second, because small groups have relatively few people among whom to divide the rewards of policy success, members of the group may each get thousands or even millions of dollars in benefit from government spending or regulation; this gives them powerful incentives to lobby and to influence elections through campaign contributions and direct advertising. On the other hand, the costs to the taxpayers of any particular program are typically only pennies per person, which means that no one has the financial incentive to work against them. By the same logic, initiatives where costs are concentrated among the few are unlikely to succeed if the benefits are widely distributed— even if the aggregate benefits are much larger than the aggregate costs.

So, how are these arguments related to families and health policy, particularly since both the benefits and the costs of health care are widely distributed? Even though health care is very broad-based, many interest groups in the health area face either highly concentrated benefits or costs associated with different policy initiatives. For instance, the demise of the Clinton administration's Health Security Act was seen by many to be the result of an effective advertising campaign by private health insurance companies. Another example is the American Medical Association (AMA), who for decades dictated policy on medical education, licensing, and treatment (Barzansky & Etzel, 2002; Gonzales, 2000; Jaklevic, 1997; Pearson, 2002). With the help of regulatory policy that suppressed competition from other types of providers and sharply limited the number of medical school slots in the country, physicians became the highest paid professionals in the country, and American families ended up footing the bill. Finally, since the overwhelming success of AIDS activists in dramatically increasing federal support for AIDS research, interest groups related to specific diseases have been increasingly successful at appealing directly to Congress for "earmarked" funds for particular disease initiatives, thereby circumventing the priority-setting role of the National Institutes of Health.

In sum, a central political problem for families is that there are too many of them. Policies that have a family component to them are going to be characterized by small, incremental benefits to a wide swath of people—not large benefits to a few. For reasons discussed earlier, the large numbers of people interested in family well-being may give some power at the ballot box, but if the policy initiatives supported by families run counter to the concentrated interests of insurers, providers, or hospitals, they will likely fail. Furthermore, health policy initiatives have to compete not only with the organized interests in health care, but with all the policy initiatives in other areas as well, including education, the environment, agriculture, national defense, and a host of others.

The Conflict of Ideologies

In addition to battling concentrated interests, advocates for a pro-family policy agenda are far from unified in their policy objectives. Underneath the rhetorical, pro-family veneer lie some of the deepest ideological divisions in American politics. On the right, a variety of associations exist that extol the traditional norms regarding the family. They define themselves as pro-family because they want strong marriages that promote the welfare of children. Their policy agenda grows out of a reaction to the social upheaval of the 1960s and 1970s and is best described by what they are opposed to: legalized abortion, pornography, nonmarital sexual activities, gay rights, forced racial integration of schools, and nonparental day care for children.

The left, on the other hand, has a family policy agenda that seeks to sanction and validate the feminist, egalitarian goals underlying the same social upheaval the right condemns. They see the family values of the right as exclusive, hierarchical, and discriminatory.

Given the easy rhetoric of protecting the welfare of children and dependent adults that is present in both major U.S. political parties, one might hope for significant common ground to emerge in the debate on families. Indeed, the area of child health and welfare is one that can be defended from libertarian, egalitarian, and communitarian value systems. Conservatives are more likely than liberals to pay homage to "traditional" families, but (in America, at least) many liberals want to support traditional families through government policies, such as health insurance for children or subsidized health care. In general, liberals will support a greater role for government programs than conservatives, but disagreements over the appropriate size and scope of government are less of a challenge when it comes to dependent family members. The conflict is not over whether children or dependent adults should have important standing in policy evaluation or even over whether parents should have special privilege in making decisions for their children. The fight is about how to address nontraditional family structures and departures from conservative sexual mores and other traditional values. The concept of family is tightly interwoven with sexuality, gender, and religion. Analyzing health policy in the context of the family, therefore, attaches these highly divisive issues to the health-family nexus. Should we allow adoption by homosexual couples? Should cohabiting parents receive the same benefits for their children as married parents? Should abortion be available to minors? Should stay-at-home parents receive the same kinds of day care subsidies as working parents?

Thus far, the public debate over health policy typically neglects discussion of the relationship between families and health, though the easy rhetoric of protecting the welfare of children and dependent adults is evident. Analyzing health policy in the context of the family will interweave issues related to sexuality, gender, religion, parenting practices, and child welfare into the already complex array of issues related to health, which makes enacting any policy that touches on issues of family even more difficult.

One might hope that the public health profession, particularly academics, might provide the impetus for integrating the family into health policy. However, the public health community is significantly left of center, at least in terms of the American political scene, and the activist approach they take to family issues polarizes the debate. As Cole, Delzell, and Rodu (2000) argue, "we have nearly converted the school of public health from an institution committed to developing the scientific bases for disease prevention into one of the many arenas for advancing social justice, or some people's idea of social justice," (p. 87) where social justice involves radically restructuring the market economy to eliminate poverty, racial and gender discrimination, and any remnants of social class. Conservatives and moderates will find little common ground with the public health community when it comes to the family.

Interestingly, the social justice movement relies critically on social epidemiological studies that have documented large disparities in health according to race, ethnicity, education, income, and social class. Scholar-activists have used these studies to fundamentally reshape epidemiological research and to propose radical structural changes to all aspects of society.

However, the very same types of studies have shown the widespread benefits of marriage to children and adults (both male and female). But no equivalent response to strengthen marriage has come from the public health community in general. Indeed, quite the opposite has occurred. Timmreck (2002) recently noted, "For the past decade or so the field of public health and epidemiology has slowly and continually excluded and diminished the role of marital status and family status in overall implications on health status of individuals and society" (p. 326).

FAMILIES AND THE FUTURE OF HEALTH POLICY

The political issues discussed in the previous section are highly fluid. Interest groups come and go; elections shift the partisan composition of Congress, and the attention of the media and the public swings from one issue to another. However, certain deep-seated social trends deserve discussion, particularly as they relate to the goal of family-centered policy.

Demographics

In the coming decades, one social force will come to dominate all others—the graying of the population. In 1950, 8.1% of the population was over age 65. In 2000 it was 12.4%, and it will be 20.3% in 2050 (Hobbs & Stoops, 2000; U.S. Census Bureau, 2000). Population aging in other industrialized countries is even more pronounced due to the relatively high birth rate in the United States and the continual inflow of immigrants. Kotlikoff and Burns (2004) refer to the policy showdowns that are brewing as the "coming generational storm." It is unclear what types of adjustments in taxes or benefits will occur, but ending or seriously weakening these programs is a political impossibility, regardless of the political party in power. Questions such as "Can Medicare be saved?" hardly deserve discussion. A better question is this: "To what extent will we continue to transfer billions of dollars from working families (many of whom are financially strapped) to finance the health care and income needs of the elderly (many of whom are wealthy)?" The demographic forces are so intense that eventually

a new public conception of social insurance must emerge. The current deceit—the accounting fallacy that Medicare and Social Security "trust funds" exist that contributors will draw upon in later life—must eventually give way to a more realistic conception of these programs as public welfare programs, and (barring some phenomenal and unlikely increase in worker productivity) the size and nature of these entitlements must change, either through means testing or through other changes to the tax and benefit structure.

Even though the financing of formal health care receives most of the public attention, the crisis in informal care is equally daunting, but the recognition of the importance of informal care is not yet widespread. The crisis—which is an increasing risk of institutional care because of the lack of a family caregiver—is due to three demographic forces. First, the boom in divorce that began in the1960s means that an increased percentage of seniors, particularly women, will lack a healthy spouse to provide care for them. Second, because of sharply declining fertility after the baby boom, the next generation of elderly will have far fewer middle-aged children to provide care for them. And third, daughters and daughters-in-law (who have typically been the primary caregivers of elderly parents) are in the labor force at higher rates than ever before. These working women will be less likely to provide significant care to their parents and in-laws.

Longer life spans have led demographers and chronic disease epidemiologists to question whether longer life means worsening health (Gruenberg, 1977; Verbrugge, 1984). But most evidence over the past two decades points to falling, or at least stable, rates of disease and disability at all ages (Manton, Corder, & Stallard, 1997). However, Freedman, Martin, and Schoeni (2002) recently conducted an extensive review of the literature and found that decreases in disability are largely concentrated among less severe indicators of disability and that the most thorough studies show very mixed (and generally negative) results for severe disability.

Furthermore, Crimmins and Saito (2000) find that the prevalence of most chronic diseases has also been rising among the elderly in the past decade. The consensus view is that in general, the elderly are becoming healthier over time, which is good news. But even if the average person becomes healthier, this does not mean that national medical expenditures will fall. Indeed, a major reason for improving health is the high levels of medical care utilization (at ever-increasing prices). Because there is no evidence that per capita demand for medical care will decline in the future, the inevitable swelling of Medicare costs will not be avoided unless Medicare benefit levels decline significantly.

The Industrialization of Medical Care

Managed care involves bringing costs and benefits explicitly into the medical decision-making process. Whereas most public policy analysts are trained to make policy recommendations based on the social consequences of policy, executives of health care companies typically consider neither the broader social consequences of their decisions nor consequences borne by families of patients. For example, an important part of controlling health care costs for a managed care organization is keeping expensive hospital stays to a minimum.

While this objective may save on hospital costs faced by the health care company, it also may drastically increase the costs borne by family members when patients come home still in need of significant care.

Competitive forces in health care markets constrain prices and promote quality improvements. Indeed, health care companies compete for customers just as firms do in other industries. However, because most health care in the U.S. is paid for by third parties (government and employers, primarily), patients end up sharing the benefits of cost-containment with the third-party payers. For instance, when an employer gets a better deal on a health plan, some of the benefits are passed on to workers, but some accrue to the firm's shareholders. Furthermore, because individuals with high expected medical costs are the most eager to buy medical insurance and because insurers often cannot distinguish high-risk enrollees from low-risk ones (a type of market failure known as "adverse selection"), the prices of individual insurance policies are often so high that they are unattainable for many families. This leaves low-income families who lack employer-provided benefits with no option other than government programs (such as Medicaid or CHIP) or to go without health insurance.

In addition to the growth of managed care, a second important trend in medicine is the ever-increasing pace of technological advancement. Medical technology (including knowledge, equipment, and drugs) has surely contributed to longer and healthier lives among many. It has also surely increased the cost of medical care. While some new technologies will have widespread beneficial effects, many others will bring only incremental improvements to quality or length of life, but at a high price tag. If medical decisions were made solely on the basis of an individual's willingness to pay, then new technology would not be a problem, but because of the strong egalitarian norms many people hold about access to health care, our society has chosen to publicly fund a large amount of our health care costs. So the question becomes, which new technologies should governments employ, and what kinds of research and development should government fund through the allocation of medical research grants? Most government programs are forced to ration in some way the use of expensive technologies—either by not providing the technology at all or by creating long waiting times to use particular services.

Like other decisions, technology decisions should take into account that individuals live in families who share in the health-related decisions of the individual. The benefits of reducing disability, for instance, accrue to the members of the disabled person's family and should, therefore, be considered part of the decision calculus. Private firms are likely to invest in those technologies that have high potential profits. These will be technologies that can be restricted in their distribution and sold to people who are willing to pay for them. It is important for the state to promote the development of technologies where potential profits are low, but where gains to society are high. Improved knowledge about disease prevention would be but one example.

CONCLUSION

The rationale for considering the family in health policy analysis is compelling. Health decisions of individuals—from questions of diet to choice of health care plan—are made in a family context, and family networks, in turn, shape society and determine the effectiveness of public health programs. It is somewhat surprising, therefore, that families are not a bigger part of the scholarly and public discussion of health policy. In this chapter, I have attempted to begin a discussion of how the highly integrated nature of health and family life can be reflected in the types of analyses we conduct in the area of health policy.

Despite the obvious importance of these issues, the immediate political future for family-centered health policy is not particularly bright. Organized interests are not promoting a pro-family agenda; there is considerable discord on what types of "family values" we, as a research community, really want to support; and the nature of representative democracy is such that narrow, concentrated interests are much more likely to be protected than broad interests, such as the welfare of families. The ray of hope is the power of good ideas. It is up to those interested in the health of our families to see that those ideas keep proliferating.

Finally, at the outset of this chapter I noted that definitions of family are highly controversial in today's political climate. But while we can discuss the family and health using a variety of different definitions of family, at some point researchers may want to make stronger claims about the types of families (including different types of family structures) that best promote the interests of their members and the interests of the larger community. Families have a potential to do both tremendous good and tremendous harm to the health of their members. A better understanding of these positive and negative forces can improve not only family life, but ultimately, public health.

REFERENCES

Asbridge, M. (2004). Public place restrictions on smoking in Canada: Assessing the role of the state, media, science, and public health advocacy. *Social Science and Medicine, 58*(1), 13–24.

Bardach, E. (2000). *A practical guide for policy analysis: The eightfold path to more effective problem solving.* New York: Chatham House.

Barnett, R. (1998). *The structure of liberty: Justice and the rule of law.* New York: Oxford University Press.

Baron, S., Field, J., & Schuller, T. (Eds.). (2001). *Social capital: Critical perspectives*. New York: Oxford University Press.

Barry, B. (1990). *Political argument: A reissue with a new introduction*. Berkeley: University of California Press.

Barzansky, B., & Etzel, S. (2002). Educational programs in U. S. medical schools, 2001–2002. *JAMA: The Journal of the American Medical Association, 288*(9), 1067–1072.

Bernstein, R. A. (1995). Directing electoral appeals away from the center: Issue position and issue salience. *Political Research Quarterly, 48*(3), 479–505.

Biblarz, T. J., & Raftery, A. E. (1999). Family structure, educational attainment, and socioeconomic success: Rethinking the "pathology of matriarchy." *The American Journal of Sociology, 105*(2), 321–365.

Black, D. (1958). *The theory of committees and elections*. London: Cambridge University Press.

Blumberg, L. J., Dubay, L., & Norton, S. A. (2000). Did the Medicaid expansions for children displace private insurance? An analysis using the SIPP. *Journal of Health Economics, 19*, 33–60.

Bolin, K., Jacobson, L., & Lindgren, B. (2001). The family as health producer: When spouses are Nash-bargainers. *Journal of Health Economics, 20*, 349–362.

Bolin, K., Jacobson, L., & Lindgren, B. (2002). The family as health producer: When spouses act strategically. *Journal of Health Economics, 21*, 475–495.

Cassell, J. (1976). The contribution of the social environment to host resistance. *American Journal of Epidemiology, 104*, 107–123.

Chandola, T. (2001). The fear of crime and area differences in health. *Health and Place, 7*, 105–116.

Cherlin, A. (1999). *Public and private families: An introduction* (2nd ed.). Boston: McGraw Hill.

Cobb, S. (1976). Social support as a moderator of life stress. *Psychosomatic Medicine, 38*, 100–115.

Cole, P., Delzell, E., & Rodu, B. (2000). Moneychangers in the temple. *Epidemiology, 11*, 84–90.

Crimmins, E. M., & Saito, Y. (2000). Change in the prevalence of diseases among older Americans: 1984-1994. *Demographic Research, 3*, Article 9. Retrieved from http://www.demographic-research.org

Crimmins, E., & Saito, Y. (2001). Trends in healthy life expectancy in the United States, 1970–1990: Gender, racial, and educational differences. *Social Science and Medicine, 52*, 1629–1641.

Freedman, V. A., Martin, L. G., & Schoeni, R. F. (2002). Recent trends in disability and functioning among older adults in the United States: A systematic review. *Journal of the American Medical Association, 288*, 3137–3146.

Fukuyama, F. (1995). *Trust: The social virtues and the creation of prosperity*. New York: Free Press.

Gonzales, A. (2000). Fighting back. *Modern Physician, 4*(10), 28.

Green, E., Courage, C., & Rushton, L. (2003, March). Reducing domestic exposure to environmental tobacco smoke: A review of attitudes and behaviours. *Journal of the Royal Society of Health*, 46–51.

Gruenberg, E. M. (1977). The failure of success. *Milbank Quarterly, 55*, 3–34.

Haveman, R., & Wolfe, B. (1995). The determinants of children's attainments: A review of methods and findings. *Journal of Economic Literature, 33*, 1829–1878.

Hippisley-Cox, J., Coupland, C., Pringle, M., Crown, N., & Hammersley, V. (2002). Married couples' risk of the same disease: Cross-sectional study. *British Medical Journal, 325*(7365), 636.

Hobbs, F., & Stoops, N. (2002). *Demographic trends in the 20th century: Census 2000 special reports.* Washington, DC: U.S. Government Printing Office.

Jaklevic, M. C. (1997). AMA accreditation debut. *Modern Healthcare, 27*(47), 30–31.

Jonsson, J. O., & Gahler, M. (1997). Family dissolution, family reconstitution, and children's educational careers: Recent evidence for Sweden. *Demography, 34*(2), 277–293.

Kamerman, S., & Kahn, A. J. (1978). *Family policy: Government and families in fourteen countries.* New York: Columbia University Press.

Kawachi, I., & Berkman, L. F. (2003). *Neighborhoods and health.* New York: Oxford University Press.

Kmietowicz, Z. (2003). Pressure mounts to ban smoking in public places. *British Medical Journal, 327*(7406), 69.

Kotlikoff, L. J., & Burns, S. (2004). *The coming generational storm: What you need to know about America's economic future.* Cambridge, MA: MIT Press.

Lau, E. M. C., Lee, P., Lynn, H., Sham, A., & Woo, J. (2003). The epidemiology of cigarette smoking in Hong Kong Chinese women. *Preventive Medicine, 37*(5), 383–388.

Law, D. D., Crane, D. R., & Mohlman-Berge, J. (2003). The influence of marital and family therapy on high utilizers of health care. *Journal of Marital and Family Therapy, 29*(3), 353–363.

Lee, R. D. (1994). Population age structure, intergenerational transfers, and wealth: A new approach with applications to the United States. *Journal of Human Resources, 29*(4), 1027–1063.

Leighley, J. E., & Nagler, J. (1992). Individual and systemic influences on turnout: Who votes? 1984. *The Journal of Politics, 54*(3), 718–740.

Li, C., Unger, J. B., Schuster, D., Rohrbach, L. A., Howard-Pitney, B., & Norman, G. (2003). Youths' exposure to environmental tobacco smoke (ETS): Associations with health beliefs and social pressure. *Addictive Behaviors, 28*(1), 39–53.

Litman, T. J., & Robins, L. S. (1997). *Health politics and policy* (3rd ed.). Albany, NY: Delmar.

Longest, B. B., Jr. (2002). *Health policymaking in the United States.* Chicago: Health Administration Press.

Manton, K., Corder, L. S., & Stallard, E. (1997). Chronic disability trends in elderly United States populations. 1982–1994. *Proceedings of the National Academy of Sciences of the U. S. A.: Medical Sciences, 94,* 2593–2598.

Miller-Tutzauer, C., Leonard, K. E., & Windle, M. (1991). Marriage and alcohol use: A longitudinal study of "maturing out." *Journal of Studies on Alcohol, 52,* 434–440.

Monden, C., de Graaf, N. D., & Kraaykamp, G. (2003). How important are parents and partners for smoking cessation in adulthood? An event history analysis. *Preventive Medicine, 36*(2), 197–203.

Nozick, R. (1974). *Anarchy, state, and utopia.* New York: Basic Books.

Oleckno, W. A. (2002). *Essential epidemiology: Principles and applications.* Long Grove, IL: Waveland Press.

Olson, M. (1971). *The logic of collective action: Public goods and the theory of groups.* Cambridge, MA: Harvard University Press.

Patel, K., & Rushefsky, M. E. (1999). *Health care politics and policy in America.* New York: M.E. Sharpe.

Patton, C. V., & Sawicki, D. S. (1993). *Basic methods of policy analysis and planning* (2nd ed.). Englewood Cliffs, NJ: Prentice Hall.

Pear, R. (2003, October 6). Medicare plan raises the cost for the affluent. *New York Times,* p. 1.

Pearson, L. (2002, January). How each state stands on legislative issues affecting advanced nursing practice. *The Nurse Practitioner, 27,* 10–22.

Philipson, T., & Posner, R. (1993). *Private choices and public health.* Cambridge, MA: Harvard University Press.

Pickett, K. E., & Pearl, M. (2001). Multi-level analyses of neighborhood socioeconomic context and health outcomes: A critical review. *Journal of Epidemiology and Community Health, 55,* 111–122.

Preston, S. (1984). Children and the elderly in the United States. *Scientific American, 251,* 44–49.

Putnam, R. D. (2000). *Bowling alone: The collapse and revival of American community.* New York: Simon & Schuster.

Rawls, J. (1971). *A theory of justice.* Cambridge, MA: Harvard University Press.

Ribar, D. C. (2004). What do social scientists know about the benefits of marriage? A review of quantitative methodologies. *IZA Discussion Paper No. 998.*

Robert, S. A. (1999). Socioeconomic position and health: The independent contribution of community socioeconomic context. *Annual Review of Sociology, 25,* 489–516.

Ross, C. E., & Mirowsky, J. (2001). Neighborhood disadvantage, disorder, and health. *Journal of Health and Social Behavior, 42,* 258–276.

Schneiderman, N. (2001). *Integrating behavioral and social science with public health.* Washington, DC: American Public Health Association.

Stecklov, G. (1997). Intergenerational resource flows in Cote d'Ivoire: Empirical analysis of aggregate flows. *Population and Development Review, 23*(3), 525–553.

Stone, D. (1997). *Policy paradox: The art of political decision making.* New York: W.W. Norton.

Timmreck, T. (2002). *An introduction to epidemiology* (3rd ed.). Sudbury, MA: Jones & Bartlett.

U.S. Census Bureau. (2000). *Projections of the resident population by age, sex, race, and Hispanic origin: 1999 to 2100.* Washington, DC: U.S. Government Printing Office.

Verbrugge, L. M. (1984). Longer life but worsening health? Trends in health and mortality of middle-aged and older persons. *Milbank Quarterly, 62,* 475–519.

Waite, L. J., & Gallagher, M. (2000). *The case for marriage: Why married people are happier, healthier, and better off financially.* New York: Doubleday.

Wallerstein, J., Lewis, J., & Blakesee, S. (2000). *The unexpected legacy of divorce: A 25-year landmark study.* New York: Hyperion.

Wilkinson, R. G. (1996). *Unhealthy societies: The afflictions of inequality.* London: Routledge.

Wilson S. E. (2001). Socioeconomic status and the prevalence of health problems among married couples in late mid-life. *American Journal of Public Health, 91,* 131–135.

Wilson, S. E. (2002). The health capital of families: An investigation of the interspousal correlation in health status. *Social Science and Medicine, 55,* 1157–1172.

CHAPTER 17

Using Agent-Based Modeling to Simulate the Influence of Family-Level Stress on Disease Progression

William A. Griffin

This volume, in its depth and breadth, reflects the ubiquitous appreciation among scientists and health practitioners that the health of an individual is tightly embedded within the social matrix of his or her family. Numerous recent publications have forwarded plausible links between the health of an individual and his or her immediate familial setting. Following from the pioneering work of Kiecolt-Glaser and her colleagues (Kiecolt-Glaser & Newton, 2001; see also Burman & Margolin, 1992) on marital dyads, many of these investigations have expanded to include entire families (e.g., Miller, Cohen, & Ritchey, 2002; Vitaliano, Zhang, & Scanlan, 2003). The common axes of this area of research are the intersection of health, immunological

response, and stress (e.g., Cohen, Miller, & Rabin, 2001; Zautra, 2003; see Sapolsky, 1998, for a nontechnical overview). Individuals under sustained physical or psychological stress are susceptible to suppressed immunological response, thereby providing opportunistic diseases the setting to invade and manifest themselves in the host.

Being in a family with an ill spouse or child is obviously stress inducing (Greene & Griffin, 1998; Miller et al., 2002). This reverberating process of stress and illness is well documented, yet the processes binding the health of a family member or members to the psychosocial milieu of their family awaits delineation (see Vitaliano et al., 2003, for a good discussion). Thinking about this highly complex reciprocal interaction between

AUTHOR'S NOTE: Support for this work comes from National Science Foundation grants NSF-0339096 and NSF-0338864. The author would like to thank Shana Schmidt and Melissa Herzog for reviewing earlier drafts of this chapter. Comments or questions about the material presented in this chapter can be obtained by contacting the author at william.griffin@asu.edu.

immediate familial illness, omnipresent stress, and physiological vulnerabilities induces a rich intellectual feast for the scientist, but at a cost: conceptualized in its fullest embodiment, this putative process creates a methodological nightmare. How, for example, do you demonstrate the reciprocal health impact of one or more family members on another family member as stresses and illnesses evolve over time, where the evolution is influenced by endogenous and exogenous factors? Endogenous factors might include the genetic predisposition to a specific illness or various illnesses distributed among family members, or something as simple as accepted hygiene in the household. Exogenous factors, those coming from outside the household, might range from the cost of health insurance to the distance needed to travel for medical care. This immense combinatorial explosion of influences—some being lagged, others simultaneous, and some anticipated—makes trying to decipher any cause and effect relationship impossible. Instead, as contemporary scientific models examine dynamical systems, based on the realities of true complex processes (Shalizi, in press), traditional analytic data strategies provide only very limited mechanisms for investigating and modeling the evolving trajectories of individuals, couples, and families. This chapter describes, illustrates, and advocates for the use of a recently developed computer-based simulation methodology: agent-based modeling (ABM) that allows the investigator to articulate and model, in very precise terms, the putative features assumed to capture the dynamics of complex biopsychosocial processes. Beyond merely applying to biopsychosocial processes, this methodology allows investigators to examine general "what if" scenarios about couples and families. Possible areas of research range from the influence of the death of a parent on family dynamics to how the birth of a child might alter marital

processes. In effect, any scientific question that addresses social processes, especially among tightly knit groups, such as families or kinship networks, are especially appropriate for agent-based modeling.

AGENT-BASED MODELS

Did you every wonder how birds flock, or how schools of fish emerge and then, when necessary, demonstrate fluid synchronicity as they react to a predator? Or closer to home, how do ants know how to find the food in the picnic basket? In 1954, Bryon Haskin directed the movie *The Naked Jungle,* and aside from the romantic entanglement of stars Charlton Heston and Eleanor Parker, the movie was about a horde of army ants, "2 miles wide and 20 miles long," cutting a swath through the jungle, eating everything in their path, and headed directly toward Heston's South American plantation. Although the movie is more melodramatic fiction than science, the coordinated and predatory action of army ants has fascinated biologists for decades: each day, as many as 150,000 to 200,000 nearly blind individuals can sweep over a 1,500 square meter area to capture and retrieve tens of thousands of mobile prey items (e.g., crickets, spiders) without a plan or leader (Camazine et al., 2001; Franks, 1989). This raiding system may be 15 or more meters wide and move across the ground at speeds up to 0.2 meters per minute. At the front of the raid is a densely packed mass of ants, darting to and fro in front of the leading edge, and immediately behind this undulating heap, at about 1 meter, is a web of variegated pheromone-laden tracks eventually converging to a single pathway back to the bivouac. How do they do it? Although many details certainly remain to be solved, investigators in this area are confident about the basic dynamics of this complex system: it can be explained—and simulated—using very simple interaction rules based on ant density, pheromone concentrations, and prey distribution (see Brown, 2004; Deneubourg et al., 1989; Sole, Bonabeau, Delgado, Fernandez, & Marin, 2000). Biologists can now reproduce raids with characteristics consistent with those seen on the forest floor using computers to implement the simple array of rules thought to form the social interactions. An excellent example of an agent-based model simulating this fascinating sociobiological process can be found at the Web site of Tim Brown (http://www.dandelion.org/ant/model).

Whether it's birds flocking or ants raiding or family members eating dinner, these coordinated social processes are composed of elemental actions, each contributing to the emergent sociality. There are numerous ways to test and refine models of social processes. The most common is the "statistical approach" (Gilbert & Troitzsch, 1999); it uses inductive or deductive reasoning or both to pair the observed behavior with some quantitative assessment of the system (e.g., correlations, variance, covariance) measured at a single point in time (Gilbert & Troitzsch, 1999; Kohler, 2000). Another recently developed method of testing models of social dynamics is computer simulation (Axelrod, 1997; Hannon & Ruth, 1997; Gilbert & Troitzsch, 1999; Kohler & Gumerman, 2000; Morrison, 1991). Axelrod (1997) referred to this latter method as the third way of doing science (inductive and deductive being the first two). Like deduction, it starts with a set of explicit assumptions, but it does not prove theorems. This method instead generates simulated data that can be analyzed inductively. But unlike the inductive method, the simulated data come from a rigorously specified set of rules rather than direct measurement of the real world. Induction seeks to find patterns while deductive methods

want to determine the consequences of assumptions, whereas computer simulations allow experimentation and aid intuition (Axelrod, 1997; Hannon & Ruth, 1997). Kohler (2000) views simulations as generators of a phenomenon that demonstrate possible causal pathways, and Axelrod (1997) views simulations as tools to enrich our understanding of fundamental processes. Either of these complimentary positions clearly states the need and value of computer simulations of social processes (Kohler & Gumerman, 2000; Belew & Mitchell, 1996).

Without going too far from the purpose of this chapter, it should be noted that this third way of doing science brings with it a new, or more accurately termed "rediscovered," logical method of examining data and generating scientific hypotheses. This method is referred to as *abduction*, meaning, literally, *inference to the best explanation* (Lipton, 1991). Abduction refers to the process of explaining phenomena by inferring the generative mechanisms underlying the processes associated with the object of study. The philosopher Charles Sanders Peirce is credited with distinguishing abductive (or *reductive* by some writers) from inductive and deductive inference (see Borgelt & Kruse, 2000 for a thorough discussion). Why should anyone interested in ABMs care about abduction? It relates to agent-based modeling in the following way: If we assume that biopsychosocial processes evolve according to rules governing the complex recursive interactions among all levels (e.g., individuals, families, and environment) of the monitored system, then an estimate of the underlying process will generate an outcome of some approximation to the realized processes. The similarities and differences between generated results and the actual process forces the investigator to evaluate the postulated rules, draw inferences about their truthfulness, modify them according to the conclusions drawn, and rerun the generator (i.e., computer model). In effect, the investigator infers *to the best explanation* about process. This explanation for the generative mechanisms forms the premises that inform rule construction in the subsequent iteration of the computer model, and so on over time, as the scientist attempts to gain insight into the opaque rules governing a system. In essence, abduction is the scientific foundation for the way agent-based modeling occurs.

What is an Agent-Based Model?

An agent-based model is one that has agents implementing social interactions according to a set of rules constructed by the investigator consistent with either theory or observed data. Agents are processes implemented on a computer that have autonomy and the ability to interact with other agents and their environment; their actions are goal directed and they evolve. These characteristics permit the agents to engage in complex social interactions unguided by the investigator. A model usually contains many agents, ranging from tens to thousands, with each being slightly different from the other on the attributes considered relevant by the investigator. This ensemble of autonomous heterogeneous agents allows social interaction to be computationally constructed and its outcomes observed based on internalized social norms, internal behavioral rules, and data acquired on the basis of agent experience (Macy & Willer, 2002). Using a complex systems paradigm, the analyst is able to explore the possible generative mechanisms underlying the observed phenomena (Holland, 1995). Most importantly, this creation of complex adaptive systems in an artificial world permits the analyst to explore emergent macro phenomena—structural patterns not reducible to or evident in the properties of the micro-level agents (Rocha, 1999). It is the recursive agent-to-agent and agent-to-environment interaction

over time, each modifying and co-adapting to the other, that creates the critical and continuously evolving macro patterns that social and behavioral scientists study.

For example, over the past two years we have been developing PlayMate, an agent-based modeling program that simulates playgroup formation in children ages four to six years (Griffin, Hanish, Martin, & Fabes, 2004). In the fall of each year, new and returning children come together in our child development lab where many eventually settle into groups of semi-stable play partners. Factors contributing to the formation of these playgroups are currently unknown. The children's social environment differs slightly each year because of variation in playgroup formations, and these formations derive from the stability of who plays with whom. Both the groupings and the resulting structures evolve as the year progresses. To keep the model simple and results tractable, PlayMate uses static (e.g., sex) and dynamic (e.g., sociability) child attributes to modify the likelihood of interacting with another child (Griffin, Cree, Martin, Fabes, & Hanish, 2002; Griffin, Hanish, et al., 2003; Griffin et al., 2004). The effects modeled for these traits or attributes can be modified to represent postulated developmental shifts. Agent-based modeling provides a mechanism for simulating this type of evolution (Griffin, 2003). In modeling the emergent behavior, we assume that individual child attributes influence the quality and subsequent likelihood of peer interactions. It is framed around a state transition model, where a child is always in one of four states: (1) playing with another child; (2) playing with an adult (a teacher); (3) playing alone after (1); or (4) playing alone after (2). Early in our work it became obvious that solitary play, either (3) or (4), occupies about 20–25% of a child's time, and the propensity to enter and exit this state varies according to (1) or (2). Analyses comparing the simulated and the realized data indicate that the current implementation of PlayMate effectively captures the general formation of specific groups within the classroom (Griffin et al., 2004).

Our investigation of children forming playgroups incorporates the key assumptions, objectives, and goals of agent-based models. These fundamental features of an ABM are

- Abduction, rather than induction or deduction, is used to infer the plausible relationship between the artificial world created by rule-generated agent behavior and the real world.
- Putative theoretical assumptions are converted to a set of rules—a computer program—outlining the behavior of the agents to each other and the environment.
- Each agent possesses a strategy set that is invoked during the interaction with another agent; agent-to-agent interaction determines and is reciprocally influenced by the emergence of structure as agent and structures co-evolve within the environment.
- Multiple interactions among heterogeneous agents are studied to examine the emerging structures that evolve for the particular set of rules implemented by the agents.
- As exchanges and interactions occur in the simulation, agents and the rules they carry evolve, producing complex social processes analogous to those found in the real world.

Numerous books, articles, and Internet sources are available that detail the theoretical, methodological, and controversial aspects of ABMs. Good introductions are offered by Casti (1997); Conte, Hegselman, and Terna (1997); Epstein and Axtell (1996); Gilbert and Troitzsch (1999); Holland (1995); Macy and Willer (2002); and Rocha (1999). More advanced works include those of Axelrod (1997) and Kohler and Gumerman (2000), and in addition, there is an excellent e-journal (Journal of Artificial Societies and Social Simulation, http://jasss.soc.surrey.ac.uk/JASSS .html) and Web site (http://www.econ.iastate.edu/ tesfatsi/ace.htm, hosted by Leigh Tesfatsion).

Well-developed areas that use agent-based modeling include political science (e.g., Cederman, 1997), economics (e.g., Tesfatsion, 1997) biology (e.g., Camazine et al., 2001) and anthropology (e.g., Kohler & Gumerman, 2000). For example, and very relevant to the work described herein, is the work by Alam (in press) who is using this methodology to compare network dynamics in Eastern (South Asian subcontinent) and Western families. Similarly relevant is the work by Todd and colleagues (e.g., Simão & Todd, 2003), who have modeled mate selection scenarios using agent-based modeling. These works represent the forefront of the incorporation of family dynamics into social science research.

What is an Agent?

Agent Properties. An agent is a small piece of computer code—an algorithm—that has agency. These encapsulated algorithms, acting as unique and discrete entities, typically have (1) a memory, (2) a goal, and (3) a set of action rules. In general, an agent is capable of independent action (i.e., they are autonomous)—providing the mechanism for achieving a goal—and this requires possessing a representation of their current or immediate past states (i.e., memory). With a goal and memory they respond by modifying their behaviors, and in turn, the environment is modified by their response. This cycle of assess, respond, and evolve continues ad infinitum. With multiple agents acting collectively, the investigator is able to generate representations of social processes. These processes, the resultant modifications of the agents, and their reciprocal relationship to each other and the environment are considered a proxy to the actual mechanisms observed in real systems.

The agent is the critical distinction between the agent-based approach and other computer simulation methods. In traditional simulation methods (e.g., equation-based models), the propensities to engage in an act or invoke a behavior usually reflect processes implemented through variable-based differential equations (see Parunak, Savit, & Riolo, 1998). The investigator constructs these equations, and any variation in outcome occurs by varying the variable parameters embedded in the formulae. Agents, on the other hand, having rule-constructed autonomy, interact and collectively produce an outcome. And consistent with complex social processes, variability is the rule, not the exception. More importantly, the investigator does not control outcome by manipulating variables but instead allows agents to respond to local information via rules, and their collective response generates the outcome. This assumption that emergent behavior results from decentralized processes composed of local interactions among constituent agents is the most frequently cited reason for the appropriateness of agent-based modeling of complex systems.

Of course, the critical feature is the putative assumptions linking observed data and simulated data. If the simulated data approximates realized data, then the model is a candidate for explicating plausible pathways to the observed outcome. However, despite the prowess often ascribed to ABMs, prediction is not the objective. Instead, the analyst seeks to construct an ensemble of robust, theoretically plausible models that capture the dynamism inherent in micro-social evolution (Bankes, 2002). It is through the process of developing the ensemble that the researcher grasps the nuances of how slight variations in the implementation of rules across agents contributes to the manifest outcome at each run.

Relevance to Health & Families

Much of the work in this handbook discusses the dynamic reciprocal relationship between individual family members and the course and duration of an illness within a family member. Agent-based modeling allows the investigator to construct a representation of the process theorized to associate disease manifestation, familial response, and disease trajectory. Having this ability allows the researcher to systematically vary those components of the theory or model thought to influence the illness, and as the variations alter the disease trajectory, these changes can be compared to those observed in empirical data. The preeminent feature of this type of modeling is the ability to imbue each agent with a distribution of characteristics and rule-based behavior hypothesized to be critical to the evolution of disease within a network of family members, or even a network of families that share a disease within a delimited environment. For example, this implies that the trajectory of a disease is influenced not only by the immediate family members, but the influence extends to other relevant families who share a disease and have contact with each other; that is, a network is formed, and its formation modifies its constituents (Note: these would be nodes or vertices in the network literature. See Barabási, 2002). Specifically, how a family responds to a disease is affected by what they see and hear from others about the disease, in particular, how others cope with the disease and its effects on their family members. This exchange of information within families and across families (and other sources such as physicians and the media) creates a dynamic environment in which the afflicted individual occupies a secondary niche in the evolution and meaning of the disease relative to the larger network. The primary feature in such a network is an aggregated phenomenon composed of differential responses of individuals in the environment to their interpretation of the meaning of the disease, and the sway of the idiographic response on the subsequent unfolding of the disease. This reciprocally generated unfolding can be modeled by having multiple agents, each responding to local information, generate actions thought to be representative of the population under study.

AN AGENT-BASED MODEL

As noted above, numerous texts and articles exist that provide clear overviews of agent-based modeling (see Gilbert & Troitzsch, 1999; Macy & Willer, 2002). To illustrate how ABMs are useful for studying the psychosocial context of disease, I have written a small model that simulates a two-year period of information acquisition, incorporation, and influence on the health of family members where one individual has a diagnosed illness. Of course, because it was developed only for illustrative purposes, I have incorporated numerous assumptions, and most are clearly noted. It is not, however, as fully developed as an ABM that an invested researcher would construct over multiple iterations of modification.

Model Structure and Objective

An agent-based model is constructed to assess the assumed rules underlying the process being investigated. It is assumed that interesting phenomena, generated through continuous iteration of the explicit rules defining the behavior among interactants, spontaneously emerge from the collective implementation of the rules. This description of ABMs contains two factors: rules and agents. Rules, reflecting the assumptions of the investigator, are made explicit and put in algorithmic form. Agents, as rule implementers, can be smart, somewhat smart, or simple. Most agent-based modelers prefer the latter condition, whereas most Artificial Intelligence (AI) modelers prefer smart agents. AI investigators try to develop agents that accomplish complex tasks at the individual level (e.g., robotics) using complex algorithms; conversely, the agent-based modeler uses the amalgamated consequences of very simple decisions (e.g., I will or will not go to work today), implemented by numerous agents, to produce complex social, psychological, and environmental processes (e.g., traffic flow based on individual decisions).

If we assume simple agents, then the intellectual task is rule development. Rules, in their simplest form, always direct the agent to take action X if Y conditions are met; the conditions being assessed are almost always at the local level, that is, in the immediate environment. These rule-resultant actions typically range from modifying spatial or temporal behavior in response to environmental cues (e.g., traffic flow, social interaction) to modifying the rules themselves. Stated differently, at its core, ABM is the collective action of hundreds or thousands of independently implemented if-then statements that use predominantly local information at each increment of time.

How might this be translated into a method to study illnesses and families? The first question would be, do I assume that the disease X is affected by psychosocial factors? Second, how does the psychosocial process occur; that is, what happens at the person-to-person level that permits or allows this process to be implemented? Third, can the answer to the second question be put in an algorithmic form as a rule for interaction between two or more agents? If we assume that all questions have been answered, and a skeleton set of rules has been developed that reflects the assumptions of the investigator, then attention would turn to the construction of the agent. The agent has to be able to carry out the rule(s). And if the rule(s) and the agent are simple, the dynamic process that emerges can be tractable; if either becomes too complex, the outcome is generally uninterruptible.

Objective

Create an agent-based model of the relationship between illness and stress. Let this relationship be modified by ecological feedback using agents (i.e., individuals within families) to distribute information. And finally, show plausible scenarios of illness outcomes across a network of families.

First Assumptions

Let the simulation consists of multiple families with each family containing one ill child between the ages of 6 and 12, where the illness condition can be mild and require only prophylactic measures to very severe and requiring occasional hospitalizations (e.g., asthmatic child; see e.g., Griffin, Cree, et al., 2002; Griffin, Parrella, Krainz, & Northey, 2002). The scientific objective is to model the reciprocal relationship between the disease morbidity and symptomatology and the psychological and physical manifestations of stress distributed among family members. We assume (1) the disease has a natural course that can be summarized by distribution of outcomes; (2) patient stress can modify those outcomes; (3) other family members influence patient stress; (4) other family members experience stress from an ill family member; and (5) stress derived from (4) increases psychological distress and susceptibility to physical illness among nonpatient family members.

Second Assumptions

For this simulation, assume that *physical health, psychological distress* (modeled as stress), and *reactivity to information* are categories characterizing each family member. These characteristics are modified by the ecology of the family. Modifications to the ecology are continuous and provided via *information* from outside the immediate family and distributed among family members. Let

information consist of three features, *perception of disease severity, cost,* and *inconvenience,* and assume all dynamically influence each characteristic simultaneously. Although estimates of cost and inconvenience are based on tangible economic or physical constraints, each also has a psychological component; this aspect of information about a disease is calculated relative to expectations, desires, and other sociopsychological features of living in a family with an ill individual. For example, a sense of cost reflects the dollar amount combined with the notion of how the money could have been spent elsewhere or having to change jobs because of better insurance benefits. Additional clarity and discussion of *information* is addressed below.

Any individual is equally likely to get information and bring it back into the family, and once brought into the family, it is equally likely to be distributed to all family members. Information about disease severity is obtained from two sources, physician and non-physician (i.e., other families, media). From whom information is most likely retrieved depends on time since diagnosis, perceived state of the illness, and perceptions about treatment effectiveness. Moreover, as time increases, families are more likely to meet, form networks, and distribute information (Watts & Strogatz, 1998). If we assume that the information is slightly less accurate coming from either the media or another family than from the physician, then the resulting health of the individual should decrease—especially if the individual getting the information is highly reactive. We are, in effect, proposing a simulation that examines the influence of an illness-based network on subsequent changes in the disease at the level of the individual via information exchange among the nodes of the network. Of course, it should be apparent to the reader that the aforementioned assumptions were constructed for illustration, and actual implementation would require other assumptions as needed to address theoretical questions pertinent to the research question.

What is Information?

Imagine a family as being encapsulated by a semi-permeable membrane, and the membrane allows such things as ideas, notions, and facts to enter and leave the family. These things are information, and families with an ill member use this information to assess the illness—especially its meaning within the family. (It is possible to conceptualize information entering a family in the Shannon (1948) sense, but for this illustration we will refer to it in the general, colloquial sense.) For the agent-based modeler, information—its source, composition, and content—provides the basis for rule construction. To construct rules, the modeler minimally needs to address the following: What is the mechanism of information influence in the family? Do we allow some proportion of the information content to be good, some neutral, and some bad? What action is taken in response to each type of information? Imagine a family getting some tidbit of information about the disease from some source on a weekly basis, and the content of the information affects perception and action within the family and modifies interaction with other families. For example, consider the following as prototypical of the content types:

- *Good:* good prognosis, insurance coverage, minimal doctor visits.
- *Neutral:* average for age and gender, some coverage, regular visits (in effect, this is a balanced condition—it could go either way depending on the other characteristics of the family).
- *Poor:* worsening condition or poor prognosis, no or inadequate insurance coverage, and frequent doctor visits or hospitalizations.

If we further reduce the content areas into their structural features, three themes emerge: perception of the illness severity, cost, and inconvenience. The latter two features are clearly related, but they also can differentially influence individual and family behavior, and thus uniquely modify the influence of the disease on the family. Although information is composed of three features, perceived severity of the condition is most likely to be the source of inaccurate information, especially coming from other families.

Next, given the classification of information as delineated above, the modeler must decide on the basis of some theoretical assumption or empirical support how inter-agent rules might answer the following questions.

- How does idiosyncratic reactivity use information to modify stress?
- What is the numerical relationship between stress and health; as stress increases by x, health decreases by y?
- Is this ratio consistent across all family members?
- What is the relationship between family level stress and disease progression?

Answering questions such as those above allow the investigator to address the "what ifs" in his or her research domain, an opportunity not afforded researchers using traditional methodologies but a key feature of agent-based modeling (Axelrod, 1997).

Model Description

Allow each individual i to be characterized by a set of attributes $\epsilon = \{1, 2, 3 \ldots, x\}$, where $i \in l$ is the collection of all individuals. The set ϵ should be kept small, and include only those elements that are thought to be theoretically relevant, quantifiable, and interpretable. For this work, at least one element of ϵ should consist of an estimate of the *physical health* of the family member, and one element

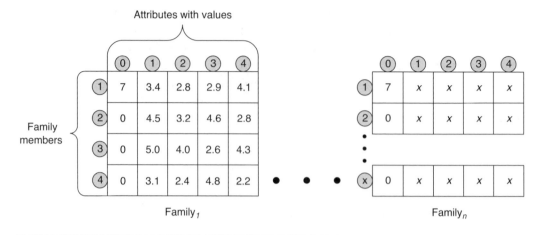

Figure 17.1   This illustration shows the structure of family-level matrices. Each row represents a family member and each column represents an attribute. Each cell within a column contains the associated attribute value for the family member. The value in the first cell of the first row indicates the illness level of the ill individual

should represent the *psychological distress* of that individual. The former is influenced by two factors: preexisting condition and response to psychological distress. *Distress* is determined by its preexisting level and modified by an indigenous general reactivity to health-related information. Information is an interpretation of the disease (e.g., mortality, morbidity, cost, inconvenience) that is generated either within the family or from the outside. Each family *f* is composed of multiple family members (between 2–5, randomly assigned) and $f \in F$, each family is in the set of all families. Thus an individual can be characterized as fi_e, that is, any individual can be viewed as being from family *f*, and having the set of attributes *e*. A $n \times m$ matrix represents a family; each row indicates the set *e* for family member *i*, and the column values reflect the magnitude of *e* across the family members. For our simple simulation, only one family member is designated as ill. This is indicated by a value > 1 in location 0 (i.e., column 1) of $e\{ \ldots \}$; the value also indicates time since diagnosis. For example, if the

ill member of the family was diagnosed with lupus seven months ago, the value in the first column in the first row of the matrix would be 7. An example of this matrix setup is illustrated in Figure 17.1. A matrix describes each family; Family 1–Family *n* can be represented by a collection of such matrices (see Figure 17.1).

To quantify change, and more importantly, to add stochasticity to individual responses within the simulation, a series of exponential distributions were constructed specifying the mean and the number of entries in each distribution. Means for each distribution were selected relative to the range of values used to initialize the attribute levels. *Small* effects are randomly drawn from an exponential distribution with a mean of .01 and 25 entries. *Moderate* effects are randomly drawn from an exponential distribution with a mean of .1 and 25 entries, and for *large* effects, the mean is 1.0 with 10 entries. These distributions are newly created on each invocation.

An important decision for the agent-based modeler given the structure detailed above is whether the individual or the family is the agent. Either choice is technically correct, but critical decisions about rules and outcome interpretation force the investigator to concentrate on one level or the other. It is generally best to focus on and construct rules for the most basic element in the system—the individual (see Conte, Edmonds, Moss, & Sawyer, 2001, for a good discussion). However, we are generating the model to demonstrate the ecology of the illness: the illness, the illness carrier, intra-familial influences on the illness, and information exchange within illness-defined networks. Consequently, model interpretations are at the macro level; we demonstrate the influence of rules on initial conditions (i.e., individual attribute sets) within each family and then examine the evolution of the illness as encapsulated by families. In essence, individual family members are the agents, but the scientific interest is how the illness is expressed in families over time.

Model Implementation

This agent-based model was constructed to illustrate the methodology and to be generic enough to allow the reader to envision how this type of modeling might be useful to his or her work. To aid explanation and convey a sense of realism, we assume the disease is childhood asthma. Asthma has increased dramatically in the past two decades (Air Pollution and Respiratory Health Bureau, 1996); its symptomatology is influenced by psychological factors including stress (Bender & Klinnert, 1998; Klinnert, 1997), and its presence affects family interaction (Griffin, Parrella, et al., 2002). These prototypic characteristics are not unlike other diseases reported in the literature, making it ideal for modeling.

At the beginning of each simulation run, 50 families are created, and individual-level attribute sets are filled with random values (range: 3.001–5.001) for health, reactivity, stress, perceived severity, cost, and

inconvenience. For the ill individual, time since diagnosis is randomly assigned to range 3–11 months, and is initialized to have, on average, a lower health score than other family members. Each simulation run is intended to estimate the effects of information—either perception of disease severity or cost or inconvenience—on the health of family members over a two-year epoch (104 weeks), where new information weekly enters the family via a randomly selected individual (see Figure 17.2).

An additional attribute, Physician Ratio, is also created that estimates the likelihood of soliciting or receiving information from a physician versus another family or media. It is assumed that the general propensity is to acquire more information from a physician than other sources. This relationship between physician versus other acquired information is given as a ratio ranging from 1 to 2; a value of 1 implies complete dependence on non-physician sources and 2 represents sole dependence on physician information. This variable reflects the perception made by family members that the health of the asthmatic child in their family is better or worse than comparable individuals; if worse, the ratio drops (non-physician information used), or if better, the propensity to adhere to physician-recommended protocols increases. In short, if the asthmatic child appears to benefit from traditional treatment relative to others, adherence continues; conversely, other sources are consulted (and valued) if the asthmatic child member seems below expectation or average.

How does it Work? Algorithm Outline

Rather than provide a detailed overview of the computer code generating the simulation, I provide a diagrammatic overview (see Figures 17.2 to 17.5) of what occurs during a typical simulation run. Again, the purpose of this simulation is to illustrate the methodology and is not based on a specific theory but simply reflects the intent of the author to show the usefulness of this tool. Additional or detailed information about the simulation can be obtained from the author.

Initially a family is drawn in a round robin fashion (this can be easily modified to selectively or randomly pick families), and a family member is randomly selected (see Figure 17.2). The selected person is knowledgeable about the illness level of the asthmatic child relative to others with a similar illness (acquired via physician and non-physician sources); this general impression is based on the health of the individual and the duration of the disease. Of course, the selected individual can also be the afflicted person. From this knowledge, the asthmatic child is categorized into one of three groupings: Severe, Moderate, and Good. These clusters provide approximate guidelines for how to respond to any received information. After being selected, this individual has equal opportunity (.33, randomly selected) to have received information about cost, inconvenience, or perceived severity of the disease. Notice that what is being modeled is not the content of the information but its influence on relevant individual level variables that, in composite, alter family dynamics.

Procedures outlined in Figure 17.3 are invoked if the information received is either cost or inconvenience. Depending on the level of disease category, one of the three methods of modifying either cost or inconvenience is implemented. (Since no theoretical reason is given to differentiate cost and inconvenience, their methods are the same; an investigator in this area could easily modify this assumption.) A couple of features are common across all the levels of categorization. First, effects are either normal or invoke extreme perturbations; these occur in a 9 to 1 ratio. On average, about 10% of the time, with a perturbation

the general magnitude of the effect is 10 times greater than the expected effect; this is indicated by the *large* versus *moderate* effect observed during 90% of the occurrences. The magnitude and derivation of *small, moderate,* and *large* are discussed above in the Model Description section. Beside the magnitude value in each box is the @ symbol followed by a fraction; this fraction indicates the probability of the action taken using the value being invoked with this magnitude. For example, a "moderate @ .5" indicates there is a 50% chance (on average) that this action will occur (either increase or decrease) using a value from the *moderate* distribution to modify the information source (i.e., cost or inconvenience).

It should be noted that the procedure discussed in this section typifies the action often used in agent-based modeling. Specifically, if X, then Y; in this case, for example, if information is cost and if the asthmatic child is categorized as severe, then 90% of the time the likelihood is .66 of increasing cost by a moderate value, compared to a .33 likelihood of decreasing the level of cost by a similar amount. Notice that the rule is deterministic but values used and the likelihood of invocation are probabilistically determined. This inherent variability is used to reflect the inherent ambiguities observed in complex biological systems (Camazine et al., 2001); agent-based models that deal with lesser complex agents or physical systems typically utilize less variability in response to action rules. In effect, with complex agents, the same environmental stimulus will have varying, though similar, responses across agents, and even with the same agent, given multiple exposures.

A second feature in Figure 17.3 is the symmetrical relationship between the Severe and the Good categories for cost and inconvenience. In general, the odds are greater that information about either cost or inconvenience will be associated with an increase in these

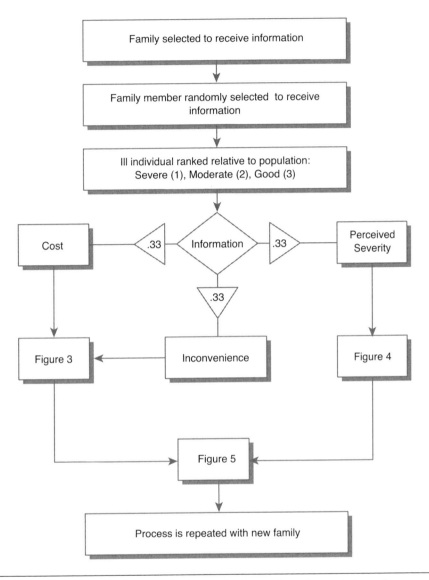

Figure 17.2 Diagrammatic overview of subject selection and routing path dependent on information type

attributes if the asthmatic child is in the Severe category; the situation is reversed for those in the Good category. Those individuals with an asthmatic child in the Moderate category experience about equal amounts of increases and decreases.

The value obtained from the process shown in Figure 17.3 is re-inserted into the attribute matrix of the individual selected. This value is subsequently used in calculating Stress level, and eventually Health (see Figure 17.5). If, instead of cost or inconvenience, incoming information addresses perceived severity, the simulation moves through the algorithm shown in Figure 17.4.

If the information is about perceived severity, the selected individual ignores the trichotomy seen in Figure 17.3, and to reflect the more general or gross perception typically associated with subjective information, the

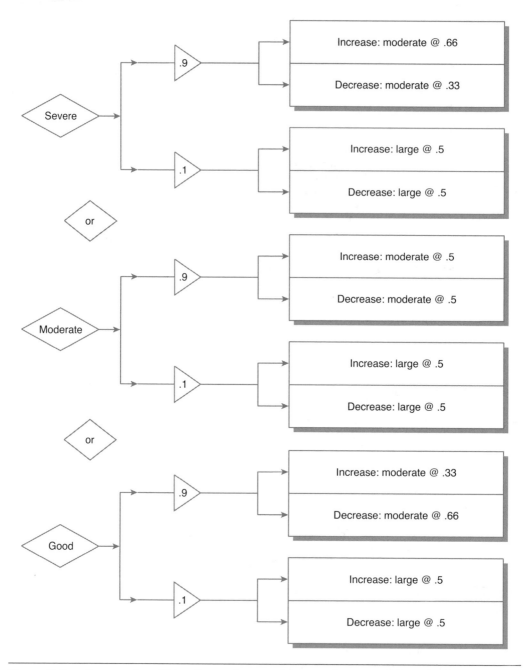

Figure 17.3   Process of modifying Cost or Inconvenience as a function of illness level

asthmatic child of the family is simply viewed as better or worse than most asthmatic children. Technically, the asthmatic child is determined to be below or above the mean for all asthmatic children in the simulation pool; this dichotomy is used to determine the action of the agent. Although current implementation assesses all asthmatic children, who gets compared to whom can be easily modified depending on researcher objective or theoretical tenets (e.g., those with similar family composition or access to health care). In the initial section of Figure 17.4, the "Above | Below Mean Ill" diamond shows the odds and distribution used to increase or decrease the perceived severity value as a function of distributional location of the asthmatic child relative to the larger network of families. The vertical bar symbol (|) indicates values associated with change above | below the mean. The newly modified perceived severity value is then entered into the calculation of the Physician Ratio. It is assumed that the subjective impression of severity modifies from whom subsequent information is solicited— either the physician or another source.

Unlike cost or inconvenience, perceived severity, being more personal, is uniquely bound to reactivity. Moreover, as structured in this simulation, the absolute value of severity has less impact than its level of change per information intake. This change, along with the change induced in the Physician Ratio, is used to calculate the new value of reactivity (most of the time, probability = .95 that this procedure will be invoked). These summed change scores are then divided by values associated with the trichotomy shown in Figure 17.3 (i.e., Severe = 1; Moderate = 2; Good = 3); those in the Good category are influenced least by new information-induced change (i.e., divided by 3) whereas those in the Severe group are most reactive to information. Score derivation for Reactivity can be seen in the section associated with the "Reactivity" diamond in Figure 17.4.

After calculating the effect of the respective information source, and adjusting Reactivity level, the simulation begins its estimation of Health and Stress. Because simple rules manifest through a complex dynamical system make interpretation of any single rule difficult, it is imperative to use simple estimation methods for critical attributes. Consequently, interpretation of the effects of modifying rules can only be understood if the rules are simple

and the output (i.e., attribute score) is decipherable. Stress, for example, combines all sources of information and adds variability via stochastic noise (i.e., inconsistent responses that have some regularity; see Figure 17.5). Of course, what constitutes stress and how its elements combine is dependent on investigator assumptions and justification. In this simulation, cost and inconvenience are multiplied and their reciprocal taken, producing a fraction; the inverse of the fraction is taken and multiplied by Reactivity. And then noise is added. Although this simple formula includes all sources of information, it separates the influence of perceived severity by using Reactivity. Recall that Reactivity is composed of changes in Perceived Severity and Physician Ratio.

After Stress is determined, its influence on Health is estimated, reflecting, of course, the assumption that Stress and Health are interdependent. Again, the estimation of influence is kept simple: if Stress goes up, Health goes down, and vice versa. Note the implications of this: with Health being modified for the particular person selected—and that person may or may not be the asthmatic child—the average health of the family, and possibly the ill child, is altered. Another family is then selected and the process begins anew. In the next iteration, the actions of the subsequent family are, in part, determined using this modified health value to classify their predicament (e.g., Severe, or Above the mean) relative to others in the network.

ILLUSTRATION OF RESULTS

Because of the complexity in the data and the volume of numerical output, investigators using this methodology depend on visual tools to interpret the effects of rules and rule changes, at least in the initial stages of model development. These visual tools usually consist of two- or three-dimensional graphs

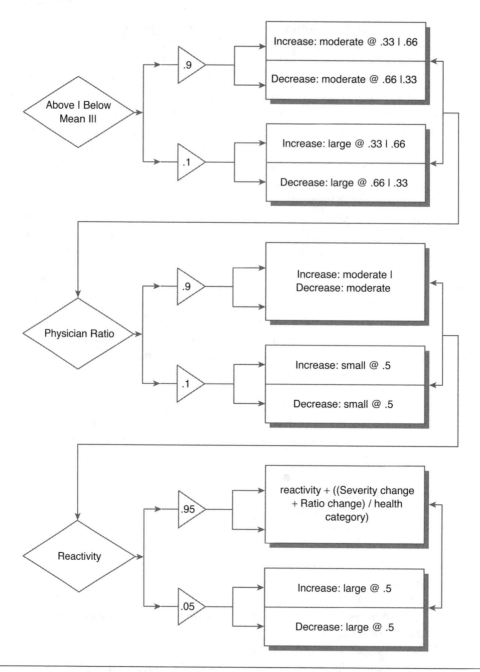

Figure 17.4   Process modifying Perceived Severity, Physician Ratio, and Reactivity dependent upon the health of the ill individual

and animations (Griffin, 2000); most agent-based modeling packages have a visual interface. Simulations always produce a lot of output. For example, using the current simulation, a typical 50-family run representing 2 years (104 weeks) produced 5,200 lines of data, each 9 columns wide. These data represent the average for each attribute (e.g., Health) per family. Depending on the needs of the investigator, it is possible to track

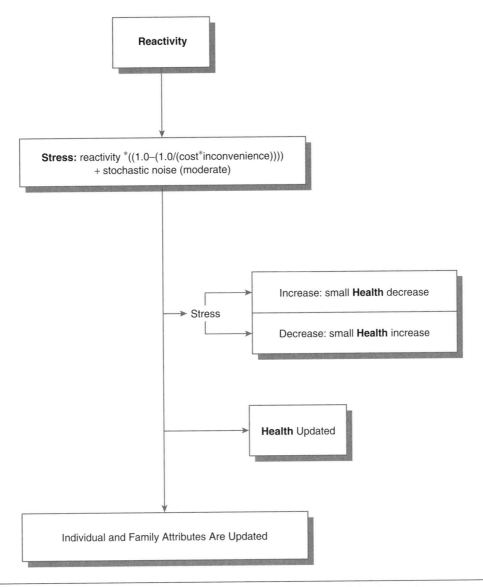

Figure 17.5   Construction of Stress and Health values for the selected family member

individual family members, but this would obviously expand the output. As was noted throughout the discussion and explanation of the model, stochasticity is added at multiple points where action is taken by the agent. Consequently, to estimate the influence of a rule, a rule change, or a formula, a collection of runs is needed to determine effects. In a simple illustration of the simulation described herein, five runs were combined into a single dataset. This 26,000-line dataset could be considered five independent implements of the same experiment. To get an accurate and confident appraisal of the model, combined runs of 25, 50, 100, or more are often needed depending on the variability in the model, rule complexity, and interpretability of output. Since these simulations were intended to introduce the methodology of agent-based modeling, no testing was done on the inherent

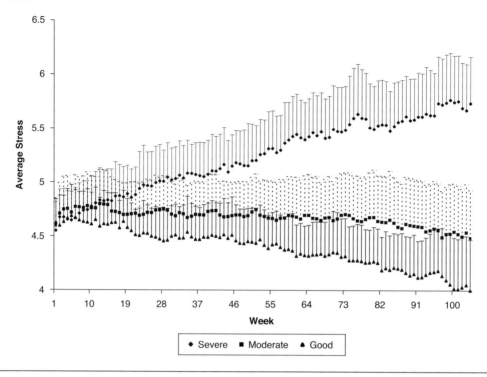

Figure 17.6   Simulated family level Stress and standard deviation upper bounds averaged over 5 runs

assumptions built into the model nor were any hypotheses forwarded.

A central tenet underlying the construction of this illustrative simulation model, and this book, is the assumed relationship between the illness of a family member, its ubiquitous influence on stress among all family members, and the reciprocal relationship between stress and health. To examine this relationship, we first look at the averaged family Stress levels as a function of the health category of the ill child (see Figure 17.6). Data in Figure 17.6 show the estimated average family stress levels over a two-year period; upper standard deviation bars are added to show variability. There are two noteworthy features about this plot: (1) all three groups show ample variability with considerable overlap, especially during the first year; (2) at about year two, families in the Severe category show increasingly higher rates of Stress, whereas families with members

in the categories of Moderate and Good show only minimal or modest declines in Stress. In other words, Stress across categories (e.g., Severe and Good) is asymmetrical; the high-risk group accelerates over time. Although this interpretation is general and speculative, from the perspective of agent-based modeling, it should be noted that these trends were evident even though individuals were not bound to a single category over time. In fact, in these data, about 20–25% of the ill individuals were in different health categories at the end of the two-year trajectory. This percentage would be higher if we consider the movement in and out of categories throughout the run. One of the primary strengths of agent-based modeling is this ability to visualize, interpret, and speculate about trends at the macro level. It allows the investigator to discuss general patterns that emerge from local rule-based (agent-level) interactions.

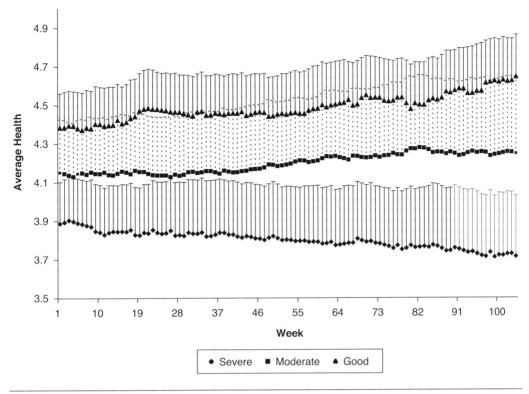

Figure 17.7 Simulated family level Health and standard deviation upper bounds averaged over 5 runs

Moving from Stress to Health, Figure 17.7 shows the average estimated Health of families across the three health categories. Figure 17.7 shows an interesting reversal from the Stress data. On average, families with an ill member in the Moderate and Good category show a very moderate gain in health whereas having an ill family member in the Severe category is associated with only a slight decrease in family health. More importantly, all groups, especially families with an ill member in the Moderate category, show a wide range of variability. In effect, differences appear to be minimal, but it is better for the health of the family if the asthmatic child is categorized as Moderate or Good relative to other asthmatic children in the network.

Next, it is apparent from Figure 17.8 that the averaged Health score for the asthmatic child follows a pattern similar to average family Health seen in Figure 17.7. This is not surprising; the only major difference is the magnitude of the average standard deviation— only among individuals in the Moderate category is there a wide range of variability. Although the findings shown in Figures 17.7 and 17.8 are somewhat intuitive, it should be reiterated that these are simulated—not empirical—data. They reflect the conceptualization and algorithmic implementation of the process envisioned by the investigator, and yet they map onto a pattern that is interpretable and similar to processes thought to exist within real families.

Finally, it is possible to follow the attribute trajectory of a single individual or agent over the course of the simulation. In Figure 17.9, all attributes are shown for one asthmatic child followed over a two-year period.

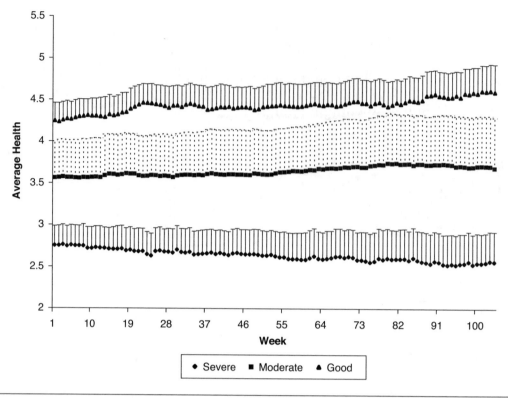

Figure 17.8   Simulated asthmatic child Health and standard deviation upper bounds averaged over 5 runs

Although this graph is crowded and a little messy because we are trying to convey too much information in a single visual representation, all relevant attributes were retained to illustrate the complex intra-individual interactions among the sources of influence for a single person. This is only a small portion of the dynamics that occur in this constructed world. We have, for example, ignored the immediate family and the other families in the network. Imagine that to visually capture the complexity of influences upon this individual we would need a complete representation of the network with all of its interconnections showing changes over time and how each family influences another, and another, and another, and so on—all reciprocally. The reader is encouraged to examine the details of Figure 17.9; its prototypical inter-associations among the

assorted attributes provide bountiful fuel for speculation and interpretation. Note, for example, that although the child began the year in the Moderate category of health (2), he or she quickly moved to the Good category (3) as Cost and Inconvenience dropped. However, very soon thereafter Perceived Severity and Reactivity began to move upward, roughly corresponding to the variability in Stress, and concurrent with a downward slide in Health. It should be remembered that any individual in any simulated family can be examined in the detail of Figure 17.9; however, the purpose of simulations is not to examine the trajectory of a single agent but to examine the collective consequences of implementing the basic rules that determine the behavior of the agent. Interpretation should be at the level of families and networks.

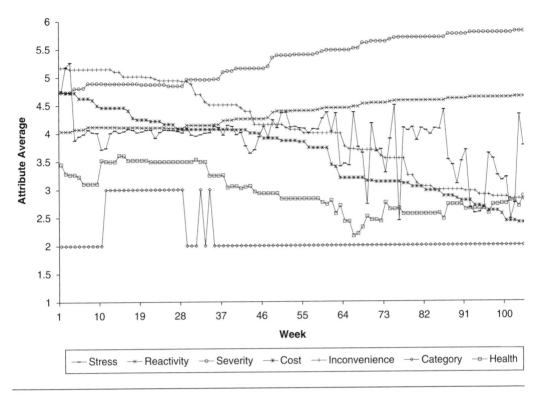

Figure 17.9   This illustrates the trajectory of major attributes for a single simulated asthmatic child over a two-year period

DISCUSSION

This chapter sought to introduce the methodology of agent-based modeling to investigators interested in studying the influence of complex social interactions on the course of a disease. At first blush, an ABM appears as complex as the phenomena that it tries to model; however, when reduced to its constituent parts, this methodology is a simple computational and logical extension of the theoretical shifting seen among social and behavioral scientists for decades. Specifically, science has moved beyond the belief in linear processes and simple explanations for complex social phenomena (Fogel, Lyra, & Valsiner, 1997; Newell & Molenaar, 1998). For the behavioral scientist using an ABM, this implies two concrete changes in studying process. First, instead of broad strokes of

intuition being used to interpret change processes, the researcher is forced to specify the details of interaction among the smallest units under study: individuals. *And these specifications must be simple.* Second, individuals are secondary to the process engendered by the implementation of actions taken collectively. In effect, it is the process that carries the scientific information and not the individual.

What does this imply for a social scientist wanting to learn agent-based modeling? Initially, the investigator must have an idea of *how* processes occur, or at least how they think they occur, among the individuals in the population of interest. In its simplest form, this would be: if *X*, then *Y*. Next, learn how to implement this {If : Then} statement in a computer program that simulates conditions consistent with the research question. The author, for example, used Python (http://www.python.org), a high-level scripting language, to write the simulation program used in this chapter, but writing your own program is not feasible or necessarily desirable for most investigators. Unlike several years ago, there are currently numerous programs available; most are free or open-source, and range from simple (e.g., Wilensky, 1999) to complex (e.g., Collier, 2002; Swarm (http://www.swarm.org); Ascape (http://www.brook.edu/es/dynamics/models/ascape/); MadKit (http://sourceforge.net/projects/madkit); or MASON (Luke, Balan, Panait, Cioffi-Revilla, & Paus, 2003)). Although these can be implemented off-the-shelf, most are on the complex end of the continuum and quick use of the program may require access to someone with computer programming expertise. However, once the program is constructed and running, the investigator can continuously ask "what if" questions by changing agent and environmental scenarios, modifying agent rules, and comparing simulated outcomes to actual data.

REFERENCES

Air Pollution and Respiratory Health Bureau, Division of Environmental Hazards and Health Effects, National Center for Environmental Health, Centers for Disease Control. (1996). Asthma mortality and hospitalization among children and young adults–United States, 1980–1993. *Morbidity and Mortality Weekly Report, 45*(17), 350–353.

Alam, S. J. (in press). On understanding the complex behavior of an Eastern family network. In M. North & D. Sallach (Eds.), *Proceedings of the workshop on social agents: Challenges in social simulation.* Chicago: University of Chicago & Argonne National Laboratory.

Axelrod, R. (1997). *The complexity of cooperation: Agent-based models of competition and collaboration.* Princeton, NJ: Princeton University Press.

Bankes, S. (2002). Tools and techniques for developing policies for complex and uncertain systems. *Proceedings of the National Academy of Sciences, 99*(3), 7263–7266.

Barabási, A. L. (2002). *Linked: The new science of networks.* Cambridge, MA: Perseus.

Belew, R. K., & Mitchell, M. (1996). *Adaptive individuals in evolving populations: Models and algorithms.* Reading, MA: Addison-Wesley.

Bender, B., & Klinnert, M. D. (1998). Psychological correlates of asthma severity and treatment outcome in children. In H. Kotses & A. Harver (Eds.), *Behavioral contributions to the management of asthma* (pp. 63–88). New York: Marcel Dekker.

Borgelt, C., & Kruse, R. (2000). Abductive inference with probabilistic networks. In D. M. Gabbay & R. Kruse (Eds.), *Handbook of defeasible reasoning and uncertainty management systems: Vol. 4. Abductive reasoning and learning* (pp. 281–314). Dordrecht, NL: Kluwer.

Brown, T. (2004). *Research interests.* Retrieved December 4, 2004, from www.infiniteworld.org

Burman, B., & Margolin, G. (1992). Analysis of the association between marital relationships and health problems: An interactional perspective. *Psychological Bulletin, 112,* 39–63.

Camazine, S., Deneubourg, J., Franks, N., Sneyd, J., Theraulaz, G., & Bonabeau, E. (2001). *Self-organization in biological systems.* Princeton, NJ: Princeton University Press.

Casti, J. L. (1997). *Would-be worlds: How simulation is changing the frontiers of science*. New York: Wiley.

Cederman, L. E. (1997). *Emergent actors in world politics: How states and nations develop and dissolve*. Princeton, NJ: Princeton University Press.

Cohen, S., Miller, G. E., & Rabin, B. S. (2001). Psychological stress and antibody response to immunization: A critical review of the human literature. *Psychosomatic Medicine, 63,* 7–18.

Collier, N. (2002). *RePast: An extensible framework for agent simulation*. Retrieved December 4, 2004, from http://repast.sourceforge.net/projects.html

Conte, R., Edmonds, B., Moss, S., & Sawyer, K. R. (2001). Sociology and social theory in agent-based social simulation: A symposium. *Computational & Mathematical Organization Theory, 7,* 183–205.

Conte, R., Hegselmann, R., & Terna, P. (1997). *Simulating social phenomena*. Berlin: Springer.

Deneubourg, J. L., et al. (1989). The blind leading the blind: Modeling chemically mediated army ant raid patterns. *Journal of Insect Behavior, 2,* 719–725.

Epstein, J. M., & Axtell, R. (1996). *Growing artificial societies: Social science from the bottom up*. Cambridge, MA: Brookings Institution/MIT Press.

Fogel, A., Lyra, M. C., & Valsiner, J. (1997). *Dynamics and indeterminism in developmental and social processes*. Mahwah, NJ: Erlbaum.

Franks, N. R. (1989). Army ants: A collective intelligence. *American Scientist, 77,* 139–145.

Gilbert, N., & Troitzsch, K. G. (1999). *Simulation for the social scientist*. Buckingham, UK: Open University Press.

Greene, S., & Griffin, W. A. (1998). The influence of marital satisfaction on symptom expression in Parkinson's disease. *Psychiatry, 61,* 35–45.

Griffin, W. A. (2000). A conceptual and graphical method for converging multisubject behavioral observational data into a single process indicator. *Behavior Research Methods, Instruments, and Computers, 32*(1), 120–133.

Griffin, W. A. (2003, April). *Agent-based models and computer simulation as a methodological aid for the study of micro-social behavior*. Paper presented to the Society for Research in Child Development, Tampa, FL.

Griffin, W. A., Cree, W., Martin, C., Fabes, R., & Hanish, L. (2002, May). *Emergent structure in children's play group formation*. Paper presented at Lake Arrowhead Conference on Computational Social Science and Social Complexity, University of California at Los Angeles Center for Human Complex Systems, Lake Arrowhead, CA.

Griffin, W. A., Hanish, L. D., Martin, C. L., & Fabes, R. A. (2003, October). *Modeling playgroups in children: Determining validity and veridicality*. Paper presented at the Agent 2003 Conference on Challenges in Social Simulation, Chicago, IL.

Griffin, W. A., Hanish, L. D., Martin, C. L., & Fabes, R. A. (2004). Modeling playgroups in children: Determining validity and veridicality. In M. North & D. Sallach (Eds.), *Proceedings of the workshop on social agents: Challenges in social simulation* (pp. 93-111). Chicago: University of Chicago & Argonne National Laboratory.

Griffin, W. A., Martin, C., Fabes, R., Hanish, L., Anders, M., Leonard, S., et al. (2003, March). *A multi-agent computational model of the evolution in children's playgroup formation*. Paper presented at the Lake Arrowhead Conference on Computational Social Science and Social Complexity, University of California at Los Angeles Center for Human Complex Systems, Lake Arrowhead, CA.

Griffin, W. A., Parrella, J., Krainz, S., & Northey, S. (2002). Behavioral differences in families with and without a male asthmatic: Beyond the psychosomatic family model. *Journal of Social and Clinical Psychology, 21*(3), 223–252.

Hannon, B., & Ruth, M. (1997). *Modeling dynamic biological systems.* New York: Springer.

Holland, J. H. (1995). *Hidden order: How adaptation builds complexity.* Reading, MA: Addison-Wesley.

Kiecolt-Glaser, J. K., & Newton, T. (2001). Marriage and health: His and hers. *Psychological Bulletin, 127*(4), 472–503.

Klinnert, M. D. (1997). The psychology of asthma in the school-aged child. In P. F. Kernberg & J. R. Bemporad (Eds.), *Handbook of child and adolescent psychiatry: Volume II. The school-aged child: Development and syndromes* (pp. 579–594). New York: John Wiley.

Kohler, T. A. (2000). Putting social sciences together again: An introduction to the volume. In T. Kohler & G. Gumerman (Eds.), *Dynamics in human and primate societies* (pp. 1–18). New York: Oxford University Press.

Kohler, T. A., & Gumerman, G. J. (Eds.). (2000). *Dynamics in human and primate societies.* New York: Oxford University Press.

Lipton, P. (1991). *Inference to the best explanation.* London: Routledge.

Luke, S., Balan, G. C., Panait, L., Cioffi-Revilla, C., & Paus, S. (2003). *MASON.* George Mason University Center for Social Complexity. Retrieved December 1, 2003, from http://socialcomplexity.gmu.edu/ and http://cs.gmu.edu/~eclab/

Macy, M. W., & Willer, R. (2002). From factors to actors: Computational sociology and agent-based modeling. *Annual Review of Sociology, 28,* 143–166.

Miller, G. E., Cohen, S., & Ritchey, A. K. (2002). Chronic psychological stress and the regulation of pro-inflammatory cytokines: A glucocorticoid-resistance model. *Health Psychology, 21*(6), 531–541.

Morrison, F. (1991). *The art of modeling dynamic systems.* New York: Wiley.

Newell, K. M., & Molenaar, P. C. (1998). *Applications of nonlinear dynamics to developmental process modeling.* Mahwah, NJ: Erlbaum.

Parunak, V., Savit, R., & Riolo, R. (1998). Agent-based modeling versus equation-based modeling: A case study and users' guide. In *Proceedings of workshop on multi-agent systems and agent-based simulation* (LNAI 1534, pp. 10–25). Berlin: Springer.

Rocha, L. M. (1999). *From artificial life to semiotic agent models.* LANL Technical Report: LA-UR-99-5475.

Sapolsky, R. M. (1998). *Why zebras don't get ulcers: An updated guide to stress, stress-related diseases, and coping.* New York: Holt.

Shalizi, C. R. (in press). Methods and techniques of complex systems science: An overview. In T. S. Deisboeck, J. Y. Kresh, & T. B. Kepler, (Eds.). *Complex systems science in biomedicine.* Dordrecht, NL: Kluwer.

Shannon, C. E. (1948). A mathematical theory of communication. *Bell System Technical Journal, 27,* 379–423, 623–656.

Simão, J., & Todd, P. M. (2003). Emergent patterns of mate choice in human populations. *Artificial Life, 9,* 403–417.

Sole, R. V., Bonabeau, E., Delgado, J., Fernandez, P., & Marin, J. (2000). Pattern formation and optimization in army ant raids. *Artificial Life, 6*(3), 219–226.

Tesfatsion, L. (1997). How economists can get a life. In W. B. Arthur, S. Durlaf, & D. Lane (Eds.), *The economy as an evolving complex system II* (pp. 533–564). Reading, MA: Addison-Wesley.

Vitaliano, P. P., Zhang, J., & Scanlan, J. M. (2003). Is caregiving hazardous to one's physical health? A meta-analysis. *Psychological Bulletin, 129*(6), 946–972.

Watts, D. J., & Strogatz, S. H. (1998). Collective dynamics of "small-world" networks. *Nature, 393,* 440–442.

Wilensky, U. (1999). *NetLogo.* Center for Connected Learning and Computer-Based Modeling, Northwestern University, Evanston, IL. Retrieved December 5, 2004, from http://ccl.northwestern.edu/netlogo

Zautra, A. J. (2003). *Emotions, stress, and health.* Oxford, UK: Oxford University Press.

CHAPTER 18

Research on the Historical Demography of Families and Health

GERALDINE P. MINEAU, KEN R. SMITH, AND LEE L. BEAN

Demographic studies of health, morbidity, and survival, with rare exception, ignore the reciprocal effects of family on health and health on family. The reason for this limitation is that demographic statistics for mortality are based on individual events that are aggregated into general categories representing individual characteristics, such as gender, age, or geographic units. There are two critical caveats to this broad critical generalization. First, the analysis of marital status has been demonstrated in a wide range of studies to be related to mortality. Second, the past few decades have seen the development of extensive data resources using historical records within which the family is the central analytical unit. These historical data include family records organized as family or village reconstitutions or families appearing directly in genealogies. In addition, family history data have been extended through linkage to other records in order to extend the historical record into more current time periods and to add critical explanatory variables.

In this chapter, we use such a historical data set exploiting the inherent family structure to study the interaction of family and health where health is represented as the mortality (survival) experience within families. In the first section, we describe the Utah Population Database, highlight some examples of previous research and define the data that are used. In the second section, we study the effects of individual events on family structure. Specifically, we examine the stability or disruption of the family unit during the time when couples are having and raising children. Using patterns of infant mortality, childhood mortality, and maternal mortality over a long time period, we can examine the increasing likelihood that the families survived "intact" as health conditions improved. In the third section, we reverse our orientation to study the effects of familial events on the survival of both mothers and fathers. For example, we

AUTHORS' NOTE: We wish to thank the Pedigree and Population Resource funded by the Huntsman Cancer Foundation, University of Utah for providing the data and valuable computing support. The work was supported by NIH grant AG 12748 (Kinship and Socio-Demographic Determinants of Mortality).

examine the specific fertility characteristics that are associated with better survival of mothers and fathers at older ages and whether these patterns are similar over time.

UTAH POPULATION DATABASE (UPDB)

Our mortality studies draw upon the Utah Population Database (UPDB) for information on a range of family and religious characteristics and their influences on the risk of mortality over the past 150 years. The UPDB contains over seven million records. It includes the genealogies of the founders of Utah and their Utah descendants. These records were computerized in the mid to late 1970s (Skolnick, Bean, Dintelman, & Mineau, 1979) and have been linked to other data sets, including birth and death certificates, cancer records, driver's license records, census records, and records from the Social Security Death Index.

These genealogical records originated as "Family Group Sheets" filled out by members of the Church of Jesus Christ of Latter-day Saints (LDS or Mormon). These records were selected from the Family History Library of the LDS Church in 1975–76 and again in 1978–79, and computerized (see Bean, Mineau, & Anderton, 1990, pp. 70–74 for more explanation). The criterion for selection was that one or more family members was born or died on the Mormon Pioneer Trail across the western United States or in Utah. The purpose was to represent migrants to Utah and their Utah descendants. The initial settlements in Utah occurred in 1847, and the genealogy records for early migrants represent birth cohorts dating back to about 1760. These 170,000 Family Group Sheets (containing about 1.6 million individuals) have been linked across generations and, in some instances, the records encompass as many as seven generations. While these records may be similar to those available on the Web with *FamilySearch* or other publicly available genealogical databases, it is not the same database and it has been maintained as a resource only for biomedical and health research.

The UPDB is a dynamic database and receives annual updates for Utah births, deaths, cancer records, and driver's licenses. Several projects have computerized and linked older sets of vital records (Herman et al., 1997), and these data are now part of the UPDB. The database now includes approximately 1.8 million Utah birth certificates from 1947–2001 and 653,000 death certificates from 1904–2001. Much of the value of this resource depends on the ability to match records on individuals from two or more data sets, known as record linking, and create longitudinally linked data that are able to capture many events associated with an individual. These record linking activities have allowed quality control for demographic information and eliminated duplicate records in the genealogical data.

Studies in population genetics have shown that the population is relatively homogeneous genetically and has a low inbreeding rate that is similar to that of the U.S. population (Jorde, 1989; O'Brien, Rogers, Beesley, & Jorde, 1994). This can be attributed to a large initial founding population, high rates of immigration from diverse groups of outside populations, and active avoidance of close consanguineous marriage. These genetic studies indicate that the population represented in the UPDB is biologically representative of a broad spectrum of the U.S. population and Western and Northern European populations. This population is not representative of the entire population of Utah or heterogeneous subpopulations in the U.S.

The Utah Resource for Genetic and Epidemiologic Research (RGE) administers access to these data through a review process of the project proposal. The protection of privacy and confidentiality of individuals represented in these records has been negotiated with agreements between RGE and the data contributors. All research projects require approval from an Institutional Review Board and RGE Review Committee (Wylie & Mineau, 2003).

Death Information

Death dates and places are available from the genealogy whether the death occurred in Utah or in other states or countries and are nearly complete through the 1960s. Additional follow-up information comes from either the Utah death certificates or the Social Security Death Index that begins in the mid-1960s. That file provides death dates and places outside of Utah.

Fertility Information

Complete fertility histories are available in the genealogy, including the birth date and place of each child. Calculations of number of children, age at first birth, and age at last birth have been made from these records.

Religious Affiliation

The UPDB contains individual religious information relating to the LDS Church, specifically dates of baptism and endowment. Baptism occurs at about age eight and for converts it could be at any later age. Endowment is a "temple" religious rite that usually takes place early in adulthood before an individual goes on an LDS mission, at the time of a "temple" marriage, or later for converts and reactivated members. Individuals who have records containing either baptism or endowment dates (but not posthumously) are treated as affiliated with the LDS Church. Records in the genealogy that do not contain these dates are classified as having less or no affiliation with the LDS Church. Religious

commitment is based on a classification scheme developed by Mineau (1980) and Bean and associates (Bean, Mineau, & Anderton, 1983; Bean et al., 1990) using the timing of an important religious rite, endowment. Individuals who have records containing endowment dates before age 40 are treated as religiously committed to the LDS Church; all others are less committed or non-LDS members.

Occupational Information

For a portion of the sample, occupational data are available from Utah death certificates. Analysis is limited to marriages from 1875 and after where the rate of record linking between family records and death certificates was 67 percent. The linkage rate was lower (45%) for the earlier marriage cohort. Occupations were coded to the 1980 U.S. Census categories and assigned a socioeconomic status score based on Nam and Powers (1983).

PREVIOUS RESEARCH USING THE DATABASE

The representativeness of the genealogy file has been demonstrated in a variety of demographic studies on infant mortality (Bean, Smith, Mineau, Fraser, & Lane, 2002; Lynch, Mineau, & Anderton, 1985) that have compared Utah rates and patterns to other populations. Other studies have analyzed fertility (Bean et al., 1990), birth spacing (Anderton & Bean, 1985), and widowhood (Mineau, 1988; Mineau, Smith, & Bean, 2002).

We examined the widely held observation that recently widowed individuals have higher rates of mortality than their married counterparts. When we compared couples married in 1860–74 with those married in 1895–1904, we found that widowers have higher risks of death than their married counterparts at all ages and across time. However, widows in the earlier period had lower or comparable mortality rates, probably because married women experienced a higher risk of mortality associated with childbearing. It was only in the more recent marriage cohorts that young widowed women experienced a significantly higher risk of mortality. "Thus, the risks of mortality for widowed versus married have changed as adult mortality rates and causes of death have changed" (Mineau et al., 2002, p. 253).

INTACT FAMILIES: THE EFFECTS OF INFANT, CHILD, AND MATERNAL MORTALITY

In recent years, demographers have decomposed the classical western demographic transition theory to focus on two separate processes: the fertility transition marked by the decline of average family size and the mortality transition marked by systematic decline in overall mortality and its concomitant increase in average life expectancy. There are a number of competing theories offered to explain the Western European fertility transition, and central to many is a focus on family dynamics (Mason, 1997). The various microeconomic theories of contemporary fertility behavior subsumed broadly under the title of "new home economics" takes the family as the central theoretical focus. The reverse causal relationship, the consequence of declining family size on family relations, underpins many arguments related to the role of women (and in fewer cases, men) in the modern small family.

Less attention has been devoted to studies of the relationship between declining mortality and the family. Nevertheless, critical historical demographic studies in England have demonstrated that the classical image of the

extended family household is more myth than reality because high mortality rates limited the likelihood of survival of three overlapping generations. In addition, Kingsley Davis has argued marital dissolution from 1865 through the early 1970s in the United States was relatively constant, with the declining rate of early husband or wife deaths offset by rising divorce (Davis, 1972).

UPDB provides sufficient historical data to explore in significant detail the relationship between declining mortality and specific forms of family stability, defined in this study as the "intact family." Our analysis focuses on mothers and their children and poses the following question. Of women who commenced childbearing in 1865–69 through 1930–34, what is the likelihood that mothers and all of their children survive until all of the children reach age 16? Families meeting these conditions are defined as "intact families."

Three types of mortality are studied to measure changing levels of disruption of intact families: infant mortality, childhood mortality, and maternal mortality. In addition, we describe in general terms the implications of declining fertility because we have shown previously that the risk of infant mortality is related to the age of the mother, parity (number of births), and birth spacing (Bean, Mineau, & Anderton, 1992).

It is important to recognize that a family unit often will survive the death of one parent as well as the death of one or more children. The loss of a parent or a child will, however, change the basic structure of the family. It is the persistence of the basic family structure—albeit one modified with additional births of children—that is emphasized in this study. Therefore throughout we refer to the loss of a mother or child as *disrupting* the intact family.

This analysis is restricted to women who married only once and had at least one child. The sample is restricted further to those

Table 18.1   Percentage of Intact Families by Date of Mother's First Birth

Date of First Birth	Intact Families Percent	All Mothers Total
1865–69	31.1	3214
1870–74	31.8	3557
1875–79	31.4	4273
1880–84	34.9	4914
1885–89	37.2	5231
1890–94	39.9	5281
1895–99	46.2	5664
1900–04	50.1	6583
1905–09	57.4	6968
1910–14	60.6	7026
1915–19	66.1	7136
1920–24	70.8	7441
1925–29	77.0	7707
1930–34	80.8	7607

women whose children were born in Utah territory adjusted to current state boundaries or Utah after its federal recognition. There are 82,602 families that meet these criteria. The mother is used as the reference person for the family, and each mother is classified by the date when her first birth occurs. We refer to each of these groups of women commencing childbearing within a five-year interval as "fertility cohorts."

Data presented in Table 18.1 indicate that among our sample of women whose first birth occurred during the half-decade intervals of 1865–69 through 1880–84, approximately only one-third survived as intact families; that is, all children survived to age 16 and the mother survived until all children reached age 16. From 1885–89 onward, the percentage of intact families increases, yet among the women who began childbearing in the 1930s, approximately one of five families still experienced the loss of a child before the age of 16 or the mother died before each of her children reached age 16.

Deaths of Infants and Children

Data presented in Table 18.2 detail the disruption of intact families due to the loss of an infant who died in the first year of life and the disruption of intact families due to the loss of at least one child under the age of 16. The percentage loss of children includes infant deaths as well as deaths between ages 1 and 16. That is, the difference between the percentages of infant deaths and child deaths represents deaths between ages 1 and 16. Deaths of infants and children are counted regardless of the age of death of the mother in these tabulations. Maternal mortality certainly may not be independent of the early death of an infant, but for purposes of analysis the death of a mother before all children reach age 16 is treated analytically as a separate event.

Among the earliest fertility cohorts, approximately two out of three mothers experience the death of at least one child before the age of 16. It was common for women to experience the loss of two or more

Table 18.2 Percentage of Once Marrierd Mothers Experiencing the Death of Infants and the Death of Children Under Age 16, and Average Number of Children Ever Born (CEB), by Date of Birth of the First Child.

Date of First Birth	Died before Age 1 1 + Infants	Died before Age 16 1 + Children	CEB
1865–69	42.7	66.4	9.0
1870–74	42.0	65.8	9.2
1875–79	42.6	66.7	9.1
1880–84	40.8	63.2	8.6
1885–89	41.2	60.6	8.2
1890–94	38.9	57.9	7.7
1895–99	35.0	52.4	7.2
1900–04	32.2	48.3	6.8
1905–09	28.1	41.4	6.3
1910–14	25.3	38.0	5.9
1915–19	21.6	33.2	5.4
1920–24	19.2	28.4	4.7
1925–29	15.3	22.5	4.3
1930–34	13.3	18.7	4.0

Table 18.3 Estimated Percentage of Maternal Deaths by Time of Death and Date at First Birth

Date of First Birth	Time of Death After Last-Born Child			
	30 Days	30 to 60 Days	3 to 12 Months	Total
1865–69	5.2	0.5	1.8	7.5
1870–74	4.5	0.6	1.9	7.0
1875–79	4.3	0.6	2.2	7.1
1880–84	4.4	0.5	2.0	6.9
1885–89	3.9	0.7	1.7	6.3
1890–94	3.7	0.5	2.0	6.2
1895–99	3.4	0.7	1.9	6.0
1900–04	3.7	0.5	1.5	5.7
1905–09	3.0	0.4	1.6	5.0
1910–14	1.9	0.3	1.6	3.8
1915–19	1.4	0.3	1.6	3.3
1920–24	1.5	0.2	0.8	2.5
1925–29	1.1	0.2	0.5	1.8
1930–34	1.1	0.1	0.4	1.6

children rather than simply one (not shown). For example, 40.9 percent of the 1865–69 fertility cohort lost two or more children while 25.5 percent lost one only (Bean et al., 2002). This is not an unexpected finding in view of the fact that with an average of over nine births to women in these early fertility cohorts, all of the children would have been exposed to the same conditions accounting for high rates of infant and early childhood mortality—contaminated water and milk, for example. In addition, the larger the number of children in the family the greater is the possibility of contagion. Elsewhere we have shown that during periods of diphtheria epidemics, temporal clustering of children's deaths was not uncommon (Bean et al., 2002). We have also shown that the great flu epidemic of 1918, and the significant rebound in 1920 that was higher in Utah than in other states, slowed the long-term secular decline in infant mortality. Infant mortality rates did not rise with overall mortality rates during these flu epidemics because of its well-known more significant impact on adults and especially males (Kolata, 1999; Noymer & Garenne, 2000).

The gap between the proportion of infant deaths and children's deaths decreases across sequential fertility cohorts, but the proportion of deaths in the first year of life accounts for roughly two-thirds of all children's deaths regardless of the date of the fertility cohort. In addition, (not shown) as the proportion of families losing children declines, the proportion of families losing two or more children falls dramatically. For the 1930–34 fertility cohort, 11.1 percent of mothers experience the death of one child only and only 2.4 percent experience the loss of two or more children. A contributing factor to these changes is the fact that in this late fertility cohort, there are, on average, fewer children in the family exposed to risk. Yet more important may be the fact that morbidity and mortality risks declined substantially

with improved water supplies, more effective elimination of sewage, extensive immunization programs, and expanding access to medical facilities (Morrell, 1956; Richards, 1953). Of some interest is the fact that it was among the 1890–94 fertility cohort that the crossover occurred from the majority of disrupted families experiencing two or more deaths of children to the majority of disrupted families experiencing the loss of one child only. This is a critical time period. Women who initiated childbearing in the 1890s did so when prophylactic measures for diphtheria became available, and the state's first public health officer encouraged the development of improved water systems and immunization programs. Additionally, as Preston and Haines (1991) have documented, it was near the turn of the century when sanitary procedures became more common in American households.

The Early Death of Mothers

In the absence of reliable statistical information, some historians assume that maternal mortality was very high during the latter half of the 19th century in Utah. For example, Blanche E. Rose wrote in her study of early medical practices in Utah,

> Brigham Young, traveling over the vast expanses of his newly founded empire, could not but be impressed with the trials and tribulations of womankind generally, particularly when they must go down into the Valley of the Shadow of Death to bring forth the new citizens who were so badly needed to develop the land of Zion. (Rose, 1939, p. 28)

In the absence of cause of death data for our earliest fertility cohorts, we have estimated maternal mortality by calculating the number of mothers who die within one month, one to two months, and three to twelve months after the date of birth of the woman's last-born child.[1] We have summarized these maternal deaths across the fertility cohorts of 1865–69 through 1930–34 in Table 18.3.

Relative to the proportion of families disrupted by the death of children, maternal deaths account for few disruptions. Among mothers who began childbearing in 1865–69, 7.5 percent died within 12 months after the birth of their last child and two-thirds of those deaths occurred within 30 days of the birth of the last child. The proportion of family disruptions associated with estimated maternal mortality declines consistently over time from 7.5 percent to 1.6 percent of the 1930–34 fertility cohort.

Disruption of the family as defined in this study arises not simply from child mortality and maternal deaths shortly after the last births but also deaths among mothers before all surviving children reach age 16. The proportions of family disruptions arising from premature deaths of mothers—including maternal mortality as estimated—are presented in Table 18.4. If one considers orphanhood as the loss of at least one parent before a child reaches age 16, the data presented in Table 18.4 indicate extreme values yet minimal potential estimates of orphanhood because we do not consider the loss of fathers. Even with this minimal estimate, slightly more than one of five disrupted families will have at least one child under the age of 16 at the time the mother dies. Among the 1930–34 fertility cohort, 7.5 percent of the families experienced the early loss of the mother.

It is important to note that the proportions of family disruptions due to the death of children and the death of mothers are not additive. Many of the mothers who died before surviving children reached the age of 16 may have experienced an early death of a child. The important point is that the data presented in Table 18.4 confirms that the trend of family disruptions arising from a relatively early death of a mother is consistent with the trends evidenced in the data for child mortality. Nevertheless, for all fertility cohorts the proportion of disruptions due to the early death of a mother is much smaller than the disruptions arising from the death of a child. The difference is not unexpected because mothers, by definition, are survivors of the higher risks of mortality in infancy and early childhood.

Changes in Family Disruption

It is not possible to confirm exactly Kingsley Davis's assertion that the modern level of family disruption arising from divorce is the demographic equivalent of family disruption arising from high rates of parental loss, but our data confirm that family disruption was very common in the 19th century. Our analyses, however, consider family disruption not simply in terms of parental loss—death of mothers only in this study—but also family disruption due to the early death of children. In this broader view of family disruption, it is clear that the decline in family disruption began most dramatically late in the 19th century and accelerated during the first three decades of the 20th century. These changes parallel expansion of public health programs and the increasing adoption of sanitary procedures in households. These changes also reflect, in turn, a parallel decline in fertility—children ever born in Table 18.2. There were increasingly fewer births at very young and very "old" ages of mothers and increased intervals between births. These factors—early and late childbearing as well as short birth intervals—have been demonstrated in a variety of studies to result in increased risk of infant mortality primarily and maternal mortality secondarily (National Research Council, 1989). Yet one must also consider a reciprocal effect. During periods of high, uncontrolled fertility the early loss of a child removes the "protective" effect of lactation,

Table 18.4 Percentage of Mothers Dying Before All Surviving Children Reach Age 16 by Date of First Birth

Date of First Birth	Percent
1865–69	21.4
1870–74	21.6
1875–79	21.8
1880–84	20.8
1885–89	19.5
1890–94	19.9
1895–99	19.4
1900–04	18.3
1905–09	18.0
1910–14	15.1
1915–19	12.2
1920–24	9.0
1925–29	7.8
1930–34	7.5

resulting in reduction of the length of post-partum amenorrhea.

The importance of family size as a factor in infant and child mortality has been explored by examining the relationship between religious commitment and infant mortality, controlling for family size. In those analyses (data not shown), we assumed that active membership in the Church of Jesus Christ of Latter-day Saints provided certain health advantages due to the extensive network of Church-sponsored nurse midwives and community support. Using religious data as recorded in UPDB, we classified mothers in the study using procedures described above. Our analysis indicates that once parity—number of live births—is held constant there are no significant infant mortality rate differences among the religious groups. Loss of children increases with the number of children ever born, but religious differences are minimal regardless of the number of children ever born.

FERTILITY AND POST-REPRODUCTIVE LONGEVITY AMONG MEN AND WOMEN

Children affect the health of their parents. This fundamental association has long been recognized in humans and nonhuman species alike and for reasons directly related to child-bearing as well as child rearing. In this section, we examine how fertility behavior affects the life span of mothers and fathers after age 60. This section summarizes previous work described in detail by Smith, Mineau, and Bean (2002).

We know that individuals with greater access to social support have better health and lower levels of mortality (House, Landis, & Umberson, 1988; Ross, Mirowsky, & Goldsteen, 1990). Except for spouses, children are regarded as the most important component of an adult's social network (Logan & Spitze, 1996; Lye, 1996; Wolf, 1994). Assistance and resource exchange between adult children and their parents flow in both directions, but they largely migrate from parents to children. When the flow of resources (social support and income) moves from children to parents it is small for contemporary U.S. families (Hogan, Eggebeen, & Clogg, 1993) and pre-industrial societies (Lee, 1997). If children receive more resources than they provide to their parents, then the cost of children to parents may serve to reduce parental longevity. Of course, adult children are themselves rearing offspring of their own, which would serve to reduce the ability of adult children to provide instrumental support to grandparents. This argument suggests that during periods of natural fertility, parents with high parity will be adversely, rather than beneficially, affected since their own high-parity children will be devoting resources to their own child rearing.

Parents bearing their first children at younger ages are more likely to invest their limited economic resources in child rearing rather than in their own health, employment, or savings (Waldron, Weiss, & Hughes, 1998). This logic suggests that individuals bearing children later in life, with other things being equal, would also experience adverse health consequences given the extended period of time over which the demands of child rearing would accumulate.

Evolutionary biology provides a potentially useful addition to demographic analyses of the interrelationships between fertility and longevity. Evolutionary theory argues that there are trade-offs that each organism makes between investing resources into somatic or physical growth and investing in reproduction (Kirkwood, 1977). The idea of a trade-off between reproduction and longevity is called the disposable soma theory (Kirkwood, 1977). This theory predicts that for females, young age at first birth and high parity will be associated with a shorter post-reproductive life span because early or high levels of fertility exact high physical (somatic) costs to such mothers which, in turn, shorten women's lives.

Evolutionary scientists (Hamilton, 1966) have therefore theorized that forces that prolong the ages during which female reproduction occurs will postpone aging and increase female longevity. This line of reasoning suggests that increasing ages at last birth should be associated with greater post-reproductive female longevity.

Table 18.5 summarizes these perspectives in terms of specific predictions for the association between fertility and post-reproductive longevity.

The empirical evidence on humans is mixed for these predictions. Westendorf and Kirkwood (1998) reported that women listed in genealogies of the British aristocracy who survived to age 60 died earlier if they had higher parity and a younger age at first birth compared to women with fewer children and later ages at first birth. Doblhammer (2000) reported that women lived somewhat longer if they had few children and if their age at first birth occurred after age 20. Friedlander (1996) found that parous women had lower survivorship than nulliparous women, and among parous women, those with higher parity lived shorter lives than those with lower parity. Conversely, some investigators (Lund, Arnesen, & Borgan, 1990) reported that nulliparous women have lower survival than their parous counterparts. A positive association has been reported between late female fertility (Doblhammer, 2000; Perls, Alpert, & Fretts, 1997) or late menopause (Cooper & Sandler, 1998; Snowdon et al., 1989) and longevity.

Other factors may explain an association between fertility and post-reproductive longevity. Religion, socioeconomic status (SES), and secular trends in fertility and mortality may confound the association between longevity and fertility. Religious affiliation may also promote an association between fertility and longevity. Couples committed to the LDS Church, for example, are more likely to live longer (Enstrom, 1978, 1989) and to have more children (Bean et al., 1990) than other couples. A family's SES may also encourage an association between fertility and longevity. High-status marriages are more likely to experience lower levels of fertility and mortality. For women married in the latter half of the 1800s, their status is

Table 18.5 Predictions for the Association Between Fertility and Post-Reproductive Longevity

Reproductive Characteristic	Association with Post-Reproductive Longevity	Social/Economic Explanation	Evolutionary Biology Explanation
Age at First Birth	Positive	Older first-time parents will have invested more in their own economic status and employment before assuming parenting duties. More asset accumulation leads to better survival	In times of natural fertility, women who are less fecund and begin childbearing later may have genes that reduce fertility and that also increase longevity
Parity	Positive	Children provide labor when young and social support as adults	
	Negative	Wealth flows mostly from parent to child; children also have offspring themselves, which reduces their support	More resources invested in reproduction instead of personal health and physical growth
Age at Last Birth	Positive		Genes associated with late reproduction, suggesting more robust ovaries and later natural menopause, forecast slow rates of aging
	Negative	Extended period over which demands of child rearing would accumulate	

best represented by their husbands' SES; accordingly, we rely on husbands' SES in this analysis.

Finally, secular trends in fertility and mortality are considered. Our investigation spans an historical period that includes patterns consistent with natural fertility for the majority in the Utah population during the late 19th and early 20th centuries (Bean et al., 1990). Couples marrying from 1860–79 make up the earliest period in this study and reflect a period of natural fertility on a frontier while the marriage cohort of 1880–99 represents the beginning of the fertility transition.

Dataset

From the UPDB, 13,897 couples have met the following selection criteria and comprise our analysis sample. Monogamous couples were selected who married between 1860 and 1899. This time interval generally excludes childbearing during the well-known fertility decline of the Great Depression. Overall, the UPDB data on marriages established during the latter half of the 19th century are particularly advantageous for testing both social and evolutionary theories given that fertility control was limited and mortality risks later in life were relatively high. Cox proportional hazard rate models are estimated separately for husbands and wives.

Measures

The fertility variables addressed in this analysis include wife's age at first birth, total number of children born, wife's age at last birth, and total number of children who died before they reached age 18. Wife's age at first birth, age at last birth, and religious status were strongly correlated with the husband's values of these measures. We have elected to use the wife's values in both husband and wife equations. Wife's age at marriage is not used as it is strongly correlated ($r = 0.96$) with wife's age at first birth. Number of children, year of marriage, age difference between spouses, and number of deceased minor children are couple-level variables by definition.

For the fertility variables, we categorize individuals so that they fall into one of five percentile categories: below the 10th, between the 10th and 25th, the middle 50 percentage, between the 75th and 90th, and above the 90th. The middle 50 percent of the distribution was used as the control or comparison group. For wife's age at last birth, we further divided the highest percentile category into two categories: between 90th and 95th and above the 95th percentiles.

Results

The findings reported below are based on models that include measures of age at first and last birth, parity, year of marriage, age difference between spouses, mortality of offspring, and commitment to the LDS Church. Mean age at first birth was 21.73 for wives and 25.58 for husbands. Wives gave birth to their last child at a mean age of 40. Families averaged 8.24 children with 1.3 dying before the children reached age 18. Nearly 70% of couples are committed to the LDS Church. All models are based on Cox proportional hazards regressions and logistic regressions. Effects for each reproductive factor reported here are adjusted for the influence of the remaining reproductive measures.

Most of our findings are presented as survival curves that show the proportion of individuals who, having lived to age 60, are alive at each subsequent age. Comparing survival curves across groups with different fertility histories is a useful way to summarize a great deal of information. However, survival curves can look similar even when substantial differences exist. To illustrate this point, we present data on the survival among men and women in Utah for 1890. Gender is perhaps one of the best predictors for survival. In Figure 18.1, we see that women (the higher survival curve) live longer than men, as expected. If we look at the age at which half of the subjects have died for each gender, we find that the mean difference in life span between men's and women's survival is about 3.5 years. We take this as a representative measure of a large and well-established survival difference between two groups at the population level.

Age at First Birth. Age at first birth was not associated with female mortality. It was for male mortality but to a small degree.

Parity. Past age 60, women with fewer children experienced better survival than those with more children (Figure 18.2). Mothers with few children (1 to 3) lived an average of 1.6 years more past age 60 than mothers with average parity (7 to 11 children) and approximately 3 years more than mothers who gave birth to 15 or more children. Male survival was not associated with parity (Figure 18.3).

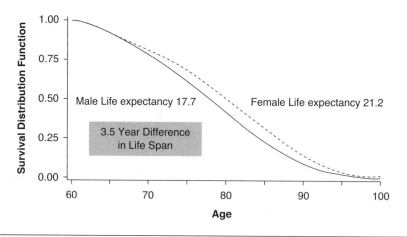

Figure 18.1 Survival Past Age 60 by Sex, Among Married Couples, Utah, 1890.

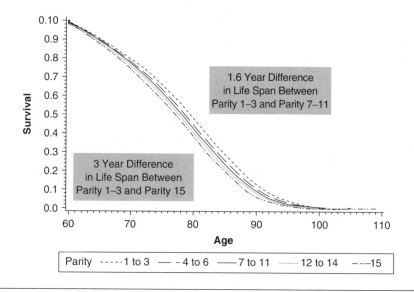

Figure 18.2 Survival Rates of Wives by Parity

Age at Last Birth. Mothers whose last birth occurred at age 46.5 or later (i.e., beyond the 95th percentile for the age-at-last-birth distribution) had an annual mortality rate that is 15% lower than women whose last child was born between ages 37.7 and 43.1 (i.e., the middle 50% of the age-at-last-birth distribution). These mothers who were fertile at advanced ages lived three years longer than mothers who ended childbearing at a young age (under 33.3) and about two years longer than mothers with modal ages at last birth (between ages 37.7 and 43.1) (Figure 18.4). There is suggestive evidence that men married to women who are fertile late in life experience some longevity benefits, but this association is substantially weaker than it is for women (Figure 18.5).

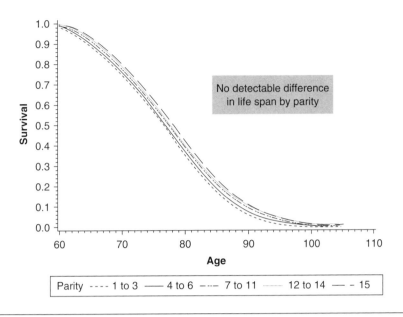

Figure 18.3   Survival Rates of Husbands by Parity

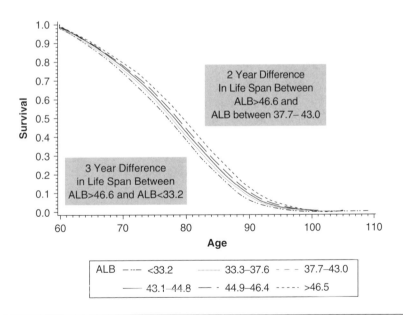

Figure 18.4   Survival Rates of Wives by Age at Last Birth (ALB)

Socioeconomic Status, Fertility, and Longevity. To address the possibility that socioeconomic status may account for the association between fertility and longevity, we incorporated husband's occupational status, measured from death certificates, into the analysis of both husbands' and wives' longevity. The influence of fertility patterns

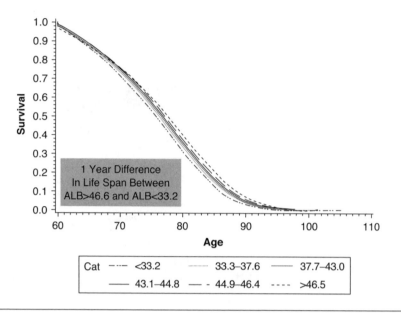

Figure 18.5   Survival Rates of Husbands by Age at Last Birth (ALB)

on maternal and paternal longevity is not affected by the introduction of statistical controls for husband's occupation.

Religion, Cohort and Longevity. We conducted this analysis by two broad marriage cohorts that reflect conditions during an earlier settlement period (married between 1860 and 1879) as well as a time when Utah became more economically developed with better transportation and infrastructure (married between 1880 and 1899). Survival is not affected by being affiliated with the LDS Church among women in either marriage cohort once fertility history is controlled for in the analyses. For men, affiliation with the LDS Church is significantly associated with better survival but only for the latter marriage cohort. This protective influence appears to extend to contemporary men in the United States (Enstrom, 1989).

Reproductive Experience and Longevity. For individuals surviving to age 60, identified in the UPDB during a period of natural fertility, we find mixed support for hypotheses that

link reproductive history with later-life longevity. The age at which individuals initiate childbearing had no impact on the longevity of fathers, controlling for parity and age at last birth. It is the latter reproductive behaviors that were strongly associated with longevity. For both parity and age at last birth, the association with survival was greatest for women. Specifically, as women increased their parity, they experienced death at younger ages. This finding supports the hypothesis that mothers with many children have devoted both physical and socioeconomic resources to their offspring, resources that could have been used to enhance a mother's own survival. Larger numbers of children do not create a bank of social support from which a mother can draw upon at older ages, in the hopes of lower mortality at older ages. Finally, we find support for the idea that fertility at advanced reproductive ages enhances female longevity, suggesting that slower ovarian aging is associated with overall aging. Other things being equal, women who bear children at late ages do not experience deleterious health effects, as indicated by their longevity.

CONCLUSION

Understanding the close association between family structure and the survival of individual family members tells us a great deal about the role that mortality plays in affecting social structure. We have shown how the intact family, with living parents and children, in the late 19th century was greatly affected by the death of infants and children, which were determined in large part by fertility patterns, the quality of life in pioneer Utah, and infectious diseases. The same reproductive behaviors that create large families and elevated infant mortality rates also adversely affect the "intact family" by increasing the risk of maternal mortality. The legacy of childbearing extends beyond the early and middle adult years to the latter third of the life span. With children fully grown, mothers, and to a lesser extent fathers, still encounter risks of reduced survival that can be attributed to bearing children. Even when parents and children survive intact so that all the children live to their late teens with living parents, the detrimental effects of having many children arises as the parents age into their elderly years. We showed that in some cases, a parent's fertility history foretells a rosy future, as is the case with women who bear children at advanced reproductive ages. In this instance, women who were fertile later in life lived longer. This life span dividend was partially shared by men married to such women. Moreover, siblings of these exceptionally late mothers also appear to benefit in terms of survival, suggesting a possibility that genes that promote late reproduction also elevate survival probabilities in later life.

Because genealogies provide data about family structure and family change spanning many generations, we continue to have the opportunity to examine how broader social changes affect family-level patterns in fertility and mortality. This type of information is needed for the study of kinship and its changes over time by focusing on the life course of an individual and the increments and decrements to her or his kinship network. It is possible to study the family circumstances into which a child is born, the survival of parents and siblings, the timing of marriage and fertility, and the proximity of relatives (Smith et al., 2002).

NOTE

1. One cannot compute normal maternal mortality ratios to compare with recorded ratios that became available after 1910 because we do not have an accurate count of the required ratio denominator, the number of all live births for all women.

REFERENCES

Anderton, D. L., & Bean, L. L. (1985). Birth spacing and fertility limitation: A behavioral analysis of a nineteenth-century frontier population. *Demography, 22,* 169–183.

Bean, L. L., Mineau, G. P., & Anderton, D. L. (1983). Residence and religious effects on declining family size: An historical analysis of the Utah population. *Review of Religious Research, 25,* 91–101.

Bean, L. L., Mineau, G. P., & Anderton, D. L. (1990). *Fertility change on the American frontier, adaptation and innovation.* Berkeley: University of California Press.

Bean, L. L., Mineau, G. P., & Anderton, D. L. (1992). High risk childbearing: Fertility and infant mortality on the American frontier. *Journal of Social Science History, 16,* 337–363.

Bean, L. L., Smith, K. R., Mineau, G. P., Fraser, A., & Lane, D. (2002). Infant deaths in Utah 1850–1939. *Utah Historical Quarterly, 70,* 158–173.

Cooper, G. S., & Sandler, D. P. (1998). Age at natural menopause and mortality. *Annals of Epidemiology, 8,* 229–235.

Davis, K. (1972). The American family in relation to demographic change. In C. Westoff & R. Parke, Jr. (Eds.), *U.S. commission on population growth and the American future: Vol. 1. Demographic and social aspects of population growth.* Washington, DC: Government Printing Office, Table 8.

Doblhammer, G. (2000). Reproductive history and mortality later in life: A comparative study of England and Wales and Austria. *Population Studies, 54,* 169–176.

Enstrom, J. E. (1978). Cancer and total mortality among active Mormons. *Cancer, 42,* 1943–1951.

Enstrom, J. E. (1989). Health practices and cancer mortality among active California Mormons. *Journal of the National Cancer Institute, 81,* 1807–1814.

Friedlander, N. J. (1996). The relation of lifetime reproduction to survivorship in women and men: A prospective study. *American Journal of Human Biology, 8,* 771–783.

Hamilton, W. D. (1966). The moulding of senescence by natural selection. *Journal of Theoretical Biology, 12,* 12–45.

Herman, A. A., McCarthy, B. J., Bakewell, J. M., Ward, R. H., Mueller, B. A., Maconochie, N. E., et al. (1997). Data linkage methods used in maternally-linked birth and infant death surveillance data sets from the United States, Israel, Norway, Scotland, and Western Australia. *Paediatric and Perinatal Epidemiology, 11,* 5–22.

Hogan, D. P., Eggebeen, D. J., & Clogg, C. C. (1993). The structure of intergenerational exchanges in American families. *American Journal of Sociology, 98,* 1428–1458.

House, J. S., Landis, K. R., & Umberson, D. (1988). Social relationships and health. *Science, 241,* 540–545.

Jorde, L. B. (1989). Inbreeding in the Utah Mormons: An evaluation of estimates based on pedigrees, isonymy, and migration matrices. *Annals of Human Genetics, 53,* 339–355.

Kirkwood, T. B. L. (1977). Evolution of ageing. *Nature, 270* (5635), 301–304.

Kolata, G. (1999). *Flu: The story of the great influenza pandemic of 1918 and the search for the virus that caused it.* New York: Farrar, Straus & Giroux.

Lee, R. D. (1997). Intergenerational relations and the elderly. In K. Wachter & C. Finch (Eds.), *Between Zeus and the salmon: The biodemography of longevity* (pp. 212–233). Washington, DC: National Academy Press.

Logan, J. R., & Spitze, G. D. (1996). *Family ties: Enduring relations between parents and their grown children.* Philadelphia, PA: Temple University Press.

Lund, E., Arnesen, E., & Borgan, J. K. (1990). Patterns of childbearing and mortality in married women: A national prospective study from Norway. *Journal of Epidemiology and Community Health, 44*(3), 237–240.

Lye, D. N. (1996). Adult child-parent relationships. *Annual Review of Sociology, 22,* 79–102.

Lynch, K. A., Mineau, G. P., & Anderton, D. L. (1985). Estimates of infant mortality on the western frontier: The use of genealogical data. *Historical Methods, 18,* 155–164.

Mason, K. O. (1997). Explaining fertility transitions. *Demography, 34,* 443–454.

Mineau, G. P. (1980). *Fertility on the frontier: An analysis of the nineteenth century Utah population.* Unpublished doctoral dissertation, University of Utah.

Mineau, G. P. (1988). Utah widowhood: A demographic profile. In A. Scadron (Ed.), *On their own: Widows and widowhood in the American southwest 1848–1939* (pp. 140–165). Chicago: University of Illinois Press.

Mineau, G. P., Smith, K., & Bean, L. L. (2002). Historical trends of survival among widows and widowers. *Social Science and Medicine, 54,* 245–254.

Morrell, J. R. (1956). *Utah's health and you: A history of Utah's public health.* Salt Lake City, UT: Deseret Book.

Nam, C. B., & Powers, M. G. (1983). *The socioeconomic approach to status measurement.* Houston, TX: Cap and Gown Press.

National Research Council. (1989). *Contraception and reproduction: Health consequences for women and children in the developing world.* Washington, DC: National Academy Press.

Noymer, A., & Garenne, M. (2000). The 1918 influenza epidemic's effects on sex differential mortality in the United States. *Population and Development Review, 26,* 565–581.

O'Brien, E., Rogers, A. R., Beesley, J., & Jorde, L. B. (1994). Genetic structure of the Utah Mormons: A comparison of results based on DNA, blood groups, migration matrices, isonymy, and pedigrees. *Human Biology, 66,* 743–759.

Perls, T. T., Alpert, L., & Fretts, R. C. (1997). Middle-aged mothers live longer. *Nature, 389,* 133.

Preston, S. H., & Haines, M. R. (1991). *Fatal years: Child mortality in late nineteenth-century America.* Princeton, NJ: Princeton University Press.

Richards, R. T. (1953). *Of medicine, hospitals, and doctors.* Salt Lake City, UT: University of Utah Press.

Rose, B. E. (1939). *The history of medicine in Utah.* Unpublished master's thesis, University of Utah.

Ross, C. E., Mirowsky, J., & Goldsteen, K. (1990). The impact of the family on health. *Journal of Marriage and the Family, 52,* 1059–1078.

Skolnick, M., Bean, L., Dintelman, S., & Mineau, G. (1979.) A computerized family history database system. *Social Science Research, 63,* 506–523.

Smith, K. R., Mineau, G. P., & Bean, L. L. (2002). Fertility and post-reproductive longevity. *Social Biology, 49*(Special Biodemography Issue), 3–205.

Snowdon, D. A., Kane, R. L., Beeson, W. L., Burke, G. L., Sprafka, J. M., Potter, J., et al. (1989). Is early natural menopause a biologic marker of health and aging? *American Journal of Public Health, 79,* 709–714.

Waldron, I., Weiss, C. C., Hughes, M. E. (1998). Effects of multiple roles on women's health. *Journal of Health and Social Behavior, 39,* 216–236.

Westendorf, R. G. J., & Kirkwood, T. B. L. (1998). Human longevity at the cost of reproductive success. *Nature, 396,* 743–746.

Wylie, J. E., & Mineau, G. P. (2003). Biomedical databases: Protecting privacy and promoting research. *Trends in Biotechnology, 21,* 113–116.

Wolf, D. A. (1994). The elderly and their kin: Patterns of availability and access. In L. G. Martin & S. H. Preston (Eds.), *Demography of aging* (pp. 146–194). Washington, DC: National Academy Press.

CHAPTER 19

Study of Family Health and the NIH: The Search for Research Support

V. Jeffery Evans

Family researchers are sometimes surprised and often confused by the way in which research on the family is supported by the National Institutes of Health (NIH). The first surprise is that the NIH is not a seamless organization in which there is a comfortable niche for family research. The NIH is a collection of 27 Institutes and Centers that support biomedical and health care research. They have many things in common but also are characterized by important differences. All institutes and centers support research and use the same set of application forms, review procedures, and funding mechanisms. On the other hand, there are significant nuances among them that can be very important to understand for eventual funding success. A second surprise is that the concept of family is used in different ways throughout the NIH. Not all of these ways will be satisfying to a researcher who is interested in family structure, process, or system. For example, family studies may include purely biomedical research, such as accumulating the genetic and health histories of related individuals.

The purpose of this chapter is to examine how a family researcher might approach health research in general and seek research support from the NIH in particular. The term "family researcher" refers to someone who is primarily interested in how families are structured and function within a system and how families affect the lives and well-being of family members. I write this chapter from a personal perspective, and not as an official representative of the NIH. I do bring 28 years of service to the NIH directly into the analysis. I am part of the NIH community. I work at the National Institute of Child Health and Human Development (NICHD). I have spent the large part of my career trying to use the tools of social science to illuminate the question of how families produce healthy children and facilitate their development to become productive adults. My view of the NIH may be different from other colleagues within the organization, but the fact that differences abound and thrive within the NIH is an important insight.

OVERVIEW OF THE NIH

The customary way to describe a federal agency is from the top down. If you are so inclined, start at the main NIH Web site (http://www.nih.gov/). Everything an applicant needs can be obtained from this gateway. The NIH community divides into several important domains: Institutes and Centers (I/C), The Center for Scientific Review (CSR), Offices of the Director of NIH, and support units for research community. This chapter will not address support units. I will devote much of the chapter to I/Cs and CSR.

The Offices of the Director are growing in importance within the NIH community, and even though these units do not directly support research, they influence funding in critical indirect ways. Most notable for family researchers are the following: The Office of Behavioral and Social Science Research (OBSSR), The Office of Research on Women's Health (ORWH), and Office of AIDS Research (OAR). These offices have budgets that are used to initiate, enhance, and coordinate research that is administered by the I/Cs. They can initiate important trans-NIH research initiatives or help an I/C fund or supplement individual research grants. Researchers usually do not deal with these offices directly, but it is wise to understand that they exist and can influence research funding.

The best way to understand the NIH is to realize that its creative processes are bottom up. Ideas begin with individuals in the larger scientific community. Colleagues at the NIH sort through these ideas and fund the best. The NIH staff works hard to maintain a system that respects individual creativity as its most important principle. Most grant money is disbursed through the unsolicited grants process that is an open system for researchers to propose their best ideas unfettered by any outside influence. Funding priorities are set by the I/Cs, but the I/Cs try to respect the scientific rankings established through the peer review system. The CSR is entrusted with maintaining the peer review system. The CSR relies on non-NIH basic researchers to provide the important peer review through its system of study sections. There is a creative tension between the program priorities of the I/Cs (where I serve) and those of the Scientific Review Officers (SRA) of the CSR, who are charged with keeping the peer review system in the hands of the scientific community and operating in a fair manner. The outcome of this system is a competitive scientific process that values the excellence of individual ideas above all else. This is the heart of the NIH system.

Applicants should understand that the system is constructed so that applicants can submit an application and the system will find an appropriate funding I/C and study section if the proposal is relevant to the NIH funding mission. If there is more than one I/C interested in the topic, then dual assignment is arranged with a designated primary institute and one or more secondary institutes. A wise applicant will have investigated funding I/Cs and study sections before submitting a grant application and will recommend a funding and review assignment in a cover letter. The system will try to accommodate an applicant's wishes as long as the request does not violate its operating procedures.

THE PEER REVIEW SYSTEM: CSR

The Center for Scientific Review (CSR) maintains the peer review system within the NIH system. Applicants can find everything they wish to know about CSR by accessing the Web site (http://www.csr.nih.gov/). When an application is submitted to the NIH, its first stop is review for scientific merit by one of the study sections supervised by CSR. It takes approximately four months after submission of the application to be reviewed by a study section. The end products of this process are the following: (a) a summary of the review (called a summary statement) and (b) a priority score. The summary statement will reveal what the study section thought of the basic scientific merit of the application and the score will determine the ranking of the application on decision lists that are used to make funding plans.

The top researchers in each particular field populate the study sections. They meet three times a year. A Scientific Review Administrator (SRA) supervises each group to make sure the process is fair and obeys the NIH rules. Three or more members of the study section read each application intensively and present their reviews to the entire study section. Then, in a general discussion, each member of the study section assigns a score indicating his or her rating of scientific merit. The summary statement contains the written reviews of the reviewers and a summary of the discussion.

Before the review session addresses individual applications, each member of the study section is asked to identify applications to be rated in the bottom half of the distribution. Such applications have no chance to win funding and are nominated to be placed in a "not scored" category. If everyone agrees, the applications are not discussed or scored. The summary statement consists only of the written reviews. This procedure allows the available time to be spent on discussing the top-rated applications so that fine distinctions that may affect their priority scores can be fully discussed.

Applicants should be mindful of several key points. The reviewers pledge to keep the review confidential. Reviewers are warned not to discuss proposals with applicants whose applications are reviewed. It is a very bad idea for applicants to query reviewers about the review. If an applicant must discuss the review process before the review, it should be done through the SRA. After the review, the applicant should ask the project officer (i.e., someone like me). The project officer of the grant sends a copy of the summary statement, in which the project officer

is identified, to the applicant as soon as it is available. Researchers should not make assumptions about anything in the review process until they have discussed it with the project officer. Even very experienced investigators often make inaccurate assumptions about what the review means and what may happen next. It is the job of the project officers to talk with applicants, and they can give a candid assessment of where the proposal stands after the review.

The Institutes and Centers (I/C)

Institutes and Centers are numerous, diverse, and dynamic within the NIH system. They usually have both extramural and intramural functions. Most of the support to organizations outside of the NIH is coordinated through extramural activities. Intramural science will sometimes procure help through contract, and it is possible that a family researcher may find research support in this way. Many I/Cs are organized to address research related to a specific disease or health issue. The National Cancer Institute is a good example of a disease-oriented institute. Other I/Cs are organized to study particular organ systems. The National Eye Institute is a good example of this type of institute. Others are oriented toward a medical specialty or technology. The National Institute of Nursing Research is an example of this type of institute. Family researchers are likely to find most support from two groups of I/Cs. It is important to realize how they are related.

The National Institute of Child Health and Human Development (NICHD) was established to understand how humans develop over the life course, with special attention to children. The National Institute on Aging (NIA), spun off from NICHD, also examines the life course with special attention to the elderly. Taken together, these two institutes support research on the life course and support family-oriented projects. The second group contains the National Institute of Mental Health (NIMH) and two spin-off institutes: The National Institute of Drug Abuse (NIDA) and the National Institute of Alcohol Abuse (NIAA). This group supports family research that illuminates mental illness or substance abuse.

Each institute or center has its own orientation toward science, which brings important nuances to the funding process. Applicants should shop around. If a family researcher has not contacted at least two institutes to assess their interest in an application, then a mistake has been made. Happy is the researcher who has two institutes fighting over his or her research. As a project officer, I respect an applicant who understands the process and deals with the system in a straightforward manner.

HOW CAN FAMILY SCIENCE RELATE TO THE NIH?

There are several ways family scientists can engage the scientific programs of the NIH. Often this requires family scientists to connect with researchers in another discipline to explain health-related topics. There is no I/C devoted specifically to the study of family.

At the NIH, *family* often means the source of genetic background, rather than a unit of study. This may be difficult for family researchers because there may appear to be not much need for understanding the family system or process. Family researchers can occasionally win support for projects using a genetic strategy. For example, researchers at the University of Utah won grants from both the NCI and NICHD to computerize the famous Mormon Genealogy Database. After many years of support, we learned much about family background and cancer as well as family structure. This is a special case, but it does indicate other possibilities. A very important new area is arising that focuses on

the genetic/environmental interaction as a critical ingredient in the developmental process. The family is an important institution for moderating gene/environment interactions. In these studies, family process and system are directly involved in the research design.

The NIH also characterizes the family as the source of important forms of social support. Social support is important in caretaking, compliance with clinical regimes, disease prevention, and health promotion. Such research could find support widely within the NIH. Often this type of research does not involve a family scientist, but there is a growing opportunity to reach out to health research in this way.

Another way that family research is supported is as an important unit of analysis in population research and as a social unit of analysis for understanding family relationships such as parent/child interactions. The National Institute of Child Health and Development (NICHD) is especially interested in supporting family research such as this, and we have learned much about family structure and its implications for family members. The current policy emphasis on using public incentives to strengthen families and promote marriage should give family researchers much to study, and NICHD is quite willing to fund research to examine these issues.

Family systems research has not really found a funding niche within the NIH system. Is there a way of illuminating health and developmental issues using a family systems approach? It should be possible to conceive a research agenda that does this, but to date this remains an area that needs development.

APPROACHING THE NIH FOR THE FIRST TIME

How does one begin to seek support from the NIH? A good way is to start with the Web site and end with a person. The

National Institutes of Health are readily accessible through the Internet, but one should always find at least one person to deal personally with the many nuances of the funding process. One can find information on funding opportunities through the *NIH Guide for Grants and Contracts* (http://grants2 .nih.gov/grants/guide/index.html). The guide is the official source of information about opportunities and policies affecting the extramural programs of the NIH. Alternatively, one can visit the Web site of any of the I/Cs and explore the descriptions of the various funding programs. In the end, one should always find a program person who understands the specific project. These people are easily approached by telephone or e-mail.

Investigators should always have a clear idea of what they want to do. An investigator should have at least a brief concept paper that states the goals and hypotheses of the project and outlines the methods and financial requirements of the project. Sending such a concept paper via e-mail and following up with a phone call is the approach that I prefer as a project officer. The e-mail communication allows a program person to determine how best to help an investigator, to engage other colleagues in the discussion, and to make quick referrals. This sets the stage for productive phone conversations. A successful search will uncover at least one funding program that finds the concept of your project relevant to its funding mission. Ideally, the researcher will find more than one program interested in the work and, perhaps, even a special funding opportunity that might enhance chances of funding.

The National Institute of Child Health and Development (http://www.nichd.nih.gov/) is a good place to start looking for interest in supporting research involving the family. There are two branches of NICHD that are heavily involved in family research. The first is the Demographic and Behavioral Sciences Branch (my home), which supports research on population topics (http://www.nichd.nih .gov/about/cpr/dbs/). The family and household are important units of measure in population research, and much work has been supported to learn about how families and households are formed, function, and dissolve. The second is the Child Development and Behavior Branch (http://www.nichd.nih .gov/crmc/cdb/cdb.htm), which supports research on the full spectrum of child development topics. In addition, there are several other branches that support research on child health and rehabilitation topics, and all support research involving the family. NICHD is the one institute within the NIH that studies the normal development from preconception through adulthood. Much family research fits reasonably into this environment.

Choose a Funding Mechanism

The NIH is an agency that offers many funding mechanisms, and investigators should choose the best mechanism for their projects. Investigators can learn about mechanisms and application forms at the following site: http://grants1.nih.gov/grants/oer.htm. Some type of *R* mechanism typically supports research. The R01, the regular research grant, is the workhorse mechanism. The application form for the R01 and other R variations is the PHS 398 (http://grants1.nih .gov/grants/funding/phs398/phs398.html).

A good rule of thumb is to conceive the project as an R01 and switch to another mechanism only for a very good reason. The only real way of assessing whether your idea is ready for the R01 competition is to try to write as an R01. Why start with an R01? It is the most flexible of all of the R mechanisms and all of the I/Cs invest most of their money in R01-type research. The R01 can probably serve your research needs throughout your entire career. The R01 is created so that investigators can propose research with a minimum of conditions imposed by the mechanism. The PHS 398 format is quite formal and follows an idealized scientific presentation in which an investigator proposes hypotheses and methods of testing these hypotheses. Many investigators start a line of research with R01 support and renew that support every three to five years for the duration of their research career. Investigators should be aware that when they request more than $500,000 of direct cost support in any year they must receive advance permission from an I/C.

What constitutes a good reason to choose a mechanism different from the R01? It may be that the project needs preliminary work in order to be competitive, and in this case an investigator may need a small grant (R03) to do a small project or initiate a new line of research, or an Exploratory/Developmental grant (R21) to create a foundation for an innovative new line of research. Another good reason to depart from the R01 is if a special competition specifies a mechanism other than a R01. Applicants should be aware that these types of mechanisms vary in the way that they are reviewed and in other types of restrictions across I/Cs in the NIH system. The differences are usually very important.

New investigators face special problems because they are inexperienced and lack records of achievement that would buttress their request for support. There are several popular routes for such investigators to travel en route to their ultimate destination of being fully independent investigators supported by R01 grants. These are the R03, F32, and K01 mechanisms. The R03 is ideal for taking the first step from supervised training to independent status. At NICHD, we try very hard to give new investigators a break with such mechanisms. F-type mechanisms are training mechanisms and the F32 supports individual post-doctoral fellowships that allow fellows to find a mentor and tailor a post-doctoral experience to fit their individual needs. The K-type mechanisms are

hybrids incorporating research and training objectives. The K01 enables a new assistant professor to find a mentor and launch a line of research while accumulating extra dimensions to research capabilities under the guidance of the mentor. At NICHD, these mechanisms have worked well for family researchers. There are differences in how these are used across the NIH so investigators should be alert to them.

When the application is ready to be submitted, the applicant should send a cover letter advising which I/Cs are preferred for funding. The wise applicant will also have contacted his or her prospective project officer to have an ARA (Awaiting Receipt of Application) filed laying claim to the application for the I/C.

Find a Review Group

When an application is submitted to the NIH, the applicant should have a clear idea which study section will review the application. Applicants can even request an assignment to a particular study section in their cover letter. The assignment of an application to a study section is the single most important decision regarding the application's eventual success in the NIH system. The wise applicant will leave nothing to chance on the assignment of the application to a study section.

The CSR makes the policy by which all study sections operate within the NIH system. The CSR also controls a large number of study sections. These typically review all unsolicited R01 applications and other individual-level applications. The I/Cs also control study sections that usually review institutional level applications, RFAs, and other types of applications. They all function under the same set of rules and procedures.

The study section is a very interesting organization. The standing study sections meet three times a year in face-to-face meetings. The members usually serve staggered four-year terms. The study sections are designed not only to represent the highest standards of excellence in a field but also to debate what constitutes cutting edge science in a field and to apply these standards in the review process. It is not surprising that each standing study section develops its own culture and ideas of what constitutes cutting edge science. The wise applicant will appreciate this fact and tailor the application to the expectations of a study section. Standing study sections will be found both at CSR and I/Cs. How does one find out about study sections? The best way is to discuss the probable assignment of one's application with prospective project officers. We observe study section behavior and have definite ideas about how various study sections are likely to react to ideas. Family researchers should be aware that there is no single study section set up to solely review family science. Rather, there are several study sections that normally have members with expertise on the family. Careful thought should be given to which review audience is best for individual cases.

Sometimes a special, one-time-only study section is set up. These are called Special Emphasis Panels (SEP). SEPs are used for very special cases and are usually smaller in size than a standing study section. The most prominent type of SEP happens when a Request for Applications (RFA) or a Program Announcement with Review (PAR) is reviewed. These are highly tailored study sections convened to focus on a relatively narrow topic.

PA, RFA, or RFP?

What is a PA, RFA, or RFP anyway? On occasion, one or more I/Cs will target a special area of research and issue a special announcement that signals to the research community that we are interested in supporting research in a topic and specifies special conditions outlining what the I/C(s) will do

to promote such research. The announcement of these opportunities is always published in the *Guide*.

It is important to understand that I/Cs are always ready to support research grants relevant to their mission through the regular unsolicited research grant process. The unsolicited grants process is the backbone of the NIH. Only announcements about special areas and new opportunities appear in the *Guide*.

So far, we have been discussing developing an application for the unsolicited process. Now we can consider what to do if one sees a special opportunity announced in the form of PA, RFA, or RFP. As a general rule, it is not a good idea to enter a new area of research just because there is a special announcement in the area. There is always the opportunity to compete in the unsolicited competition to support your best idea and you will often hurt yourself if you abandon the pursuit of your best ideas to chase someone else's idea. You should consider applying to a special announcement if you can pursue your idea without making any crippling compromises.

A Program Announcement (PA) is only intended to inform the research community that I/Cs are interested in supporting a research topic. The PA might address a new area, seek to clarify which I/Cs are taking the lead in an established area, or remind the field that a longstanding interest is still there. A PA brings no special commitment to the topic. It is purely informational. There is a special type of PA that does commit the system to some special course of action to promote a topic. This is the Program Announcement with Review (PAR) and it confers the benefit of a special review.

A Request for Proposals (RFP) is the most targeted form of announcement because it will use the contract mechanism. To reply to an RFP there are special formats for contract proposals and successful offerors will be working under the direction of a federal employee. This is quite restrictive and one should only apply after careful thought about the implications of working for the federal government. Most RFPs are published in the *Guide*, but to fully access the world of contracts one should check http://fedbizopps.gov. In the past, NICHD has used contracts to lay the foundation for large surveys such as the National Survey of Families and Households. Recently, NICHD awarded another contract to find a model for new work that examines how better to understand family change and variation. The model research and data collection program integrates previously disparate streams within family research, including research on fertility, marriage and cohabitation, sexual behavior, and parenting, and has the potential to significantly advance understanding of the factors and processes that drive family change at both the individual and societal levels.

A Request for Applications (RFA) targets a research topic but uses some form of assistance mechanism, namely a grant rather than a contract. This is a much less constraining approach than an RFP, and is the approach commonly used by the NIH to stimulate specific research areas. In an RFA, the I/C(s) issuing it specifies how much funding is set aside to fund applications and a special study section (SEP) is set up to review it. If an applicant can fit his or her project comfortably into an RFA, it usually enhances the chances of winning an award. Usually, the SEP is set up by the I/C issuing the RFA but for some RFAs, CSR runs the SEP. The major benefit of an RFA is that the applicant is guaranteed that there will be a review group that is both knowledgeable and sympathetic to the research topic, and there is funding available to support worthy proposals. Many times RFAs specify special mechanisms and conditions to the award. All of the necessary information is contained in the RFA announcement. In the recent past, NICHD and NIA collaborated on a RFA titled "Intergenerational Family Resource Allocation" and have funded 16 projects on this topic. The rationale for this RFA was to focus the attention of the research community on a very policy-relevant topic. It is expected that many more projects on this topic will be funded in the future through the unsolicited research program.

WHAT MAKES AN IDEA COMPETITIVE?

It is often said that no amount of grantsmanship can compensate for the lack of a good idea, but that bad grantsmanship can destroy a good idea. There is no magic presentation format that guarantees success without a good idea behind it. The NIH system is just too competitive to think that presentation alone will carry the day for any applicant.

What constitutes a good idea? Theory-driven research is paramount in the NIH system. Projects predicated on ideas that are grounded in interesting theory and tested in a definitive manner are afforded the highest priority in the system. The existence of a good idea is revealed early in an NIH proposal in the Specific Aims section. The aims should unveil a set of theory-driven hypotheses. Many reviewers turn to the specific aims section first to see what the application is focused on. If a crisply stated set of interesting hypotheses pops out of the specific aims, they set a positive tone for the rest of the review. Family research often features descriptive and qualitative approaches. How do these ideas compete with theory-driven research? Unless a descriptive project is focused on a new phenomenon or is clearly part of a larger program of research leading to testing a theory-driven idea, it is usually not as highly rated as a true theory-driven project. The same can be said of qualitative research. It should be tied to a program of research that will quantify and test important ideas. Mixed method approaches in which qualitative and quantitative approaches are blended can generate much enthusiasm in the NIH system.

Newcomers to the NIH are often uncertain whether they should be the principal investigator on a study and whether they should add famous consultants or collaborators to the project. If the idea driving the projects belongs to you then you should be the Principal Investigator. There are special benefits and responsibilities that belong only to the Principal Investigator. The NIH system is structured to give new investigators the benefit of the doubt, so there is no real reason for a young investigator not to be the Principal Investigator. Moreover, only add consultants and collaborators if there is a real role in the project for them. Window dressing in the proposal is not helpful and can be held against the project. In my experience, there is nothing more exciting than to see a young investigator propose a new idea and give a credible outline of how he or she will develop the idea. Reviewers will respond favorably to such individuals.

WHAT CAN HURT
A COMPETITIVE IDEA?

In the application process, clarity is your friend and confusion is your enemy. Theory and methods should be clearly articulated and tied together seamlessly. Make the presentation in terms of the work for which you are requesting assistance, and avoid talking about end products such as monographs or sabbaticals. The application should not only state what will be done in the project but also explain why a problem is posed and an analytic method is chosen. Sophisticated researchers always know the limits of their data and methodology, and reviewers look for indications that applicants recognize these limitations and know what to do about

them. It should be clear who performs the various tasks and roles in the project, and each person's role should be justified. The budget request should match the scope of the work proposed. If someone is donating effort or if some other source is supporting parts of a project that are critical to the success of the proposed work, then it ought to be clear that the needed support is in place. A good practice is to have consultants, subcontractors, and outside collaborators submit letters that spell out what they will do.

The NIH system is a most stylized system. The NIH has specific formats of presentation for applications, and reviewers are quite accustomed to sorting through ideas using this format. Don't deviate from the format. The PHS 398 is the format for the gold standard R01 grant application. All other formats derive from this format in some way. Do not try to use a National Science Foundation (NSF) format in the NIH system. Do not try to use a format that one might use to sell a book to a publisher. The NIH is strict about page limits and related matters. The NIH requires that applicants address specific issues, such as the inclusion of women and children and minorities in research designs. Even if the answer is obvious, there must be some response in the application in regard to these issues. Human subject issues should be described and defended even if the local Institutional Review Board has already approved the design. The NIH reviewers respect professionalism. Make sure the presentation meets the highest professional standards. Wise applicants will refer to http://www.nichd.nih.gov/about/cpr/dbs/appls.htm for help in preparing an application headed toward NICHD.

When the application has been clearly written according to the NIH format, investigators should ask themselves whether they have sold the importance of the idea to the reader. Ideas are important because they extend a theory in some important way or have a practical importance to clinical practice or public policy. They can sometimes derive importance because they will improve measurement or methodology or illuminate an emerging area. Don't forget to point out why your project is important.

HOW TO INTERPRET FEEDBACK FROM THE NIH

The NIH peer review system assembles the cream of the scientific talent crop to make up its study sections, and the reviewers work hard to understand researchers' ideas. Rarely will anyone find an opportunity to entice so many top-flight scientists to focus on an idea and render meaningful criticism. The summary statement is the official report of these deliberations, and the program staff has probably witnessed the review first hand. Both should be consulted to understand the criticisms.

Consider the context of the review. Each study section member is assigned 5–10 applications to read intensively and to prepare a critical analysis and recommendation for the whole study section. In addition, they may read all of the other applications with a reduced level of intensity and thoroughness. A typical study section may review 75 applications over a two-day meeting. Before the meeting, the SRA asks each reviewer to nominate applications that they judge to be in the bottom half of the distribution of priority scores. These nominations are presented to the whole study section as nominations for "not scored" status. This means that the application is just not competitive and no more discussion will occur. If anyone in the study section objects to giving the application "not scored" status, then the application is discussed. At the meeting of the study section, each application that will be scored is discussed independently. The primary, secondary, and tertiary reviewers will present their criticisms and recommendations to the entire study section. Then a general discussion occurs, and if the recommendations are generally favorable, the debate often resembles a gauntlet. The wise applicant will write an application that gives plenty of ammunition to any reviewer who might champion the application. Program staff observes the study section meeting, but cannot intervene in any way. They become astute listeners and can fill the nuances of the debate that may not be captured by the summary statement. Applicants should consult with their project officer for his or her perspective on the review.

The summary statement yields a score for the competitive applications. The score is in two parts: a priority score and percentile. The priority score is the arithmetic mean of the reviewer's scores multiplied by 100. Reviewers are asked to score applications with numbers ranging from 1.0 to 5.0 in multiples of 0.1 with 1.0 representing the highest scientific merit. Generally speaking, scores ranging from 1.0–1.5 are outstanding and are nearly perfect. Scores in the 1.5–2.0 range are excellent and are very solid applications without any significant flaw. Scores worse than 2.0 have a flaw of some severity. Because there are many study sections, and each has its own scoring culture, the NIH has found it necessary to produce a relative score that can afford comparisons across study sections. This is called the percentile and represents the percentile ranking that an application has in the distribution of applications reviewed over a full year of study section experience. "Not scored" applications are imputed a score of 5.0 in this process. A 0.0% means that the application is at the absolute top of the distribution. A 20.0% means that 80% of the distribution is ranked below the application. I/Cs use percentiles to make funding lists, on which all of the applications assigned to a program are ranked according to percentile. Normal practice in the grants program is to fund applications on the funding list in rank order. If applications are funded out of order then the program staff must make a strong justification for so doing. RFAs follow a similar practice, except that the priority score is used to create the rank order on the funding list. Funding out of rank order occurs more frequently for RFAs because there are usually program goals specified in the RFA announcement and staff may fund out of rank order to accomplish these goals.

Applicants should always consult with their project officers to determine funding probabilities of their proposals. Funding probabilities vary with the amount of funding available and the dollar amount of competing applications. It is too difficult to predict in advance what the probabilities are because the research community has a tendency to overreact to news concerning the budget prospects of the federal government. Sometimes bad fiscal news will discourage the field more than is warranted and create a favorable funding environment for those brave enough to apply.

REVISE AND RESUBMIT?

Often an application is not funded the first time it is reviewed. This situation forces the applicant to consider whether to submit a revised application. It is useful to consider the funding decision process to understand when to make this decision. The study sections meet approximately four to five months after the application deadline. Thereafter, the application will have a priority score, and the score is used to position the application on funding lists. Sometimes the ranking is based on the raw score given by the study section. Often the score is converted into a percentile ranking that indicates the relative ranking of the application within the group of applications reviewed by the study section. The percentile is then used to establish a ranking on funding

lists. Whether a raw score or percentile is used depends on many factors, and applicants should check with their program officers to determine what is used in their case.

Once the priority score is established, the fate of some, but not all, applications is fairly clear. Applications not scored are out of the running for funding. Applications with outstanding priority scores are very good bets to be funded. However, there is usually a large zone in the priority range that cannot be accurately forecasted with respect to funding. These applications must wait until formal decisions are actually made.

Formal funding decisions are usually made after the second stage of review at the National Advisory Council meetings. These occur approximately eight months after the application deadline. Sometimes it takes longer than this because of delays in approving a federal budget. After these Council meetings, the project officer should be in a good position to determine whether the project will be funded, and formal notification will come at the very end of the process. A few applications may dangle in a zone of funding uncertainty for months as the program staff tries to find the funds to support the project. These few applicants are often quite torn as to whether to resubmit or not. This is because a resubmitted application will substitute for the old application on funding lists after a study section reviews it. If money arrives after an application has disappeared from one funding list and before the new funding list takes effect, then an opportunity may be missed. Careful consideration of the odds of adverse consequences should be weighed before resubmitting such an application.

NIH summary statements tend to be quite substantive and usually spell out the flaws that need correction in detail. If it is possible to correct the flaws, then the wise applicant will resubmit. This means starting the application process over from the beginning. Consultation with the project officer can be very helpful in making this decision. The most important element of a resubmission strategy is to be responsive to the criticisms of the previous review. This cannot be over-emphasized. The revised application is sent back to the study section that did the first review. The summary statement of the first review is attached to the revised application, and is used as the point of departure for the review of the revised application. Revisions should be self-contained proposals that include a brief roadmap of how the applicant has responded to the criticisms. The responses should be highlighted in the text to show where the changes have occurred. Applicants get two chances to revise. This is a rather collegial process by which science is sharpened to a fine cutting edge. Unscored applications can be revised successfully, and the more complicated the project, the more likely it will be critiqued and need revision. One of my very favorite projects once received a summary statement over 50 pages long! The criticisms made the project much better and much more expensive. As the project officer, I felt rather daunted in negotiating the budget knowing that the study section felt strongly about the design. In the end, the review process really helped make the project better and made a strong case for increasing the financial support of the project.

I should mention that there is an official appeals system in the NIH. It is set up to remedy malfunctions in the peer review system in which something happens that overtly prejudices a review. This happens rarely, and the opportunity is not available for an applicant to argue with the scientific judgment of the study section.

Negotiating a Budget With the NIH

The NIH is always in the position of trying to stretch available funds. It is quite common to cut projects, and the larger the project budget the greater the cut is likely to be. Let's consider the roles of the parties in the budget

negotiation process for assistance mechanisms (I will skip the contracting process because it has a very formal negotiation process that requires an extended discussion). Once the applicant has been given official notification that the NIH intends to make an award, two key people enter into the negotiation process. They are (a) the Grants Management Officer (GMO) and (b) the Project Officer (PO). The I/C will establish budget guidelines that will serve as a framework for the negotiations. The GMO is the only person who has the delegated authority to make an award. Nothing is official until the GMO says so. The GMO, or someone working for the GMO, ensures that NIH grants policy is followed and tries hard to avoid any budget overlap in the project with some other source of support. The PO is charged with protecting the substantive interests of the government, namely science. The applicant must deal with both the GMO and PO in coming to a final budget agreement.

Grantees should always get to know the PO and GMO assigned to their projects. These two people will be their companions throughout the life of the grant. Any decision relating to the administration of the grant necessarily involves the agreement between these two people and the applicant. When we are at our best, we can help grantees solve problems that arise during the course of investigation. Personally, I like this aspect of my job and my colleagues in grants management feel the same.

SUMMARY AND CONCLUSION

It is important to remember that the NIH system is predicated on the assumption that the research community is the source of innovative ideas and that there should always be room for supporting exciting new ideas. There is always room for good ideas at the NIH. Even in times of extreme budget tightness, the NIH finds ways to protect the investigator-initiated system. The purpose of this chapter is to help investigators with good ideas to find the best audience for their work and to avoid the pitfalls of poor grantsmanship that can obscure a good idea.

The NIH is a very dynamic place. Program emphasis is quick to change in response to scientific developments. Potential applicants should not be dismayed by these changes. Just remember to make sure that you find at least one program with an interest in your work and find a program officer to advise you. Pick an appropriate mechanism and find the best review audience for your work. Make sure that your application not only explains your idea but also sells its importance.

FURTHER READING

Because the best material about the grants process is produced for the various Web sites in the NIH community, I will stick with material on the Internet. There are some very

elaborate and imaginative Web sites. One of the best is maintained by the National Institute of Allergy and Infectious Diseases (NIAID) (http://www.niaid.nih.gov/ncn/). From this site, one can obtain a tutorial on writing a grant application (http://www.niaid.nih.gov/ncn/grants/default.htm) and an annotated model application (http://www.niaid.nih.gov/ncn/grants/app/default.htm). Also, it is possible to find projects that are currently supported by the NIH through the CRISP system (http://crisp.cit.nih.gov/). This system allows one to search the abstracts of funding grants. Also, one can find information on success rates throughout the NIH at http://grants1.nih.gov/grants/award/success.htm. Detailed information about grants policy can be found at http://grants1.nih.gov/grants/policy/policy.htm. Since we are now in the electronic research administration age, no set of bookmarks is complete without the ERA system (http://grants1.nih.gov/grants/era/era.htm).

CHAPTER 20

Developing Partnerships in Commissioned Research: A Perspective From England

JOHN CARPENTER

This chapter will describe, with the help of examples from the work of the Centre for Applied Social Studies (CASS) at the University of Durham in England, some principles for developing partnerships in applied social research concerning families and health. These partnerships include collaborations with (a) service organizations, professionals, and clients in order to design research proposals and win grant funding from government, regional health and social welfare agencies, and charitable foundations; (b) service managers, practitioners, and clients in order to carry out studies that are relevant and useful to the services examined; and (c) service organizations and funders to disseminate and apply the findings of research in order to influence policy and improve practice.

APPLIED SOCIAL RESEARCH

The Centre for Applied Social Studies (CASS) engages in applied social research, meaning that our research is directed primarily toward practical use, rather than to the development and testing of hypotheses as part of a process of constructing a body of theoretical knowledge, as in basic research. Both basic and applied research should adhere to the same fundamental principles and methods of social science. The difference between the two, as Rossi and colleagues pointed out in a classic paper on the subject, is partly a matter of working practices; "the theories, methods, and procedures of basic and applied research are quite similar but the style of work encountered in each camp is not" (Rossi, Wright, & Wright, 1978, p.171). A central element of the style of applied social research is the principle and practice of partnership.

The kinds of applied research that CASS undertakes encompass the three broad types identified by Rossi and associates (1978). Some of our work is *descriptive*. For example, in a current project, which I will discuss in detail, we are attempting to identify and describe the barriers that families from minority ethnic groups experience in gaining access to, and effective support from, services for their children with disabilities. Our research may also be *analytical* in the sense that we are attempting to model empirically the social phenomenon under investigation. For example, one of our projects focused on understanding the relationship between the organization of service provision and stress experienced by family caregivers of people with severe mental illness (Schneider, Carpenter, Wooff, & Brandon, 2001). But much of our work is essentially the *evaluation* of services and interventions. In our Centre, one example is the evaluation of a number of social programs intended to enhance the lives of families in socially and economically disadvantaged neighborhoods and to promote preschool children's chances for success when starting school. Another project concerns the comparative cost-effectiveness of therapeutic services for families that are provided by state and charitable agencies. Note that here we are interested not so much in whether therapeutic interventions work, but rather in what works best, for whom, and at what cost.

Funding Applied Social Research

In England, much applied social research in the field of families and health is funded directly by central government through the national Department of Health, and indirectly by the requirement that initiatives in health and social care, which are sponsored by government, be independently evaluated. In addition, local health and social welfare commissioners and providers may themselves commission descriptive and evaluative research on services. Other main sources of funding are charitable foundations, the most important of which, the Joseph Rowntree Foundation and the Nuffield Foundation, have the specific goal of sponsoring research designed to influence policy and practice (Lewis, 2000).

RESEARCH AND POLICY MAKING

Research funded by the Department of Health is itself intended to have an impact on policy. The Department's Policy Research Division supports a number of research units in universities with which it negotiates programs of research designed to inform policy development and to carry out evaluations of policy. In addition, it launches regular invitations to researchers nationally to propose research projects on topics of current policy interest. For example, the research project mentioned above, on the comparative cost-effectiveness of therapeutic services for families, was funded as one of a number of projects concerned with investigating the costs and outcomes of social welfare services for children. Invitations to propose research projects may suggest fairly broad topics in which the Department is interested or, as increasingly seems to be the case, may actually pose questions for descriptive or evaluative research. In these cases, it is reasonable to suppose that someone at least wants to know the answers—always an encouraging sign for researchers who do not want the report of their findings to be left untouched on the shelf in the office of an overworked bureaucrat.

It may be helpful to observe some differences between the United States and the United Kingdom and Europe in terms of policy implications of research findings. In an interesting paper subtitled "reflections on the relation of knowledge to policy in the United States and abroad," Wilensky (1997) argued that social scientists in the United States have less influence on policy than researchers in other Western democracies where there are tighter relations between knowledge and power. This, Wilensky suggests, is a consequence of "corporatist" European national systems in contrast to the decentralized political economy in the U.S. Wilensky further contended that much evaluation research in the United States focuses on short-term effects and is used for political leverage rather than long-term policy planning. I am not qualified to judge the merits of these observations about the situation in the U.S., but it is true to say that there have been some strong statements from government in the United Kingdom about the importance of "evidence-based" policy and practice. Thus, in an address to a meeting of academics, the then-Minister for Education stated

> Social science should be at the heart of policy making. We need a revolution in relations between government and the social research community—we need social scientists to help determine what works and why, and what types of policy initiatives are likely to be effective. (Blunkett, 2000, cited in Nulty & Webb, 2002)

Partnerships in applied social research should include its commissioners and, in the case of research commissioned by government, the people who actually make the policy. Ideally, policymakers should be involved as partners throughout the research.

Designing Policy-Relevant Research

At the risk of stating the obvious, *the* essential step in developing research proposals that are likely to attract support from government or agencies concerned with policy development or evaluation, or from charitable foundations seeking to influence policy, is to ask appropriate questions. Such questions are grounded in experience and have been formulated to address the concerns of service managers, practitioners, and service users (clients) as well as policymakers.

Case Example: Study of South Asian children with disabilities and their families

One case example is an account of the development of a research proposal to explore the experiences of minority ethnic families with children with disabilities. The project began as a response to a call for proposals issued by the regional health authority for research on improving the quality of communication between people from minority ethnic groups and health services. The director of the social services department in Newcastle upon Tyne approached me and explained that he and colleagues in the local health and education departments had resolved to reorganize services for families in the area with severely disabled children in order to meet their expressed needs more effectively. He was particularly concerned that families from the local Pakistani and Bangladeshi populations were not being served effectively. He wondered if the research funds available might provide an opportunity to investigate the reasons for what he believed was a relatively low uptake of services by these families.

Representing the health service on the interagency joint planning group was a pediatrician who is also the professor of pediatric neurology at Newcastle University. The pediatrician shared these concerns and, as a practicing clinician, felt confident in asserting that access to services by these Pakistani and Bangladeshi families was hampered by problems in communication. In that respect, an investigation of the factors involved would fit the funder's call for research proposals.

The first step in developing a proposal was to check the assumption that Pakistani and Bangladeshi families were indeed underrepresented in the numbers of children with disabilities who were using health and welfare services. To do this, the physician drew on published national epidemiological surveys to estimate the numbers of children with severe and complex disabilities in the city. Knowing the size and structure of the minority ethnic populations from census data, she estimated the numbers of Pakistani and Bangladeshi children who should be known to services. These figures were then compared to those on the social services department database, revealing that only about half the predicted number was actually known to the department. Since welfare system social services departments in the U.K. control the budget for community support services for people with disabilities and their families, this was strong evidence in support of our assumption.

The next step was to confer with *Dek Bhal,* a self-help group for south Asian mothers of children with disabilities, which operated in the city with some financial support from the social services department. The director of social services and a Pakistani researcher working at CASS attended a meeting of *Dek Bhal* in order to listen to members' views. The mothers attending were generally well-engaged with community services. Nevertheless, they readily identified families with children with severe disabilities who they believed received little or no support. The group members suggested a number of possible reasons for this lack of engagement:

- Services do not provide accessible and helpful information. Parents lack understanding and knowledge of services, how they relate to one another, and how to access them.
- Services and professionals are not sensitive to needs, particularly of South Asian families who may encounter personal and institutional racism.
- Families may encounter professional beliefs (stereotypes) about disability (e.g., "Asian people have lower thresholds of pain") and caring (e.g., "They look after their own"). Conversely, professionals may underestimate families' strengths and coping abilities.
- Linguistic and cultural barriers exist that impair communication between professionals and families. Cultural barriers may include different beliefs about disability and its causes, the place of religion, and the role of professionals. Linguistic barriers are exacerbated by the limited availability of interpreters with relevant knowledge about disability and sensitivity to parents' concerns.
- Parents' fear and experience of stigma and discrimination in the minority community as well as in wider society may mean that some parents and children have minimal contact with the outside world.

These possibilities were supplemented by a list derived from discussion with health and social services professionals working in the field:

- Services provided by different agencies are not well co-coordinated and professionals are not well-informed about services provided by other agencies.
- Interagency and interprofessional communication is fraught with conflict (e.g., over responsibility for provision of resources).
- Services do not take a holistic approach to the social and health needs of children but rely on a narrow medical model that restricts families' abilities to present their needs and limits the scope of services provided.

My own task was to relate these factors to the limited research literature and to formulate a set of hypotheses for the research study and propose how they might be investigated. Briefly, I proposed a qualitative study designed to elicit the views of parents and their children with disabilities as well as their siblings. I suggested comparing two groups of families, classified according to their level of engagement with services. One group would be known to and engaged with services; the other group would have little or no involvement, being known only to the primary care physician (almost everyone in the U.K. is registered with a general practitioner) and to the schools service. The aims would be to identify barriers to access and to discover how they might be overcome. We recognized that social class and the experience of living in relative poverty were likely to influence access to and use of services. Pakistani and Bangladeshi families are among the most disadvantaged minority ethnic groups in the U.K., and generally live in a poor area of the city. Consequently, we proposed comparison groups of white children and families living in the same area. Again, we would seek to interview subgroups of service users and non-users. This would enable us to distinguish factors associated with living in the area from those associated with ethnicity.

So far, I have described partnerships with service users and professionals in the formulation of research hypotheses or questions. Table 20.1 shows other partners in the research project and the purposes of these partnerships. It should be noted that the research team itself constituted a partnership between academic researchers from different disciplines (applied social research, medicine, community studies, and educational psychology) and between academics and practitioners (social work, pediatrics, and community nursing). Further, in the team of eight members, we comprised four South Asian and four white people, one of whom had a disability. The team was, therefore, able to share different academic, service, and cultural perspectives. Since the desirability of multidisciplinary collaboration and collaboration between practitioners and academics were two of the factors stressed in the research call for proposals from the Regional Health Authority, I am sure that the composition of the team contributed to the successful application for funding.

Table 20.1   Purpose of Partnerships with Families, Professionals, and Agencies (Study of South Asian Children with Disabilities and Their Families)

Partnership	Purpose
Research Team	1. Contributing different professional and academic perspectives
Self-help group of mothers of disabled children (Dek Bhal)	1. Developing study hypotheses 2. Finding research participants 3. Interpreting data 4. Disseminating findings to minority ethnic community
Primary Health Care Services	1. Finding research participants 2. Agreeing to interview professional staff 3. Implementing recommendations
Parents and disabled children	1. Participating in the study through interviews (with informed consent) 2. Agreeing to review assessments
Social Services, Health, and Education services	1. Agreeing to interview professional staff 2. Assessing unmet needs of families in the study 3. Implementing recommendations
Professional, community, and family experts (Project Advisory Group)	1. Advising on conduct of research 2. Interpreting findings 3. Advising on dissemination
Joint Executive Group	1. Reviewing existing services in the light of research finding and making recommendations
Regional Health Authority	1. Funding 2. Considering implications of findings for regional and national policy development.

PARTNERSHIPS IN THE CONDUCT OF RESEARCH

Since partnerships with professionals will be discussed in a later example, I simply note here the necessity of collaboration in gaining access to research participants. In the United Kingdom, the ethics committees, which govern the conduct of research with health services patients, do not allow researchers to contact research participants directly. This must be done through the responsible clinician, who has the authority to decline access in cases where he or she considers that family members might be distressed by contact with researchers. This, in itself, can cause problems in research design, particularly representativeness of the sample, especially if individual clinicians apply different exclusion criteria. In this study, we had an unexpected problem when one team of community-based practitioners initially refused our request to distribute letters to families, apparently on the grounds that the research project was considered "racist." In this case, it was necessary to explain that the intention of the study was not to pathologize the South Asian families but rather to promote changes to improve effectiveness of service delivery.

As with all of our projects, we have established a Project Advisory Group to support the research team by advising on the conduct of the research, the interpretation of its findings, and on the dissemination of its results. Group members are invited on the basis of their expert knowledge as researchers, practitioners, service managers, and clients of services, or as influential people who may be able to lead the implementation of the research findings. The standard terms of reference we use are shown in Figure 20.1.

They are modeled on those used by the Joseph Rowntree Foundation, a major research funder in this field, which has strongly promoted the contribution of expertise from clients alongside that of the technical experts commonly found in advisory groups. The composition of the Project Advisory Group is shown in Table 20.2.

Before leaving this example, I would like to note the potential for the impact of research on local policy. The city social services and education departments and the health authority have explicitly recognized the need for change and have made a commitment to reconfigure services, extend funding, and to develop a joint approach to meeting the needs of the children based on a social model of disability. This new approach is intended to be informed by the research evidence about the needs of children and their families drawn directly from the families themselves.

The second objective of the project has therefore been designed so that the emerging research findings will be reported to a subgroup of an interagency Joint Executive Group (JEG). This group comprises family representatives and service providers, including two newly appointed development officers from health and social services. Its task will be to review existing services in light of the findings and to make specific recommendations for coordinated and responsive services. One of the researchers will monitor the success of this process by attending JEG meetings, recording decisions, and tracking their implementation. The researcher will maintain contact with key people and interview them in order to establish their understanding of the contribution of various factors, including the research findings, on decision making and on the outcomes of these processes. Thus, through this case study, we hope to obtain evidence of the potential long-term impact of partnership-based research.

PARTNERSHIPS IN PROGRAM EVALUATION

As indicated, CASS is often invited to evaluate programs that have been funded by central or regional government agencies. A requirement of such programs is that they are independently evaluated. In preparing our research proposal, we follow two general considerations. The first consideration is how the evaluation can be useful to the participants in the program, including its clients. The second factor is the opportunity for us to advance our understanding of social interventions, their processes, and outcomes. In other

University of Durham
Centre for Applied Social Studies

Being a Member

Members of this group are chosen to achieve a spread of knowledge and experience which can contribute to the research project. CASS encourages the involvement of carers and clients as Project Advisory Group members. A senior member of CASS will chair the group.

Your Contribution

Project Advisory Groups are set up to help projects succeed. As a member of this group you can contribute in a number of ways:

- Provide support for the research project workers as a whole
- Advise on the overall structure of the project
- Provide information about other work in progress
- Provide information about policy and practice development
- Help with specific aspects (such as research access)
- Ensure the project maintains a focus on how the findings will be used and shared
- Advise on how the findings are presented
- Share responsibility for taking the messages from the research to relevant groups
- Use your own networks to publicize findings

Ground Rules

Project Advisory Group members are expected to act in a personal capacity and not just as representatives of their organizations.

- *Respect* – the Project Advisory Group needs to allow for a diversity of opinions and discussion will always be encouraged.
- *Clarification* – to ensure that participants understand each other, we must feel free to ask for explanations.
- Project Advisory Groups are *advisory*, and do not have a management responsibility for the project, its staff, and its finances.
- *Confidentiality* – the research project is in process, so all papers are confidential. There may be matters arising in meetings which are important for participants to share with others—please use discretion in doing so.
- Findings may be informally disseminated in advance of publication only if CASS agrees that it is appropriate to do so.

The Meetings

There will be four Project Advisory Group meetings during the course of the _____ research. The meetings will be held in _____. These meetings provide milestones in the progress of the research project, and the times are chosen for the best input from the group members.

Honoraria and Expenses

We will pay travel and subsistence expenses to anyone whose participation is not supported by their employing organization. In addition, service users and carers are entitled to an honorarium as an acknowledgement of their time and effort.

Thank you

We are grateful to those who give up their time to take part in Project Advisory Groups. Project Advisory Group members usually find that they learn and benefit from membership in the group as well as making a contribution. We hope all participants gain some satisfaction from meeting with fellow group members and from helping in the progress and conclusion of the _____ Research Project.

Figure 20.1   Guidelines for Members of a Research Project Advisory Group

Table 20.2   Example: Membership of a Project Advisory Group (Study of South Asian Children with Disabilities with Their Families)

Director of Social Services Department (Chair)

Two members of Dek Bhal self-help group (one Pakistani, one Bangladeshi)

Muslim religious leader from local community

Clinical psychologist, specialist in learning disability

Community pediatrician

Community nurse

Social worker (children's services)

Education manager of services for disabled children

Plus members of the research team

words, the proposed evaluation must be relevant and useful to the program and to the advancement of research-based knowledge.

In setting up and carrying out program evaluations, we have learned from Patton's *Utilization-Focused Evaluation* (1997), with its emphasis on ensuring that evaluations are constructed from the beginning with a primary concern for their usefulness. Patton asserts that the best way to ensure utilization is through partnership with the people he calls "stakeholders." A stakeholder is potentially anyone who has an interest in the findings of an evaluation; however, as Patton (1997, p. 42) points out, stakeholders typically have diverse and often competing interests, and the evaluation is unlikely to be able to answer all questions. Consequently, he suggests narrowing the list of potential stakeholders to a specific group of primary intended users. This, Patton says, is beyond the traditional recommendation of evaluation texts to identify the audience. A particularly useful comment is that "people, not organizations, use evaluation information" (p. 147).

To illustrate how utilization-focused evaluation works in practice, I refer to current work in which we are evaluating a set of local programs funded as part of a national initiative known as *Sure Start*. Sure Start has the overall goal of helping preschool children from disadvantaged neighborhoods, but each local program is expected to develop its own methods to suit particular local circumstances. Local Sure Start programs are themselves partnerships between health and local government agencies and members of the community. Thus, proposals for program funding must demonstrate interagency partnerships and show how parents and community have been involved. The evaluation of these programs should logically be based on the same partnerships.

Partnerships In Formative Evaluation: The Sure Start Project

The first four Sure Start programs in our locality formed a consortium that invited proposals for a linked evaluation over three years. Evaluators were asked to present their approach to a mixed audience of program staff, partner agencies, and parents who had been involved in drawing up the program specification. This meant that from the beginning, the evaluation had to be framed in terms that could readily be understood and seen as relevant by all partners. But there was also a personal factor. We subsequently received feedback after one such presentation that the parent representatives had been pleased when the slick media presentation had failed to work and the evaluators had to use an informal, conversational style.

In addition to the many local evaluations that have been or are being commissioned all over England (approximately 160 individual programs), central government has commissioned an overall evaluation of the outcomes of Sure Start. This evaluation will be using a quasi-experimental design, monitoring inputs in the form of service contacts and comparing outcomes between Sure Start and non-Sure Start areas. At a local level, stakeholders are interested in both formative and summative evaluation. Yes, they want to know whether the elements of the program are effective, but in the words of one participant, "We don't want to wait for three years only for you to tell us that we got it all wrong, and that we should have done it differently." Rather, participants want feedback on process as well as outcomes; they want to be able to change what they are doing if the mechanisms they are using do not seem to be working.

For example, one of the key principles of Sure Start is to involve parents in the management of programs. In order to evaluate the extent to which this was being achieved, our researcher attended management meetings and interviewed parent representatives, program staff, and agency representatives. She found that in general, while professionals believed that they were successful in involving parents, the parents themselves said that they had great difficulty in meetings because of the jargon used in discussion and because they did not understand how decisions were made. These problems were raised at a program meeting of parents and professionals convened especially to discuss a report of the findings and to consider their implications.

The result was an agreed set of guidelines for meetings designed to ensure full participation of all members.

Parents have also contributed to the formulation of questions for the Sure Start evaluations. In some projects, parents have chosen to work with the evaluators in separate groups from staff. In others, parents and staff have joined in workshops together. Patton (1997, p. 100) pointed out "participatory evaluation" involved participants in learning the logic of evaluation and something about its methods. Figure 20.2 offers an example of a flyer designed for parents for a first workshop. All participants, including parents, have to learn how to ask questions, which questions can be answered by empirical evidence, and which are a matter of opinion and conjecture. They need to check whether the answer is already known and if not, who wants to know and what difference it would make if the answer could be found. These last points are especially important in a utilization-focused approach: if no one wants to know, or cannot say what use the information would be, then it is a waste of time and effort to ask in the first place.

The approach we use to generate and focus questions in a participatory evaluation is described by Patton (1997). We begin by asking participants to work in small groups to generate questions using the formula, "I would like to know X about Y (some aspect of the program)." They test these questions against the criteria discussed, consider who would be interested in the answers, and determine how the answers would be used. The task of the evaluators is to focus and collate the questions and propose methods by which they might be answered. These are then fed back to a second workshop at which the proposals are discussed and a protocol developed. An example from one of the projects is shown in Figure 20.3. Through this approach, parents as well as staff may become involved in data collection; for

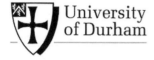

University
of Durham

Asking Questions

In our evaluation of Sure Start, we want to help programmes find out what's going well and what could be going better.

To do this we will be looking at some Sure Start activities more closely. We need parents and Sure Start staff to help decide which projects to choose and what questions we should ask about them.

In the spring we will have an open meeting so that parents can come and help choose the projects for us to look at. Below are some questions and answers you may find helpful:

Do I need to know a lot about Sure Start to come along?

No, all you need is an interest in Sure Start and a child under 4.

What if I can't think of questions?

Don't worry, we'll help you, and everyone will be sitting in groups of just three or four people to share ideas.

What will happen next?

We will take the questions away and see how we can answer them.

We will then come back to you to see what you think of our ideas.

If you want to know more, please talk to Jill on 333 3333

We would be very grateful if you could come along

Figure 20.2   Flyer for Parents Invited to an Evaluation Workshop (Sure Start Evaluation)

1. How many parents know about Sure Start?

2. Why don't Dads come to the group?

3. What do Moms think of the family support workers?

4. How well does the multi-professional team work?

5. Do the *Learning through Play* groups help children learn?

6. What will happen when the money runs out?

7. Is Sure Start cost-effective?

Figure 20.3   Questions Generated Through Participatory Evaluation Workshop (Sure Start Project)

example, mothers may give questionnaires to other mothers they know who have not engaged in the project, or staff may agree to collect and supply information gathered during routine visits. Some participants may even be willing to assist in the data analysis, but all are motivated to engage in its interpretation and in formulating recommendations. The development of guidelines in response to the identification of a problem in parents' participation in Sure Start management meetings, described above, is an example of this process.

Key principles in participatory evaluation have been proposed by Patton (1997, p. 100):

- Participants own the evaluation. They make the decisions about the questions to be asked, the methods used and how the findings are used.
- All aspects of the evaluation should be as open as possible. Methods and findings should be understandable and meaningful to participants.
- The process involves participants in learning the logic of evaluation and about evaluation methods.
- Evaluators recognize and value the perspectives and knowledge of all participants. They work to help all participants recognize their own and others' expertise.

While these principles provide a helpful guide in working with projects such as Sure Start, where we have been commissioned by the program itself, it is important to remember that as a university research center, we also have a stake in the evaluation. That is, we have a responsibility to generate knowledge that may be generalized or extrapolated. Consequently, we acknowledge explicitly that we have our own aims in participating in the research and strive to reconcile these with program partners. Thus, what is particularly interesting to us as academics is the ability to make comparisons between the seven Sure Start programs in the county where we are engaged. They all have the same overall aims and objectives, but are using markedly different methods to achieve these ends. As Pawson and Tilley (1997) have argued, it is inappropriate to treat social initiatives (like Sure Start) as "independent variables," or as "treatments." Instead, we must appreciate that they work "through a process of reasoning, change, influence, negotiation, battle of wills, persuasion, choice increase (or decrease), arbitration, or some such like" (p. 17). The Sure Start evaluations provide an excellent opportunity to understand these processes as well as to measure the outcomes. After all, it is not much use knowing that something has worked if we don't know *why* it worked.

PARTNERSHIPS WITH PRACTITIONERS

It would be quite wrong to imply that partnerships in research are uncomplicated, especially when professional practice is being evaluated. Some of the difficulties that can arise are well-illustrated in a current project, funded by the Department of Health, which aims to assess the comparative cost-effectiveness of therapeutic services for children provided by local authorities and by charitable (not-for-profit) agencies. This is an important national policy matter. The

Department has promoted these services strongly because it considered that too much effort was being spent on policing families suspected of child abuse and neglect and not enough on supporting them in the difficult tasks of parenting. However, such services are thought to be expensive, there are some concerns about their effectiveness, and disputes arise about which agencies should provide them. These issues were also of obvious interest to senior managers of both types of organization, and we did not have too much difficulty in recruiting for the study from relevant agencies. The managers agreed to explain the study to their staff and assisted us in organizing a series of workshops for professional staff and administrators. In these we introduced the methods by which we were to assess the outcomes for families and to estimate the costs of the services provided.

During the workshops, we explained to the professionals that we had selected a number of standardized measures that we believed would help them as practitioners in assessing child and family problems and strengths as well as provide us with a comprehensive set of baseline data. These were all instruments that have been used extensively elsewhere and included those which were promoted by the Department of Health as part of a new assessment framework for use in children's services. The approach we proposed, which had worked well in a previous project, was that the practitioners should explain the research to families entering the service and, if they agreed to participate, collect an initial set of data using some of the measures. Our researcher would then visit a few weeks later to confirm the families' participation in the research and to collect further data, including views on the quality of the service they had experienced thus far.

We had taken pains to explain to the practitioners the significance of the research, observing that the Department of Health had commissioned it because so little was known about therapeutic services for families: here was the chance to provide the evidence to support what they were doing. There was the opportunity for discussion as part of each workshop, during which various concerns were raised and reassurances given. We returned to the university and waited for the first sets of data to arrive. Unfortunately, we had underestimated the strength of practitioners' resistance to participation, and the data have been very slow to come in, with some projects in the study failing to provide a single referral to the research. Some of the reasons given by practitioners were the following:

- The research will upset the children and/or their families.
- The measures are inappropriate for families in crisis—and by the time they are ready to complete them, they have changed.
- The instruments do not assess the changes I think are important.
- The research will be used to shut down the service—whatever the results.
- Whatever they say, this research is about evaluating my practice.
- I haven't got time to do all these assessments and form filling. (I'll put them aside and the project will go away.)
- I don't really understand what it's all about. It's too complicated.
- I did explain to a couple of families, but they were not interested, so I gave up.

We have tried various approaches to stimulate participation, which are described in detail elsewhere (Tidmarsh, Carpenter, & Slade, 2003). These include a booklet of "Frequently Asked Questions," which seeks to address practitioner concerns. We have run supplementary workshops and have followed up with team managers to identify new referrals to their projects who met the inclusion criteria for the study. So far, and in spite of senior managers' renewed expressions of support, we have had limited success. This may not be one of our more successful projects. It is only a little reassuring to discover that similar problems have been experienced elsewhere (see Draper, 2001).

PARTNERSHIPS IN THE DISSEMINATION AND APPLICATION OF RESEARCH

Dissemination and the application of research findings deserve a separate chapter in their own right. It is easy to find reasons for pessimism about the possibility of research ever having an impact on policy and practice. However, I have suggested earlier in this chapter how we might enhance its potential: by ensuring through partnership with practitioners and clients that researchers ask relevant questions. In this final section, I will share two examples of ways in which we have attempted to promote the use of research in practice.

First, I should be clear that I am discussing one aspect of research utilization among the many identified by Weiss (1979) in her influential categorization. This Weiss calls the decision-driven or problem-solving model. As applied to policy making, this model begins when policymakers identify a problem and look for research to help them reach an informed decision. This is the model explicit in the Policy Research program of the Department of Health which, in theory at least, commissions research for this purpose. Of course, in many cases, the Department has already decided and may even have implemented the policy before the research project even begins. However, rather than extend this discussion, I will switch to the level of practice.

Project Examples

The "Making Research Count" Project. Making Research Count is a project in the north east of England led by colleagues at York University. It involves a partnership of local authority social services departments and health authorities whose members are asked to agree on a series of key topics concerning service developments in the area of collaborative care for children and adults. Workshops are set up by the university at which researchers present a synthesis of research findings. For example, we have presented a workshop on assertive community treatment for people with severe mental illness. This was in response to a decree from the Department of Health that all areas should implement such services within twelve months. However, the exact form these services should take was left up to local managers. Our task at the workshop was to present evidence from existing studies and to discuss with those practitioners and managers how these findings might inform decisions about the configuration and operational policies of their new services. Of course, there would be other influences on their decisions, such as the level of funding provided and the availability of appropriately qualified staff.

"Research-Informed Practice" Project. This project, which was established following a discussion with the director of another local social services department, aims to increase the use of research evidence to inform decision making in individual cases held by children and family social workers. Again, it is a problem-solving approach. Rather than presenting seminars on research into best practice, the project works from issues of concern to practitioners. Teams of social workers meet twice monthly in "practice development groups." Team members present a case from their practice and a researcher helps them to formulate questions. The answers to these questions may help them to understand more about the case and to take decisions about intervention that are grounded in research evidence. The researcher aims to teach them how to find relevant research evidence, for

example by using the Internet, and helps them to evaluate the evidence. The group considers the implications of the evidence for the case, leaving the caseworker to take the decisions.

Both *Making Research Count* and *Research-Informed Practice* are being evaluated and early findings show promise. In both cases, the principle of partnership is an important element in their success.

CONCLUSION

In this chapter, I have tried to show how partnerships between researchers and policymakers, practitioners, and clients can be of mutual benefit. The benefits to researchers are clear: such partnerships help us to design research which is relevant to policy and practice, thereby enhancing the prospects of winning grants from funders of applied social research. As indicated, the projects themselves are often complicated and challenging to carry out, but they never fail to be interesting and are usually great fun. There is also the satisfaction of knowing that if all goes well, there are others committed to the project and to making use of its findings. When these findings can be used to support or inform the development and implementation of best policy and practice, then we may have a realistic hope that research can contribute to making the world a better place for families, which is surely the point of the whole exercise.

REFERENCES

Blunkett, D. (2000). *Influence or irrelevance: Can social science improve government?* Lecture given to the Economic and Social Research Council, Department for Education and Employment, London, UK.

Draper, L. (2001). Being evaluated: A practitioner's view. *Children and Society, 15,* 46–52.

Lewis, J. (2000). Funding social science research in academia. *Social Policy and Administration, 34,* 365–376.

Nulty, S., & Webb, J. (2002). Evidence and the policy process. In H. Davies, S. Nulty, & P. Smith (Eds.), *What works? Evidence-based policy and practice in public services* (pp. 13–41). Bristol, UK: The Policy Press.

Patton, M. Q. (1997). *Utilization-focused evaluation* (3rd ed.). Thousand Oaks, CA: Sage.

Pawson, R., & Tilley, N. (1997). *Realistic evaluation.* London, UK: Sage.

Rossi, P., Wright, J., & Wright, S. (1978). The theory and practice of applied social research. *Evaluation Quarterly, 2,* 171–191.

Schneider, J., Carpenter, J., Wooff, D., & Brandon, T. (2001). Carers and community mental health services. *Social Psychiatry and Psychiatric Epidemiology, 36,* 604–607.

Tidmarsh, J., Carpenter, J., & Slade, J. (2003). Practitioners as gatekeepers and researchers: Assessing the outcomes of family support services. *International Journal of Sociology and Social Policy, 23,* 59–79.

Weiss, C. (1979). The many meanings of research utilization. *Public Administration Review, 39,* 426–431.

Wilensky, H. (1997). Social science and the public agenda: Reflections on the relation of knowledge to policy in the United States and abroad. *Journal of Health Politics, Policy and Law, 22,* 1241–1265.

CHAPTER 21

Swirling Waters: History and Current Choices for Families to Navigate Health Care Financing

HARVEY HILLIN

The cost of health care is a growing concern for American families. In the United States we spend about $1.2 trillion per year on health care: two to four times per capita what other industrialized countries spend. Although there is not agreement on how routine health care costs should be managed, there is agreement that catastrophic illness or injury not only threatens the life of the family member, but the economic survival of the family as well. As co-pays and deductibles replace the historic "fee for service" payments, the decision to seek health care at all is becoming an economic one. Indeed, most "prescriptions" for change in the health care system of the United States are focused on the dollar.

In April of 2003, a national survey found that the cost of health care and insurance eclipsed most other economic worries for U.S. residents (Kaiser Family Foundation, 2003). Over one-third of the poor (designated by an income of $28,256 or less for a family of three in 2001) and one-fourth of those in the next economic bracket lack health insurance coverage (Kaiser, 2003). In an exhaustive review of 25 years of research on the consequences of not having health insurance, Hadley (2003) found the following: uninsured persons have fewer preventive services, tend to be more severely ill when diagnosed, and receive less care. All of these factors result in higher premature death rates. Mortality estimates for the uninsured people range from 4% to 25%.

By 1979, employer-based insurance coverage peaked, providing benefits to two-thirds of the workforce. In 1983, almost half of employers offering health insurance paid 100% of the costs for employees, but by 1998, only one quarter of employers did this. Today, growing unrest about health care costs drives labor union skirmishes with management in many industries as those cost increases get passed along to erode wages (Appleby, 2003). Family coverage costs more than three times what individual coverage costs—and this is the case only when coverage is available through employers. The number of uninsured persons in the United States is about 41 million people. The demographic makeup of this group includes 16%

of non-elderly Americans, mostly adults; half of Hispanic adult males; and one-third of black adult males, although the number of uninsured children in this population is decreasing. Health care spending per capita rose 10% in 2001, but employment-based health insurance cost rose 12.7% and hospital cost rose 12% (Strunk, Ginsburg, & Gabel, 2002).

It was believed that fee-for-service payments (in combination with oversupply of specialty care in urban areas) drove over-utilization and drove up health care costs. Despite common beliefs to the contrary, the "graying of America" (aging baby boomers) is also not a primary driver of rising health care costs—though this is controversial because of the shift of aged and disabled adults out of private sector health coverage and into public sector coverage (Strunk & Ginsburg, 2002). Managed care and assignment of primary care physicians for gate-keeping to specialty care brought some savings, but pressures from consumers, providers, and lawyers soon expanded the complexity and costs of health care in new ways.

The true costs of health care rose 15% in 2001, as benefit buy-downs became common practice, and large insurers refused to spread the cost of unreimbursed and under-reimbursed care. The hydraulic pressure of cost shifting changed dramatically with the advent of managed care, under-reimbursement of Medicare and Medicaid, and large insurer discounting in markets where there are multiple providers of health care. The migration of medicine to specialization and the filling of urbanized areas with an over-capacity of services and hospital beds fueled over-utilization of services. Pharmacy advancements that are marketed directly to consumers have also worked to increase health care costs for families.

Costs for unreimbursed care have always been shifted to those who can pay (Dobson,

DaVanzo, & Sen, 2002). In fact, virtually all hospitals had some affiliation with or as charitable organizations less than half a century ago. Another way to shift cost includes limiting care to the seriously ill or culling them out of a plan, because the sickest of the sick (perhaps 2% of a typical risk pool) easily require 30% or more of the costs. The cost of employment health insurance has shifted from employer to employee, so that the number of workers actually taking health insurance options declined by 1996 to about 80% of those eligible. Of particular interest are younger workers who are in relatively good health, with low risk, for whom the "price" of health insurance is becoming prohibitive. These persons help carry the economic costs for the seriously and chronically ill in shared-risk pools, but are being priced out of the pool. The percentage of workers or families with employment-based insurance did not increase between 1997 and 2001, while public program enrollment did, primarily through the State Children's Health Insurance Program (SCHIP) for low-income children (Strunk & Reschovsky, 2002). The net effect for children in 2001 was a modest decline in the number of uninsured.

What can rural and urban families do to manage health care costs, and how does this differ from what families have done in previous generations? How does Medicaid enter into the picture as a "payer of last resort"? Just as importantly, what can health care and service professionals do to help families navigate health care financing?

HISTORY OF HEALTH CARE FINANCE

Until a century ago health care, if available at all, was performed for a fee. Physicians acted as small businesses, operating independently. As recently as the 1940s, the fee for labor and delivery was about $50 to the hospital (for about a week's care) and $25 to the physician. Medical records consisted of paper charts hanging on the end of the bed, or index cards kept in a pocket of the nurse's uniform (E. Platt & K. Platt, personal notes, 1979). Families paid the fee in installments of several dollars a month. No interest was charged, and banks, financial institutions, insurers, and lawyers were out of the loop. In rural areas, bartering items such as garden vegetables, poultry, and eggs for health care with rural physicians who made house calls was common. This was a dyadic system of physician-patient that operated for perhaps 30 centuries and that has transformed within the last 50 years into a triangular one of three parties, the third being "payer" (Starr, 1982). Patients were transformed into "consumers" (the object of "ask for it by name" direct marketing from pharmaceutical companies), and physicians became "providers" (an anathema to the profession). What part the "payer" plays in the triangle is less clear.

Although sickness insurance was available in Massachusetts, with the Massachusetts Health Insurance Company of Boston, as early as 1847, compulsory contributions from seamen's wages to health costs date to 1789 with the U.S. Marine Hospital Service. By 1853, the French Mutual Aid Society of San Francisco offered hospital care, and by 1863 the Travelers Insurance Company of Hartford, Connecticut offered accident insurance. By 1866 there were about 60 companies offering health insurance. One of the early group policies was Montgomery Ward's health insurance for employees in 1910. Most policies were "loss of income" policies providing benefits for specified diseases such as typhus, scarlet fever, smallpox, diphtheria, and diabetes. Between 1915 and 1920, 16 state legislatures debated compulsory health insurance, but all bills failed. In the 1970s through the 1990s the idea of "national health insurance," with emphasis on models from Canada, England, Germany, Sweden, Norway, and other industrialized countries, entered and exited from the national political stage on several occasions. Of the 25 major industrialized countries today, only 2 do not have national health insurance: South Africa and the United States.

What we now call "health insurance" is the product of two distinct movements in health care. The first was organization based or "company doctors" who served large mining, railroad, and manufacturing industries, a carry-over from military doctors stationed with posts and naval ports. The second was the banding together of physician groups or labor organizations (which later became shared-risk pools) that began in the Great Depression of the 1930s. In 1929, Dallas teachers organized to arrange care at Baylor Hospital, which was the forerunner of Blue Cross and Shield Plans. Also in 1929, Farmers Union established the first Health Maintenance Organization (HMO). In 1930 only 2% of workers had health insurance (White, 2001). Today, HMOs have two forms. Delivery system HMOs have medical groups and hospitals working for defined populations giving prepaid care (Enthoven, 2003). More numerous, however, are carrier HMOs (insurance companies negotiating with physicians), which is really a "pass through" fee-for-service system of discounted fees that attempts to control utilization.

Publicly funded versions of health insurance appeared through two venues: movements and shared-risk health insurance. The movements include: military, Veterans Administration, and Indian Health Service. Shared-risk health insurance, which was a 1960s extension of the Social Security Act of 1935, includes Medicare, Title XVIII and Medicaid, and Title XIX. Since both venues originally reimbursed using a "cost-based" method and added millions of persons to the insured groups in a short period of time (with no concurrent increase in the number of health care providers), health care costs became wildly inflated. Less than one year after inception, Congress had to immediately raise the Social Security tax by an additional 25% to pay for it.

Two other significant federal laws affecting health coverage before the 1960s were tax related: the Revenue Act of 1939, which excluded insurance compensation from income; and the Revenue Act of 1954, which excluded contributions to health plans. This made it possible for companies to insure workers in ways advantageous to both. Favorable tax treatment of insurance premiums and payments means that untaxed dollars have greater value than out-of-pocket dollars paid after taxes in purchasing health care.

Today there are three major sources of health coverage of interest to families. The largest of the three is private, usually employer-based, health insurance with over 600 companies nationally. In the early stages of employer-based coverage, insurance evenly spread costs among the covered persons, everyone was covered, and no one suffered severe loss in the pool. Then companies discovered some groups (young people, for instance) spent very little on health care. "Experience-rated" policies, which offer lower premiums based on age, demographics, and other factors followed. This discovery—that covering lower-risk people made profits—created new pressures. Unfortunately, experience-rated risk pools create situations where acutely or chronically ill people can't get coverage, and where healthy people avoid coverage because of costs. Medicare was created to balance the system, but it did not succeed.

Although people are concerned about health care costs (when polled), they tend not to be equally concerned about health insurance costs, for one major reason: eighty-five percent of the insured public gets that health insurance from employer-based plans, and typically only pay 20% of the total premium costs. When spending "someone else's" money in the medical market there are no

incentives to conserve expenses, creating a kind of "free lunch fantasy." This is fueled by the likelihood most want the best health care for themselves and perhaps the economy package for others. The more recent antidotes to free-lunch pressures are steadily rising co-payments and deductibles to try to shift the balance back to the consumer. But in reality, most insured people don't even ask about cost anymore.

The other two major sources of health insurance are Medicare and Medicaid. From 1980 to 1990 Medicare spending grew 352% and Medicaid spending grew 287%. By the 1950s, industrialized countries spent 4% of Gross National Product (GNP) on health care. In 1960, the U.S. spent 5.3%. By 1970 this spending rose to 7.3%; by 1980 it rose to 9.2%, and by 1990 it reached 12.2%. Today it approaches 20% in the United States. Anderson, Reinhardt, Hussey, and Petrosyan (2003) noted that per capita spending on health care that doubles that of other countries is traced in terms of share of the Gross Domestic Product, public/private spending, pharmacy, nurse/physician workforce, hospital bed capacity, and technology. Health care worker salaries, hospital costs, and the highly fragmented complex payment system in the U.S., requiring much higher administrative costs, are cited as culprits. Interestingly, those authors do not cite pharmacy among primary cost inflators; or lawyers, the fourth party to the "triangle" with litigious demands for defensive medicine practices that further increase costs; or liability insurers, the fifth party, demanding up to $300,000 annual premiums for obstetricians in states such as Nevada; or widely practiced fraudulent over-billing, although many other researchers do mention these as cost drivers. Politicians arrive in the mix as well, and the "broth is already spoiled."

There were stark changes in the 1970s through the 1990s in health care finance. Most efforts were aimed at cost containment, such as rate negotiations, initiation of state and local planning councils to "certify need" for proliferation of hospitals and beds, and Professional Standards Review Organizations (PSRO). Health Maintenance Organization programs were created to fix fees and reduce procedure-based billing. The Tax Equity and Fiscal Responsibility Act of 1982 set limits on Medicare reimbursement. The Prospective Payment system of 1993 established predetermined rates based on diagnostic groupings, and Resource Based Relative Value measures were introduced in physician reimbursement.

HEALTH CARE FINANCE TODAY

There are numerous philosophies of health care finance on the street today. They include: free-market ideology (although health care does not fit the criteria for a free-market system), single government control in a national health care model (comparison models in other countries provide basic care but offer less advancement of practices or technologies in health care, and are not immune to inflationary pressures), health planning approaches by regulatory control, public utility approaches, managed care approaches, managed competition hybrids, and incremental tinkering (Blakeslee, 2003). Among these, "managed competition," which claims to avoid the poles of socialized medicine or of free markets through the transformation of insurers into managers of health care delivery, has growing influence in large markets. Prototypes for managed competition are the Federal Employees Health Benefits Program and similar programs for public employees in California, Minnesota, and elsewhere. However, the legitimacy of insurers as managers of health care delivery is controversial.

Key players in the politics of health care finance are physicians, nurses, other health care providers, large insurance companies, hospitals, employers, and pharmaceutical companies. Although organized labor appears on the radar screen occasionally in these debates, patients (consumers) have little voice. Patients can exercise control in health care to the extent that they can decide whether to be in or out of voluntary insurance plans, and are known to hop from plan to plan when better options (health or economic) are available. Plan "hopping" guarantees that there are no economic advantages to really offering preventive care by the payer. Plan "churning"—change of plans by company, payer, or agent between payers—defeats the purpose of preventive care and creates a lack of consistent "medical home" physician who is familiar with one's health. Intense lobbying, lack of consensus among voting citizens, and strong ideological differences were the demise of national health insurance proposals by Presidents Truman, Nixon, Ford, Carter, and Clinton.

RURAL HEALTH CARE IS NOT URBAN

No discussion of the uninsured or underinsured would be complete without a discussion of rural areas, where larger proportions of uninsured live in comparison to urban areas. Much of the national debate regarding health care and finance options has focused on models of care that presume overabundant and competing resources as well as inappropriate utilization of care. Rather than these issues, the major problem in rural health care concerns access. Although 20% of people live in rural areas, fewer than 11% of physicians practice in rural areas (Office of Rural Health Policy, 1997). In addition, existing safety net services in areas of declining population density are particularly vulnerable to policy changes in health care finance (Geller, 1998). Characteristics of rural areas that create difficulty with health care finance include: lack of proximity to a central place, sparse population density, low total population, unstable economies, and social factors (Hewitt, 1989). Rural areas can also be characterized by harsh climate changes, difficult terrain, lack of water, long distance to metropolitan areas, few resources, low tolerance for systems (government mandates in particular), and independence born of necessity, at least until one has a health care issue.

The single economic base of these areas, often composed of agriculture or mining, makes earning a consistent living difficult, and makes migration of young people in search of work likely. When the economic base is depressed or collapses, an inevitable chain reaction of other business reversals occurs because of the fragile nature of these linkages. Rural health care, like every other rural enterprise, demonstrates the impact of few people and long miles on the system. Because of isolation and access issues, the economic feasibility of health services (much less specialty services) in frontier and many rural areas is in question. Laboratory results go back and forth by delivery truck, and advanced technology care resources are rare. When compared with urban areas, where competition and discounting are factors in health care costs, costs are higher for health care in rural areas—just as they are for other goods and services.

Though not all rural areas are homogeneous, a trend in the Great Plains has been out-migration of young people and an increasing average age of remaining residents. There has been steady decline of population in many rural areas since the 1900 census, when agriculture depended on many workers. For example, Kansas' biggest export is now people, not wheat. Telephone disconnections and deaths outnumbering births are commonplace in smaller rural communities. Rural satellite office infrastructure requires greater resources than health

plans are generally willing to make. Operability of centrally managed care concepts like strong provider network, high volume of services, and significant market share is dubious in rural areas. The managed care literature generally asserts that a critical population mass of at least 300,000 persons is minimal for economic viability (National Rural Health Association, 1999).

Rural hospitals are linked to the attraction and retention of physicians and other health care professionals to rural communities (Langwell, Czajka, Nelson, Lenk, & Berman, 1985). Rural health care professionals provide much larger amounts of uncompensated care than their urban counterparts, and cannot avoid or cost-shift risk as readily as urban health care professionals. In some cases, when Medicaid is available, rural health care professionals are working with rate structures that have not increased in 12 years. As group practice buyouts and management group models take over rural practice, the personal altruism and commitment of physicians to care for the poor are replaced by bottom line practices, dwindling the pool of those who participate as Medicaid-enrolled providers. National surveys indicate that from 1978 to 1983 the proportion of pediatricians "limiting" their Medicaid participation increased from 26% to 35% (Perloff, Kletke, & Neckerman, 1987). In some states, vaccinations for children are diminishing in the context of managed care. In one state, they decreased almost 50% from 1995 to 1999.

Across the nation, the number of providers willing to serve Medicaid patients is dropping consistently (Fox, Weiner, & Phua, 1992). The replacement of independent practices with group practice is not increasing access for the poor, disabled, or children of working poor. Reimbursement levels are among the issues cited in the decline. Rural state legislatures are also less likely to capitalize on the buying power of state funds mixed with federal matching funds to improve state resident health or to develop state economic infrastructure. Hence there is typically greater outflow of funds to Washington than inflow of funds in return. This further erodes the fragile health care sector within the fabric of rural communities.

Numerous policy concerns emerge beyond insurance status for rural and frontier areas. These include support of existing networks from further erosion, integration of services, the classic outreach approaches (circuit riders, satellite/mobile clinics, telemedicine, use of natural helpers and resources—like Alaska's medical services within indigenous communities), and connections with technology for diagnostic service with triage when needed.

Access to care in rural areas remains a barrier to service (Weisgrau, 1995). Short of increasing fee payment levels (in some cases rates haven't increased since the inception of the programs, while related costs of meeting requirements have), there are no viable ways of increasing physician participation in Medicaid (Perloff, Kletke, & Fossett, 1995).

MEDICAID AS THE "PAYER OF LAST RESORT"

Although federal and state governments pay 40% of health care claims, they provide virtually all of the medical school education and most of the research and development dollars in health care. In many states, the majority of post-World War II public and private hospitals were built with Hill/Burton Act funds for construction. Most state legislatures view Medicaid as a vehicle to insure low-income persons, secondary to meeting the growing needs of persons with disabilities and the elderly. Few legislators understand the connectedness of decisions about Medicaid and the economic viability of health care services in their own communities to health care infrastructure. There is often a "disconnect" between their vote to cut Medicaid and

the impact of hospital or nursing home closures in their community.

Medicaid (and Medicare for that matter) requires, whenever possible, that recipients use other funding sources to obtain needed care. When states get a waiver for this provision, there is the obligation to recover third party reimbursement after the state pays a Medicaid claim. These are known in Medicaid circles as "pay and chase," which is the philosophical opposite of "pay as last resort."

Pay and chase usually refers to seeking other insurance coverage for health care but can also include going after insurance by a noncustodial parent charged with support (Child Support Enforcement); workers compensation; health, injury, and tort related claims; and other resources. Since Medicare regulations have similar provisions, the Health Care Financing Administration has allowed Medicaid to be secondary to Medicare. Medicare is secondary to any other insurance, as well as to all of the "assets and income" tests of recipient status itself in Medicaid. Since 1988, the Medicaid Act has prohibited states from asserting payer of last resort rules in regard to special education. There is a growing body of case law involving reimbursement of augmentative and alternative communication (AAC) devices (*Daubert v. Merrill Dow Pharmaceuticals* 1992 & remand 1995); *Fred C. v. Texas Health and Human Services Commission* 1996; *Meyers v. Mississippi* 1995).

Generally speaking, the state general fund (SGF) is the final "downstream" resource for persons in state institutions. The exceptions are persons with developmental disabilities receiving "active treatment" services and inpatient psychiatric treatment, specifically excluding vocational or education expenses. The prohibition of Federal Financial Participation (FFP) was revised in the February 21, 1990 Federal Register (55 FR 6015–6018), concerning intermediate care facilities for the mentally retarded (ICF/MR), reiterating that the Medicaid program is fundamentally for medical assistance and a payer of last resort.

The concept of "payer of last resort" refers to the state's obligation to discover and use third party insurance reimbursement for services *prior* to payment by Medicaid (in USC s. 1396b[o]). The state must exhaust other payment sources before drawing from state and federal tax dollars to meet medical bills of beneficiaries. The words "payer of last resort" do not appear in the United States Code (USC Search Engine, Cornell Law) but do appear in review sections of the Federal Register with reference to Medicaid, Part H, and in the Indian Health Service (IHS) regulations promulgated by publication in the Federal Register in February of 1990. However, this does not mean the states have historically felt bound by the federal trust responsibility, particularly with respect to state matching funds, or to maintaining separation of services offered.

Military personnel and dependents are covered in CHAMPUS/TRICARE insurance, whereas other federal, and most state, employees have private health insurance coverage options. The Veterans Administration considers itself as downstream from private insurance, Medicare, and Medicaid, but not from the Indian Health Service.

The picture for adults is also complicated by the presence of end-stage renal disease (Medicare), various disabilities (Medicare or Medicaid), venereal diseases and tuberculosis (public health statutes), pregnancy (Medicaid higher-eligibility cutoffs), breast or cervical cancer (Medicaid higher-eligibility cutoffs or services provided by CDC-approved Health Department screenings), immigrant status (Medicaid one-time emergency medical services required by federal law), or HIV/AIDS (Ryan White Act). There are also implications not covered in this chapter for pharmacy "point of sale" requirements that pharmacists discover and bill other insurance prior to billing Medicaid.

Health Care for Adults

For adults, with regard to health care services that are medically necessary and prescribed in an individualized treatment plan by a licensed health care professional, the issue of who pays as a last resort is more straightforward. A metaphor comes to mind: a waiter (health care provider) presents a person with the bill for a very expensive meal, and everyone else is hiding or won't make eye contact. Figure 21.1 accounts for the more common (but not all) possibilities faced by adults who are seeking health care.

Health Care for Children

The question of who is payer of last resort in matters of services to children is decidedly more complex. In fact, if the decision tree under handicap were expanded, Figure 21.2 would go over a page. The responsibility for payer of last resort depends on what services are provided, the age of the child, and any handicapping conditions that are present. Of course, the presence of a disabling condition raises the stakes for all interested parties.

In 1975, the Education for all Handicapped Children Act (PL 94–142, or Part B of the Education of the Handicapped Act) required all children with disabilities to be provided a "free appropriate public education" at no cost to the parents. In 1977, regulations appeared that allowed states to use state, private, local, and federal resources to meet these requirements, with the proviso that no third party insurer was relieved of otherwise valid obligation to pay for services.

Many insurers bailed out anyway, many employers structured benefits pools to avoid persons with disabilities, and many states enacted policies to not allow Medicaid to pay for services written in the Individual Education Plan (IEP), even though a child was otherwise eligible.

By 1980, the Office of Special Education and the Office of Civil Rights of the U.S.

Is the person an adult?	N	See children's chart		
Y				
In a state institution?	Y	Receives active treatment	N	State pays
N		at ICF/MR or psychiatric?	Y	If eligible, insurance,
Medically necessary?	N	No health care payment		Medicare, or Medicaid pays, in that order.
Y				
Is there private insurance?	Y	Insurance pays		
N				
Workers compensation?	Y	Worker comp pays		
N				
Accident, tort or court related damage award?	Y	Court award pays		
		If pending, recovery by Medicare or Medicaid, but not provider		
N				
End stage renal disease?	Y	Medicare pays, retaining recovery rights to third party liens, insurance		
N				
Medicare eligible?	Y	Medicare pays, retaining recovery rights to third party liens, insurance		
N				
Medicaid eligible?	Y	Medicaid pays, retaining recovery secondary to Medicare recovery		
N				
Pregnant, cancer of cervix or breast, disabled, or waiver?	Y	Expanded Medicaid eligibility		Medicaid pays
N				
VA eligible?	Y	VA provides the care, but is not a payer except in some long term care		
N				
Indian Health Service?	Y	Indian Health Service provides service		
N				
Provider at risk		Unless illegal alien under SOBRA provisions		

Figure 21.1   Adult Health Care Financing Decision Tree

Department of Education published a Notice of Interpretation about an education agency's authority to require parents of a disabled child to file insurance claims and use the proceeds to pay for services under Part B of PL 94–142 or Section 504 of the Rehabilitation Act of 1973. Up through the 1980s, HCFA (now CMS) philosophy was that all services under state and federal education laws were excluded from Medicaid reimbursement and a state's responsibility. This changed with *Bowen v. Massachusetts* (1988) in which the Supreme Court upheld a Massachusetts district court opinion that the nature of the service determines whether it is education, not the state's method of administering the service. PL 99–457 Education of the Handicapped amendments of 1986 complicated matters further by addressing Medicaid funding and expanding special education and related services to children aged three to five years, not normally in public school. The

Is the person a child?	N	See adult chart		
Y				
In a state institution?	Y	Receives active treatment at ICF/MR or psychiatric?	N	State pays
N			Y	Insurance, Medicare or Medicaid if eligible
Medically necessary?	N	Educational service?	Y	Education pays
Y		N		
		No payment		
Is there private insurance?	Y	Insurance pays (includes non-custodial parent insurance)		
N				
Foster child, or adoption?	Y	Medicaid pays foster, and in some cases adoption support		
N				
Handicap, disability or waiver?	Y	Insurance, Medicare or Medicaid if eligible		
N				
Child of working poor?	Y	Possible SCHIP coverage		
N				
Indian Health Service?	Y	Indian Health Service provides		
N				

Figure 21.2   Health Care Financing Decision Tree for Children

unfunded mandate hit state Medicaid budgets when it amended section 203 of PL 94–142 to the following:

> This paragraph shall not be construed to limit the responsibility of agencies other than educational agencies in a state from providing or paying for some or all of the costs of a free appropriate public education to be provided to handicapped children in the state.

Section 613 (a)(13) further stated:

> This act shall not be construed to permit a state to reduce medical or other assistance available or to alter eligibility under titles V or XIX of the Social Security Act with respect to the provision of a free appropriate public education for handicapped children within the state.

The act also made amendments to Part B of the Education of the Handicapped Act (EHA), and added toddlers and early intervention programs (Part H), encouraging early intervention and services at no cost except where federal or state law provides for a system of payments by families, including a schedule of sliding scale fees. There was a provision of additional federal funds indirectly for this purpose. States were charged to coordinate services of the following:

1. Title V of the Social Security Act (Maternal and Child Health)

2. Title XIX of the Social Security Act—Medicaid and especially Early and Periodic Screening and Diagnosis (EPSDT)

3. The Head Start Act

4. Parts B and H of EHA

5. Subpart 2 of Part D of Chapter I of Title I of the Elementary and Secondary Education Act of 1965

6. The Developmentally Disabled Assistance and Bill of Rights Act (PL 94–103)

7. Other federal programs (34 CFR 303.522)

PL 99–457 indicated that Part H funds were to be used as a payer of last resort, in the following words:

> Funds under this part may not be used to satisfy a financial commitment for services that would otherwise have been paid for from another public or private source but for the enactment of Part H of the Act. Therefore, funds under this part may be used only for early intervention services that an eligible child needs but is not currently entitled to under any other federal, state, local, or private source. (34 CFR, 303.527 (a))

The federal government uses a "non-supplanting" principle in framing much of its legislation, and generally is wary of use of funding in one bill to satisfy commitments of other governmental agencies at the state, local, or federal level. These escape clauses are integral to virtually all of the federal legislation, for fear that states, or other governmental agencies at the federal level, will bail out of costs or maintenance of current effort. For instance, section 411(k)(13) of the Medicare Catastrophic Coverage Act of 1988 (PL 100–360) cites HCFA intent as "to insure that services that would ordinarily be provided or paid for by other agencies for handicapped children would be continued."

The act also provides that state Medicaid programs are responsible for covered "related services" (such as speech-language pathology or physical therapy) included in a child's IEP plan or an infant or toddler's individual family service plan, independent of service site (in many cases, at school). The providers of service are also obliged to meet the conditions of participation in Medicaid. Another example is CFR 55, February 21, 1990, 6015–6018, clarifying the prohibition of vocational training or educational activities at ICF/MR facilities.

COST SHIFTING

For the purposes of this chapter, cost shifting includes the fear in the Congress that promulgated rules to have Medicaid be a payer of last resort. That fear was integral to the federal legislative debates framing the Social Security Act of 1935 because the Congress did not want the burden of persons in state institutions shifted to the federal budget level. Modern statistical methods and computerization allow most insurance companies and employers to refine the practice of cost shifting persons with catastrophic and chronic illnesses or disabilities out of the risk pools of covered persons. Because Medicaid and Medicare often pay below costs, they also now serve as principal reasons cost shifting occurs in hospital care, nursing home care, and other health care. In health care financing, cost shifting is usually defined as charging one subset of patients higher prices to offset losses of unreimbursed and underreimbursed care (Showalter, 1997). Often the term is restricted to what is charged to private payers to offset public and insurance reimbursements. It usually refers to hospitals but also refers to doctors and dentists. In hospital care, it often implies a private paying patient will pay for his or her own hospital expenses plus from 30% to 50% to cover unpaid or underpaid expenses (which are composed of free care, Medicaid, Medicare, and contracted care at negotiated rates) of other patients. As traditional insurers balked at these surcharges and negotiated better rates, the shift escalated to 71% or greater levels on remaining players.

Cost shifting varies geographically, based on market power of providers, public payer levels or reimbursement (Medicaid and Medicare), and the levels of uncompensated care in relation to access to other revenue sources (Dobson et al., 2002). The correlation of lack of insurance and low hospital operating margins has a profound impact on access to care (and health care infrastructure and community economies), especially in rural states. When it refers to doctors (often to practice groups), it usually reflects limited acceptance of Medicaid or Medicare patients. It also may mean that people without insurance receive bills for higher charges than insurers pay for covered persons for the same service. The poor may be charged more. They may also be placed in peril of aggressive collection practices, including garnishments, compared with those with insurance and negotiated discounts from insurers.

In government health care financing, cost shifting might as easily refer to cost avoidance directly by Medicaid and many other methods:

1. Avoidance (delay pay or no pay)

2. Recovery or pay and chase (post-pay searches for third party liability payers to reduce Medicaid liability)

3. Narrowing of what costs will be reimbursed

4. Direct cost limitations (TEFRA 1982)

5. Managed care switches to other methods of reimbursement such as negotiated and discounted rates, benefits, management, capitation, and shared-risk schemes

In state budgets, cost shifting can also refer to the shifting of state general fund (SGF) liability for needy disabled populations historically in institutions (asylums or correctional institutions) to community-based services through mechanisms such as the Home and Community Based Services (HCBS) waivers. For states, the policy implications of cost

shifting in Medicaid are profound, given growth in caseloads and health care costs. For states and for the nation, cost shifting means the real costs of health care are almost always hidden. As cost shifting continues in both public and private arenas, the impact of discounting prices can have devastating economic effects on the poor and uninsured when bills go to collection and recovery.

There is growing evidence the uninsured are charged at more than double (about 139%) what is charged to insurers, and the working poor make up a large portion of private-pay visits (Wielawski, 2000).

Some hospitals are also becoming aggressive about charges: wasting no time in using collection agencies, liens, and garnishments, despite the fact that over-billing can be detected at audit on the majority of itemized bills.

Utilization of Medicaid maximization strategies makes a lot of sense. These strategies operate for the benefit of the state, health care beneficiaries and providers, and the community. Yet programs to serve the poor face an uphill battle, as public concern for those less fortunate continues to ebb. In an economy that has experienced 30 years of unparalleled growth and abundance, the gap between wealthy and poor has widened. In 1980, the richest 1% of households had 24.8% of the nation's wealth. By 1997, they had 40.1% of the nation's wealth (Wolf, 2000). The time to address interrelated health and social problems is now. Unless Medicaid reimbursement levels are raised, there will be continued erosion of the willing service provider base, decreasing access to care, losses of safety net services, and ultimately public health consequences with respect to the risks of communicable diseases. The public health consequences of a trip to the mall or grocery store could begin to mean exposure to the consequences of low immunization rates and increasing exposure to diseases such as tuberculosis.

In urban areas where there are plan choices for the employed, there is strong statistical evidence of plan hopping based on rate structures. This occurs even when employment is maintained. There is also a growing trend of turnover of employees in jobs which traditionally had stable workforces. This means that managed care providers are increasingly aware that preventive care does not pay off for the plan. Avoidance of preventive care makes short-term profit (though not for individual health or public health).

Employers, stunned by over half a decade of annual double-digit inflation in health costs, are dropping plans and options, which makes employees more sensitive to medical prices. The future public health consequences could be substantial. The managed care notion of a "medical home" for individuals or families will escape many. The health and social problems families face today will not go away easily.

FOR FAMILIES, CONSUMERS, AND ADVOCATES

The average family can work to control health costs through lifestyle management, preventive care, good nutrition, avoiding high-risk behaviors, practicing self-examination, and taking an active role in health decisions. It is also important to know what health care coverage one has, and to avoid over-utilization. Save emergency room visits for emergencies. In non-emergencies, review insurance coverage (especially for exceptions and exclusions) and know what is covered beforehand. Find out what the room charges are at the hospital and what is included. If tissues aren't covered, bring your own. Ask physicians for estimates of what the charges will be and whether regular prescriptions can be brought from home. Make sure that everyone who treats your family, or plans to

treat you, is included in the coverage of the health insurance plan. Keep a log of what happens, or have a family member do so. Assertive, talkative people with solid social or family networks have better health outcomes than those without those characteristics. Ask lots of questions. Avoid "defensive" medicine services and tests. Demand itemized bills. Every state now requires this be available. When receiving the bill, read it carefully and compare it to the log and to estimates you received.

Establish a medical "home" and avoid most specialized services unless unresolved health issues persist in the face of primary care. A recent survey by the Kaiser Foundation found 33% of people had changed health plans within the last year (Kaiser, 2003). Switching usually means changing physicians, delays in appointments, transferring records, and substituting medications (which poses risks, especially for persons with hereditary risk for chronic diseases like diabetes).

The plan that takes the smallest paycheck deduction isn't necessarily the plan with the lowest total cost. Out-of-pocket expenses should be factored in. If one can carry the load of front-end expenses, overall costs and premiums will often be lower in the long range. Some things might best be paid out of pocket rather than using insurance, even if covered, when it is affordable to do so. This includes purchase of certain drugs to treat depression or anxiety and the use of counseling or psychotherapy, because insurance companies have linked computerized records systems that "factor in" health issues regarding one's future insurability. Even the federal government avoids enlisting persons in military service who have certain treatment histories—in the same way they consider asthma, HIV, and injuries to tendons. No organization willingly exposes itself to possible higher health care costs. Everyone is getting into the act of using statistical methods to cost avoid or cost shift.

In evaluating plans, (1) estimate expenses on health care; (2) check for differences in preventive care; (3) for prescriptions, assess use of brand names for substitution with generics; (4) rethink HMO's cost in relation to quality; (5) consider the risks of serious illness; (6) take advantage of "calculators" provided by companies or available on the Internet (Elders, in particular, will need to do this for the Medicare Modernization Act of 2003 for their prescription drugs in comparing Medicare pharmacy discount plans at www.medicare.gov); (7) consider split coverage rather than family coverage, which is often the most expensive option, when there is the possibility of employer coverage;

(8) use flexible medical spending accounts offered by employers; and (9) make necessary lifestyle, dietary, and exercise changes to reduce risks.

It is hoped this overview gives readers ideas about when, where, and how families handle health care finance, depending on age, poverty, geographic location, or disability, as compared to decades ago. Special attention has been given to Medicaid as the payer of last resort in most health crisis scenarios and how other resources must be exhausted when this is the case. Understanding the current choices families face can help them and those serving them know how they can best navigate health care financing.

REFERENCES

Anderson, G. F., Reinhardt, U. E., Hussey, P. S., & Petrosyan, V. (2003). It's the prices, stupid: Why the U.S. is so different from other countries. *Health Affairs, 22,* 89–105.

Appleby, J. (2003). Health insurance costs fire up unions. *USA Today.* Retrieved January 8, 2003, from www.usatoday.com/money/industries/health/2003–01–08-workers-strikes_x.htm

Blakeslee, A. (2003). *Overview of U.S. healthcare systems.* Class notes, Business Department, Broome Community College, State University of New York.

Bowen v. Massachusetts, 484 US 1003, 108 S. Ct. 693, 98 L.Ed. 2d 645 (1988).

Daubert v. Merrell Dow Pharmaceuticals, 113 S.Ct. 2876 (1992), and remand, 43F3d, 1311 (9th Cir. 1995).

Dobson, A., DaVanzo, J., & Sen, N. (2002, November 13). *Cost shifting: An integral aspect of U.S. health care finance.* The Lewin Group.

Enthoven, A. C. (2003, May). Employment-based health insurance is failing: Now what? *Health Affairs, 22(3),* 237–248.

Fox, M. H., Weiner, J. P., & Phua, K. (1992). Effect of Medicaid payment levels on access to obstetrical care. *Health Affairs, 11(4),* 150–161.

Fred C. v. Texas Health & Human Services Commission, 924 F. Supp. 788 (W.D. Tex. 1996).

Geller, J. M. (1998*). The role of primary care providers in the provision of mental health services: Voices from the plains* (Letter to the Field #10). Denver, CO: University of Denver, Frontier Mental Health Services Network.

Hadley, J. (2003) Sicker and poorer—the consequences of being uninsured: A review of the research on the relationship between health insurance, medical care use, health, work, and income. *Medical Care Research and Review, 60*(2, Supplement), 3S-75S.

Hewitt, M. (1989). *Defining rural areas: Impact on health care policy & research.* Washington, DC: Health Program, Office of Technology Assessment, Congress of the United States.

Kaiser Family Foundation. (2003, March/April). Health care worries in context with other worries. *Health Security Watch,* 1.

Langwell, K., Czajka, J. L., Nelson, S. L., Lenk, E., & Berman, K. (1985). Young physicians in rural areas: The impact of service in the National Health Service Corps: Vol. 1. County characteristics. *Office of Data Analysis & Management Report* (pp. 3–86). Rockville, MD: Public Health Service.

Myers v. Mississippi, NO 3: 94-CIV-185LN (S.D. Miss., June 23, 1995).

National Rural Health Association. (1999, May). *Access to health care for the uninsured in rural and frontier America.* Kansas City, MO: Author.

Office of Rural Health Policy (DHHS). (1997). *Fact sheet. Rural physician: facts about rural physicians,* 1–4.

Perloff, J. D., Kletke, P. R., & Fossett, J. W. (1995). Which physicians limit their Medicaid participation, and why. *Health Services Research, 30,* 7–26.

Perloff, J. D., Kletke, P. R., & Neckerman, K. M. (1987). Physicians decisions to limit Medicaid participation: Determinants and policy implications. *Journal of Health Politics, Policy, and Law, 12,* 221–235.

Showalter, M. H. (1997). Physicians' cost shifting behavior: Medicaid versus other patients. *Contemporary Economic Policy, 15*(2), 74–84.

Starr, P. (1982). *The social transformation of American medicine.* New York: Basic Books.

Strunk, B. C., & Ginsburg, P. B. (2002, September 23). *Aging plays limited role in health care cost trends.* Washington, DC: Center for Studying Health System Change.

Strunk, B. C., Ginsburg, P. B., & Gabel, J. R. (2002). Tracking health care costs: Growth accelerates again in 2001. *Health Affairs,* W299–310.

Strunk, B. C., & Reschovsky, J. D. (2002, August). Working families, health insurance coverage, 1997–2001. *Results from the community tracking study, No. 4.* Washington, DC: Center for Studying Health System Change.

Wielawski, I. (2000, Sept/Oct). Gouging the uninsured: A tale of two bills. *Health Affairs, 19*(5), 181.

Weisgrau, S. (1995). Issues in rural health: Access, hospitals, & reform. *Health Care Finance Review, 17*(1), 1–14.

White, B. (2001, January). The future of health care financing. *Family Practice Management.* Retrieved from www.aafp.org/fpm/20010100/31thef.html

Wolf, E. (2000, February 21). U.S. Department of Labor statistics, data analysis. *US News & World Report,* 42.

Part IV

INTERVENTIONS TO IMPROVE FAMILY HEALTH

CHAPTER 22

Improving Health Through Family Interventions

Thomas L. Campbell

A large body of research has demonstrated that families have a powerful influence on physical health, including overall morbidity and mortality (Burman & Margolin, 1992; Campbell, 1986; Campbell & Patterson, 1995; Kiecolt-Glaser & Newton, 2001). Numerous epidemiological studies have demonstrated that social support, particularly from the family, is associated with improved health (Berkman, 1995, 2000). In an article in 1988 in the journal *Science*, sociologist James House reviewed this research and concluded:

> The evidence regarding social relationships and health increasingly approximates the evidence in the 1964 Surgeon General's report that established cigarette smoking as a cause or risk factor for mortality and morbidity from a range of disease. The age-adjusted relative risk ratios are stronger than the relative risks for all cause mortality reported for cigarette smoking. (House, Landis, & Umberson, 1988, p. 542)

Family support affects the outcome of many chronic medical illnesses. Berkman and colleagues found that after suffering a myocardial infarction, women who are isolated and have few family or social supports experienced two to three times the mortality rate compared to other women (Berkman, Leo-Summers, & Horwitz, 1992). Many stresses within the family, such as loss of a spouse and divorce, significantly impact morbidity and mortality.

Marriage is the family relationship that has the strongest influence on physical health. Even after controlling for other factors, marital status affects overall mortality, mortality from specific illnesses (e.g., cancer and coronary disease), and morbidity (Burman & Margolin, 1992; Kiecolt-Glaser & Newton, 2001). Married individuals are healthier than the widowed, who are in turn healthier than either divorced or never-married individuals. Many large studies have shown that bereavement or death of a spouse increases mortality, especially for men (Martikainen & Valkonen, 1996; Osterweis, Solomon, & Green, 1984). Separation and divorce are also associated with increased mortality.

The quality of marital relationships can influence the outcome of chronic medical illnesses. Marital stress has been shown to worsen coronary artery disease in women (Orth-Gomer et al., 2000). Coyne and colleagues (Coyne et al., 2001) found that marital quality, measured by a composite of self-report and observation of marital interaction, predicts survival from congestive heart failure, even after controlling for the initial severity of the heart failure. Dyadic negativity has been shown to shorten survival in women on dialysis with end-stage renal disease (Kimmel et al., 2000). Women with early breast cancer who do not confide in their spouses have higher recurrence rates than those who do have a confiding relationship (Weihs, Enright, Simmens, & Reiss, 2000). These findings suggest that loss of a spouse has the greatest health effects on men, but the impact of poor marital quality may be greater for women.

Hostile or negative marital and family relationships have a stronger influence on health than positive or supportive relationships. Family criticism is strongly predictive of relapse and poor outcome with smoking cessation (Mermelstein, Lichtenstein, & McIntyre, 1983), weight management (Fischmann-Havstad & Marston, 1984), diabetes (Klausner, Koenigsberg, Skolnick, & Chung, 1995; Koenigsberg, Klausner, Pelino, & Rosnick, 1993), asthma, and migraine headaches. Physiological studies have shown that conflict and criticism among family members can raise blood pressure (Ewart, Taylor, Kraemer, & Agras, 1991) and worsen diabetes control (Minuchin, Rosman, & Baker, 1978).

Although there is strong observational research demonstrating that family relationships influence physical health, there are few studies examining whether family interventions improve physical health. This chapter will review the evidence that family interventions are beneficial in the prevention or treatment of physical disorders. While it has been clearly demonstrated that family therapy can improve the emotional health of family members and family functioning, there is much less evidence that family interventions can improve the physical health of family members. Studies, mostly randomized controlled trials of family interventions, are reviewed using the family life cycle as an organizing theme. After reviewing studies on the prevention of chronic illness, research on chronic illness in children, adults, and the elderly will be reviewed. Finally, recommendations for future research and implications for family clinicians are presented.

FAMILY INTERVENTIONS FOR PHYSICAL DISORDERS

Many types of family interventions have been developed and tested for a wide range of physical disorders.

Prevention of Chronic Disease

Over one-third of all deaths in the United States can be directly attributable to unhealthy behaviors, particularly smoking, lack of exercise, poor nutrition, and alcohol abuse, and are potentially preventable. These unhealthy behaviors account for much of morbidity or suffering from chronic illnesses such as heart disease, cancer, diabetes, and stroke. Health habits usually develop, are maintained, and are changed within the context of the family. Unhealthy behaviors or risk factors tend to cluster within families, since family members tend to share similar diets, physical activities, and use or abuse of unhealthy substances, such as tobacco. The World Health Organization (1976) has characterized the family as "the primary social agent in the promotion of health and well-being" (p. 17).

Nutrition and Prevention of Cardiovascular Disease. Despite some societal changes, families still tend to eat together, share the same diets, and consume similar amounts of salt, calories, cholesterol, and saturated fats (Doherty & Campbell, 1988; Nader et al., 1983). If one family member changes his or her diet, other family members tend to make similar changes (Sexton et al., 1987). However, most dietary interventions are directed toward individuals, with little or no attention to the rest of the family.

Family intervention can change diet and promote a healthier lifestyle, but family interventions have not been compared to individual interventions. In the British Family Heart Study, over 12,000 middle-aged couples received family-based counseling from a nurse about healthy lifestyles and cardiac risk reduction (Graham, Senior, Dukes, & Lazarus, 1993). At one-year follow-up, the couples receiving the intervention had reduced their smoking, blood pressure, and cholesterol level and had a 16% reduction in their overall cardiac risk score. Other studies have found similar results with small but significant improvements in healthy behaviors (Knutsen & Knutsen, 1991; Perry et al., 1989).

Weight Reduction. Over 30% of the population is considered obese (more than 20% over ideal body weight), which contributes to numerous chronic illnesses, including diabetes, hypertension, coronary heart disease, and arthritis. Obesity is a major public health problem. Overeating and obesity can play important homeostatic roles in families. The parents of obese children are less likely to encourage exercise and more likely to encourage their children to eat than other parents (Hanson, Klesges, Eck, & Cigrang, 1990; Waxman & Stunkard, 1980). The family plays an important role in both the development and the treatment of eating disorders such as anorexia nervosa and bulimia (Campbell & Patterson, 1995).

In obesity treatment programs, spousal support predicts successful weight loss (Streja, Boyko, & Rabkin, 1982) and spousal criticism or high expressed emotion is associated with little or no weight loss (Fischmann-Havstad & Marston, 1984). There are ten randomized controlled trials of spouse or partner involvement in weight reduction programs

(Black, Gleser, & Kooyers, 1990). These interventions are based upon individual cognitive behavioral approaches in which a spouse is viewed as reinforcing desired behaviors. The results of the couple interventions were mixed. In approximately one-half the studies, the intervention groups were able to maintain the weight loss for up to three years. A meta-analysis of these studies (Black et al., 1990) concluded that couples interventions had a small but significant improvement in weight loss at the end of the programs, but the differences were no longer apparent at two- and three-year follow-up.

There was little or no increase in supportive behaviors by the partners in these studies. Obese subjects who reported higher marital satisfaction lost more weight (Dubbert & Wilson, 1984). In one study, the greatest weight loss occurred in the group in which the spouses were asked not to nag, criticize, or otherwise participate in their partner's efforts at weight reduction. These studies suggest that blocking partner criticism and addressing marital conflict and dissatisfaction may be more important than trying to increase supportive behaviors.

Childhood obesity is a growing problem, and family interventions for this problem are more encouraging. Parental involvement in weight reduction programs for children results in greater weight loss for both the child and the parent, with a high correlation between the parent's and child's weight loss (Epstein, Wing, Koeske, Andrasik, & Ossip, 1981). One program for obese adolescents found the best results when the adolescent and the parent received separate training, thus respecting the adolescent's growing independence (Brownell, Kelman, & Stunkard, 1983).

Cigarette Smoking. Smoking causes over 350,000 deaths in the United States per year, mostly from heart disease and cancer, and remains the number one national public health problem. Smoking is strongly influenced by the family. Adolescents are five times more likely to start smoking if a parent or older sibling smokes (Bewley & Bland, 1977). Smokers tend to marry other smokers, to smoke the same number of cigarettes as their spouse, and to quit at the same time (Venters, Jacobs, Luepker, Maiman, & Gillum, 1984). Smokers married to non- or ex-smokers are more likely to quit and remain abstinent. Support from the smoker's partner or spouse is highly predictive of successful smoking cessation. Specific supportive behaviors such as providing encouragement and positive reinforcement predict successful quitting, while negative behaviors such as nagging or criticism predict failure to quit or relapse (Coppotelli & Orleans, 1985; Mermelstein, 1986). The Agency for Healthcare Quality and Research (AHRQ) recommends family and social support interventions as components of effective smoking cessation (Fiore, 2000).

Nine randomized controlled trials involving over 1700 subjects have examined the impact of partner support in smoking cessation (Park, Schultz, Tudiver, Campbell, & Becker, 2002). These studies add a social support intervention to a traditional smoking cessation program, which includes nicotine replacement, behavioral therapy, and relapse prevention. The partner, usually the spouse, is given suggestions and feedback on helpful and unhelpful behaviors for smoking cessation.

The results of these studies have been mixed, and a meta-analysis found no overall impact of partner support on smoking cessation (Park et al., 2002). In most of these studies, the amount of partner support reported by the smokers continued to predict successful smoking cessation, but few of the interventions had any impact on partner support. These results suggest that it is difficult to increase levels of partner support for smoking cessation.

The failure of these interventions to improve partner support or smoking cessation may result from a nonsystemic view of marriage. Partner behaviors are part of a complex marital relationship influenced by the history and quality of the marital relationship. Instructing partners or spouses to be more supportive or less critical is not likely to have its desired effect. It may be easier to increase supportive behaviors in couples that have higher levels of marital satisfaction. Qualitative studies of what happens to couples when they participate in smoking cessation programs would be helpful to better understand the relationship between marital dynamics and smoking behaviors.

CHRONIC DISEASE THROUGH THE LIFECYCLE

Pediatric Chronic Illnesses

The course and outcome of childhood chronic illnesses are strongly influenced by both family structure and function. Parents are responsible for the treatment of most pediatric illnesses. Many family variables are associated with health outcomes across a broad range of chronic illnesses. For example, healthy family functioning is strongly correlated with improved control of diabetes, while family conflict, parental indifference, and low cohesion have all been associated with poor metabolic control in diabetes (Anderson & Kornblum, 1984; Gustafsson, Kjellman, & Cederblad, 1986). In a comprehensive literature review, Patterson (1991) identified nine aspects of family process that have been consistently associated with good outcomes in children with chronic illness and disabilities: (1) balancing the illness with other family needs, (2) maintaining clear boundaries, (3) developing communication competence, (4) attributing positive meaning to the situation, (5) maintaining family flexibility, (6) maintaining family cohesiveness, (7) engaging active coping efforts, (8) maintaining social supports, and (9) developing collaborative relationships with professionals.

Many of these family variables have been targeted by family interventions.

Psychosomatic Families. Salvador Minuchin, one of the founders of family therapy, developed early and well-known family interventions in childhood chronic illness. In a series of studies, he and his colleagues at the Philadelphia Child Guidance Clinic (Minuchin et al., 1975; Minuchin et al., 1978) studied poorly controlled diabetic children and their families. These children had recurrent episodes of diabetic ketoacidosis, but when hospitalized, the diabetes was easily managed. Stress and emotional arousal within the family appeared to affect the child's blood sugar. Minuchin described a specific pattern of interaction in these "psychosomatic families," characterized by enmeshment (high cohesion), overprotectiveness, rigidity, and conflict avoidance.

Minuchin (Minuchin et al., 1975) studied these diabetic children's physiologic responses to a stressful family interview to determine how these family patterns can affect diabetes. During the family interview, the children from psychosomatic families had a rapid rise in free fatty acids (FFA), a precursor to diabetic ketoacidosis. Minuchin hypothesized that in psychosomatic families, parental conflict is detoured or defused through the chronically ill child, and the resulting stress leads to exacerbation of the illness. Minuchin was the first investigator to demonstrate a link between family and physiologic processes.

Minuchin and his colleagues (Minuchin et al., 1978) successfully treated psychosomatic families using structural family therapy to help disengage the diabetic child and establish more appropriate family boundaries. In 15 cases, the pattern of recurrent ketoacidosis ceased and insulin doses were reduced. However, these early case reports lacked any standardized outcome measures or control groups. The psychosomatic family model has been criticized as blaming families

for the child's illness and lacking empirical validation (Coyne & Anderson, 1989). Wood and colleagues (Wood et al., 1989) proposed a more systemic and comprehensive biobehavioral model of childhood chronic illness.

Insulin-Dependent Diabetes Mellitus. Several different types of family interventions have been more carefully studied in childhood (Type 1–insulin dependent) diabetes. Family education and support groups (Anderson, Wolf, Burkhart, Cornell, & Bacon, 1989; Dougherty, Schiffrin, White, Soderstrom, & Sufrategui, 1999; McNabb, Quinn, Murphy, Thorp, & Cook, 1994; Wing, Marcus, Epstein, & Jawad, 1991) and more intensive psychoeducational programs that address collaborative problem solving and problematic family interactions (Galatzer, Amir, Gil, Karp, & Laron, 1982; Wing et al., 1991) have been examined. Mendenhall identified 12 randomized controlled trials of family interventions for childhood diabetes, 10 of which used hemoglobin A1C (HBA1C) as an outcome measure, an excellent measure of chronic blood sugar control (Mendenhall, 2002). Seven of ten studies demonstrated a significant improvement in diabetic control with a family intervention. Blood sugar control worsened in two studies. These interventions were effective in improving diabetic control, but which interventions were more effective is not clear.

Asthma. Asthma has been strongly associated with psychosocial distress, depression, and disturbed family relationships (Liebman, Minuchin, & Baker, 1974). The only randomized controlled trials of family therapy for a childhood illness have been conducted for severe childhood asthma. Two studies involved a total of 55 children with moderately severe asthma and were based on structural family therapy models. Strengthening of boundaries between generations and addressing hidden conflicts were used to alter dysfunctional patterns of interaction. Both interventions improved asthma symptoms and a number of measures of lung function. A recent Cochrane review of these studies concluded that "there is some indication that family therapy may be a useful adjunct to medication for children with asthma" (Panton & Barley, 2002).

In a review of the literature, Bernard-Bonnin and associates (Bernard-Bonnin, Stachenko, Bonin, Charette, & Rousseau, 1995) identified 11 well-designed randomized controlled trials of family psychoeducation for asthma. In their meta-analysis, they found a significant improvement in several measures of asthma severity. Although the overall effect sizes were small (<.2), the results of these interventions were significantly better when limited to children with more severe asthma. This is an important issue worth highlighting across all chronic disorders. Family interventions are more likely to improve health outcomes with more severe illness. Patients with mild disease are unlikely to need or benefit from family interventions.

Cystic Fibrosis. Cystic fibrosis (CF) is a genetic disorder of children in which a missing enzyme in the lungs results in progressive deterioration in lung function over several decades and eventual early death. Complex treatment programs involving frequent chest physical therapy, aggressive use of antibiotics, and synthetic enzymes have dramatically improved the survival of these young adults. These treatments are very demanding on families. Patterson showed that family variables (especially family organization) predict the rate of decline of pulmonary function over a 10-year period (Patterson, Budd, Goetz, & Warwick, 1993). Bartholomew and colleagues developed separate psychoeducational groups for children and adolescents with CF and their parents (Bartholomew & Schneiderman, 1982) and found that the

children and adolescents who received the intervention reported improved knowledge, self-efficacy, self-management of the illness and overall health status. Family psychoeducation may actually be able to extend the lives of those who suffer from this disorder.

Congenital Heart Disease. Two studies have studied the impact of family interventions to reduce the psychological morbidity associated with surgery for congenital heart disease (Campbell, Kirkpatrick, Berry, & Lamberti, 1995; Campbell Clark, & Kirkpatrick, 1986). Both interventions provided informational and skills training separately to the child and one parent before cardiac surgery. The children in the intervention group were better adjusted at home and had higher functioning at school after the procedure. The parents in the intervention group felt more competent in caring for their child, but there were no differences in the parents' reports of anxiety.

Childhood Cancer. A few studies have used family interventions to reduce the psychological morbidity associated with diagnosis and treatment of childhood cancers. Two interventions to improve parental coping failed to reduce parental distress (Hoekstra-Weebers, Heuvel, Jaspers, Kamps, & Klip, 1998; Jay & Elliott, 1990). Working with children with leukemia and their families, Kazak and her colleagues were able to reduce the child's distress related to painful procedure using a cognitive-behavioral, family-oriented intervention (Kazak et al., 1996). In another study, Kazak piloted a multi-family group intervention for survivors of childhood cancer to reduce the post-traumatic stress symptoms related to the diagnosis and treatment of the cancer. In a pre-post test design, they were able to show a decrease in post-traumatic stress and anxiety in the survivors and their family members (Kazak, 1989).

Adult Chronic Diseases

There are very few family or marital intervention studies in adult physical illness despite the evidence that marital quality affects disease outcomes. Most of this research has focused on the role of the spouse as the primary caregiver. Gonzales, Steinglass, and Reiss (1989) developed an innovative multifamily psychoeducational group intervention for families with chronic medical illnesses. Based upon their clinical work, they found that chronic illness tends to dominate family life and take over a family's identity. The goal of their groups is to help families balance the needs of the illness with the needs of the family by putting the illness in its appropriate place in family life. It is currently being studied as an intervention with a wide range of illnesses, including HIV/AIDS, adult cancer, and end-stage renal disease.

Non-Insulin-Dependent Diabetes. Non-insulin-dependent diabetes (NIDDM or Type 2) afflicts over 15 million adults in the United States and is 10 times more common than insulin-dependent diabetes, a disease of children and young adults. Most patients with NIDDM are overweight, and the major challenge for these patients is adherence to recommended diet, exercise, medication, and blood sugar monitoring. Only two studies have examined the impact of a couple's intervention on diabetes outcomes. Gilden (Gilden, Hendryx, Casia, & Singh, 1989) included the wives in a six-week diabetes education program. Patients with participating spouses showed greater improvement in knowledge, increase in family involvement, and improved diabetic control. Wing and colleagues enrolled diabetic patients and their obese spouses in a behavioral weight reduction program (Wing et al., 1991). Patients and their spouses were randomly assigned to an individual or couples program. At one-year follow-up, there was no difference in overall weight loss in the two groups, but the women lost more weight in the couples groups and the men lost more weight when treated alone. This study emphasizes the importance of examining gender effects with couple interventions, which are likely to have very different effects on women than men.

Cardiac Rehabilitation. Spouses of heart attack patients have high levels of depression, anxiety, and guilt, and experience similar levels of overall distress as the patients (Bedsworth & Molen, 1982). Many male cardiac patients feel overprotected by their wives (Fiske, Coyne, & Smith, 1991). Emotional support provided by a family member (usually spouse) or confidante is a strong predictor of survival after a myocardial infarction, stronger than physiologic measures.

Several studies have examined the impact of spouse involvement in cardiac rehabilitation on psychosocial outcomes. In one clever study, wives of heart attack patients walked on the treadmill at the same workload as their husbands, three weeks after their husband's heart attack (Taylor, Bandura, Ewart, Miller, & DeBusk, 1985). These wives were much more confident and less anxious about their husbands' health and capability than wives in the control group who merely observed their husbands' tests. When these women actually experienced what their husband were capable of doing, they were less overprotective and the husbands had improved cardiac functioning 11 and 26 weeks after the heart attack. Of the three studies that included couple counseling as part of cardiac rehabilitation (Dracup, Meleis, Baker, & Edlefsen, 1984; Gilliss, Neuhaus, & Hauck, 1990; Thompson & Meddis, 1990), only one was able to show any improvement in the spouses' emotional health (Dracup et al., 1984). Patient outcomes were not examined. Although observational research suggests that spouses play an important role in recovery from heart attacks, few couple or family interventions have been tested, and those that have report mixed results.

Hypertension. Less than one-half of adults with elevated blood pressure take their medication as directed. Medication compliance is correlated with marital satisfaction in hypertensive patients (Trevino, Young, Groff, & Jono, 1990). In experimental studies, blood pressure reactivity has been linked to marital interaction and conflict (Gottman, 1994). Ewart and colleagues taught communication skills to 20 hypertensive patients and their spouses to help them reduce conflict and emotional reactivity during arguments (Ewart, Taylor, Kraemer, & Agras, 1984). These couples showed less hostility, fewer combative behaviors, and a significant reduction in systolic blood pressure.

Two randomized controlled trials have examined the impact of a family intervention on hypertension compliance. Morisky and colleagues compared three psychoeducation interventions (brief individual counseling, counseling the spouse during a home visit, and patient support group) to improve blood pressure treatment in an inner city population (Morisky et al., 1983). The family intervention was added after a patient survey indicated that 70% of the hypertensive patients at the clinic wished that their spouse or other family members knew more about their illness and were more involved. Educating and counseling the spouse improved treatment adherence and lowered both blood pressure and overall mortality. Overall, the experimental groups had a 57% reduction in mortality, and the family intervention seemed to have the greatest effect. A similar study (Earp, Ory, & Strogatz, 1982) failed to demonstrate any benefits from involving a family member during a home visit, but the follow-up may not have been long enough to detect a difference.

CHRONIC DISEASES IN THE ELDERLY

With the aging of the general population, the rising incidence of degenerative and disabling conditions, and fewer resources for professional caregiving, a growing percentage of older individuals must rely on family members for care. It is estimated that over 40% of the elderly over the age of 85 have some form of dementia, and one half of those individuals are cared for by family members in their own communities (Biegel, Sales, & Schulz, 1991). Caregiving exacts a heavy toll from family members. Family caregivers have higher morbidity and mortality than age-matched controls. Caregivers over age 65 who are experiencing emotional strain are 63% more likely to die than age-matched non-caregivers over a four-year period (Schulz & Beach, 1999). Caregivers suffer higher rates of physical illnesses, depression, and anxiety. One-half of family caregivers of dementia patients are clinically depressed (Gallagher, Rose, Rivera, Lovett, & Thompson, 1989). These caregivers often restrict their social activities and reduce their time at work. The financial impact of caregiving on families can be enormous, both in terms of decreased wages and the high cost of providing equipment and services in the home for the patient.

Family caregivers are essential members of the health care team. They provide clinical observation, direct care, case management, and a range of other services. In chronic illnesses, such as Alzheimer's disease, these caregivers may devote years of their own lives to caring for a loved one. Unfortunately, our current health care system offers little institutional support for families who are burdened with caregiving. Managed care has shifted many of the burdens of caregiving from professionals in the hospital and other institutions to family members at home, without providing adequate support. As hospital stays have shortened, elderly patients are being discharged home sicker and with more health care needs than in the past.

Family support groups for caregivers of patients with Alzheimer's disease have become common and are promoted by advocacy groups. These are usually open-ended groups that are professionally or peer led and provide information and emotional support to families. Studies of these groups suggest that participants learn new information and report high levels of satisfaction, but the impact on the caregivers' emotional distress and sense of burden is inconsistent (Haley, Brown, & Levine, 1987; Kahan, Kemp, Staples, & Brummel-Smith, 1985; Orleans, George, Houpt, & Brodie, 1985).

Family psychoeducational programs provide more intensive skills training to help family caregivers manage many of the common problems presented by elders with dementia (Chiverton & Caine, 1989; Gallagher et al., 1989; Goodman & Pynoos, 1990; Marriott, Donaldson, Tarrier, & Burns, 2000; Mittelman, Ferris, Shulman, Steinberg, & Levin, 1996; Toseland, Labrecque, Goebel, & Whitney, 1992; Toseland et al., 2001). These interventions usually include weekly group sessions led by a trained professional and typically last for 8 to 10 weeks. In randomized controlled trials, they have consistently reduced depressive symptoms, emotional distress, and the sense of burden of family caregivers.

An effective family psychoeducational intervention for family caregivers of patients with Alzheimer's disease (AD) was developed by Mittelman and tested in a randomized controlled trial (Mittelman et al., 1996). These families attended individual and group instructional and problem-solving sessions where they learned how to manage many of the troublesome behaviors of patients with AD. They also attended an ongoing family support group and used

crisis intervention services to help with urgent problems. The caregivers who received the intervention were less depressed and physically healthier than those who did not, and patients with AD were able to remain at home for almost a year longer than patients in the control group. The savings in nursing home costs were several times the cost of the interventions.

Sorensen and colleagues (Sorensen, Pinquart, & Duberstein, 2002) conducted a meta-analysis of 78 caregiver intervention studies representing six different types of interventions for different illnesses. They found a significant improvement across all six outcome variables (caregiver burden, depression, subjective well-being, perceived caregiver satisfaction, ability/knowledge, and patient symptoms). The effects were the smallest for caregivers of patients with dementia and most consistent with the psychoeducational interventions. Caregiver ability and knowledge improved more than subjective burden and depression. Group interventions had smaller improvements than individual interventions.

These studies of family interventions for family caregivers suggest that providing education and support for family caregivers is necessary but not sufficient to reduce their burden and improve their emotional health. Family caregivers need more intensive interventions that include skills training and assistance with problem-solving. Similar results were found in a study of caregivers of stroke patients (Evans, Matlock, Bishop, Stranahan, & Pederson, 1988). Family psychoeducational programs for family caregivers are effective in improving both the physical and emotional health of the caregiver and can be cost effective. These programs have many similarities with psychoeducational programs that have been developed and tested for schizophrenia and can be used as models for family interventions for other physical disorders.

FUTURE DIRECTIONS
FOR RESEARCH

Much more research on family interventions for physical disorders needs to be done. This area of research is still in its infancy, at the stage where research on families and schizophrenia was 30 years ago. This situation creates many opportunities for new family researchers to become involved in this exciting area of research.

Few family interventions for physical disorders have been designed by family researchers or based on family science. Medical and nursing researchers have been the principal investigators in most of these studies. Rarely is a particular family characteristic or variable targeted by the intervention, and family assessment is usually absent. There are only a few trials of family therapy for any physical disorders. Family researchers and therapists need to become involved in research on families and health and help design and implement family interventions for physical disorders.

Although there is a large body of non-interventioned research on families and health, more observational studies are needed. Few family variables have been consistently shown to be predictive of health outcomes. The most promising research has focused on the impact of family criticism, family conflict, and expressed emotion on physical health.

Family and health research needs to be based on family theories and family science. Most existing studies are atheoretical. Intervention strategies should be guided by theoretical models that hypothesize relationships between family and health variables and then measure these family variables before and after the intervention. For example, studies of spouse involvement in smoking cessation and weight loss should measure marital satisfaction or quality as well as helpful and harmful behaviors before and after the interventions. Pre-intervention family assessment will also

allow researchers to determine which families are likely to benefit.

Most family intervention studies target a single disease with little generalizable to other illnesses. Family interventions should be developed for several chronic diseases that have some commonalities. Interventions that have been shown to be effective for one disease (such as family psychoeducation for caregivers of patients with Alzheimer's disease) should be tested with other similar disease (such as stroke or Parkinson's disease).

These intervention studies should measure multiple outcomes, including patient physical and emotional health, family members' physical and emotional health, family functioning, marital satisfaction or quality, and both health care and overall costs. Many of the benefits of a family intervention may not be captured by traditional measures. For example, a family intervention may improve the health of family members other than the identified patient and reduce their use of health care services. Family interventions need to be adaptable to meet the specific needs and characteristics of individual families. Families in which there is conflict, disengagement, or dissatisfaction will need a different and more intensive approach than more functional families. The cost of family interventions and potential financial benefits should be more carefully studied.

In this research, the family interventions need to be described in more detail, so that they can be replicated and the most effective ingredients can be identified. This will help determine why one and not another intervention is effective. Researchers need to pay close attention to gender effects. As noted earlier, marriage has very different effects on the physical health of men and women (Kiecolt-Glaser et al., 2001). Marriage is often the primary source of social support for men, whereas women's health is most influenced by the quality of many social relationships. Couple interventions will have different effects on men and women's health. The only one intervention study to examine gender effects found that women had better outcomes (weight loss) in couples treatment and men did better alone.

Finally, family intervention studies need to include more diversity. Most of current research involves white middle class families. Future studies should include different family types (e.g., single-parent families, gay families) and families from different racial, ethnic, and socioeconomic backgrounds.

CONCLUSION

This chapter reviews the research on family interventions for chronic psychosocial disorders. There are effective family interventions for some physical disorders and promising ones for others, but family interventions have not been developed or tested for many chronic physical illnesses. Family psychoeducation is the most commonly studied and effective type of family intervention, and it is widely applicable to numerous disorders. Whether family psychoeducation provided in a group setting is more effective than family psychoeducation for individual families is not known and needs study. There is insufficient research on family therapy for physical disorders to comment on its effectiveness, although family therapy is likely to be most effective with dysfunctional families.

Family involvement in health promotion and disease prevention programs offers great promise. Family-centered nutrition and cardiovascular risk reduction programs are effective in improving the health of multiple members, but have not been directly compared with individually oriented programs. Family-based programs for obesity in children are clearly more effective than individual programs, but their effectiveness for adults is unclear. Partner or spouse involvement for smoking cessation has been shown to be ineffective.

Family psychoeducation for the caregivers of patients with dementia appears to be the most effective type of family intervention. These family interventions improve the physical and mental health of the caregivers, and are cost effective. Mittelman's comprehensive intervention for family caregivers of patients with AD can be adapted to other chronic disorders (Mittelman et al., 1996). Family interventions for childhood disorders, especially diabetes and asthma, are effective in improving medical (e.g., HBA1C levels and pulmonary function) as well as psychosocial outcomes. Not surprisingly, family interventions are most effective at each end of the life cycle, when much of the care is provided by family caregivers.

This research suggests that marriage and family therapists have an important, but unmet, role in the treatment of physical illness. Family therapists should be a part of most health care teams, offering a family and systemic perspective that is so often missing. Much has been written about family therapists working in primary care settings, helping family physicians, pediatricians, and primary care internists care for patients and their families. There are also opportunities for working with medical specialties, especially rehabilitation medicine, reproductive health, oncology, cardiac rehabilitation, and geriatrics (Seaburn, Lorenz, Gunn, & Gawinski, 1996).

Family therapy training programs need to provide the knowledge and skills for all new family therapists to work in medical settings and with families with health problems. These programs should offer courses on medical family therapy, collaboration with medical providers, and psychopharmacology. Family therapy trainees should be provided with opportunities to work in medical settings under supervision during graduate school and internship. Only by better understanding how important families may be as a resource in medical care will our health care system become more family-oriented and higher quality.

REFERENCES

Anderson, B. J., & Kornblum, H. (1984). The family environment of children with a diabetic parent: Issues for research. *Family Systems Medicine, 2*(1), 17–27.

Anderson, B. J., Wolf, F. M., Burkhart, M. T., Cornell, R. G., & Bacon, G. E. (1989). Effects of peer-group intervention on metabolic control of adolescents with IDDM: Randomized outpatient study. *Diabetes Care, 12,* 179–183.

Bartholomew, L., & Schneiderman, L. J. (1982). Attitudes of patients toward family care in a family practice group. *Journal of Family Practice, 15,* 477–481.

Bedsworth, J. A., & Molen, M. T. (1982). Psychological stress in spouses of patients with myocardial infarction. *Heart & Lung, 11,* 450–456.

Berkman, L. F. (1995). The role of social relations in health promotion. *Psychosomatic Medicine, 57,* 245–254.

Berkman, L. F. (2000). Social support, social networks, social cohesion, and health. *Social Work in Health Care, 31,* 3–14.

Berkman, L. F., Leo-Summers, L., & Horwitz, R. I. (1992). Emotional support and survival after myocardial infarction: A prospective, population-based study of the elderly. *Annals of Internal Medicine, 117,* 1003–1009.

Bernard-Bonnin, A. C., Stachenko, S., Bonin, D., Charette, C., & Rousseau, E. (1995). Self-management teaching programs and morbidity of pediatric asthma: A meta-analysis. *Journal of Allergy & Clinical Immunology, 95,* 34–41.

Bewley, B. R., & Bland, J. M. (1977). Academic performance and social factors related to cigarette smoking by schoolchildren. *British Journal of Preventive & Social Medicine, 31,* 18–24.

Biegel, D. E., Sales, E., & Schulz, R. (1991). *Family caregiving in chronic illness: Alzheimer's disease, cancer, heart disease, mental illness, and stroke.* Newbury Park, CA: Sage.

Black, D. R., Gleser, L. J., & Kooyers, K. J. (1990). A meta-analytic evaluation of couples weight-loss programs. *Health Psychology, 9*(3), 330–347.

Brownell, K. D., Kelman, J. H., & Stunkard, A. J. (1983). Treatment of obese children with and without their mothers: Changes in weight and blood pressure. *Pediatrics, 71,* 515–523.

Burman, B., & Margolin, G. (1992). Analysis of the association between marital relationships and health problems: An interactional perspective. *Psychological Bulletin, 112,* 39–63.

Campbell L. A., Clark, M., & Kirkpatrick S. E. (1986). Stress management for parents/children undergoing cardiac catheterization. *American Journal of Orthopsychiatry, 56*(2), 234–243.

Campbell, L. A., Kirkpatrick, S. E., Berry, C. C., & Lamberti, J. J. (1995). Preparing children with congenital heart disease for cardiac surgery. *Journal of Pediatric Psychology, 20,* 313–328.

Campbell, T. L. (1986). The family's impact on health: A critical review and annotated bibliography. *Family Systems Medicine, 4,* 135–328.

Campbell, T. L., & Patterson, J. M. (1995). The effectiveness of family interventions in the treatment of physical illness. *Journal of Marital and Family Therapy, 21,* 545–583.

Chiverton, P., & Caine, E. D. (1989). Education to assist spouses in coping with Alzheimer's disease. A controlled trial. *Journal of the American Geriatrics Society, 37,* 593–598.

Coppotelli, H. C., & Orleans, C. T. (1985). Partner support and other determinants of smoking cessation maintenance among women. *Journal of Consulting and Clinical Psychology, 53*(4), 455–460.

Coyne, J. C., & Anderson, B. J. (1989). The "psychosomatic family" reconsidered II: Recalling a defective model and looking ahead. *Journal of Marital and Family Therapy, 15,* 139–148.

Coyne, J. C., Rohrbaugh, M. J., Shoham, V., Sonnega, J. S., Nicklas, J. M., & Cranford, J. A. (2001). Prognostic importance of marital quality for survival of congestive heart failure. *American Journal of Cardiology, 88,* 526–529.

Doherty, W. A., & Campbell, T. L. (1988). *Families and health.* Beverly Hills, CA: Sage.

Dougherty, G., Schiffrin, A., White, D., Soderstrom, L., & Sufrategui, M. (1999). Home-based management can achieve intensification cost-effectively in type I diabetes. *Pediatrics, 103,* 122–128.

Dracup, K., Meleis, A., Baker, K., & Edlefsen, P. (1984). Family-focused cardiac rehabilitation: A role supplementation program for cardiac patients and spouses. *Nursing Clinics of North America, 19,* 113–124.

Dubbert, P. M., & Wilson, G. T. (1984). Goal-setting and spouse involvement in the treatment of obesity. *Behaviour Research and Therapy, 22*(3), 227–242.

Earp, J. A., Ory, M. G., & Strogatz, D. S. (1982). The effects of family involvement and practitioner home visits on the control of hypertension. *American Journal of Public Health, 72,* 1146–1153.

Epstein, L. H., Wing, R. R., Koeske, R., Andrasik, F., & Ossip, D. J. (1981). Child and parent weight loss in family-based behavior modification programs. *Journal of Consulting and Clinical Psychology, 49,* 674–685.

Evans, R. L., Matlock, A. L., Bishop, D. S., Stranahan, S., & Pederson, C. (1988). Family intervention after stroke: Does counseling or education help? *Stroke, 19,* 1243–1249.

Ewart, C. K., Taylor, C. B., Kraemer, H. C., & Agras, W. S. (1984). Reducing blood pressure reactivity during interpersonal conflict: Effects of marital communication training. *Behavior Therapy, 15*(5), 473–484.

Ewart, C. K., Taylor, C. B., Kraemer, H. C., & Agras, W. S. (1991). High blood pressure and marital discord: Not being nasty matters more than being nice. *Health Psychology, 10,* 155–163.

Fiore, M. C. (2000). A clinical practice guideline for treating tobacco use and dependence: A U.S. Public Health Service report. *Journal of the American Medical Association [JAMA], 283*(24), 3250–3254.

Fischmann-Havstad, L., & Marston, A. R. (1984). Weight loss maintenance as an aspect of family emotion and process. *British Journal of Clinical Psychology, 23*(4), 265–271.

Fiske, V., Coyne, J. C., & Smith, D. A. (1991). Couples coping with myocardial infarction: An empirical reconsideration of the role of overprotectiveness. *Journal of Family Psychology, 5*(1), 4–20.

Galatzer, A., Amir, S., Gil, R., Karp, M., & Laron, Z. (1982). Crisis intervention program in newly diagnosed diabetic children. *Diabetes Care, 5,* 414–419.

Gallagher, D., Rose, J., Rivera, P., Lovett, S., & Thompson, L. W. (1989). Prevalence of depression in family caregivers. *Gerontologist, 29,* 449–456.

Gilden, J. L., Hendryx, M., Casia, C., & Singh, S. P. (1989). The effectiveness of diabetes education programs for older patients and their spouses. *Journal of the American Geriatrics Society, 37,* 1023–1030.

Gilliss, C. L., Neuhaus, J. M., & Hauck, W. W. (1990). Improving family functioning after cardiac surgery: A randomized trial. *Heart and Lung, 19,* 648–654.

Gonzalez, S., Steinglass, P., & Reiss, D. (1989). Putting the illness in its place: Discussion groups for families with chronic medical illnesses. *Family Process, 28,* 69–87.

Goodman, C. C., & Pynoos, J. (1990). A model telephone information and support program for caregivers of Alzheimer's patients. *Gerontologist, 30,* 399–404.

Gottman, J. M. (1994). *What predicts divorce? The relationship between marital processes and marital outcomes.* Hillsdale, NJ: Lawrence Erlbaum.

Graham, H., Senior, R., Dukes, S., & Lazarus, M. (1993). The introduction of family therapy to British general practice. *Family Systems Medicine, 11*(4), 363–373.

Gustafsson, P. A., Kjellman, N. I., & Cederblad, M. (1986). Family therapy in the treatment of severe childhood asthma. *Journal of Psychosomatic Research, 30,* 369–374.

Haley, W. E., Brown, S. L., & Levine, E. G. (1987). Experimental evaluation of the effectiveness of group intervention for dementia caregivers. *Gerontologist, 27,* 376–382.

Hanson, C. L., Klesges, R. C., Eck, L. H., & Cigrang, J. A. (1990). Family relations, coping styles, stress, and cardiovascular disease risk factors among children and their parents. *Family Systems Medicine, 8*(4), 387–400.

Hoekstra-Weebers, J. E., Heuvel, F., Jaspers, J. P., Kamps, W. A., & Klip, E. C. (1998). Brief report: An intervention program for parents of pediatric cancer patients: A randomized controlled trial. *Journal of Pediatric Psychology, 23,* 207–214.

House, J. S., Landis, K. R., & Umberson, D. (1988). Social relationships and health. *Science, 241,* 540–545.

Jay, S. M., & Elliott, C. H. (1990). A stress inoculation program for parents whose children are undergoing painful medical procedures. *Journal of Consulting and Clinical Psychology, 58,* 799–804.

Kahan, J., Kemp, B., Staples, F. R., & Brummel-Smith, K. (1985). Decreasing the burden in families caring for a relative with a dementing illness. A controlled study. *Journal of the American Geriatrics Society, 33,* 664–670.

Kazak, A. E. (1989). Families of chronically ill children: A systems and social-ecological model of adaptation and challenge. *Journal of Consulting Clinical Psychology, 57,* 25–30.

Kazak, A. E., Penati, B., Boyer, B. A., Himelstein, B., Brophy, P., Waibel, M. K., et al. (1996). A randomized controlled prospective outcome study of a psychological and pharmacological intervention protocol for procedural distress in pediatric leukemia. *Journal of Pediatric Psychology, 21,* 615–631.

Kiecolt-Glaser, J. K., & Newton, T. L. (2001). Marriage and health: His and hers. *Psychological Bulletin, 127,* 472–503.

Kimmel, P. L., Peterson, R. A., Weihs, K. L., Shidler, N., Simmens, S. J., Alleyne, S., et al. (2000). Dyadic relationship conflict, gender, and mortality in urban hemodialysis patients. *Journal of the American Society of Nephrology, 11,* 1518–1525.

Klausner, E. J., Koenigsberg, H. W., Skolnick, N., & Chung, H. (1995). Perceived familial criticism and glucose control in insulin-dependent diabetes mellitus. *International Journal of Mental Health, 24,* 64–75.

Knutsen, S. F., & Knutsen, R. (1991). The Tromso Survey: The Family Intervention study—the effect of intervention on some coronary risk factors and dietary habits, a 6-year follow-up. *Preventive Medicine, 20,* 197–212.

Koenigsberg, H. W., Klausner, E., Pelino, D., & Rosnick, P. (1993). Expressed emotion and glucose control in insulin-dependent diabetes mellitus. *American Journal of Psychiatry, 150,* 1114–1115.

Liebman, R., Minuchin, S., & Baker, L. (1974). The use of structural family therapy in the treatment of intractable asthma. *American Journal of Psychiatry, 131,* 535–540.

Marriott, A., Donaldson, C., Tarrier, N., & Burns, A. (2000). Effectiveness of cognitive-behavioural family intervention in reducing the burden of care in carers of patients with Alzheimer's disease. *British Journal of Psychiatry, 176,* 557–562.

Martikainen, P., & Valkonen, T. (1996). Mortality after death of spouse in relation to duration of bereavement in Finland. *Journal of Epidemiology & Community Health, 50,* 264–268.

McNabb, W. L., Quinn, M. T., Murphy, D. M., Thorp, F. K., & Cook, S. (1994). Increasing children's responsibility for diabetes self-care: The In Control study. *Diabetes Educator, 20,* 121–124.

Mendenhall, T. J. (2002.). *Family-based intervention for persons with diabetes.* Unpublished dissertation, University of Minnesota.

Mermelstein, R. (1986). Social support and smoking cessation and maintenance. *Journal of Consulting and Clinical Psychology, 54*(4), 442–453.

Mermelstein, R., Lichtenstein, E., & McIntyre, K. (1983). Partner support and relapse in smoking-cessation programs. *Journal of Consulting and Clinical Psychology, 51*(3), 465–466.

Minuchin, S., Baker, L., Rosman, B. L., Liebman, R., Milman, L., & Todd, T. C. (1975). A conceptual model of psychosomatic illness in children: Family organization and family therapy. *Archives of General Psychiatry, 32,* 1031–1038.

Minuchin, S., Rosman, B. L., & Baker, L. (1978). *Psychosomatic families: Anorexia nervosa in context.* Cambridge, MA: Harvard University Press.

Mittelman, M. S., Ferris, S. H., Shulman, E., Steinberg, G., & Levin, B. (1996). A family intervention to delay nursing home placement of patients with Alzheimer disease: A randomized controlled trial. *Journal of the American Medical Association [JAMA], 276,* 1725–1731.

Morisky, D. E., Levine, D. M., Green, L. W., Shapiro, S., Russell, R. P., & Smith, C. R. (1983). Five-year blood pressure control and mortality following health education for hypertensive patients. *American Journal of Public Health, 73,* 153–162.

Nader, P. R., Baranowski, T., Vanderpool, N. A., Dunn, K., Dworkin, R., & Ray, L. (1983). The family health project: Cardiovascular risk reduction education for children and parents. *Journal of Developmental and Behavioral Pediatrics, 4,* 3–10.

Orleans, C. T., George, L. K., Houpt, J. L., & Brodie, H. K. (1985). How primary care physicians treat psychiatric disorders: A XX national survey of family practitioners. *American Journal of Psychiatry, 142,* 52–57.

Orth-Gomer, K., Wamala, S. P., Horsten, M., Schenck-Gustafsson, K., Schneiderman, N., & Mittleman, M. A. (2000). Marital stress worsens prognosis in women with coronary heart disease: The Stockholm Female Coronary Risk Study. *Journal of the American Medical Association [JAMA], 284,* 3008–3014.

Osterweis, M., Solomon, F., & Green, M. (1984). *Bereavement: Reactions, consequences, and care.* Washington, DC: National Academy Press.

Panton, J., & Barley, E. A. (2002). Family therapy for asthma. Cochrane Airways Group. *Cochrane Database of Systematic Reviews, 3.*

Park, E. W., Schultz, J. K., Tudiver, F., Campbell, T., & Becker, L. (2002). Enhancing partner support to improve smoking cessation. Cochrane Tobacco Addiction Group. *Cochrane Database of Systematic Reviews, 2.*

Patterson, J. M. (1991). Family resilience to the challenge of a child's disability. *Pediatric Annals, 20,* 491–499.

Patterson, J. M., Budd, J., Goetz, D., & Warwick, W. J. (1993). Family correlates of a 10-year pulmonary health trend in cystic fibrosis. *Pediatrics, 91,* 383–389.

Perry, C. L., Luepker, R. V., Murray, D. M., Hearn, M. D., Halper, A., Dudovitz, B., et al. (1989). Parent involvement with children's health promotion: A one-year follow-up of the Minnesota home team. *Health Education Quarterly, 16,* 171–180.

Schulz, R., & Beach, S. R. (1999). Caregiving as a risk factor for mortality: The Caregiver Health Effects Study. *Journal of the American Medical Association [JAMA], 282,* 2215–2219.

Seaburn, D. B., Lorenz, A. D., Gunn, W. B. J., & Gawinski, B. A. (1996). *Models of collaboration: A guide for mental health professionals working with health care practitioners.* New York: Basic Books.

Sexton, M., Bross, D., Hebel, J. R., Schumann, B. C., Gerace, T. A., Lasser, N., et al. (1987). Risk-factor changes in wives with husbands at high risk of coronary heart disease (CHD): The spin-off effect. *Journal of Behavioral Medicine, 10,* 251–261.

Sorensen, S., Pinquart, M., & Duberstein, P. (2002). How effective are interventions with caregivers? An updated meta-analysis. *The Gerontologist, 43,* 356–372.

Streja, D. A., Boyko, E., & Rabkin, S. W. (1982). Predictors of outcome in a risk factor intervention trial using behavior modification. *Preventive Medicine, 11,* 291–303.

Taylor, C. B., Bandura, A., Ewart, C. K., Miller, N. H., & DeBusk, R. F. (1985). Exercise testing to enhance wives' confidence in their husbands' cardiac capability soon after clinically uncomplicated acute myocardial infarction. *American Journal of Cardiology, 55,* 635–638.

Thompson, D. R., & Meddis, R. (1990). Wives' responses to counselling early after myocardial infarction. *Journal of Psychosomatic Research, 34,* 249–258.

Toseland, R. W., Labrecque, M. S., Goebel, S. T., & Whitney, M. H. (1992). An evaluation of a group program for spouses of frail elderly veterans. *Gerontologist, 32,* 382–390.

Toseland, R. W., McCallion, P., Smith, T., Huck, S., Bourgeois, P., & Garstka, T. A. (2001). Health education groups for caregivers in an HMO. *Journal of Clinical Psychology, 57,* 551–570.

Trevino, D. B., Young, E. H., Groff, J., & Jono, R. T. (1990). The association between marital adjustment and compliance with antihypertension regimens. *Journal of the American Board of Family Practice, 3,* 17–25.

Venters, M. H., Jacobs, D. R., Jr., Luepker, R. V., Maiman, L. A., & Gillum, R. F. (1984). Spouse concordance of smoking patterns: The Minnesota Heart Survey. *American Journal of Epidemiology, 120,* 608–616.

Waxman, M., & Stunkard, A. J. (1980). Caloric intake and expenditure of obese boys. *Journal of Pediatrics, 96,* 187–193.

Weihs, K. L., Enright, T. M., Simmens, S. J., & Reiss, D. (2000). Negative affectivity, restriction of emotions, and site of metastases predict mortality in recurrent breast cancer. *Journal of Psychosomatic Research, 49,* 59–68.

Wing, R. R., Marcus, M. D., Epstein, L. H., & Jawad, A. (1991). A "family-based" approach to the treatment of obese type II diabetic patients. *Journal of Consulting and Clinical Psychology, 59,* 156–162.

Wood, B., Watkins, J. B., Boyle, J. T., Nogueira, J., Zimand, E., & Carroll, L. (1989). The "psychosomatic family" model: An empirical and theoretical analysis. *Family Process, 28,* 399–417.

World Health Organization. (1976). *Statistical Indices of Family Health* (Rep. No. 589). Geneva, CH: WHO Press.

CHAPTER 23

Does DNA Determine Destiny? A Role for Medical Family Therapy With Genetic Screening/Testing for Breast Cancer and Other Genetic Illnesses

Susan H. McDaniel

Health care is being transformed by the mapping of the human genome and the resulting promise of genetic testing for many illnesses with genetic components. Mapping the human genome now enables clinicians to find out who is genetically "at risk" for a particular genetic illness. But who is at risk emotionally? What is the risk to family relationships? Similarly, genetic testing allows us to discover who is "affected" genetically by a particular mutation. But who is affected psychologically or interpersonally? In addition to these psychological issues, many other ethical, legal, philosophical, and social issues face us as we confront the rapidly changing science involved in the human genome studies (McDaniel & Campbell, 1999): What is the essence of being human? How much will we try to control the sex, the temperament, the genetic heritage of our children? The family component of genetic illness makes it

a natural venue for family therapists to participate in the evolving practice of helping patients understand their risk for genetic illness: how to cope with this information and that of other family members; what decisions to make regarding testing, preventive measures, or treatment; and how to increase individual coping and improve family relationships in the face of these challenges.

Traditionally, clinical genetics related primarily to prenatal testing for relatively common single-gene disorders like Down syndrome, or adult testing for rare single-gene dominant disorders like Huntington's disease. Evidence of these genetic mutations means that an affected person will inevitably develop the illness. More recently, cracking the genetic code has led to the discovery of more complex, multifactorial disorders which are the genetic components of common disorders. Mutations of these genes often require some interaction of a mutation and an environment that leads to the development of a disorder, such as cardiovascular disease, cancers, and mental illness. Different illnesses have different components related to genetic versus environmental factors. Most genetic inheritance involves multiple genes acting at once, each with small effects. Some multifactor illnesses require multiple genetic mutations. Some of these disorders require mutations of more than one gene. All may have some environmental influence.

Genetic information is likely to become part of primary health care. Some genetic illnesses can be successfully treated or managed; for others, no treatment exists. Clearly, genetic testing is most helpful when the identification of genetic risk can lead to a targeted intervention with presumptive benefit and a chance for an improved health outcome. Already new diagnostic tests proliferate in the marketplace and predict, to a greater or lesser extent, the risk of disease. This raises the possibility that prevention and treatment can be tailored much more specifically to personal risk factors that depend on a patient's genetic blueprint and environmental situation.

The public has reacted strongly to these scientific discoveries. A belief that the secrets of life will soon be revealed by genetic discoveries has evolved over the past decade in American media, fiction, and popular culture. However exciting the evolving discoveries related to mapping the human genome, understanding DNA does *not* equal controlling one's destiny. Much of the significance of the information in DNA sequences is largely unknown and will take decades of study to understand (Acheson, 2001). At this time, many genetic tests do not lead to a clear recommendation about changing our behaviors once the outcome is known. There are new uncertainties. With any positive test, it can be very difficult to tell just when a condition will occur and what its course will

be. This means that it may be possible to diagnose a genetic predisposition at birth for a condition that may not be manifest until old age.

In addition, each human carries several deleterious as well as several potentially beneficial genetic variations or mutations. Whether genetic variations are beneficial or harmful depends on the environmental circumstances. Wynne and colleagues' research on schizophrenia in Finland shows that the mutation for schizophrenia is actually a responsivity mutation: those with the mutation who have an environment full of resources do much better than mutation-free controls; those with the mutation who have too many challenges in their environment are much more likely than those without it to develop one of the schizophrenia-spectrum disorders (Wahlberg et al., 1997).

This chapter proposes a biopsychosocial, family-sensitive approach to genetic screening and genetic testing. This approach includes the family therapist as part of an interdisciplinary health care team. The chapter begins with a review of the literature that reveals a growing consensus about individual factors and how little is known about family and interpersonal factors that relate to genetic screening and testing.

WHAT IS KNOWN NOW ABOUT PSYCHOLOGICAL AND INTERPERSONAL RESPONSE TO FAMILIAL ILLNESS

Research to date on psychosocial aspects of genetic testing has demonstrated that most people do not develop significant distress or mental health problems as a result of testing results, whether those results are positive or negative (Lerman, Croyle, Tercyak, & Hamann, 2002). However, this research paints broad strokes about a picture that is complex and varied. Much still needs to be studied to understand that minority of people who are psychologically at risk—with what illnesses and under which circumstances? It only makes sense that the impact of testing positive for Huntington's disease is a very different experience than testing positive for the BRCA1 genetic mutation for breast cancer. Huntington's is a single-gene disorder with high penetrance, so that having the gene means that one will inevitably develop the illness at middle age. It is a slow, progressive, terminal neurological disorder. Indeed, research on Huntington's disease showed significant discrepancies for at-risk people between their intentions to get tested and their actual test behavior (or test uptake). Only 10–20% of at-risk individuals seek testing (Quaid & Morris, 1993). Breast cancer, on the other hand, is a multifactorial genetic illness. People who test positive for the BRCA1 mutation have a 70–80% chance of developing breast cancer at some point in their lives, but it is not inevitably a terminal illness. Studies of large families with known BRCA1 mutations found test uptake of 35–43% (Lerman et al., 1996; Nash et al., 1999).

Recent studies clearly demonstrate that it is the patient's *perceived risk,* rather than scientific risk, that predicts whether or not someone chooses to have a genetic test, and then the psychological outcome and distress after genetic testing (French, Kurczynski, Weaver, & Pituch, 1992; Marteau et al., 1991). Patients often overestimate their personal cancer risk (Andrykowski, Mumm, & Studts, 1996), and many experience relief if they test negative. Of those who may be vulnerable to adverse psychological effects are people with information-seeking coping styles (Lerman et al., 2000). Several studies found that baseline distress scores are the best predictors of post-testing distress, with genetic status only marginally predictive (Codori, Slavney, Young, Miglioretti, & Brandt, 1997). Interestingly, a breast cancer testing study found the highest distress scores for those women who had the highest pre-test scores of stress and did *not* choose to get tested (Lerman et al., 1998).

As will be demonstrated in the subsequent interview, these early studies also point to a disconnect between genetic testing and health surveillance behaviors. Early studies of high-risk individuals indicated that psychological distress may lead to avoidance of surveillance behaviors or screening (Kash, Holland, Halper, & Miller, 1992). Also, most women who test positive for the BRCA1/2 mutations do not pursue prophylactic mastectomy or oophorectomy, and only 15% had the recommended ovarian cancer screening (Lerman et al., 2000). Similarly, genetic counseling as part of smoking cessation to assess an individual's increased susceptibility to lung cancer did not lead to a higher quit rate than standard smoking cessation counseling (Lerman et al., 1997).

Research on psychosocial factors involved in genetic testing is still at an early stage. Little is known of the factors that influence perceived risk and how emotional and interpersonal aspects of premorbid functioning and the disease itself influence outcome. Even less is known about how family factors affect perception, decision making, and response to testing (Lerman et al., 2000).

Genetic illness is by definition a family issue. How do family members communicate about familial illness? One preliminary study of mothers who received BRCA testing showed that a little over half these women told their children under age 18 about the results (Tercyak, Peshkin, DeMarco, Brogan, & Lerman, 2002). Disclosure was related to a prior style of open communication in the family. Little else is known about why parents do or do not disclose, how couples manage the information, and what patterns of communication occur across the extended family.

In addition, the clinical tradition of health care targeting individuals is challenged by familial illness. What is the practitioner's duty to inform first-degree relatives, for example, of a patient's genetic mutation for colon cancer? This information has the potential for radically altering family relationships—subdividing families and creating new family alignments. There is much work to be done by family researchers.

A ROLE FOR FAMILY THERAPISTS

Given the implications for families of genetic screening and testing, family therapists and other family clinicians and family researchers can play an important role in the evolving research and clinical care for genetic illness. Expertise in family dynamics is valuable in understanding and helping patients with decision making, disclosure, and the unforeseen repercussions of test results on the individual and the family. With primary care professionals, geneticists, and genetic counselors, family-oriented mental health professionals can play a role in guiding and communicating with families and vulnerable patients as they work to understand the lifelong impact of genetic information on them and their relationships. Especially for those illnesses like Huntington's, for which there is no cure, some patients want information to inform their life planning. Others do not. Even with multifactorial illnesses, individuals in the same family will respond to the possibility of testing very differently, as in a recent case of sisters at increased risk for breast cancer. The older sister is considering preventive mastectomy after testing, whereas the younger sister is uninterested in testing or preventive measures. Some people want to try to control their biology; others wish to turn it over to fate.

When people do desire testing, the timing of the testing often coincides with developmental changes in the life of a family. A decision to marry or to have a child can produce a

flurry of questions about family health history that can lead to genetic screening or testing.

To accomplish the many tasks involved in screening and testing for genetic illness, an interdisciplinary team provides the range of skills needed by patients and families (McDaniel, Johnson, & Sears, 2004). This team includes the primary care physician or nurse practitioner, the genetic counselor, the geneticist, and a family therapist.

> The primary care clinician initially takes the detailed family history, and decides if further assessment or testing is warranted. He or she then presents the situation to the patient. It is the primary care doc that will follow the patient after testing, through adaptation and anticipation, and then with the early and later courses of the illness. (McDaniel, Campbell, Hepworth, & Lorenz, 2004)

Genetic counselors are generally very well-informed about the genetic science involved in their area. They provide prenatal and genetic screening counseling, discuss what it means if a test is positive or negative, and discuss the advantages and disadvantages of knowing the test results. Typically they provide one session before the test and one for the results to be shared. In rural areas, the primary care professional is likely to provide this service.

The geneticist is often the specialist who analyzes and provides the test results to patients. He or she is the scientist/clinician who provides the information; puts it in context; explains its biological meaning; and describes options for monitoring, prevention, or treatment.

The role of the family therapist, or family-oriented mental health professional such as a family nurse practitioner, is yet to be well-developed or widely accepted. The possibilities are numerous. Such professionals can help patients with the lifestyle changes and surveillance behaviors that are likely to decrease their risk with multifactorial genetic illness. They can provide a forum for more extensive discussions of whether to test or not, the meaning of test results, who to inform, as well as offer post-test services such as psychoeducational groups for families who test positive. While the primary care physician can provide long-term medical follow-up, other health care professionals can provide long-term psychological follow-up. They can also provide valuable consultation to primary care clinicians, geneticists, and genetic counselors who deal with the difficult issues of familial illness on a daily basis. Each of these professionals played an important role in the case below.

CASE ILLUSTRATION: A YOUNG WOMAN'S DECISION-MAKING PROCESS REGARDING GENETIC TESTING FOR THE BREAST CANCER MUTATIONS

Given the many questions that remain in the research literature about psychosocial factors and genetic screening/testing, it is important to continue to pay close attention to single case and qualitative studies of patients who relate their experiences with the new testing technology. Another paper (McDaniel, Johnson, et al., 2004) reports an interview with three generations of a family coping with a single-gene dominant disorder, myotonic dystrophy. This chapter will use a young woman's decision regarding genetic testing for breast cancer as an example of a multifactorial genetic illness. Many of the issues faced by this articulate young woman are common to patients and families facing decisions about genetic illness.

This is an interview with Sharon, a 28-year-old young woman who is considering genetic testing for the BRCA1/2 mutations. Actually she first considered testing about five years ago, soon after her mother died of

breast cancer rather suddenly. Her maternal aunt had breast cancer in her thirties and survived. Now Sharon is engaged to be married and thinking about having children, so these issues are at the forefront of her thoughts again. As a family therapist, I conducted the interview as an exploration of the factors involved in deciding whether or not to be tested. I also felt a responsibility to focus on the importance of surveillance behaviors for women at risk for breast cancer. Sharon's genogram (see Figure 23.1) is marked with those who have a history of breast cancer. No one in her family has yet been tested for the mutation. Sharon has sought genetic counseling twice. Her name is changed for confidentiality. She has given permission for portions to be used in this chapter. The interview was filmed in December, 2000.

The following dialogue describes Sharon's first experience at age 23, one year after her mother's death, in which her primary care internist told her she might be at risk and may want to consider genetic counseling.

Addressing the Illness the First Time: Grief Issues

Sharon: It was quite overwhelming for me at the time. I don't think actually I was quite ready psychologically, emotionally ready to hear what they had to say at the time. So, I had sort of gone because intellectually it seemed like a good idea and because the physician had suggested it. But the experience was not very positive. I mean, basically I think I ended up feeling more uncertain about what I should do and what I shouldn't do, in terms of my own making decisions about my own health care and health, sort of, surveillance. And also just overwhelmed

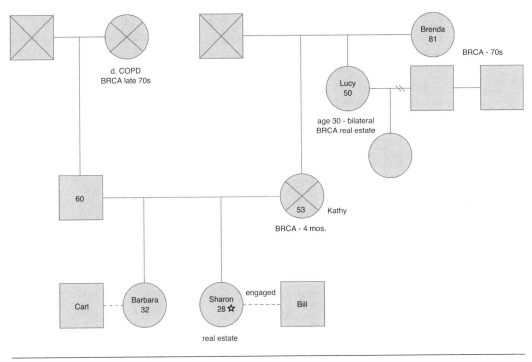

Figure 23.1   Family Genogram

because the amount of information was . . . There is a lot of information and a lot of it so ambiguous that. . . .

Dr. M.: There was no clear direction? They weren't telling to go this way or to go that way?

Sharon: There was really no clear direction. Right. And also, the oncologist that was part of the team was . . . zealous. And I really found her a little too . . . I found that some of the recommendations that she made were uncomfortable for me.

Dr. M.: Like?

Sharon: Like having a mammogram every year starting at . . . starting the age that I was then. Actually she said, "You really should have started a couple of years ago, but we can start now."

Dr. M.: "Thank goodness we caught you now."

Sharon: Right, which wasn't very assuring. And, you know, just talking to me about, you know, prophylactic surgery and things that I just couldn't, I was not ready to hear.

Dr. M.: I'd be curious if you have thoughts about how your family doctor or whatever might have picked up that this wasn't the right time for you yet?

Sharon: Yeah, that's a good question. I think she did what she could or what most, probably what most internists are trained to do . . . But she also did not, um . . . she really didn't ask, I don't think.

I can't remember her asking any questions about my emotional state and, you know, where I was in the process of grief. Um, you know what the experience was like for me of losing my mom. Did I have fears? Did I have concerns?

Dr. M.: The missing component was the emotional assessment.

Sharon: Right.

The importance of a biopsychosocial approach to genetic assessment cannot be overstated. Helping primary care clinicians understand this is an important educational and consultative role for family therapists and other mental health professionals. Next Sharon tells about the second time she had genetic counseling. This time she was more ready to hear what health care professionals have to say.

Addressing the Illness the Second Time: Uncertainty, Ambiguity, and Development

Dr. M.: And how did you come to the place of being sort of young and scared, to being able to tolerate the ambiguity [involved in genetic testing results for breast cancer mutations]?

Sharon: [You mean,] to being older and scared?

Dr. M.: Okay . . . well, fair enough.

Sharon: In the course of less than a year, I had two separate breast lumps. Neither of them ended up being a problem. But on some level for all these years, that concern, that heightened concern . . . Maybe this is something, this a disease that is going to befall me, like it did my mom and my aunt. At that

point, I was just much more emotionally ready to go and get some additional information. I ended up getting a lot of the same information, or similar information that I had gotten the first time. But I could hear it, I could digest it more.

Dr. M.: And why do you think that was the case?

Sharon: Um, because I had gone through a lot more of my own grief process, and also just growth. And I was older . . . I felt less overwhelmed by the information. I was also more . . . skeptical isn't quite the right word, but I was much aware of the ambiguity of . . . really all the information they have to this area. How new it is. How, you know, there are some contradictory studies.

Sharon is quite articulate about the way the uncertainty and ambiguity of the test information was difficult for her to handle. Individual differences in tolerance for uncertainty or desire for information may be one of the predictors of how patients respond to test information (Croyle, Dutson, Tran, & Sun, 1995; Miller, 1995).

Sharon: [Genetic testing is] . . . really out of season for me . . .

Dr. M.: Uh huh.

Sharon: Well, you know, a sense of being a young woman and really having no . . . certainly no . . . same-aged peers who were going through anything like this. So, being kind of thrust into this world that I really felt was kind of beyond me . . . I really felt that I was too young to be having to face this kind of . . . these kind of questions.

Sharon makes clear in this part of the interview how genetic testing pushes younger people to face issues that feel developmentally out of sync. At one point, she said, "I'm not mature enough to deal with this." I am not sure any of us is, but certainly in one's twenties it is that much harder to contemplate. In the past, most of us did not have to face serious illness until later in our lives.

Testing for a multifactorial illness like breast cancer is a very different proposition, scientifically and emotionally, than testing for a single-gene disorder. A positive test for a dominant, single-gene disorder is a diagnosis. A positive test for a multifactorial disorder is a probability, a statement of increased risk. Sharon is very well-informed about all of this. Here she talks about how she would react to test results.

Considering Testing: What if the Results Are Positive? What if They're Negative?

Sharon: When one considers being tested, one always thinks about what would I do if it were positive? What would it feel like, how would I, and what would I do with the information? It is very difficult for me to know how I would feel. It is very difficult for me to project into a potential future outcome, and to know how I would feel and what choices I would make. I think that there will be some practical things that I would probably do differently if I had positive test results. In terms of just more vigilant surveillance. How it would be emotionally to sort of live with the knowledge that I had this very high likelihood of contracting this disease. It is really hard for me to know what that would feel like. I

imagine that it would be challenging in some ways, it would be difficult, maybe more difficult at first, and then possibly become something that is a little more just part of who I am and part of what I live with. Just like there are so many other risks factors that we all have to live with. . . . The question I have asked myself is, would I actually be reassured by a negative result?

Dr. M.: Uh huh.

Sharon: And I am not sure that I would. Plus I also know that a very small percentage of breast cancers are actually, you know, linked to those two gene mutations.

Dr. M.: So it feels sort of like you dodged one bullet, or two bullets.

Sharon: Right.

Dr. M.: But . . .

Sharon: But there's a whole firing squad out there!

Surveillance is very important for women at risk for breast cancer, whether or not they are ever tested. As mentioned earlier, surveillance behaviors and screening or testing are not necessarily related. A woman can avoid surveillance behaviors and still want to be tested, and vice versa. In the next section, Sharon talks about why her surveillance is not the best.

Surveillance, Denial, and Anger

Sharon: I really do not do the kind of surveillance that I know I should be doing. I don't want to find something bad, so which, you know.

Dr. M.: So why look?

Sharon: Which makes totally no sense, intellectually? It is totally irrational. I know that it is irrational, but that is the emotional experience. I don't want to know. So, I'm not going to go looking. And the other piece of it for me has been some anger, I think, and some defiance. Some sort of defiant kind of acting out against the anger I feel at having to deal with the situation.

Similar to other issues of noncompliance, understanding the meaning and the emotions associated with the behaviors is important. Anger and grief are two emotions that frequently surface with familial illness. Next Sharon talks about how her grief affects her surveillance and screening behaviors.

The Relationship of Grief to Testing

Sharon: In terms of the relationship of my grief to my thoughts and feelings about being tested, I am more anxious because I have seen people very close to me suffer and I have seen up close and personal what this disease can do to someone . . . I want to avoid that for myself.

Following are some final words from Sharon, in which she talks about what physicians can do to help:

How Physicians Can Help

Sharon: I mean, I've had conversations with physicians who, you know, who I really like and trust and respect who have said, "I don't know much more about this than you do, you know. Here is what I know or here is where you can go and find out more. Or let me find out some more for you and get you some articles to read. And, we can try to, you know, puzzle this out a little bit together." And that's been probably the most helpful . . . The person that I am seeing currently, who actually has . . . Her own family history is almost exactly the same as mine.

Dr. M.: How did you find that person?

Sharon: Isn't that interesting?

Dr. M.: Yes.

Sharon: She told me the first visit because I brought it up. I said, "Look, I have this history, I have these concerns. This is where I am in the process of trying to figure out what to do about it." And she said, "Oh yeah, I have the almost the same exact situation in my family."

None of us is immune. We all have genetic mutations; most of us are just unaware of which ones.

CONCLUSION

The road ahead promises massive change in the way health care is delivered because of advances in the science of genetics. Family therapists and other care providers have important roles to play in understanding and shaping clinical applications of this information, from helping individuals like Sharon and her family to decide about testing, to providing post-testing services such as a psychoeducational group for patients who test positive for the BRCA1/2 mutations (McDaniel &

Speice, 2001; Speice, McDaniel, Rowley, & Loader, in press). With other members of the professional genetic team, family therapists and family researchers have a unique opportunity to make a contribution to these new patient problems that sit at the interface of technology, ethics, health, and the family.

REFERENCES

Acheson, L. (2001, March). The family physician's perspective. Part of the plenary: L. Acheson, S. McDaniel, & J. Rolland, *Does DNA determine destiny? Patient perceptions and family processes involving genetic information.* Paper presented at The Family in Family Medicine 21st Annual Conference of the Society of Teachers of Family Medicine, Kiawah Island, South Carolina.

Andrykowski, M. A., Mumm, R. K., & Studts, J. L. (1996). Interest in learning of personal genetic risk for cancer: A general population survey. *Preventive Medicine, 25*(5), 527–536.

Codori, A. M., Slavney, P. R., Young, C., Miglioretti, D. L., & Brandt, J. (1997). Predictors of psychological adjustment to genetic testing: Huntington's disease. *Health Psychology, 16*(1), 36–50.

Croyle, R. T., Dutson, D. S., Tran, V. T., & Sun, Y. C. (1995). Need for certainty and interest in genetic testing. *Women's Health, 1*(4), 239–339.

French, B. N., Kurczynski, T. W., Weaver, M. T., & Pituch, M. J. (1992). Evaluation of the Health Belief Model and decision making regarding amniocentesis in women of advanced maternal age. *Health Education* Quarterly, *19*(2), 177–186.

Kash, K. M., Holland, J. C., Halper, M. S., & Miller, D. G. (1992). Psychological distress and surveillance behaviors of women with a family history of breast cancer. *Journal of the National Cancer Institute, 84*(1), 24–30.

Lerman, C., Croyle, R. T., Tercyak, K. P., & Hamann, H. (2002). Genetic testing: Psychological aspects and implications. *Journal of Consulting and Clinical Psychology, 70*(3), 784–797.

Lerman, C., Gold, K., Audrain, J., Lin, T. H., Boyd, N. R., Orleans, C. T., et al. (1997). Incorporating biomarkers of exposure and genetic susceptibility into smoking cessation treatment: Effects on smoking-related cognitions, emotions, and behavior change. *Health Psychology, 16*(1), 87–99.

Lerman, C., Hughes, C., Croyle, R. T., Main, D., Durham, C., Snyder, C., et al. (2000). Prophylactic surgery decisions and surveillance practices one year following BRCA 1/2 testing. *Preventive Medicine, 31*(1), 75–80.

Lerman, C., Hughes, C., Lemon, S. J., Main, D., Snyder, C., Durham, C., et al. (1998). What you don't know can hurt you: Adverse psychologic effects in members of BRCA 1-linked and BRCA 2-linked families who decline genetic testing. *Journal of Clinical Oncology, 16*(5), 1650–1654.

Lerman, C., Narod, S., Schulman, K., Hughes, C., Gomez-Caminero, A., Bonney, G., et al. (1996). BRCA1 testing in families with hereditary breast-ovarian cancer: A prospective study of patient decision making and outcomes. *Journal of the American Medical Association, 275*(24), 1885–1892.

Marteau, T. M., Kidd, J., Cook, R., Michie, S., Johnston, M., Slack, J., et al. (1991). Perceived risk not actual risk predicts uptake of amniocentesis. *British Journal of Obstetrics and Gynaecology, 98*(3), 282–286.

McDaniel, S. H., & Campbell, T. L. (Eds.). (1999). Special issue on genetic testing and the family. *Families, Systems, and Health, 17,* 1–132.

McDaniel, S. H., Campbell, T. L., Hepworth, J., & Lorenz, A. (2004). *Family-oriented primary care: A manual for healthcare professionals* (2nd ed.). New York: Springer-Verlag.

McDaniel, S. H., Johnson, S. B., & Sears, S. (2004). Psychologists promote biopsychosocial health in families. In R. Rozensky, S. Johnson, C. Goodheart, & R. Hammond (Eds.), *Psychology builds a healthy world* (pp. 49–75). Washington, DC: American Psychological Association Publications.

McDaniel, S. H., & Speice, J. (2001). What family psychology has to offer women's health: The examples of conversion, somatization, infertility treatment, and genetic testing. *Professional Psychology: Research and Practice, 32,* 44–51.

Miller, S. M. (1995). Monitoring versus blunting styles of coping with cancer influence the information patients want and need about their disease. *Cancer, 76,* 167–177.

Nash, J. E., Dutson, D., Croyle, R. T., Smith, K. R., Baty, B., & Botkin, J. R. (1999). *BRCA1 testing uptake in a large kindred.* Unpublished manuscript.

Quaid, K. A., & Morris, M. (1993). Reluctance to undergo predictive testing: The case of Huntington disease. *American Journal of Medical Genetics, 45,* 41–45.

Speice, J., McDaniel, S. H., Rowley. P., & Loader, S. (in press). Family issues in a psychoeducational group for women with BRCA mutation. *Clinical Genetics.*

Tercyak, K. P., Peshkin, B. N., DeMarco, T. A., Brogan, B. M., & Lerman, C. (2002). Parent-child factors and their effect on communicating BRCA 1/2 test results to children. *Patient Education and Counseling, 47,* 145–153.

Wahlberg, K. E., Wynne, L. C, Oja, H., Keskitalo, P., Pykalainen, L., Lahti, K., et al. (1997). Gene-environment interaction in vulnerability to schizophrenia: Findings from the Finnish adoptive family study of schizophrenia. *American Journal of Psychiatry, 154,* 355–362.

CHAPTER 24

Interventions With Family Caregivers

Jonathan G. Sandberg

As a typical self-centered teenager, I struggled to find anything good about grandma moving in with us. Grandma required a lot of help with stairs, dressing, bathing; I noticed this brought a new kind of stress into our home. I think it was particularly hard on my mother, who provided most of the daily care for her mother-in-law. Living in a basement bedroom, I could escape from the stress if I wanted. I did not share a bathroom or hallway, I did not have to listen to incoherent talk and cries in the night as Alzheimer's disease began to take its toll. Yet, I knew that my parents and some siblings slept less, worried more, and lost some freedom.

Over time, I began to feel drawn to grandma. Though I was still angry on occasion, I also found tender moments with her. I appreciated more the few small opportunities I had to help grandma or my parents as they were helping her. I remember sitting side by side with her one Christmas Eve long after she had lost the ability to carry on a conversation—at least I thought. As a favorite hymn began to play she nudged me and said, "We better stand as we sing this one." I helped her to her feet and she proceeded to sing all three verses from memory as we stood arm in arm. At that moment I could see her; she was still in there somewhere, that deeply spiritual, strong, and committed music teacher. It was a memorable moment to connect with her on that level. I am particularly grateful for that shared experience because shortly thereafter my family made the difficult decision to move grandma to a long-term care facility. She then passed away while I was far from home.

As I reflect upon this experience, I am reminded of several ironies regarding family caregiving. The emotional and physical work of caregiving can be so burdensome, yet somehow that service and sacrifice can bind hearts together in a powerful way. Caregiving is a family affair, yet individual members can feel isolated in their own experience, even lonely when surrounded by others. Perhaps caregiving is best described as a great tension of opposites: burden and privilege, isolation and connection, pain and joy. In some ways it also represents the past, present, and future, with all its fears and dreams, rolled up in one. However described, caregiving in a family setting is a commonly experienced and well-researched phenomenon.

FAMILY CAREGIVING: PREVALENCE AND TRENDS

A number of large-scale demographic trends have greatly influenced the number of families providing daily care for an aging loved one. First, people across the world are living longer, much longer (Armas, 2003). For example, in the United States the average life expectancy has nearly doubled, from the mid-forties in 1900 to nearly 80 in the year 2000 (Corcoran, Fairchild-Kienlen, & Phillips, 2000). Because of combined trends of overall decreases in birth rates and the aging of the baby boom generation, the largest segment of the U.S. population is quickly approaching age 65. By 2030, it is estimated that the number of older adults (65 and older) will jump to 70 million, a full 20% of the overall population and twice the number in 1999 (Administration on Aging [AoA], 2000). The fastest growth during that time is projected to occur among minority older adults, a 219% growth rate as compared to only an 81% increase for the white population (AoA, 2000).

The dramatic increase in life expectancy can be attributed to many factors, perhaps chief among them the tremendous ability of modern medicine to preserve and prolong life. For this reason, many older adults are living longer with chronic and debilitating physical and mental conditions (Zarit & Zarit, 1998). These trends, prolonged life and fewer births, combine to present a staggering challenge to family caregiving. At the same time a greater number of older adults may need daily care, there are fewer family members to provide it. Research near the turn of the 21st century suggested that nearly one-quarter of all homes in the U.S. already had at least one caregiver (Corcoran et al., 2000). At that time, one national survey concluded that a typical caregiver was a married woman in her 40s, working full time and providing care for an older care recipient (average age 77). The average

caregiver provided 18 hours of care a week, with one in five providing more than 40 hours (Corcoran et al., 2000). Clearly, these trends will only increase as the population ages. Since families are always "the first line of defense ... [for providing] extensive care, often at considerable sacrifice of their own health and well-being," it is appropriate that researchers, policy makers, and clinicians pay particular attention to the issues of family caregiving (Zarit & Zarit, 1998, p. 290).

THE EXPERIENCE OF PROVIDING CARE

In the last two decades of the 20th century, over 400 empirical studies solely on the psychological effects of caregiving were published (Pinquart & Sorensen, 2003a). These papers, along with published case studies and narratives, paint caregiving as both a challenging and a rewarding task. Caregiver burden is the most researched topic among this literature. Major theorists have noted that caregivers experience stress or burden on two levels. Primary stressors are related to direct care of the recipient and the behavioral, emotional, and physical tasks required in that process. Secondary stressors are related to the impact of caregiving on other aspects of the caregiver's life, such as marriage, employment, and personal finances (Zarit & Zarit, 1998).

A meta-analysis of caregiver burden research has clearly shown that caregivers experience lower levels of physical health and subjective well-being and greater levels of stress and depression than non-caregivers (Pinquart & Sorensen, 2003b). Other studies have noted that family caregivers spend less time interacting with others in their social network, particularly outside the home, and experience increased conflict with family members regarding caregiving responsibilities (Pillemer, Suitor, & Wethington, 2003). Study after study has shown that caregivers are vulnerable to multiple physical and mental health problems and are frequently isolated in their suffering.

Researchers have also sought to identify which aspects of caregiving prove most troublesome for caregiving. Theorists have hypothesized that care recipients' impairment (cognitive, physical, or behavior problems), caregiver involvement (amount of care, duration), and perception of uplift all play a major role in determining caregiver burden outcomes (Pinquart & Sorensen, 2003a). A second meta-analysis suggested that behavior problems of the care recipient are most strongly associated with caregiver burden and depression, although levels of physical and cognitive impairment are also associated with burden and depression at less significant levels (Pinquart & Sorensen, 2003a). Clearly, interventions that can serve to decrease burden, particularly the strain of care recipient behavior problems, and help caregivers stay socially engaged are of great worth to both families and society at large.

It is also important to note that many caregivers experience satisfaction and joy as a result of their service (Kramer, 1997). Some studies report that up to 75% of caregivers report that providing care helps them feel useful (i.e., facilitates self worth, confidence) (Myers, 2003). Other studies suggest that caregiving fosters an increased closeness to the care recipient and a sense of fulfilling one's duty (Pinquart & Sorensen, 2003b). When caregivers are able to experience a sense of mastery in caregiving tasks, they can also experience a sense of accomplishment and control that may serve to offset burden (Kramer, 1997; Wilken, Altergott, & Sandberg, 1996). A quotation from one caregiver highlights how the sweet can accompany the bitter while providing care: "This year and a half [of caregiving] has been so hard, but I can honestly say my mother and I have had some of the most tender times of our lives" (Hargrave, 2002, p. 26).

THE EXPERIENCE OF RECEIVING CARE

As broad and almost overwhelming as the caregiving literature has become, there is a similarly striking absence of research on the experience of care recipients. In the majority of caregiving studies, the receiver of care is viewed objectively in terms of her or his impairment and behavior and its impact on caregiver burden (Lyons, Zarit, Syer, & Whitlatch, 2002). Even in cases where the recipient's cognitive functioning is good and her or his input is sought, few studies go beyond assessing mental health status or decisions around institutionalization (Lyons et al., 2002). Non-caregiving research related to normative physical decline and loss (e.g., retirement, change of residence) associated with healthy aging suggests that decreased autonomy and independence can be very difficult for older adults (Sandberg & Platt, 2001). Such decline and loss can make the care recipient more vulnerable to social withdrawal and inactivity as well as depression (Hargrave & Hanna, 1997; Pillemer et al., 2003).

One group of researchers integrated both caregiver and care recipient perspectives and noted givers and receivers differed little over care recipient needs, but disagreed significantly on their appraisal of caregiving difficulties (Lyons et al., 2002). Specifically, the authors noted that caregivers perceived less support and cooperation than care recipients and that this discrepancy increased as the level of caregiving difficulties increased as well. Interestingly, the authors also point out that the caregiver's appraisal of relationship strain predicted the level of discrepancy and level of caregiving difficulties, indicating that the quality and nature of the relationship between giver and recipient has an impact on caregiver experience.

A second study (Conger & Marshall, 1998) that looked at both caregivers and care recipients provides greater insight into the experience of those who receive care. Drawing upon data from a series of longitudinal qualitative interviews with caregiving dyads, the authors theorize that care recipients may enter into a redefinition period where they shift long-held views and beliefs about self and relationships. Specifically, Conger and Marshall (1998) suggested that illness often brings a change in roles and an accompanying sense of loss for care recipients. The process of redefining self is one of acknowledging change and coming to terms with new priorities and less control and autonomy in one's life. Where cognitively possible, the care recipient may also seek to redefine his or her marital relationship as the couple creates shared meaning around the multitude of changes in their lives. In cases where the process of redefining life is beyond the reach of care recipients or their caregivers, the stresses and challenges of daily caregiving may soon take their toll on the relationship.

CULTURAL AND GENDER DIFFERENCES IN THE CAREGIVING EXPERIENCE

As mentioned, the first half of the 21st century will likely be known as an age of "graying," particularly among culturally and racially diverse groups. While the non-Hispanic white elderly population will likely double by the year 2050, the African American elderly population will quadruple, the Latino elderly population will increase by 7 times, the Asian/Pacific Islander by 6.5, and the American Indian population will increase to 3.5 times its current size (Dilworth-Anderson, Williams, & Gibson, 2002). With these trends in mind, there is a clear social imperative to increase understanding regarding the needs of dependent older adults in racially and ethnically diverse groups (Dilworth-Anderson et al., 2002). Because

cultural values, norms, and perceptions influence all aspects of caregiving, from an understanding of how disease is contracted to what "good" caregivers should and should not do (Dilworth-Anderson & Gibson, 2002), it is important that helping professionals do not fall into the trap of assuming sameness across families and cultures. A "theoretical myth of sameness," or "the conventional ideology . . . that minority families are no different than non-minority families," is a common belief in the social sciences that must be challenged in order to provide competent and truly helpful assistance to a heterogeneous host of caregivers (Hardy, 1989, p. 18).

In their 20-year review of issues of race, culture, and ethnicity in the caregiving literature, Dilworth-Anderson and colleagues (2002) noted key differences among racially and ethnically diverse groups regarding social support (extended informal support networks), negative effects (burden, depression), coping (spirituality), and cultural effects (cultural rules and guidelines). Although a helpful starting point, noticing these differences in how caregiving is done and how it affects caregivers is not enough. Helping professionals must go beyond differences in outcome, seeking to understand differences in process and the meanings and intents that drive these processes. Important questions emerge that focus on both outcome (burden, depression) and process (values, meanings, intent) for caregivers: How do the concepts of responsibility and respect factor into your decision-making processes as a caregiver? What are your beliefs about the aging of a body and your role in caring for an ailing loved one? Though few, a number of exemplary studies are now focusing on these types of questions and are attempting to understand how differing cultural values and meanings drive process and outcome for caregivers (Dilworth-Anderson & Gibson, 2002).

Cloutterbuck and Mahoney (2003), studying African American caregivers, explored the cultural meaning of respect and how the application of this concept may help explain why African American caregivers seem to be able to carry a heavier caregiving load for longer periods of time with fewer reports of burden and depression than their white counterparts. Holroyd (2003) studied Chinese caregivers over a two-year period, focusing on how cultural and religious understandings of the body impact caregiving decisions. In her study, Holroyd learned that the caring for a loved one experiencing bodily illness and decay can have profound personal and social ramifications for caregivers, thereby complicating greatly the entire caregiving process. Cultural aspects of caregiving continue to be understudied among a variety of cultures, including Native Americans, for example.

Research on gender differences in caregiving has highlighted the fact that women provide the greatest bulk of caregiving service. "Women tend to provide more personal and instrumental care than men [and] are more likely to report impaired well-being than men because of their greater sensitivity to negative feelings, greater willingness to report negative feelings, and less effective coping styles" (Pinquart & Sorensen, 2003b). Research has also shown that men are more likely to engage additional helpers and less likely to refer to caregiving as emotional work (Allen, 1994; Miller & Kaufman, 1996). Because of the tremendous burden they carry and the multiple roles they attempt to fulfill on a daily basis, it is easy to understand why many female caregivers may struggle to balance tremendous family and employment responsibilities while at the same time they may also be experiencing poorer emotional health (Navaie-Waliser, Spriggs, & Feldman, 2002).

Other studies suggest that many husbands adopt a task-oriented approach to caregiving, thereby maintaining an authority position, while wives work to preserve autonomy for their husbands and connection in the relationship (Corcoran, 1992; Wilken et al., 1996). Future research, which can better identify the meanings and intent of gender-specific behavior, would serve to clarify whether men and women do focus on or prefer instrumental versus affiliative support. Wilken and colleagues (1996) suggested that caregivers who feel adept at providing both types of care might be less vulnerable to strain. In the end, it is important to note that caregiving is carried out (objective) and experienced (subjective) differently by women and men and across diverse cultures.

LEVELS OF INTERVENTION: FROM RESPITE CARE TO PSYCHOTHERAPY

Over the years, helping professionals have worked with caregivers on a number of levels. Although the intent of most interventions is similar (alleviate burden, foster coping, build support), the approaches do differ in major ways (see Sorensen, Pinquart, & Duberstein, 2002 for a comprehensive review of the effectiveness of caregiver interventions).

Respite Care

As the stressors of caregiving begin to mount, numerous caregivers have found help through the use of respite care (Zarit, Johansson, & Jarrott, 1998). Respite care takes many forms, ranging from adult day care services to in-home care to friends and family helping out (see Zarit et al., 1998 for more detailed review). The primary purpose of this formal respite care is to ease the burden of the caregiver, and where possible, provide a safe and socially engaging experience for the recipient. Research has shown that caregiver satisfaction with respite care services is usually quite high, and even though respite care can trigger emotional (guilt over leaving a loved one in the care of others) and financial struggles, many care-givers would utilize these services more often if they could (Zarit et al., 1998). Respite care provides a needed break from caregiver res-ponsibilities. Though limited by cost and availability, it appears to be a helpful coping technique (Gaugler et al., 2003; Sorensen et al., 2002). Unfortunately, research has yet to clearly link caregiver satisfaction with enduring positive change in caregiver well-being (Myers, 2003).

Support Groups

Support groups for caregivers are perhaps the most well-known and popular form of intervention. Having arisen out of a grass roots effort to support caregivers of persons with Alzheimer's disease, support groups are a key setting for providing important infor-mation, combating isolation, and fostering collaborative problem solving (Zarit & Zarit, 1998). The scant research on support group outcomes is mixed and has not yet shown that groups are effective at reducing caregiver burden (Corcoran et al., 2000; Myers, 2003). Nevertheless, support groups remain popular, likely because they are widely available, afford-able, and provide a close-knit support system of those who share a similar experience. Some researchers have cautioned that support groups may not always be monitored for accuracy of information and advice or run by leaders with training; therefore, support groups "should not be the first line of help or the only source of help for caregivers" (Zarit & Zarit, 1998, p. 314; Jacobs, 1997).

Psychoeducation/Skills Training

Providing families with education and skills regarding the course of a loved one's ill-ness and accompanying care recipient needs, specific caregiving tasks, available resources, and successful coping strategies can serve to greatly reduce avoidable struggle and conflict. Psychoeducational interventions differ from traditional support groups in that they are typically more formal and research based. Such programs are consistently led by a trained leader and can take many forms (all day sem-inar, multi-week group, lecture, distribution of written materials); whatever the format, psychoeducational interventions have proven effective in reducing caregiver burden and depression and care receiver symptoms (Sorensen et al., 2002). A simple but effective example of the potential positive impact of timely education is noted by Zarit & Zarit (1998). In their work, they cite several touch-ing examples of helping caregivers learn that a calming and reassuring response is more effective than a corrective and argumentative one when care recipients wish to engage in dangerous activities. Although there has been some disagreement over the long-term bene-fits, psychoeducational approaches to care-giver intervention consistently rate among the most effective type of interventions (Corcoran et al., 2000; Sorensen et al., 2002).

Psychotherapy

Psychotherapy as an intervention can be described as a therapeutic relationship between a caregiver and a trained mental health professional (Sorensen et al., 2002). As Sorensen and colleagues (2002) noted in their review, traditional cognitive-behavioral approaches to therapy with caregivers serve to help them "develop problem-solving abil-ities by focusing on time management, over-load, and emotional reactivity management, and help the caregiver reengage in pleasant activities and positive experiences" (p. 358). Therapy may be short or long term, strength or problem focused; in the end, therapy provides caregivers with a set time to discuss concerns and receive individual attention from a trained professional poised to help in burden management and problem resolution (Zarit & Zarit, 1998). The Zarits (1998) note that therapy may be especially helpful in situations where the caregiver environment is particularly problematic. In such circumstances, there is evidence that psychotherapy interventions with caregivers have resulted in gains related to caregiving burden and well-being (Sorensen et al., 2002).

Common Factors Among Interventions

Whether the intervention involves a support group or a professional therapist, effective interventions seem to share a few common factors. Excluding respite care, all of the above-mentioned interventions rely heavily upon three treatment strategies highlighted in a model developed by Zarit and colleagues over years of practice and research (Zarit & Zarit, 1998). In this model, the authors describe the need for interventions to provide *information*, foster *problem solving*, and provide *support*. Over time, this three-pronged approach to intervention has received consistent empirical support, regardless of the mode of intervention (Zarit & Zarit, 1998).

WHAT ABOUT THE FAMILY?

In 1989, Steven Zarit wrote a provocative editorial titled, "Do we really need another 'stress and caregiving' study?" In his paper, Zarit argued that more attention should be placed on identifying effective (both in terms of cost and suffering) interventions than on re-establishing a well-known fact, namely that caregiving can be very stressful. Apparently researchers have heeded Zarit's call, evidenced by two major meta-analyses of caregiver interventions since his original piece was published (Knight, Lutzky, & Macofsky-Urban, 1993; Sorensen et al., 2002). Although there has been a clearly marked

increase in intervention studies, most continue to focus on and intervene at the individual level. Though the language of family caregiving or providing care in a family setting is often employed, few interventions actually attempt to address and resolve specific family concerns or foster change and healing within strained family relationships (Mitrani & Czaja, 2000).

This oversight may prove costly because research on caregiving has consistently shown that the quality of the relationship between caregivers and care recipients, as well as between caregivers and other family members, directly affects caregiver outcomes (Lyons et al., 2002; Miller, 1990). In a review and commentary on caregiving literature, Miller (1990) noted numerous empirical studies have found that a significant amount of caregiver burden can be attributed to conflictual family relationships. For his support, Miller points to studies reporting that family relationship quality may predict a greater amount of perceived caregiver effectiveness than care recipient impairment (Townsend & Noelker, 1987) and level of conflict between caregiver and care recipient may predict a significant amount of caregiver strain and negative affect (Sheehan & Nuttall, 1988). A significant body of research has already demonstrated that conflict in non-caregiving couples has a negative effect on health variables ranging from immunology to daily health practices (Keicolt-Glaser & Newton, 2001). Factors in family relationships seem to have a major impact on caregiver experience, yet it is ironic that two major reviews of the caregiving experience and intervention did not include family variables related to caregiver outcomes (see Pinquart & Sorensen, 2003a; Sorensen et al., 2002).

The Family Meeting

An appealing approach to addressing family issues, particularly to fostering cooperation among family caregivers, is the family meeting (Zarit & Zarit, 1998). The guiding principles behind the family meeting are rooted in family systems theory.

> From a family systems perspective, it is [very] useful to get a sense of how a family functions, for example, who is influential and who is not, who is close to and distant from whom, and what the roles of the caregiver and care recipient have been in the family. (Zarit & Zarit, 1998, p. 310)

Guided by a trained clinician, the family meeting provides an appropriate venue to ensure all family members have the same accurate information about the loved one's illness and that each understands the level of care required. Once this occurs, the meeting can focus on what the primary caregiver wants and needs and the role of other family members in the caregiving process. The clinician can help the family form a plan for future action by being "neutral and supportive" and guiding them towards a resolution of conflict; however, "the therapist should . . . not try to change family process or treat long-standing problems or to redress the balance of power within the family" (Zarit & Zarit, 1998, p. 312). This is the role of family therapy.

Other Family-Based Interventions for Caregiving Families: Empirical Support

There are a few studies that tested the effectiveness of a structured, family-based intervention for caregiving families. Two noteworthy studies provide excellent examples of how family caregiving systems can be engaged and helped through family-based interventions. In their randomized controlled trial, Mittelman, Ferris, Shulman, Steinberg, and Levin (1996) provided four family counseling sessions as a part of their broader protocol. In those sessions, the counselor helped

families address and resolve problems regarding patient behavior, improve communication among family members, and increase emotional and instrumental support for the primary caregiver. Families who participated in the broad-based intervention were able to care for their loved one at home for longer periods of time than those in the control group, especially throughout beginning stages of dementia when placement in a care facility may not be necessary.

A second study, reported by Mitrani and Czaja (2000), demonstrates how culturally sensitive home-based family therapy may be a particularly appropriate and effective intervention. Mitrani, Czaja, and colleagues applied Structural Ecosystemic Therapy (SET), a proven family systems-based therapy, to their work with Cuban caregiving families. In their sessions, members of the SET team worked in the home with caregiving families to build a healthy and functional family structure (hierarchy, alliance, communication), foster resonance (address caregiver and care recipient enmeshment), and resolve conflict. The SET intervention was one of nine active interventions tested in the REACH multisite initiative with caregivers and the only approach that evaluated a family systems-based intervention. At six month follow-up, the SET approach had not only established itself as effective when compared to inactive groups; it was also one of two interventions that had significantly reduced depressive symptoms in caregivers (Gitlin et al., 2003).

A THEORETICAL FRAMEWORK FOR EXTENDING FAMILY-BASED WORK

In a recent paper, Pillemer and colleagues (2003) argued that although intertwined, good theory precedes quality intervention design and testing. Because of the oversight regarding and need for increased research into family-based interventions with caregivers, it is important that a solid, family-based theoretical framework is laid upon which to build an intervention framework. Perhaps a combination of developmental and relational ethics theories could serve as an initial launching point for a richer discussion of family-based theory and its implications for helping professionals on the front lines with caregiving families.

Developmental Theory

It is important to recognize a few key developmental factors that may result in strain for many caregivers and recipients. The eighth stage of Erik Erickson's (1963) theory of psychosocial development provides a useful lens through which to view the one major struggle of later-life families. According to the theory, as older adults approach death, they naturally grapple to find the meaning in their existence: Has my life mattered? Have I accomplished my goals? Have I made a difference? These are questions that may arise as older adults struggle with ego integrity versus despair (Crain, 1992; Hargrave & Anderson, 1997). This normative process of sifting through past experiences as motivated by the nearness of death has been termed life review (Butler, 1963).

Likewise, many adult children and spouses are faced with a similar process as they are drawn towards their ailing loved one because of the perceived finality of death (Carstensen, 1998). In many cases, this review of the relational landscape may not immediately yield feelings of contentment and appreciation; in fact, it may only amplify family members' struggles with past contention and inflicted hurts. The pressure to "make things right" in a short period of time can greatly complicate family processes. This stage of life and the naturally occurring process of life review places older adults and their families in a vulnerable position as they recall intense and painful interactions, wounds, and conflicts from their past (Hargrave & Anderson, 1997). It is at this stage and in this context that the bulk of caregiving often occurs. How can family members balance the opposing forces of providing care out of a sense of love and duty and a looming sense of frustration and anger over past hurts?

Relational Ethics

Boszormenyi-Nagy's theory of relational ethics, commonly known as contextual theory, provides potential answers to this difficult question and a useful lens for clinicians dealing with caregiving issues (Boszormenyi-Nagy & Krasner, 1986; see Hargrave & Anderson, 1992 for a beautiful and clear application of contextual theory to common clinical problems of aging families). Relational ethics are concerned "with the subjective balance of trustworthiness, justice, loyalty, merit, and entitlement among members of a relationship" (Hargrave & Anderson, 1997, p. 63). When family members can interact in a balanced or fair manner, where both can give and take without manipulation, trustworthiness is developed. According to this theory, trustworthiness is the key to family loyalty and strength across generations (Hargrave & Anderson, 1997). Conversely, when trust erodes, family dysfunction often follows (Anderson & Hargrave, 1990).

Symptoms of intergenerational conflict or dysfunction can be seen as a sign of an unbalanced relational account. These accounts or ledgers can be described as ongoing legacies of emotional commitments and obligations (Everett, Russell, & Keller, 1992; Spark, 1974). Simply put, multigenerational ledgers are accounts of relational charges (hurts) and credits (benefits) accrued by family members over time (Boszormenyi-Nagy, 1974).

This metaphor of families making transactions (interacting) with overdrawn accounts (unbalanced ledgers) can be readily applied to caregiving families. Imagine an adult daughter who is providing care for her ailing father. As is typical of many caregivers, she is trying to balance the demands of her own family and a job while looking after her father. Although her cultural and personal expectations are that she provides loving and dutiful care, she is often resentful and angry. As a result, she is experiencing increased conflict in her own home and feels criticized by her own siblings regarding the type of care she is providing for their father.

In a family meeting or family therapy session, would it not be common for some of the following questions to be raised? "Why was I the one selected to be the primary caregiver? I have always done more work than my brothers and sisters." "This is just like it was when we were kids; she was always in control. How are we supposed to help when she never lets us get involved?" "How can I feel loving and connected to Dad when he was never part of my life? Even when he was home from work, he was always so angry and violent. Am I supposed to forget all of that pain?" Though often ignored in the research literature, clinicians recognize that expectations regarding loyalty and fairness can drive caregiving decisions and experience (Hargrave & Anderson, 1997; Jacobs, 1997; Sandberg, 1999).

Therefore, a major task for many caregiving families is to reconcile themselves with painful issues from their past. As painful as the process may be, contextual theory claims that revisiting these encounters can prepare the way for a balancing of intergenerational accounts. Therefore, "older [adults and their] families need to do the work of communicating about, reconciling with, and forgiving the past. In these actions, the ground work for trustworthy relations[hips] is constructed" (Hargrave & Anderson, 1997, p. 65).

PRACTICAL INTERVENTIONS FOR FAMILY-FOCUSED WORKERS

There are times when family therapy is needed to address long-standing problems and address issues of power and control in caregiving families (Zarit & Zarit, 1998). Developmental and contextual theories provide a base from which the following interventions are built.

The Life Review

Life review interventions (Butler, 1963) are based upon the concept that older adults and their families will naturally undergo a period of reflection about the purpose and meaning of their existence as death approaches. Because issues of fairness, loyalty, and entitlement become evident as past experiences are recalled through the life review, important details regarding the family's intergenerational ledger can be gleaned in this process. With this increased awareness of how and when injustices first occurred, aging families are better able to understand their own relationship with both the past (their own parents) and the future (their children). This process allows family members to identify with each other in healthier ways through appreciation and understanding. It is only through these new, fairer interactions that trust is rebuilt and ledgers are balanced. The life review exercise, in the presence of family, is one action strategy to foster this healing (Spark, 1974).

In addition, the life review can be used as a simple yet powerful tool for connecting and calming when relationships have become strained in more acute, rather than chronic, ways. Hargrave (2002) described a clinical case in which an adult daughter Robin (age 60) and her mother Maggie (84) came to family therapy. Shortly after Maggie had left her long-term residence and moved to Robin's home, the relationship environment began to sour. Although Maggie was still able to function independently in a number of areas at these beginning stages of Alzheimer's disease, she felt bossed around by her daughter; Robin was frustrated over her mother's increasing dependence and angry outbursts. Perhaps in an attempt to connect and calm, Dr. Hargrave engaged Robin and Maggie in a conversation about the "good old days."

This simple looking back led Robin and Maggie into a conversation about a "good husband" and a "good father" and how they both missed him. At one point, Maggie slid her hand into her daughter's, saying, "Well, I guess you and I are what we have now." Robin came to realize that the pressures of caregiving had caused her to press too hard to get things done in a hurry. In turn, this likely frustrated her mother at a level that she could not verbalize, and so she wound up expressing herself [by throwing] a hairbrush. Robin was eager to make changes. She sought ways to connect with her mother, like sharing old pictures. Robin learned how to keep the storytelling from becoming repetitive, and picked out two personal events each week that helped bring back old times. Maggie had no more violent outbursts . . . [and during] those months, Robin had learned to connect with her mom emotionally . . . [leading her to call this period] some of the most tender times in our lives. (Hargrave, 2002, p. 26)

The Work of Forgiveness

A second approach to balancing intergenerational accounts in later life is through the work of forgiveness. Interventions aimed at forgiveness may be particularly helpful in addressing "basic questions of love and trust in the family and rebuild[ing] relationships after severe family violations have occurred" (Hargrave & Anderson, 1997, p. 68). For some individuals, increased awareness regarding their aging parent's own suffering,

although extremely beneficial, will not be enough to compensate for long-standing injustices. For such families, the work of forgiveness can provide a more structured format for resolving long-standing relational indebtedness. The ability to resolve these long-standing conflicts may be particularly valuable when the person experiencing the hurt is valiantly trying to provide care for the one who did the hurting.

Hargrave and Anderson (1997) described forgiveness as two distinct processes, exoneration and forgiveness. "Exoneration means the victim is able to lift the load of culpability from the victimizer while making significant connection and identification, whereas forgiveness means that the victim and victimizer are actually able to restore a loving and trustworthy relationship" (p. 68). Although it is not possible or wise for all individuals to achieve this definition of forgiveness (that is, in cases where a victimizer continues to make unjust demands on the victim's account), it is possible for most individuals to exonerate their ailing loved one.

The work of exoneration can be broken down into two stations (Hargrave & Anderson, 1992; Hargrave, 1994). The first station, *insight*, involves gaining a cognitive awareness of the experience of another and how past pains have been transferred to current relationships (Hargrave & Anderson, 1997). Not until the hurt party can identify relationship patterns that perpetuate pain can he or she stop the process. The second station, *understanding*, seeks to foster a level of identification with or even empathy for the victimizer's own suffering and efforts to change problematic patterns in his or her own life (Hargrave & Anderson, 1997). Both the insight and the deeper level of understanding can be facilitated in a life review intervention.

The actual work of forgiveness also involves two stations. *Giving the opportunity for compensation* is a process whereby the victim allows the victimizer to change and rebuild the relationship by demonstrating trust and love over time in an effort to erase past injustices (Hargrave & Anderson, 1997). This process allows the hurt party to test, in stages, the trustworthiness of the one who has previously inflicted pain. Only as trustworthiness is built can the ledger be rebalanced. The fourth station, *the overt act of forgiveness,* is where victim and victimizer work directly and honestly to confront and heal from past hurt through the "agreement, acknowledgement, and apology" (Hargrave & Anderson, 1997, p. 4). During this last phase, family-focused workers must help the victim and victimizer come to a ball park agreement of what the hurt is, acknowledge that the wrongdoer is responsible for the wrongs committed, and facilitate an apology that demonstrates regret and a sincere desire to do better (Hargrave & Anderson, 1997). This process, though extremely intense and only possible with two willing parties, can provide tremendous healing.

Returning to the previous hypothetical example of a family session with an adult daughter caregiver, her siblings, and an ailing father, how could a family therapist help facilitate exoneration or forgiveness and what difference would it make? A family therapist based in Contextual theory may seek to help children understand the experiences in their own father's life that might have led him to be more absent or violent than they or he wanted (insight). The family therapist might also help the children understand how the tendency to avoid or blow up surfaces at times in their own lives (understanding). The family therapist would also work to help the father, if cognitively able, to engage in a healing dialogue with his children in which he acknowledges past mistakes and takes responsibility for them (initial steps of forgiveness). Such difficult and healing dialogues between father and children and among siblings have a tremendous potential

to increase support and unity among family members and reduce subjective burden, two factors that contribute greatly to the overall experience of a caregiver.

FUTURE DIRECTIONS

To paraphrase Zarit (1989), do we really need more studies that focus on the individual experience of caregivers and treatments that intervene on an individual level? If families are truly the primary and most basic support structure for providing care for ailing loved ones, future researchers and clinicians will need to combine together to successfully address three key areas relating to family caregiving (Zarit & Zarit, 1998).

Absence of Empirical Research Regarding Family-Based Interventions for Caregivers

Though theoretically and logically sound, few studies have actually tested family-based models for caregiving families. Because of elevated divorce rates, greater distance between family members, and decreased health care coverage trends, more and more family members will be forced to face difficult issues as they struggle to provide care in a family setting. As a result, more and more practitioners will be called upon to help these families. Unfortunately, the amount of clinical research, even theoretical research, in this area is insufficient to support the looming need.

Absence of Culturally Sensitive and Effective Family Interventions with Caregivers

With exception of the work by Mitrani and Czaja (2000), very little is known about how to best intervene with families from a variety of cultural backgrounds. It is interesting to note that in a major meta-analysis of the caregiving intervention literature, race and culture is not addressed as a variable of interest (Sorensen et al., 2002). Do not racial and cultural differences impact the experience of caregiving? Should not interventions be tailored to meet the specific needs and highlight the unique strengths of specific groups? The continued under-appreciation of differences (Hardy, 1989) will prove costly in light of tremendous increases in diverse groups of the elderly over the next 50 years.

Linking Research, Policy and Practice

If researchers and clinicians are able to work collaboratively to identify and highlight culturally competent, effective family-based interventions for caregivers, there still remains the tremendous task of making those interventions available to those who need them most. For many families, treatment for any struggle related to relational, emotional, or mental health is simply out of their reach. Though demographics demand more emphasis and money be put into aging issues, such a change has yet to occur at a level that will be required. A significant shift is needed to make therapy for caregiving families readily available and truly beneficial.

CONCLUSION

In a heart-rending article, Jacobs (1997) pays homage to caregivers he works with, describing them as:

> saints and war heroes, for their devotion, unstinting selflessness, and seemingly superhuman strength . . . [as] they spoon-feed, wipe dry, undress, clothe, clean, watch over, guide and sometimes literally tote on their backs to and from the toilet [their loved ones]. They also comfort, correct, chasten, cajole, entertain, and cry with them every hour every day, for years if necessary. (p. 213)

At times it is easy to forget that behind each of the thousands of caregiving studies is a family of real people trying to do the best they can. May we, as researchers and clinicians, keep that in mind as we push forward to help decrease burdens and increase uplifts for these noble families.

REFERENCES

Administration on Aging (AoA), U.S. Department of Health and Human Services. (2000). *A profile of older Americans: 2000.* Washington, DC: U.S. Government Printing Office.

Allen, S. M. (1994). Gender differences in spousal caregiving and unmet need for care. *Journal of Gerontology, 49*(4), S187–S195.

Anderson, W. T., & Hargrave, T. D. (1990). Contextual family therapy and older people: Building trust in the intergenerational community. *Journal of Family Therapy, 12,* 311–320.

Armas, G. C. (2003). Worldwide population aging. In H. Cox (Ed.), *Annual editions: Aging* (pp. 3–4). Guilford, CT: McGraw-Hill.

Boszormenyi-Nagy, I. (1974). Ethical and practical implications of intergenerational family therapy: What is psychotherapy? *Psychosomatic, 24,* 261–268.

Boszormenyi-Nagy, I., & Krasner, B. (1986). *Between give and take: A clinical guide to contextual therapy.* New York: Harper & Row.

Butler, R. N. (1963). The life review: An interpretation of reminiscence in the aged. *Psychiatry, 26,* 65–76.

Carstensen, L. (1998). *Emotional functioning in old age.* Paper presented at Gerontological Society of America Annual Conference, Philadelphia, PA.

Cloutterbuck, J., & Mahoney, D. F. (2003). African American dementia caregivers. *Dementia, 2*(2), 221–243.

Conger, C. O., & Marshall, E. S. (1998). Recreating life: Toward a theory of relationship development in acute home care. *Qualitative Health Research, 8*(4), 526–546.

Corcoran, M. A. (1992). Gender differences in dementia management plans of spousal caregivers: Implications for occupational therapy. *American Journal of Occupational Therapy, 46*(11), 1006–1012.

Corcoran, M. A., Fairchild-Kienlen, S., & Phillips, J. H. (2000). Family treatment with caregivers of the elderly. In J. Corcoran (Ed.), *Evidence-based social work practice with families* (pp. 505–556). New York: Springer.

Crain, W. (1992). *Theories of development: Concepts and applications.* Englewood Cliffs, NJ: Prentice-Hall.

Dilworth-Anderson, P., & Gibson, B. E. (2002). The cultural influence of values, norms, meanings, and perceptions in understanding dementia in ethnic minorities. *Alzheimer Disease and Associated Disorders, 16*(Supp. 2), S56–S63.

Dilworth-Anderson, P., Williams, I. C., & Gibson, B. E. (2002). Issues of race, ethnicity, and culture in caregiving research: A 20-year review (1980–2000). *The Gerontologist, 42*(2), 237–272.

Erikson, E. H. (1963). *Childhood and society* (2nd ed.). New York: Norton.

Everett, C. A., Russell, C. S., & Keller, J. (1992). *Family therapy glossary* (pp. 1–40). Washington, DC: The American Association for Marriage and Family Therapy.

Gaugler, J. E., Jarrott, S. E., Zarit, S. H., Stephens, M. P., Townsend, A., & Greene, R. (2003). Adult day service use and reductions in caregiving hours: Effects on stress and psychological well-being for dementia caregivers. *International Journal of Geriatric Psychiatry, 18,* 55–62.

Gitlin, L. N., Belle, S. H., Burgio, L. D., Czaja, S. J., Mahoney, D., Gallagher-Thompson, D., et al. (2003). Effect of multicomponent interventions on caregiver burden and depression: The REACH multisite initiative at 6-month follow-up. *Psychology and Aging, 18*(3), 361–374.

Hardy, K. V. (1989). The theoretical myth of sameness: A critical issue in family therapy training and treatment. *Journal of Psychotherapy and the Family, 6*(1–2), 17–33.

Hargrave, T. (2002). My child, my mother. *Modern Maturity, 45*(2), 25–26.

Hargrave, T. D., & Anderson, W. T. (1992). *Finishing well: Aging and reparation in the intergenerational family.* New York: Brunner/Mazel.

Hargrave, T. D., & Anderson, W. T. (1997). Finishing well: A contextual family therapy approach to the aging family. In T.D. Hargrave & S. M. Hanna (Eds.), *The aging family* (pp. 61–80). New York: Brunner/Mazel.

Hargrave, T. D., & Hanna, S. M. (1997). *The aging family: New visions in theory, practice, and reality.* New York: Brunner/Mazel.

Holroyd, E. (2003). Hong Kong Chinese family caregiving: Cultural categories of bodily order and location of self. *Qualitative Health Research, 13*(2), 158–170.

Jacobs, B. J. (1997). In sickness and health: At the caregiver support group. *Families, Systems and Health, 15*(2), 213–220.

Kiecolt-Glaser, J. K., & Newton, T. L. (2001). Marriage and health: His and hers. *Psychological Bulletin, 127*(4), 472–503.

Knight, B. G., Lutzky, S. M., & Macofsky-Urban, F. (1993). A meta-analytic review of interventions for caregiver distress: Recommendations for future research. *The Gerontologist, 33*, 240–248.

Kramer, B. J. (1997). Gain in the caregiving experience: Where are we? What next? *The Gerontologist, 17*(2), 218–232.

Lyons, K. S., Zarit, S. H., Sayer, A. G., & Whitlatch, C. J. (2002). Caregiving as a dyadic process: Perspectives from caregiver and receiver. *Journal of Gerontology: Psychological Sciences, 57B*(3), P195–P204.

Miller, B., & Kaufman, J. E. (1996). Beyond gender stereotypes: Spouse caregivers of persons with dementia. *Journal of Aging Studies, 10*(3), 189–204.

Miller, R. B. (1990). *Building bridges between family policy, research, and practice.* Paper presented at Seventh National Forum on Aging, Lincoln, NE.

Mitrani, V. B., & Czaja, S. J. (2000). Family-based therapy for dementia caregivers: Clinical observations. *Aging and Mental Health, 4*(3), 200–209.

Mittelman, M. S., Ferris, S. H., Shulman, E., Steinberg, G., & Levin, B. (1996). A family intervention to delay nursing home placement of patients with Alzheimer disease. *Journal of the American Medical Association, 276*(21), 1725–1731.

Myers, J. E. (2003). Coping with caregiving stress: A wellness-oriented, strengths-based, approach for family counselors. *The Family Journal: Counseling and Therapy for Couples and Families, 11*(2), 153–161.

Navaie-Waliser, M., Spriggs, A., & Feldman, P. H. (2002). Informal caregiving: Differential experiences by gender. *Medical Care, 40*(12), 1249–1259.

Pillemer, K., Suitor, J. J., & Wethington, E. (2003). Integrating theory, basic research, and intervention: Two case studies from caregiving research. *The Gerontologist, 43*(SI1), 19–28.

Pinquart, M., & Sorensen, S. (2003a). Associations of stressors and uplifts of caregiving with caregiver burden and depressive mood: A meta-analysis. *Journal of Gerontology: Psychological Sciences, 58B*(2), 112–128.

Pinquart, M., & Sorensen, S. (2003b). Differences between caregivers and noncaregivers in psychological health and physical health: A meta-analysis. *Psychology and Aging, 18*(2), 250–267.

Sandberg, J. G. (1999). "It just isn't fair": Helping older families balance their ledgers before the note comes due. *Family Relations, 48*, 177–179.

Sandberg, J. G., & Platt, J. J. (2001). Family therapy and issues of aging. In M. M. MacFarlane (Ed.), *Family therapy and mental health: Innovations in theory and practice* (pp. 361–388). Binghamton, NY: The Haworth Clinical Practice Press.

Sheehan, N., & Nuttall, P. (1988). Conflict, emotion, and personal strain among family caregivers. *Family Relations, 37*, 92–98.

Sorensen, S., Pinquart, M., & Duberstein, P. (2002). How effective are interventions with caregivers? An updated meta-analysis. *The Gerontologist, 42*(3), 356–372.

Spark, G. M. (1974). Grandparents and intergenerational family therapy. *Family Process, 13*(2), 225–237.

Townsend, A., & Noelker, L. (1987). The impact of family relationships on perceived caregiving effectiveness. In T. Brubaker (Ed.), *Aging, health, and family: Long term care* (pp. 80–99). Newbury Park, CA: Sage.

Wilken, C. S., Altergott, K., & Sandberg, J. (1996). Spouses' self-perceptions as caregivers: The influence of feminine and masculine sex-role orientation on caring for confused and non-confused partners. *American Journal of Alzheimer's Disease, 11*(6), 37–42.

Zarit, S. H. (1989). Do we need another "stress and caregiving" study? *The Gerontologist, 29,* 481–483.

Zarit, S. H., Johansson, L., & Jarrott, S. E. (1998). Family caregiving: Stresses, social programs, and clinical interventions. In I. H. Nadhus, G. R. Vanden-Bos, S. Bera, & P. Fromholt (Eds.), *Clinical Geropsychology* (pp. 345–360). Washington, DC: American Psychological Association.

Zarit, S. H., & Zarit, J. M. (1998). *Mental disorders in older adults: Fundamentals of assessment and treatment.* New York: Guilford.

CHAPTER 25

Facing What Can and Cannot Be Said: Working With Families, Parents, and Couples When a Parent Has a Serious Illness

Barbara J. Dale and Jenny Altschuler

This chapter explores how focusing on the interplay between mind, body, and relationships offers a frame for thinking about parental illness with couples, children, and families. The material draws primarily on discussions in therapy from work with families where a parent has a seriously debilitating or life-threatening illness, including multiple sclerosis, motor neuron disease, celiac disease, AIDS, and various forms of cancer.

To the individual, illness is both a physical and psychological experience: what happens to us physically cannot be separated from the impact illness has on our psychological sense of ourselves. This is reflected in the increasing attention of medical science to the impact of psychological factors, such as stress, on physical health (Greer & Silberfarb, 1982; Panksepp, 1998). When one is in severe pain, nausea, or excessively fatigued, healing requires two separate activities: a physical response such as medication, dialysis, or the body's own buildup of antibodies, and a psychological response requiring a repositioning of self to deal with the emotional impact, whether alone or with the help of family, friends, and professionals.

In working with the families in which a parent had a life-risking illness, we were initially concerned that challenging therapy could exacerbate the illness by increasing stress. Over time, we have come to recognize the different levels of stress: while intense therapy at one level may cause stress, at another level it makes a positive difference to far more destructive processes. We too have needed to challenge our own beliefs about the role these links play in organizing our readiness to confront issues that parents might find distressing. In general, we now have greater concern about the overinclusive way in which emotional stress has been linked to physical health.

A SYSTEMIC APPROACH TO WORKING WITH FAMILIES FACING ILLNESS

The chapter draws on a systemic approach to working with people facing illness. The approach originally evolved from cybernetics and the idea that in order to understand how any system operates, we need to study the transactional processes occurring between members of that system, regardless of whether we are referring to a family, health care unit, school or the links between these systems (Bateson, 1972). Rather than seeing a problem, solution, or dilemma as rooted in any one person, emphasis is placed on the interactions among people, on the pattern of relating that becomes set up between two or more people. It also means that instead of seeing our sense of ourselves as relatively static, it continues to be constructed in an ongoing way through interactions with others. In order to understand what an illness might mean for any one of us, we need to have a sense of what this means for those around us and how their beliefs and actions inform the illness experience.

Influenced by social constructionism, systemic approaches have shifted more recently to embrace the wider context: rather than viewing what happens in any one family as idiosyncratic, greater emphasis is placed on trying to understand how this relates to the context in which that family is embedded (Goldner, 1991; Krause, 1998; Dwedi, 1999). This includes thinking about the way in which relationships between family members and professionals might be informed by cultural constructs of health, illness, parenting, and couple relationships. It also includes considering how constructs like this have been influenced by the gendered, racialized, and class-based discourses dominant in society.

The work also draws on the understanding that the meanings we give to events serve to explain, shape, and constrain the choices we see as possible courses of action. The chapter focuses on the stories parents and children tell of their experience, and the value of helping people uncover aspects of their stories that have been marginalized, in order to reconstruct stories that are more useful and creative in meeting the very complex challenges they face.

Time and Pace

Our experience has been that one must guard against being too concerned about the time required to undertake the work. The critical factor seems to be not attempting to accelerate the process of therapy. There can be a great pressure for urgency on the part of the sick parent or partner to say as much as possible as they may be fearful they have little time left and information may be given too fast. As we have written elsewhere (Dale & Altschuler, 1997), parents, partners, and children in particular can be overwhelmed by too much expectation of progress; less may mean more if therapy is well-balanced and inclusive of all family members.

This means recognizing that some work will be incomplete. That is the nature of untimely illness and death. Although untimely death might be relatively unfamiliar in Western countries, this is not so elsewhere in the world. We have had to explore our own Western beliefs about "certainty" and the idea that parents will live to see their children as adults.

In discussing her work with children with leukemia, Judd (1989) referred to parents acting as a "protective filter" on what is shared, a filter that allows ideas and fears to flow in both directions. So too with parental illness; it may not be about sharing everything with children but pacing what is said to acknowledge some of the fears they and their parents have. Rather than increasing separation, such sharing offers the opportunity for retaining and rebuilding connections that might have been threatened during the course of the illness.

Through not attempting to hold to a set formula of seeing all family members together, we have been able to remain flexible about whom to see. The work has comprised a combination of sessions with all family members living in the one home, couples, siblings, individuals, and grandparents, giving the message that there can be no prescribed way of addressing the complex issues people bring to this work. This can empower the family to work out its own route, and the process has been very helpful in developing a therapist and family collaborative approach. This collaboration can help to create some sense of security in the climate of uncertainty that illness brings.

Couples and Children

For this chapter we have chosen two aspects of our work with the families: children and couple's work. One of the themes that link both areas is the uncertainty about what can and cannot be said. For both groups, this raised poignant dilemmas. For the children, this uncertainty focused on the nature and seriousness of the illness and how far they felt able to risk speaking about it or asking questions. Mourning the death of their parents is particularly complicated for children who fear they may have caused the death of their parent, leaving them with an increased risk of a long-term sense of failure and blame. For the partner, uncertainty about what could be said tended to be less about the illness and more about unresolved aspects of their own relationship, or on intimate relationships with others. For some, the dilemma they faced was how far to risk talking about those issues now and possibly increasing stress, or alternately, what might it mean never to have explored those differences. Without addressing their unresolved issues, they are at risk of being unable to fully mourn and consequently less able to embrace the role of acting on behalf of them both as parents, as they both had wanted.

CONVERSATIONS AND PLAY WITH CHILDREN

The material draws primarily on discussions in therapy in the presence of parents and therapists. It reflects the way in which the children made sense of their experience in the context of the profound change their parents were undergoing. What they might have chosen to share would no doubt have been different had they been seen alone.

The process of telling any story involves both a narrator and an audience, even if the audience is primarily in the mind of the narrator. What children choose to say, ask, and show, either in therapy or at home, is inevitably connected with assumptions as to who they think may be listening. This includes their guesses of what we or their parents can bear to hear and whether their questions are likely to be answered. Children often feel responsible for their parents' emotional well-being, and hold back on what is said for fear of increasing the burden faced by their already distressed parents. For example, 11-year-old Thomas started saying that a great deal had changed since his mother became ill. When asked what he meant he said, "I forget." Similarly, Nita, aged 13, started to talk about the work of her terminally ill father. She spoke as if this only occurred in the past. She stopped to correct herself and continued in the present tense, preserving the image of him as a man engaged in paid employment outside of home.

Although many of the parents we have seen seek therapy to help them talk to their children, children often understand the reasons for referral differently. They may believe that therapy is aimed at finding ways in which they could be more helpful to sick parents, to help them take better care of themselves and increase their chances of survival. Sasha, aged 13, said, "I thought I'd better come along 'cause Mum wanted us to come along, 'cause she thinks it's going to help us, her illness, or something." These comments reflect her sense of needing to find a way of healing not only herself but her mother as well, a task well beyond her level of expertise. In many cases, one of the most important aspects of therapy is to try to explore the levels of responsibility children can really assume. Having some discrete tasks can help children retain a sense of their own agency; being asked to take on tasks that are well beyond their reach is not only unrealistic, it can impair their sense of competence, increasing the burden they already face. In many ways, they face a complex choice: acting in an unruly manner might increase parents' stress levels. However, becoming more helpful may feel equally dangerous, signifying that it is they who need to care for their parents rather than the reverse.

Illness can impose an imbalance in the caregiving system. Two systems operate side by side: one organized around developmental issues, the other around the medical condition. While receiving care from children does not preclude caring for them, an extensive imbalance in generational hierarchy can limit the extent to which parents feel able to contribute to their children. At such times it can be enormously helpful for someone outside the family to consider what might be age appropriate. In many situations, families find it impossible to hold on to a unitary idea of what is or is not age appropriate. Helping them reconnect to other contexts such as school and peer groups can be very helpful in mediating the overwhelming experience of their parent's illness.

Extending Teachers' Role "In Loco Parentis"

For some children, school provides a safe haven where they can be sure of boundaries and the expectations. For example, for six-year-old Max, whose mother had experienced a serious brain hemorrhage, her altered condition meant that the relationship between his parents had altered considerably, and his mother responded to him in ways that were quite different from before. School became the one place where he could understand the rules of how to behave, receive the attention he needed to help him progress, and separate himself from the overwhelming worries of home.

However, this is not the case for all. Thirteen-year-old Nita felt far more distress at school than at home. She found the quiet times devoted to learning created a space in which her anger and anxiety grew, anger related both to her mother's illness and issues that predated this. She struggled with her resentment at feeling different from her peers, feeling watched by both the staff and her friends, and was upset when she found herself crying at school.

Her behavior at home was extremely contained and she acted with a level of responsibility far beyond her age. Paradoxically, it was at school that she felt safe enough to illustrate her enormous distress, to show how out of control she really felt.

Work with schools formed a central part of the project. This included consultation at schools and joint meetings with teachers, children, and parents. When a parent is unwell, teachers often find themselves having to increase the extent to which they have to stand in for a mother or father who is temporarily or permanently unavailable to their child. In such cases, teachers may struggle to know what level of input to provide: while helping children study or talk may enable them to deal with what they face, stepping in too far may minimize the role of someone who is already struggling to hold on to their identity as a parent (Altschuler, Dale, & Sass-Booth, 1999).

In some situations, illness has meant that parents are pushed to share issues with teachers that they had previously kept private. For example, in a family where the parents were in a same-sex relationship, their daughter's prior experiences of being bullied at school had meant that she had decided to guard against sharing this aspect of their family life at her new school. When one of the mothers became very ill, both parents felt the school needed to know that one of her mothers was dying. An important part of the work included thinking, with all the family, what this young girl wanted to say to her peers and what help she might want from her teacher to deal with their response to these two very different situations.

Often teachers are a similar age to the ill parent, so that in helping children deal with the effect this is having on themselves and their peer group, teachers are likely to be personally affected by the illness. The work has therefore also involved meeting with teachers to think together about the impact of the illness on both staff and peer groups. This has included planning together for how the family wants the school to respond when a parent dies.

Mind-Body Interplay

Children make sense of illness at a physical and psychological level. This is evident in the way in which they speak and play about illness and in how they describe what they know about parents' illness. It shows when they choose to interrupt discussions and how they understand their own role in their parents' health. Even very young children listen carefully to what is said and demonstrate in a nonverbal way their attempts to understand what is happening. In the absence of being told, children continue to learn and develop their own stories, stories that may be more frightening than the reality they face. Lisa, aged three years, was asked why her mother was crying and she knew it was because she was "very, very sick."

The age of the child and visibility of the illness play a major part in determining what

parents tell children. In some situations, there is a close fit between what is said and shown at a nonverbal level, facilitating the process by which the child develops a sense of coherence central to resilience (Garmezy & Masten, 1994; Rutter, 1999). However, this is not always the case, and children may struggle to make sense of the conflicting messages they hear and see. This interplay seems to have a crucial role in how children learn: young children rely on visual representations in conceptualizing what illness "looks like." A six-year-old, Max, said his mother was brain-damaged; she had experienced a brain hemorrhage. He did not know if this meant she was still unwell but he knew she had a dent in her head from surgery and needed a bandage and plastic clip. He added that he did not know what color the clip was. Max illustrated what he did know at a concrete level, but this was in stark contrast to his broader uncertainty—uncertainty about his mother's condition, the meaning of the changes he had seen as a result of the hemorrhage, and whether she would hemorrhage again and die. Drawing on his more ordinary frame of minor abrasions and childhood flu, Max went on to say he was not sure if the bandage had helped, and he did not know whether this meant his mother was still brain-damaged.

So too, Lisa said her mother had needed to go to hospital " 'cause she wasn't well, 'cause she had lettuce in a lump in her tummy." Her mother had cancer of the throat. Her parents were puzzled about how she had reached this view until they recalled that she had seen her mother choke on lettuce when visiting her in hospital. In the midst of this discussion, she drew a face saying, "ET goes home," signifying her wish that going home would help her mother recover as well.

A similar process has been evident in the way in which parents explain their condition to their children. A mother with cancer put her son's hands on the "little lumps" in her neck. In the context of ongoing uncertainty, referring to what could be felt offered a concrete frame for talking to her son and helping him integrate his experience. This is particularly important when much of what is affecting the parent is invisible and therefore difficult to comprehend. For other children, drawing has been very valuable: a child who was thought too young to know about his mother's breast cancer drew a picture of a woman with a black hole in her chest as she spoke.

Body Talk

Focusing on the concrete to the exclusion of an accompanying psychological explanation can increase uncertainty and leave children unsure of their own relationship to illness. A core part of early development involves the child learning that she or he is a separate person from her or his parent. However, children's play and comments in therapy suggest that separation may prove more complex when the parent from whom one is separating is seriously ill.

Even when children have not been told parents are ill they sense the concern, often indicating this through a preoccupation with their own health. In our research, several children developed sore tummies, flu, and colds. Talking about their sore throats and flu provided a context for exploring the physical connection to their parents, comparing their condition with that of their parents, and fantasies of both cause and cure: if the doctor could cure their throat virus, surely cancer of the throat is curable too.

In a family where the father had an early stage of AIDS, his son developed complex symptoms for which no cause could be found. His father was not yet ready to disclose his condition to his son. However, recognizing his son's anxiety about his own body was a first step toward enabling him to acknowledge the boy's concerns about changes he had witnessed in his father. Some children are afraid of being left alone with seriously ill parents, and it can be difficult to separate anxiety about being attacked or contaminated by the illness from an anxiety about how they would respond should a medical emergency occur.

Again and again, children's comments and play reflect questions of personal responsibility, of their having contributed to causing or exacerbating illness. Needless to say, anxiety about personal responsibility is not unique to children: discourses of blame powerfully shape the illness experiences of adults, too (Kleinman, 1988; Sontag, 1991).

Max, whose mother had a cerebral brain hemorrhage, said, "I don't like giving Mummy a bad headache." It was important to him that his mother went for a walk when he couldn't stop his friends making noise. "Help, help," was the call of another child as he rolled his toy fire engine and crawled under a chair to sleep while his mother talked about her worries.

Though this chapter focuses primarily on making sense of the illness, this process cannot be separated from relationships that predated the illness as well. Thirteen-year-old Nita confronted her mother in therapy saying, "You blamed me for your disease, Mum, you've said it a thousand times," referring to their stormy battles. She had decided that her life would not change after her mother's diagnosis but found herself unable to concentrate at school. Everything she studied seemed to link with illness. Even at school she felt blamed for her mother's illness. Her headmistress called her in to tell her she needed to behave better for her mother's sake. She responded, "She's really annoying me by telling me what to do when she's not part of it at all."

Knowing at Two Levels

We have often been struck by differences in how the physical and psychological aspects of the illness are discussed. Thomas, aged 11, described his mother's condition as "a tumor with cancer cells (looking to his physically well parent) that blocks up or takes over, you know the flesh and stuff inside you." However, this eloquent account did not prevent him from having frightening dreams about both his parents dying and about a monster taking over inside him.

It seems as if there are two levels of knowledge about illness. One is based on definite information, on what can be seen, measured, and can be discussed openly. The other, which is less frequently shared, is the knowledge that relates to uncertainty and fear. Here as elsewhere, there seemed to be an intricate balance between the experience of Thomas and that of his mother. At first he did not remember the dream she mentioned. It was as if in her parenting role his mother could acknowledge fear as it related to her son but not in relation to herself. She tried minimizing her health worries in an attempt to protect him; the effect was to leave him isolated, holding on to the fear on behalf of all the family.

In a society where childhood is portrayed as a protected space, parents and professionals tend to be reticent about risking discussion that challenges that protection. However, the fear and anxiety do not go away but remain, albeit in an "unlanguaged" manner. Even at age 11, Thomas's fear returned in the form of an internalized monster.

Therapy is often about listening carefully to what children have seen at a concrete level to make their concerns more visible psychologically. This helps unhook children from holding on to anxiety for all.

Linking Parents' and Children's Experience

Parents who are diagnosed with a serious illness are rarely helped to think about what this means for parenting (Stein & Kroll, 1998; Burke, Barnes, Kroll, & Stein, 2000). This compounds the challenge they face in responding in this relatively uncharted territory. What children understand and the gaps they experience cannot be separated from what they have not only been told but shown.

As mentioned, discourses about illness move between the physical and psychological. In many situations, there is sufficient interplay to enable families to make sense of their shared and individual experiences. However, at others the contradictions are considerable, creating complex challenges for both parents and children alike. For example, children may be confronted with contradictory messages about prognosis. Though Adam's father talked about his illness as temporary, his mother prepared him for his father's death by reading him a story about death, *Badger's Parting Gift* (Varley, 1984). In view of the information they had been given, no single view was more correct than the other. However, this difference blocked Adam and his sister from establishing their own story, while remaining connected with what each parent could offer. Some children find themselves caught in the crossfire of rifts that predated or were exacerbated by illness. Where one parent is unwilling to support his or her ill partner, children may be torn about their role: supporting a sick parent might enable the other to disengage, but stepping into his or her shoes highlights their parent's unavailability, compounding the difficulties parents face. One young boy's way out of what had become untenable for him was to begin to cut himself.

CONVERSATIONS WITH COUPLES

A number of patterns of relationships have emerged in working with couples in which one partner has a serious or life-risking illness. While it would be mistaken to use these in a prescriptive way, noting these patterns has enabled us to explore the different belief systems influencing how the illness is understood and where the boundaries of responsibility lie within the couple relationship. The couples described here were referred initially because they had expressed concern about their children. In some instances, their concern focused on their children in relation to their illness, and in others, although illness was mentioned, they did not make a connection between the referral problem and the illness.

Our experience has been that it is important to be cautious and avoid moving too quickly in the direction of couple work before proper attention has been given to the basis of the referral. This does not only relate to the general issue of engagement and the importance of attending to the problem as defined. It makes a particular connection to the way in which these couples facing life-threatening illness conceptualize their problems in terms of their parenting. Many of the couples we saw were more connected about parenting than their couple relationship. This has been true for same-sex and heterosexual couples.

Patterns of Recognition

Some couples came to recognize the need to resolve issues in their couple relationship through exploring their hopes for their children in the future. This could arise because it became apparent that the non-ill partner was in some way held back from fulfilling his or her parenting role by entanglements in the couple relationship, which without resolution were likely to continue even in the event of the partner's death. In other couples, they became aware that the difficulties in their relationship were preventing them from changing the patterns of their parenting to adjust to the new circumstances of one of them being very seriously ill.

For example, in one couple the father Derek's relationship with his children had, in many respects, been restricted to some connection with their school work, occasional days out, and family holidays. In the light of his wife Wendy's terminal illness, his need to have a different parenting role was both very apparent and extremely difficult for the couple to achieve. In this family, Wendy was the central parent, although she also worked outside the family home. She managed her terminal breast cancer on the outside of family life. She told the family very little of what was happening to her, depending on friends for support, including frequently asking them to attend appointments with her. From Wendy's perspective, this enabled her to protect her children both from her illness and from what she saw as the inadequate parenting skills of their father. These parents appeared to have managed their own need to keep their relationship at a particular distance by a constant series of very acrimonious rows. As Wendy's illness progressed, the impossibility of keeping everything outside the family became more and more apparent. Her need for care from her family was in conflict with the definition of herself as the caregiver: their rows denied them the space to parent together.

Distance Regulation

For Derek and Wendy, what emerged was the importance of the rows. Rather than keeping distance, they enabled them to sustain a level of intimacy that was nonphysical and thus remain connected in their couple relationship. The fights were "distance regulators" (Byng-Hall, 1980). However, their conflicts were extremely detrimental to their children. These parents found it very hard to think about themselves and their relationship. It was only in reflecting on the needs of their children that they could explore their own sense of connection and disconnection.

Their relationship appeared to be based on stoicism about their feelings and experience. They sustained an adversarial culture of blame, which in turn led to evidence stored up for future rows. Wendy wept as she spoke about losing her hair, eyelashes, and brows, "It was the most awful thing, absolutely awful, I can't even think about it. I have a friend who came with me to have my hair cut off." A short time later she went on, "Anyway it is all finished now, so that is fine." It then emerged that they had fought over her not wearing her wig. Wendy says, "I got stupidly upset." The weather was very hot and the wig very uncomfortable. When it was suggested that being distressed about her hair was reasonable, she said, "Well I did, but it was only a temporary thing. No, it really does not matter. I am far more worried about Anna (her daughter)." When asked how she thought her loss of hair had affected her husband, Wendy said, "I don't know because he really does not notice things."

On being asked to take a guess about his experience she said, "Well he hasn't got very much hair, men are not bothered about those things." Derek eventually responded, "I was very upset when Wendy lost her hair, I really was." Wendy responded, "You did not mention it then. You seem to think by not mentioning things they will go away." Derek went on to explain there were practical discussions, and then with prompting he was able to say, "It was frightening when she had no hair. I mean people do look very different." Having come close to an open expression of his feelings, Derek withdrew again. When asked if the loss of hair made the illness very present he said, "Well, not particularly," at which point Wendy came in, "Yes, but for me it was a reminder every time I looked in the mirror. You can forget about it for hours on end, days even." The acrimonious pattern between them remained embedded in the process unless we anchored our ideas in their parenting roles. It was in speaking to them about the conflict of interest between their stoicism, which can be supportive in times of crisis, and their adversarial process, which forced them to keep their inner fears secret to prevent them being used in future rows, that we were able to identify the impact this process was having on their children. The more the parents suppressed their fears but made their anger toward each other visible, the more their children were restricted in their understanding and discussion of their mother's illness. They were also denied a sense of agency that can come through being able to demonstrate their undoubted care and concern because they were confused about when Wendy was ill, when angry, and on whom her anger was focused.

Thinking Tension

We found that making the distance regulation pattern visible to the couple (Erickson, 1993) was a very important part of the process. Anchoring the therapeutic discourse in the way the couple relationship interacted with the illness, and how this impacted their children, enabled this couple to make connections with their parenting responsibilities. Through this we were able to create a thinking tension in the sessions, interrupting their attacks on each other. For a significant time their rows had held them in such grip that they were unable to connect to the needs of their children or to themselves as parents. Eventually, they were able to challenge some of their own problems and recognize the contradiction between their couple relationship and their aspirations to protect and parent their children differently. It is likely that it was only in the context of the severity of the illness and their children's distress that these parents would have undertaken couple work.

Dazzle Factors

Serious illness can so embrace an individual, a family, or a couple as to make them almost invisible in other ways. As professionals working with these families, it is of the greatest importance to be able to reflect on whether we too are so dazzled by the illness we are unable to explore alternative explanations for the problems in the family. The dazzle potential of illness can affect other family members too. For example, partners who put the needs of their sick partner above their own can be perceived in a very different light. They can appear to take on a new persona, which can in turn mask relationship problems that continue to cut across their ability to respond to the new dilemmas they face.

A couple where the mother was dying of colon cancer became the center of their community. The well partner and friends continually did acts of service for the sick woman. From the woman's perspective, she felt burdened by being grateful and at the same time did not feel listened to about her wish not to be overprotected. She felt her wish to be allowed to join in an ordinary way—to have arguments, to be cross and unhappy—was never really listened to. She wanted to be herself and not to be seen as her illness. She wanted above all to maximize her space to be "real" with her children and partner.

The work with this couple was very painful when the well partner came to realize the extent of the assumptions everyone had made about his wife's needs. Tracking back in their relationship, it seemed over the period of their marriage that they had grown accustomed to his making assumptions about her needs. From his perspective, when she became ill he applied the same rules. From her perspective, her illness meant she experienced a sense of urgency for her voice to be heard, and this gave her a sense of empowerment to voice views, which in the past she would have only spoken indirectly.

A Louder Voice

When we started this project in 1991, we had an idea that if women were armed with the kind of scientific knowledge the understanding of illness potentially brings, they might change their position in the couple relationship. Our experience has been that such changes are more likely in circumstances where it is the woman who is ill. The most distinctive change is when the woman voices needs on her own behalf, when in the past she has generally spoken on behalf of others. In some circumstances, the woman's new voice is welcomed. As in the case just described, once the couple endured the pain of recognizing they had so frequently misunderstood each other and mourned the lost times, what emerged was a different quality of relationship. It made for quantifiably different levels of discussion and an ability to reconcile issues with each other on a much more mutual basis before her death. (Jordan et al., 1991).

For other couples, the woman's "louder" voice has been much less welcomed. Alan, whose partner, Eunice, had a heart-lung transplant said, "Things are going the opposite to what we thought; we argue more now than we did before she was ill. The trouble I've got, she is now a different person from before, both physically and mentally. You know the weller she becomes, the more strong willed she becomes and it's difficult." For Eunice, as for others, the near-death experience had given her a different level of urgency to express her views. For some women, their "speaking out" would still be focused on their wishes for their children. Other women spoke more clearly or were listened to in a different way about their own needs. In the example given above, this brought relationship issues to the surface that were problematic for both members of the couple. Eunice said, "I want to speak about it (her needs). For years I have kept silent."

INTENTION AND EXPERIENCE

Our work has been greatly influenced by the research on women's growth and development (Gilligan, Lyons, & Hanmer, 1990;

Jordan et al., 1997). Using the theory of the subjugated discourse of women's relational needs brought us to examine other subjugated discourses: in particular, the different ways men and women express emotions. As two women working on the project, we were very aware that male discourses could be underrepresented in our thinking. We were also aware that therapy privileges relational language. This can have the tendency to make it more sympathetic to the position of women, who more frequently discuss relationships. We attempted to actively position ourselves to listen differently to male ways of discussing emotions, particularly understanding the role of action as a language. We tried to incorporate into the process of the session the importance of not being reliant on speaking about distress in verbal language (Frosh, Phoenix, & Patterson, 2002; Erickson, 1993). In exploring these issues, we have tried wherever possible to open up the difference between intention and experience. Our hope in doing this is couples will begin to make much more use of their different languages: exploring the differences between their own intention through action or words and their partner's experience, thus moving away from insisting their partner resolve issues in the way they do themselves.

After her heart-lung transplant, as she progressively got stronger, Eunice and Alan found themselves increasingly at variance with one another. They both expressed dismay. Their expectation had been that their life would open up as Eunice got more well. A side effect of the medication was a rapid increase in weight; within six months Eunice had been transformed from an exceptionally slim woman to a much more substantial person. None of her clothes fit and she found herself in a strange new body: someone else's heart and lungs, her body constantly changing shape as she put on weight. They also had to contend with what a heart symbolizes in terms of their emotional beliefs, for example, "I give my heart to you." Alan's response

was to tell her to go to the gym and lose weight. He became impatient when she did not respond to his recommendations. He admitted that he liked her less at this size, that in the past he'd liked to be seen with Eunice and now felt this much less. Alan did not respond to discussions as Eunice wished; whenever things got very difficult he would return to his garage and repair a car.

The work focused on the difference between their intention and their partner's experience. Alan was disinclined to talk when he felt distressed; he described himself as carrying on as normal, "I would just go to work as normal, I won't mope about, I go and repair a car—I think it was Winston Churchill if he had a problem he'd go and build a wall." So for him the action, rather than talking of remaining "normal," helped him to feel he could contain his feelings, giving him a sense of things being under control, which was very important to him. Eunice explained she frequently didn't know there was anything wrong for Alan. When asked if they had very different ways of coping with sadness, Eunice said, "Yes, I want to talk about what gets me down," but Alan would shy away from this. To the suggestion that her stored-up wish to talk may ultimately mean her fears come out in a rush which takes Alan by surprise and creates in him a sense of panic she responds, "Yet he tucks himself away in a corner and won't talk to me." Eunice wished to talk to Alan about her distress and have him really understand her fears about having someone else's heart. There was an idea that she was a new person. She feared, as did Alan, that the new heart had come with someone else's affections. They both thought Eunice's upset feelings towards Alan were in some way explained by this; her "old" feelings had been lost when her heart was replaced. Alan's intention in trying to get her to slim had been that if she felt more attractive, she would not just feel but would "be" more like herself and both his and her "real" feelings would return.

"Normal" Behavior

Prior to Eunice's transplant, Alan described his own experience of his mother's breast cancer. When she was discharged from the hospital, both he and his father, with whom he worked, had said they would expect dinner on the table at the same time as usual. When we unpicked their intention in saying this, it emerged that they had thought it would be reassuring for her. They felt if she could retain her usual routine she would feel reassured and feel she too was more "normal." Their intention had been to be helpful rather than adding to the burden she was already experiencing.

Inadvertently, health professionals can create a similar confusion between intention and experience. People undergoing chemotherapy, surgery, or radiotherapy are commonly encouraged to think they can carry on their "normal" activities, including retaining full time work with minor adjustments. The intention seems to be that staying within the normal pattern of their lives will be most supportive in healing. They then will feel more like their usual selves in spite of their illness. For some, this may be extremely supportive. However for others, it has the opposite effect. The recommendation can result in their feeling guilty or even a failure because they have found the regime too exhausting and had to do far less or behave differently from "normal."

Intimacy

For many couples, the intensity, proximity, and intimacy of being cared for or being the caregiver has brought new meaning to their relationship, particularly when the couple has previously had a more distant connection. The intensity of the experience at the acute stage of the illness brought a non-languaged and more mutual physical and emotional closeness. Some had previously been unable to express or experience these feelings; in some instances this had been the case for very many years and in others, this had never been possible. This is not in any way to romanticize the dreadful physical and emotional demands of what was happening to them.

This special experience has seemed rather less likely to occur when it was the woman who was ill. For some of the women, the experience was very different. They became intensely distressed at what they perceived as a lack of concern or even neglect. This lack of a sense of being cared for may reflect the powerful way in which illness challenges gendered assumptions and seemed to occur both when the women who were ill were in heterosexual and same-sex relationships. Frequently they were distressed because they had to ask their partner for help. They explained that in their partner's shoes they would have anticipated [intuitively] the need for help, thus not waiting to be asked. Despite some changes in expectations of women's role, women's sense of self still tends to be constructed around caring for others. As such, an ill woman having to balance caring for herself with caring for others challenges the expectations for both women and men about what they can ask, offer, or have the right to receive (Altschuler & Dale, 1999; Weingarten, 1994).

Even in cases where the partner was dying, experiencing intimacy made a great deal of difference to some couples. Although very poignant—"So many wasted years," as one dying man said—it also had the potential to transform the narrative of the surviving partner. This couple's new experience of mutual respect and intimacy gave renewed strength to a wife who had profoundly doubted her ability to parent alone.

However, for other couples this change in their intimacy faded as the ill partner became healthier. Just at the stage when family and friends might expect them to be relieved and happy, they find themselves disconcertingly unhappy and rather lost. Taking time to unpick this process and detect with the couple just how their experience of each other changed and what it meant to each of them has been an important part of the work. An example is a couple where the father, Saul, was cared for at home over a prolonged period. His occupation had been very absorbing, requiring him to take high levels of responsibility, and had left him rather detached from family life. Rachel, his wife, largely ran the home and had confidence in herself as a mother. Neither of them had much confidence in themselves as partners. They had related to each other much more as parents. Saul's illness resulted in him spending long periods at home. Although that could challenge Rachel's position with Saul being more involved with his children, it also let him develop the kind of parenting she had always desired. This change in his relationship to the children, and her acceptance of it, enabled them both to be aware of each other's vulnerability and their need to be intimately cared for and respected by each other. During these acute stages, their relationship became softer and more intimate than they had experienced at any other time. Each time as Saul became stronger this closeness receded, and it was as though in greater health they were denied the understanding of their inner distress and longing for love and acceptance. This loss became expressed in anger and anguish, a situation that remained little changed until his death. For this couple, the growth in their relationship was too small to be sustained when the other pressures of their lives returned. These situations are very distressing because they had been aware of the possibility but it had not lasted. This can make their disappointment in each other and sometimes the therapy process almost unbearable.

CONCLUSION

This chapter has highlighted the importance of listening for the gaps in what is said when helping families reflect on the meaning an illness has on their everyday lives. Our experience has been that work of the kind we have described has been comparatively rarely undertaken. Although there is considerable awareness of the importance of being with children when they are sick, adult hospital wards seldom have family-friendly space. Taking children to visit their parent in the hospital can be of enormous importance to the child and the parent, and yet it is an area that is rarely accommodated in the United Kingdom. The result is that visiting with children is effectively discouraged. Seeing children distressed is thought to be unhelpful and stressful for other patients. As the facilities for visiting are so inadequate, the potential experience for children and adults alike can be very fraught. Very few of the adults we have seen have ever been asked if they were a parent. At one level, such organizational decisions might have had a supposedly practical basis. However, it may well reflect a wider difficulty for health professionals and society in recognizing that the parents of even very young children can become ill and die, and like adults, children are likely to be powerfully affected by this. Instead, decisions appear to be based on a narrow concept of caring needs, even in relation to the psychological well being in adult health.

Our work has highlighted the complex interplay among the different roles between partners, parents, and children. Creating opportunities to move between both relationships, including the experience of the children, is of the greatest importance in providing effective family care that respects all the aspects of being a sick parent.

REFERENCES

Altschuler, J., & Dale, B. (1999) On being an ill parent. *Journal of Clinical Child Psychology and Psychiatry, 4,* 23–37.

Altschuler, J., Dale, B., & Sass-Booth, A. (1999). Supporting children when a parent is physically ill: Implications for schools. *Educational Psychology in Practice, 15*(1), 25–32.

Bateson, G. (1972). *Steps to an ecology of mind: Mind and nature.* New York: Ballantine.

Burke, O., Barnes, J., Kroll, L., & Stein, A. (2000). Qualitative interview study of communication between parents and children about maternal breast cancer. *British Medical Journal, 321,* 479–482.

Byng-Hall, J. (1980). The symptom bearer as marital distance regulator: Clinical implications. *Family Process, 19,* 355–365.

Dale, B., & Altschuler, J. (1997). Different gender-different language: Narratives of inclusion and exclusion. In R. K. Papadopoulos & J. Byng-Hall (Eds.), *Multiple voices* (pp. 125–145). London: Duckworth.

Dwedi, K. (1999). Special edition: Sowing the seeds of cultural competence. *Context, 44,* 1–52.

Erickson, B. M. (1993). *Helping men change: The role of the female therapist.* Newbury Park, CA: Sage.

Frosh, S., Phoenix, A., & Patterson, R. (2002). *Young masculinities.* Basingstoke, UK: Palgrave.

Garmezy, N., & Masten, A. S. (1994). Chronic adversities. In M. Rutter, E. Taylor, & L. Hersov (Eds.), *Child and adolescent psychiatry* (pp. 191–208). Oxford: Blackwell.

Gilligan, C., Lyons, N. P., & Hanmer, T. J. (1990). *Making connections. The relational worlds of adolescent girls at Emma Willard School.* Cambridge, MA: Harvard University Press.

Goldner, V. (1991). Sex, power and gender: A feminist analysis of the politics of passion. *Journal of Feminist Family Therapy, 3,* 17–31.

Greer, S., & Silberfarb, P. M. (1982). Psychological concomitants of cancer: Current state of research. *Psychological Medicine, 12,* 563–573.

Jordan, J., Bergman, S. J., Coll, C. G., Eldridge, N., Menches, J., Baker, G., et al. (1997). *Women's growth in diversity: More writings from the Stone Center.* New York: Guilford.

Jordan, J. V., Kaplan, A., Baker, G., Miller, J., Stiver, I., & Surrey, J. L. (1991). *Women's growth in connection: Writings from the Stone Center.* New York: Guilford.

Judd, D. (1989). *Give sorrow words.* London: Free Association Press.

Kleinman, A. (1988). The illness narratives: Suffering, healing and the human condition. London: Basic Books.

Krause, I. (1998). *Therapy across culture.* London: Sage.

Panksepp, J. (1998). *Affective neuroscience.* London: Oxford University Press.

Rutter, M. (1999). Resilience concepts and findings: Implications for family therapy. *Journal of Family Therapy, 21,* 119–144.

Sontag, S. (1991). *Illness as metaphor and AIDS and its metaphors.* Harmondsworth, UK: Penguin.

Stein, A., & Kroll, L. (1998). Cancer in parents: Telling children sensitive communication can reduce psychological problems. *British Medical Journal, 316,* 880.

Varley, S. (1984). *Badger's parting gift.* London: Harper Collins.

Weingarten, K. (1994). *The mother's voice: Strengthening intimacy in families.* London: Harcourt Brace.

CHAPTER 26

Maximizing Patients' Health Through Engagement With Families

WILLIAM J. SIEBER, TODD M. EDWARDS,
GENE A. KALLENBERG, AND JO ELLEN PATTERSON

Growing evidence has shown the myriad ways that social relationships influence health. For most patients, the most influential relationships are those with family members. Yet most research on how to best treat or manage a patient's health has focused interventions on the individual and targeted a singular disease condition. This chapter will review research demonstrating the impact of social relationships on health, then focus on ways to assess and best use these relationships to maximize a patient's well-being. Concluding comments will outline the need for working models to engage a patient's family in support of health care services and then propose future directions that should be explored in a clinical research context. The focus will be on assisting medical and mental health providers who work in busy primary care settings to assess and engage families for maximal patient health.

SOCIAL RELATIONSHIPS AND HEALTH

Impact of Social Factors on Health

Research and clinical evidence indicates that the application of social interventions has helped stem the spread of disease for more than 100 years, with public health policies having the greatest impact on the health of the world's population. That is, more than 100 years ago the germ theory promoted our understanding of the social transmission of disease; individuals exposed to others with disease or social conditions associated with poverty were more likely to fall ill. More recent research has examined the specific mechanisms of the effect of social relationships on health, but the perspective most often looks at how it relates to individual health. However, there are many important problems that can be identified as *family* health issues. Examples include children with physical or developmental disabilities, bereavement, and healthy behaviors such as diet and exercise changes. Other topics include teenage pregnancy, infertility, hypertension, cardiac rehabilitation, cancer, chronic illness, depression, and family violence (Smilkstein, 1994).

Campbell (2003) provided an excellent review of the mechanisms by which one's social relationships, especially within the family, may influence health. Studies have shown that conflict in relationships influences psycho-physiological processes that result in disease. Ewart, Taylor, Kraemer, and Agras

(1991) as well as Gottman (1994) have shown that criticism between family members increases blood pressure. Kiecolt-Glaser and Newton (2001) and Kiecolt-Glaser and colleagues (1987) reported that several markers of decreased immunity are associated with marital dissatisfaction or loss of a spouse (the classic studies related to incidence of tuberculosis after loss of spouse). Another mechanism linking families to a patient's health is members' influence on adherence to medically prescribed regimens by way of general support, compliance, collaboration in therapeutic plans, and interactions with caregivers (Coppetelli & Orleans, 1985; Doherty & Campbell, 1988; Trevino, Young, Groff, & Jono, 1990; Venters, Jacobs, Luepker, Maiman, & Gillum, 1984).

Work by Larry Fisher (Fisher et al., 1998; Fisher, Term, & Ransom, 1990) has advanced our understanding of how to efficiently assess families in health care settings. Fisher and associates (1998, 2000) proposed four reasons why a patient's family should be considered critical to improving a patient's health. First, most disease management takes place in the home. Second, the family is the source of a person's most influential intimate relationships. Third, family members often simultaneously undertake new or changed health behaviors (e.g., diet, exercise, health monitoring) along with the designated patient, or such family members have partial responsibility for the patient's target behavior (for example, shopping and preparing meals are instrumental in long-term dietary changes). Fourth, the family influences a patient's behavior through cultural practices and health belief systems. For example, Fisher and colleagues (2000) demonstrated that while family coherence is associated with glycemic control in diabetic patients, family coherence was not as important in the health outcomes of Hispanic patients.

Lisa Berkman has been a leader in documenting the negative impact that a lack of social support has on a variety of health outcomes (1995, 2000; Berkman, Leo-Summers, & Horowitz, 1992). Sheldon Cohen's work has demonstrated that the increased clinical symptoms of influenza that result from a withdrawal of social support are a direct outcome of compromised immune defenses (for review, see Cohen & Underwood, 2000). Teresa Seeman and her colleagues (Seeman, 2000; Seeman, Lusignolo, Albert, & Berkman, 2001; Seeman & McEwan, 1996; Seeman, Singer, Ryff, Dienberg-Love, & Levy-Storms, 2002) as well as others (Kiecolt-Glaser & Newton, 2001) have demonstrated that emotional support, as compared to instrumental support, is predictive of allostatic load, a measure of overall propensity to develop disease and illness as we age.

The quality of one's marital relationship, a specific measure of social support, has received significant attention in the past decade. While married adults have frequently been shown to have lower mortality and morbidity at various time points than single adults (Burman & Margolin, 1992; Kiecolt-Glaser & Newton, 2001), benefits of being married may be greater for men, while positive marital quality appears most predictive of health for women (Berkman et al., 1992; Coyne et al., 2001; Martikainen & Valkonen, 1996; Orth-Gomer et al., 2000). Overall, the relationship between negative or hostile family relationships and illness is stronger than the relationship between positive family relationships and good health. For example, low scores on measures of satisfaction with one's family members are associated with poor outcomes for smoking cessation (Mermelstein, Lichtenstein, & McIntyre, 1983) as well as poorer diabetic control (Klausner, Koenigsberg, Skolnick, & Chung, 1995). In a study examining spousal support, Weihs (2002) found that breast cancer patients who were not satisfied in their marital relationships were four times more likely to have a recurrence of breast cancer than those who were satisfied.

ENGAGING FAMILIES IN HEALTH PROMOTION

In today's primary care offices chronic illness has become commonplace. In such circumstances much of the burden of care is transferred to the patient's home environment. Several social and economic forces have led to decreased availability of health care personnel and services, thus resulting in increased need for patients and their families to provide supplementary health care services as well as to encourage patients more often to engage in self-management behaviors (Ho, Marger, Beart, Yip, & Shekelle, 1997; Piette & Mah, 1997).

The goals of family-focused interventions for chronic disease include helping families manage the stresses as a team, mobilizing natural support systems (i.e., extended family, church community), coping with losses, reorganizing the family to ensure optimal patient care, and often coordinating and performing actual physical care. How these goals are achieved can vary from family to family. It is possible for a family to be too empathetic or too involved in the patient's coping. In addition, moving too quickly to solve problems, criticizing the member's choices, or catastrophizing may also be detrimental. However, moderated empathy at the appropriate time, humor, self-disclosure, and supportive behaviors can help family members cope with serious illnesses (Berg & Upchurch, 2003). The initial steps of such family-focused interventions would include some assessment strategy such as that described by Larry Fisher (Fisher et al., 1998; Fisher et al., 1990).

Another area being studied involves situations where family members are directly involved in health interventions. Some studies have targeted the caregivers of patients whereas others have focused on inclusion of other family members in the treatment of the primary patient. Most studies have reported that benefits to caregiver or patient tend to arise in those situations where the individual's

disease is moderately or significantly advanced. Patients with milder forms of disease tend not to be included to the same degree in most studies, or minimal effects are reported in these less disabled or non-terminal patient populations.

Caregivers

Parents of Sick Children. Chronic family conflict and low cohesion have been associated with poor diabetic control (Anderson & Kornblum, 1984; Minuchin et al., 1975). Bernard-Bonnin, Stachenko, Bonin, Charette, and Rousseau (1995) reviewed 11 studies related to family functioning and childhood asthma. While effect sizes were small, such studies found interventions to be most effective for children with most severe asthma. Panton and Barley (2002), after their review of studies examining the impact of family therapy as an adjunct to medication for children with asthma, concluded that significant benefits are seen episodically at best. A review by Mendenhall (2002) concluded that while family education and support improve patient outcomes in cystic fibrosis and cancer, many such interventions were time-intensive and may not be easily implemented in busy primary care settings.

Caregivers of Patients With Chronic Illness. Interventions that are more intense and effortful than support groups have shown some benefit to caregivers. Skills training, such as that reported by Mittleman, Ferris, Shulman, Steinberg, and Levin (1996) in the treatment of Alzheimer's disease, showed that six individual and family sessions in addition to a support group intervention over a four-month period was most helpful in prolonging the time caregivers were able to care for patients in the early and middle stages of the disease. Caregivers were also less depressed and physically healthier, which led to the conclusion that better health care might be delivered to the patient (Toseland et al.,

2001). Sorenson, Pinquart, and Duberstein (2002) conducted a meta-analysis concluding that the effects of interventions were least encouraging when interventions were directed toward the caregiver. Documentation of an impact on patients, as is often reported in the literature of family interventions in childhood disease, is absent when looking at elderly patients with deteriorating disease.

Spouse Involvement

Another way families are addressed as supportive change agents is by having patients' spouses engage in treatment activities with the patient. One example of enhancing the impact of a dietary change program by including spouses in treatment was reported by Wing, Marcus, Epstein, and Jawad (1991). Half the patients were treated as a group in a 20-week behavioral weight control program without their spouses attending, while spouses in the other half were treated together in an identical group intervention with their spouse as part of the group (all patients and spouses in the study were obese). While the amount of weight loss was similar in both groups immediately after the program, an interesting interaction effect was seen at one-year follow-up. Women did better when treated with spouses whereas men did better when going through the program without their spouses. This highlights the need to identify patient and family characteristics that may predict greatest benefit. Law and Crane (2000) recently summarized the cost-offset associated with these types of interventions.

ENGAGING FAMILIES AS PARTNERS IN CARE

Points of Contact

Doherty and Baird (1986), and more recently McDaniel, Hepworth, and Doherty (1992), identified five levels at which the physician may think about and interact with families. The first level is where there is minimal emphasis on the family. Level two involves communicating medical information to the patient's family members. Level three is characterized by meeting with family members, responding to their emotional needs, and facilitating referrals to mental health professionals when appropriate. Level four involves brief and limited assessment and intervention with a patient and family, encouraging problem-solving and developing specific skills that may enhance the patient's well-being. The fifth and final level involves conducting what is more often understood as family therapy, discussing issues tangentially related to the patient's medical condition and treatment. This early work has helped to clarify that in a busy primary care setting, engagement at intermediate levels may be a realistic way in which the patient's social network can be harnessed for maximum health benefit.

There are different reasons why contact between patient and physician may occur. A health maintenance visit has the purpose of assessing risk, screening, and promoting health or changing behavior. Ideally, it would include a family history, social and sexual history, and a survey of health behaviors. A visit for a serious, acute medical condition would focus on obtaining key information and assisting with immediate coping and care. For either type of visit, family members can provide additional valuable history and information.

When helping a patient to change in some way, every health care professional should keep in mind that the process of change should be consistent with how a person can maintain such behavior in a larger social context, such as within the family. That is, external reinforcement from a health professional for maintaining dietary changes is not likely to be maintained in a home environment where such reinforcements may not be viable. Thus, suggested behaviors and sources of motivation should consider whether family members may be able to reinforce such motivation and, specifically, which family members might be both available and willing to take on such assignments.

Trying to manage chronic medical conditions, as well as minimizing the emotional impact of such conditions, can be frustrating for the primary care provider. However, once aware of the power of the family in the patient's life, the care provider can begin to leverage the supportive and curative potential of the family.

MODELS OF FAMILY ASSESSMENT

Rolland (1984, 1994) has identified the following disease variables in his typology describing the family's potential responses to the course of chronic disease: onset, course, outcome, and degree of incapacitation. Onset of illness refers to whether it is acute, like stroke, or gradual, like Alzheimer's disease. A family will likely respond to an acute illness differently than to a gradual onset illness. For example, an acute illness will quickly mobilize the family and force them to create and implement crisis management skills. This rapid change will be handled better by some families. The course of a chronic disease can be progressive (Type 1 diabetes), constant (spinal cord injury), or relapsing-episodic (asthma). Relapsing illnesses create tremendous unpredictability in families. Further, they demand flexibility in the family structure due to the transitions between crisis and noncrisis periods and ongoing worry about when the next crisis will take place. The illness outcome refers to a continuum of whether it will shorten one's life span or likely cause the death of a patient. Some illnesses are non-fatal, such as arthritis, whereas others are fatal, such as Huntington's disease. Another intermediate category refers both to illnesses that shorten

the life span and those with the possibility of sudden death. Families coping with life-threatening illnesses experience anticipatory grief and the intense emotions of pulling the ill member closer for more intimacy and preparing themselves for the painful process of letting go of the ill member. Incapacitation refers to the degree of a patient's disability: incapacitating (Alzheimer's disease) or non-incapacitating (early lung cancer).

Developmental Perspectives

Family Transitions. According to Rolland (1994), when one considers the interface among the type of illness, the time phase of the illness, and the family's developmental state, one can begin to appreciate the unique and complex effects of illness on a family. Using Combrinck-Graham's (1985) Family Life Spiral as a backdrop, Rolland states that families naturally oscillate through times of greater closeness (centripetal periods), such as the birth of a new baby, and times of greater distance (centrifugal periods), such as a child leaving home following adolescence. Centripetal periods are characterized by greater family cohesion and greater focus on internal family life. Centrifugal periods display a loosening of family boundaries, allowing individual family members to pursue goals and interactions with the extra-familial environment.

Similar to the addition of a new family member, the onset of illness generally has a centripetal pull on families. An illness that emerges during a centripetal period may prolong this period or result in a family getting stuck in this phase of development. When an illness strikes during a centrifugal period, it can interrupt a family's natural developmental progression and force family members to redirect their attention back to the family. A common example is an adolescent remaining at home beyond the time she originally expected to leave in order to help care for an ill parent.

A situation of crisis can also put a patient in a very vulnerable position, but the stress experienced during this time can raise the patient's level of awareness, leaving him or her more open to change. On the other hand, there is often a tendency in crisis to revert to old response patterns that are most ingrained for a given individual or family. The difficulty in predicting which direction a family or family member will take in such a situation (i.e., greater awareness vs. old patterns), be it a chronic stressor or a chronic illness, points to the importance of assessment of the factors known to predict family coping as well as a history of this family during previous stressful developmental changes.

Sawa (1985) developed an elegant, brief, yet comprehensive model of assessment. He argued to go beyond the initial inquiry by the physician (i.e., "How are things going within the family?" "What concerns at home are coming up regularly?" "Tell me what enjoyable things the family does together?"). Sawa proposed the best snapshot of family functioning emerges by asking a series of five questions. These questions appear to be largely based on Smilkstein's earlier work on the family APGAR (Smilkstein, 1978, 1980; Smilkstein, Ashworth, & Montano, 1982). Sawa named five elements to assess family functioning: Adaptation, Partnership, Growth, Affection, and Resolve. Sawa (1985) also described a few principles that are the foundation of such an assessment. One is that the focus of any interaction with the family should be on the present, not on past events or relationships. A second principle is that responsibility for change is squarely placed on each family member and is not the responsibility of the health care provider. Another principle is that how the family interacts in the physician's office is a fairly accurate representation of how they interact outside the office, and that attending to the process of

communication and not just the content conveys a lot of information.

Sawa's work also contains several domains of family functioning that the practitioner may want to further assess, depending on resources and time available. These include (1) how connected the family members are to each other, their family of origin, and to the community; (2) where the family is in a developmental cycle (newlyweds, childrearing, divorce, retirement); (3) their "internal" functions, including their communications and ability to support each other emotionally and functionally (e.g., childrearing, finances, housework); and (4) the physical and mental health of each family member.

One of the chronic stressors on patients and families is the presence of a chronic illness. Whether it involves decreased functioning, progressive disability, instability of emotional well-being, or medical management that can be effortful and time-consuming, chronic illness challenges the resources of even the healthiest and most well-functioning families. It is the context of chronic disease management that presents perhaps the best opportunity for the primary care physician to engage the patient's family as an ally in the health care plan. However, whether these challenges require a change in health behaviors, interpersonal relationships, or in lifestyle in general, knowing how ready the family is to change is crucial to connecting with them in a health-promoting manner.

INTERVENTIONS IN PRIMARY CARE

Most often the change that occurs for a patient when interacting with a health professional is unplanned and unwanted. Unlike when a person engages in a planned and positive change, unplanned change (i.e., a recent diagnosis of a chronic disease) is beyond the control of the patient and thus experienced as negative. Such an experience is likely to lead to resistance to change for patient or family, and empathizing with this difficulty of change while pointing to potential benefits of change may be an effective strategy or response. Barriers to change may include institutional or instrumental barriers, though such overt obstacles (e.g., lack of financial resources, lack of behavioral skill) may be addressed directly and overcome to a certain extent. Social support targeted toward such changes or barriers to change can be a focus for patients who may be especially isolated, or in families where communication patterns exacerbate a patient's reluctance to change.

Intervention from the health provider can take many forms. Serving as a change agent is one of them. A change agent is someone in the patient's life who will aid in enabling the patient to progress toward his or her goal. For instance, the change agent will address disruptive behaviors, create an environment to facilitate change, or map out steps in the change process that are reasonable to the client. Proper planning for change, often not in the skill set of patient or family, is a very important intervention that can be provided by the physician or clinic staff.

While behavioral modification strategies may be useful for changing or shaping discrete behaviors, they are often limited by lack of attention to affective or cognitive domains. Realistic limitations on environmental control and extrinsic rewards for motivation make purely behavioral interventions somewhat limited in effectiveness, though with cognitively impaired populations such strategies may be effective.

Stages of Change and Motivational Interviewing. When it is not a matter of skill development or directly changing the environment, motivation for change may be the most appropriate short-term target for intervention. If this is the case, a coalescing of two models of behavior change may prove most helpful: Stages of Change emanating from

the trans-theoretical model (DiClemente and Prochaska, 1998; Prochaska & DiClemente, 1983; Prochaska, DiClemente, & Norcross, 1992), and Motivational Interviewing (Miller & Rollnick, 2002). From a family systems perspective, another consideration emerges. The health care provider must consider how to respond when different family members are at different stages of change. This can be especially problematic when the potential change involves high risks for the family. For example, a family may be considering chemotherapy, surgery, or alternative treatments for a parent's cancer. Each member may have a different perspective and be at a different point in the stages of change model. Family dynamics such as power and control, hierarchy, boundaries, hidden agendas, and trust may all influence the process. In this instance, focused effort by a mental health professional is warranted, as a physician is unlikely to have the time or the skills to adequately address such complexity, but he or she should have the clinical acumen and the established practice habit to recognize the complexity of the situation and the need to seek consultation or referral for specific needs.

Providers should not ignore racial, ethnic, and cultural differences should they exist. Such sensitivity has been shown to have an impact on patient satisfaction and a patient's willingness to report personal information. Alternatively, the patient's ethnicity has been shown to affect the physician's perception of the patient's problems, as was shown when minority women who complained of chest pain received a lower level of care. Certainly physicians should be taught to address any such discrepancies between themselves and their patient directly yet with sensitivity (Shi, Forrest, Von Schrader, & Ng, 2003).

Family Interventions. Physicians and medical therapists most often include families in the assessment and treatment process when it is a necessity, namely, when the patient cannot function alone. Another primary reason that families are included in treatment planning is that the individual patient is not the decision maker or he or she cannot perform the disease management behaviors (Weihs, Fisher, & Baird, 2002). Depending on the illness, at least part of the responsibility and burden of the illness is given to the family members.

Examples of these "required" family-based treatments include coping with illnesses of young children, adolescents, and the elderly. Other examples include adult illnesses that limit the patient's ability to provide self-care, such as loss of mental function, cancer, or serious heart disease. High-risk family situations occur when the breadwinner or family caretaker is incapacitated and no longer able to perform his or her role. While the parent's health declines, the children are also at risk because of the loss of parenting and financial support.

While most health experts theoretically understand that a decline in the health of one family member affects all family members, it is not unusual for these effects to be overlooked. In general, health care providers are looking to families to assume some of the burden and responsibility of the member's illness. They are not looking for ways to include the family's needs as part of the treatment plan.

Nevertheless, there has been some preliminary research looking at family-focused interventions for health problems. These interventions fall along a continuum of involvement. Weihs, Fisher, and Baird (2002) identify the different interventions and their goals:

- *Psychoeducational:* the most common intervention. The goal is to increase understanding of the disease in hopes that understanding will help the family cope. Behavioral changes in the family's daily functioning are targeted.
- *Family Relationship Quality and Functioning:* psychoeducation and family relationship interventions. The goals of these interventions are to reduce social isolation,

prevent the disease from consuming all the family resources, help the family cope with loss, promote communication and collaboration, improve empathy, deal with stigma, and help the family cope with conflict.

- *Family Therapy:* The goals of family therapy are often varied depending on the illness. In general, the goal in family therapy when conducted primarily in a mental health care setting is often to help reduce the duration and impact of the illness on the family's well-being, whereas in a medical setting the goal is often to improve the actual functioning level so that the family can interact with the health care team in a more effective manner.
- *Reconfiguration of the Health Care Team:* The goals of these interventions are to create health care providers who are more "family friendly" in their responses to the patient's needs. Health care workers are encouraged to consider the family's feelings and needs, not simply those of their patients.

While these interventions suggest lofty ideals, it will be easy for health care providers to continue overlooking family's needs and the impact of the illness on the family. The many competing demands on clinicians' time (e.g., managed care) may often allow little room for interventions beyond immediate treatment of the patient's physical problems, and family members often keep their needs to themselves and remain focused on the identified patient. To accurately assess the impact of an illness and offer effective family-based treatments, clinicians must be willing to expand their scope of care and have the needed skills and resources to expand.

COLLABORATIVE CARE AS THE TREATMENT OF CHOICE

Given the rediscovered "connections" among medical conditions, mental health, and social environment, the challenges of increasing chronic disease management, and an increasingly fragmented health care system with an increasingly diverse population, the challenges to primary care and family physicians may often appear overwhelming. They should not have to go it alone. In our opinions, a collaborative model of treatment that brings together all of the stakeholders, including patient, family, and health care providers, is essential to address the multitude of patient needs identified in a busy primary care practice.

There is a growing movement in health care that is committed to models of collaboration between physicians and therapists in assessing, planning, and providing patient care. These health professionals are attempting to repair both the fragmentation in health care services and the conceptual split between mind and body. In fact, there are several organizations and groups devoted to championing this model of care, especially in the United States, the United Kingdom, and Australia. Table 26.1 provides a partial list of organizations and their Web sites. Although there is much interest in the spirit of collaboration, there are continuing questions about how to collaborate with other health care professionals.

For mental health professionals, successful collaboration often demands a shift in attitude. Patterson, Peck, Heinrich, Bishoff, and Scherger (2002) summarize the differences in viewing oneself as a traditional mental health specialist versus a team member on a collaborative team. In general, the therapist relinquishes the role of

expert in the mental health and emotions of a shared patient and instead embraces a more holistic view of the patient's problems, medical and mental health. In this model, the therapist acknowledges that all areas related to health are inextricably intertwined. Mental health professionals must appreciate the larger systems that surround their patient, rather than just the clinical interaction.

In our roles as educators, we have noticed that there is little attention given to collaboration. Instead, most students are busy learning the language, skills, and paradigm of their discipline. Doherty and Baird (1986) talk about this split in training when they say that they were taught to treat "body-less minds" while their physician colleagues were taught to treat "mind-less bodies." In addition to this idea of collaborating on both mind and body, medical and mental health professionals must learn to collaborate with the family, an often under-used ally in maximizing the health of the patient. To successfully collaborate, health care professionals will have to relinquish some ideas they were taught in training and embrace new ideas and skills.

The UCSD/USD Collaborative Care Experience

At the University of California at San Diego (UCSD) Division of Family Medicine, we have developed a program in collaboration with faculty at the University of San

Table 26.1   Groups supporting collaboration among different health professions

Australian Mental Health Branch of Health Services	www.mentalhealth.gov.au/boimhc/index.htm
Collaborative Family Healthcare Association	www.cfhcc.org
Society for Behavioral Medicine	www.sbm.org
Counseling in Primary Care Trust	www.cpct.co.uk/cpct/
International Society for Behavioral Medicine	www.isbm.info
WHO Guide to Mental Health in Primary Care	www.mentalneurologicalprimarycare.org
Integrated Primary Care	www.integratedprimarycare.com
The Cummings Foundation	www.thecummingsfoundation.com

Diego that involves training our physicians in both the attitudes and skills of working better with families and mental health professionals. In this program, mental health professionals share office space with physicians and work side by side with them. This allows all professional groups to provide mutually beneficial real-time consultation services to each other, and to have frequent meetings about specific patients, their families, and the collaborative process itself. Trainees from a variety of disciplines are involved, setting an example for how to provide such collaborative care in the future. In addition to the collaboration of various service-oriented disciplines, researchers are integral to documenting the experiences and outcomes of patients and professionals alike.

CONCLUSION

Shared medical decision making and choice for families is greater than at any point in history. Questioning the physician, second opinions, and exploring therapeutic options are becoming new standards. High degrees of patient involvement, control, information-seeking, and expression of emotions (by both patient and provider) correlate with positive clinical outcomes (e.g., Golin, DiMatteo, & Gelberg, 1996).

Today's primary care physicians must be trained to participate in all levels of care and should receive training experience with family therapists and clinicians of other disciplines so they may know their roles and functions, indications for consultation, and how to participate in ongoing collaborative care of their mutual patients and families. Similarly, mental health professionals must be adequately familiar with the medical environment to provide services where they are most likely to be accessed and thus deliver the greatest good to the community at large. This review has attempted to introduce the evidence encouraging us all to collaborate more, not only with other professionals, but with patients' families with the goal to serve the greatest good.

REFERENCES

Anderson, B. J., & Kornblum, H. (1984). The family environment of children with a diabetic parent: Issues for research. *Family Systems Medicine, 2*(2), 17–27.

Berg, C., & Upchurch, R. (2003, March). *The interpersonal context of adjusting to chronic illness.* Paper presented at the annual meeting of the Society of Behavioral Medicine, Salt Lake City, UT.

Berkman, L. F. (1995). The role of social relations in health promotion. *Psychosomatic Medicine, 57,* 245–254.

Berkman, L. F. (2000). Social support, social networks, social cohesion and health. *Social Work in Health Care, 31,* 3–14.

Berkman, L. F., Leo-Summers, L., & Horowitz, R. I. (1992). Emotional support and survival after myocardial infarction: A prospective, population-based study of the elderly. *Annals of Internal Medicine, 117,* 1003–1009.

Bernard-Bonin, A. C., Stachenko, S., Bonin, D., Charette, C., & Rousseau, E. (1995). Self-management teaching programs and morbidity of pediatric asthma: A meta-analysis. *Journal of Allergy and Clinical Immunology, 95,* 34–41.

Burman, B., & Margolin, G. (1992). Analysis of the association between marital relationships and health problems: An interactional perspective. *Psychological Bulletin, 112,* 39–63.

Campbell, T. L. (2003). The effectiveness of family interventions for physical disorders. *Journal of Marital and Family Therapy, 29*(2), 263–281.

Cohen, S., & Underwood L. (2000). *Social support measurement and intervention: A guide for health and social scientists.* London: Oxford University Press.

Combrinck-Graham, L. (1985). A developmental model for family systems. *Family Process, 24,* 139–150.

Coppetelli, H. C., & Orleans, C. T. (1985). Partner support and other determinants of smoking cessation maintenance among women. *Journal of Consulting and Clinical Psychology, 53*(4), 455–460.

Coyne, J. C., Rohrbaugh, M. J., Shoham, V., Sonnega, J. S., Nicklas, J. M., & Cranford, J. A. (2001). Prognostic importance of marital quality for survival of congestive heart failure. *American Journal of Cardiology, 88,* 526–529.

DiClemente, C. C., & Prochaska, J. O. (1998). Toward a comprehensive transtheoretical model of change: Stages of change and addictive behaviors. In W. Miller & N. Heather (Eds.), *Treating addictive behaviors: Applied clinical psychology* (2nd ed., pp. 3–24). New York: Plenum Press.

Doherty, W. J., & Baird, M. A. (1986). Developmental levels of physician involvement with families. *Family Medicine, 18,* 153–156.

Doherty, W. J., & Campbell, T. L. (1988). *Families and Health.* Beverly Hills, CA: Sage.

Ewart, C. K., Taylor, C. B., Kraemer, H. C., & Agras, W. S. (1991). High blood pressure and marital discord: Not being nasty matters more than being nice. *Health Psychology, 10,* 155–163.

Fisher, L., Chesla, C. A., Bartz, R. J., Gillis, C., Skaff, M. A., Sabogal, F., et al. (1998). The family and type 2 diabetes: A framework for intervention. *Diabetes Educator, 24,* 599–607.

Fisher, L., Chesla, C. A., Skaff, M. A., Gillis, C., Mullan, J. T., Bartz, R. J., et al. (2000). The family and disease management in Hispanic and European-American patients with type 2 diabetes. *Diabetes Care, 23*(3), 267–272.

Fisher, L., Term, H. E., & Ransom, D. C. (1990). Advancing a family perspective in health research: Models and methods. *Family Process, 29,* 177–189.

Golin, C. E., DiMatteo, M. R., & Gelberg, L. (1996). The role of patient participation in the doctor visit. *Diabetes Care, 19,* 1153–1164.

Gottman, J. M. (1994). *What predicts divorce? The relationship between marital processes and marital outcomes.* Hillsdale, NJ: Erlbaum.

Ho, M., Marger, M., Beart, J., Yip, I., & Shekelle, P. (1997). Is the quality of diabetes care better in a diabetes clinic or in a general medicine clinic? *Diabetes Care, 20,* 472–475.

Kiecolt-Glaser, J. K., Fisher, L. D., Ogrocki, P., Stout, J. C., Speicher, C. E., & Glaser, R. (1987). Marital quality, marital disruption, and immune function. *Psychosomatic Medicine, 49,* 13–34.

Kiecolt-Glaser, J. K., & Newton, T. L. (2001). Marriage and health: His and hers. *Psychological Bulletin, 127,* 472–503.

Klausner, E. J., Koenigsberg, H. W., Skolnick, N., & Chung, H. (1995). Perceived familial criticism and glucose control in insulin-dependent diabetes mellitus. *International Journal of Mental Health, 24,* 64–75.

Law, D. D., & Crane, D. R. (2000). The influence of marital and family therapy on health care utilization in a health-maintenance organization. *Journal of Marital and Family Therapy, 26*(3), 281–291.

Martikainen, P., & Valkonen, T. (1996). Mortality after death of spouse in relation to duration of bereavement in Finland. *Journal of Epidemiology & Community Health, 50,* 264–268.

McDaniel, S. H., Hepworth, J., & Doherty, W. J. (1992). *Medical family therapy.* New York: Basic Books.

Mendenhall, T. J. (2002). Family-based intervention for persons with diabetes. Unpublished doctoral dissertation, University of Minnesota.

Mermelstein, R., Lichtenstein, E., & McIntyre, K. (1983). Partner support and relapse in smoking cessation programs. *Journal of Consulting and Clinical Psychology, 51*(3), 465–466.

Miller, W. R., & Rollnick, S. (2002). *Motivational interviewing: Preparing people for change* (2nd ed.). New York: Guilford.

Minuchin, S., Baker, L., Rosman, B. L., Liebman, R., Milman, L., & Todd, T. C. (1975). A conceptual model of psychosomatic illness in children: Family organization and family therapy. *Archives of General Psychiatry, 32,* 1031–1038.

Mittleman, M. S., Ferris, S. H., Shulman, E., Steinberg, G., & Levin, B. (1996). A family intervention to delay nursing home placement of patients with Alzheimer disease: A randomized controlled trial. *Journal of the American Medical Association (JAMA), 276*(21), 1725–1731.

Orth-Gomer, K., Wamala, S. P., Horsten M., Schenck-Gustafsson, K., Schneiderman, N., & Mittleman, M. A. (2000). Marital stress worsens prognosis in women with coronary heart disease: The Stockholm female coronary risk study. *Journal of the American Medical Association (JAMA), 284,* 3008–3014.

Panton, J., & Barley, E. A. (2002). Family therapy for asthma in children. *Cochrane Database of Systematic Reviews, 2.*

Patterson, J. E., Peck, C. J., Heinrich, R., Bishoff, R., & Scherger, J. (2002). *Mental health professional in medical settings: A primer.* New York: W. W. Norton.

Piette, J. D., & Mah, C. A. (1997). The feasibility of automated voice messaging as an adjunct to diabetes outpatient care. *Diabetes Care, 20,* 15–21.

Prochaska, J. O., & DiClemente, C. C. (1983). Stages and processes of self-change of smoking: Toward an integrative model of change. *Journal of Consulting and Clinical Psychology, 51*(3), 390–395.

Prochaska, J. O., DiClemente, C. C., & Norcross, J. C. (1992). In search of how people change: Applications to addictive behaviors. *American Psychologist, 47*(9), 1102–1114.

Rolland, J. (1984). Toward a psychosocial typology of chronic and life-threatening illness. *Family Systems Medicine, 2*(3), 245–262.

Rolland, J (1994). *Families, illness, and disability.* New York: Basic Books.

Sawa, R. J. (1985). *Family dynamics for physicians: Guidelines to assessment and treatment.* New York: Edwin Mellon Press.

Seeman, T. E. (2000). Health promoting effects of friends and family on health outcomes in older adults. *American Journal of Health Promotion, 14*(6), 362–370.

Seeman, S. E., Lusignolo, T. M., Albert, M., & Berkman, L. (2001). Social relationships, social support, and patterns of cognitive aging in healthy, high-functioning older adults: MacArthur studies of successful aging. *Health Psychology, 20*(4), 243–255.

Seeman, T. E., & McEwan, B. S. (1996). Impact of social environment characteristics on neuro-endocrine regulation. *Psychosomatic Medicine, 58*(5), 459–471.

Seeman, T. E., Singer, B. H., Ryff, C., Dienberg–Love, G., & Levy-Storms, L. (2002). Social relationships, gender, and allostatic load across two age cohorts. *Psychosomatic Medicine, 64*(3), 395–406.

Shi, L., Forrest, C. B., Von Schrader, S., & Ng, J. (2003). Vulnerability and the patient-practitioner relationship: The roles of gate-keeping and primary care performance. *American Journal of Public Health, 93*(1), 138–144.

Smilkstein, G. (1978). The family APGAR: A proposal for a family function test and its use by physicians. *Journal of Family Practice, 6,* 1231–1239.

Smilkstein, G. (1980). The cycle of family functioning: A conceptual model for family medicine. *Journal of Family Practice, 11*(2), 223–232.

Smilkstein, G. (1994). The family in family medicine revisited, again. *Journal of Family Practice, 39,* 527–31.

Smilkstein, G., Ashworth, C., & Montano, D. (1982). Validity and reliability of the family APGAR as a test of family function. *Journal of Family Practice, 15,* 303–311.

Sorenson, S., Pinquart, M., & Duberstein, P. (2002). How effective are interventions with caregivers? An updated meta-analysis. *Gerontologist, 43,* 356–372.

Toseland, R. W., McCallion, P., Smith, T., Huck, S., Bourgeois, P., & Garstka, T. A. (2001). Health education groups for caregivers in an HMO. *Journal of Clinical Psychology, 57,* 551–570.

Trevino, D. B., Young, E. H., Groff, J., & Jono, R. T. (1990). The association between marital adjustment and compliance with antihypertensive regimens. *Journal of the American Board of Family Practice, 3,* 17–25.

Venters, M. H., Jacobs, D. R., Luepker, R. V., Maiman, L. A., & Gillum, R. F. (1984). Spouse concordance of smoking patterns: The Minnesota Heart Survey. *American Journal of Epidemiology, 120,* 608–616.

Weihs, K. (2002, March). *Relationship quality with spouse predicts decreased disease progression in breast cancer patient.* Paper presented at the Family in Family Medicine Conference, San Diego, CA.

Weihs, K., Fisher, L., & Baird, M. (2002). Families, health, and behavior. *Families, Systems, & Health, 20,* 7–46.

Wing, R. R., Marcus, M. D., Epstein, L. H., & Jawad, A. (1991). A "family-based' approach to the treatment of obese Type II diabetic patients. *Journal of Consulting and Clinical Psychology, 59*(1), 156–162.

CHAPTER 27

Interventions With Families of an Acutely or Critically Ill Child

MARION E. BROOME AND WILMA POWELL STUART

CHILDHOOD ILLNESS: EFFECTS ON THE FAMILY

Effects of Acute or Critical Illness or Hospitalization of the Child on the Family

Acute or critical illness and subsequent hospitalization for medical treatment and nursing care have long been recognized as highly disruptive and stressful events for children and their families. Previous integrative reviews of the effects of acute or critical illness and hospitalization on children and their families have consistently documented their high stress levels, followed by long-term sequelae and effects on the total family (Broome, 1998; Thompson, 1985; Vernon, Foley, Sipowicz, & Schulman, 1965). During hospitalization of a child for an acute or critical illness, parents report feelings of disequilibrium, vulnerability, and disorganization in early stages, followed by feelings of helplessness, inadequacy, exhaustion, and irritability (Hanson, Johnson, Jeppson, Thomas, & Hall, 1994; Todres, Earle, & Jellinek, 1994). These feelings are associated with their reactions to the threat to their child's health and well-being, changes in the child's behavior and appearance, and the loss of their own parental role (Miles & D'Auria, 1994). Research has documented that parents do not know how to best support their child who is hospitalized, do not feel competent to minimize their child's fears, and do not feel they can protect him or her from pain (Melnyk & Alpert-Gillis, 1998).

Effects of Chronic Illness of the Child on the Family

Families in the United States provide care to an estimated 12 to 18 million children and adolescents with a chronic disease or chronic health condition (National Institutes of Health, 2003), with 8% of children between the ages of 5 and 17 years exhibiting changes in their activity levels related to the chronic condition (CDC, 2003). A chronic condition may vary significantly in its onset, course, and duration but is generally expected to last at least three months or more (AAP, 1993). A wide range of chronic health problems in children may evolve from genetics, illness, or injury (Miles, 2003). The most frequent chronic illness in children is asthma, with nine million children in the United States under the age of 18 affected and 44% reporting an asthma attack within the preceding 12 months (CDC, 2001). Other chronic illnesses frequently observed in children and adolescents may include, but are not limited to, diabetes, chronic kidney disease, juvenile rheumatoid arthritis, epilepsy, hemophilia, cystic fibrosis, spina bifida, congenital heart disease, cancer, sickle cell disease, HIV, obesity, autism, and attention deficit disorders. Until the mid-1990s, chronic illness was defined categorically by the particular health condition. Non-categorical definitions were subsequently developed to describe the commonalities between the experiences of the children and their families (Perrin et al., 1993). Commonalities among the chronic illnesses may be found in the impact the illness has on psychosocial responses, family life changes, and economic burdens. Parents are expected to provide complex daily care relating to disease management while maintaining a normal parenting role for the child and other children in the family. The unpredictability of the disease increases distress for the family caregivers (Garwick, Patterson, Meschke, Bennett, & Blum, 2002; Mansour, Lanphear, & DeWitte, 2000).

Chronic illness in a child provokes a variety of related issues for families. An estimated 27 million school day absences and 8.8 million annual physician contacts are attributed to children with chronic illness activity limitations (Newacheck & Halfon, 1998). Missed school days and visits to physicians are just two of many activities that necessitate responses within the family to accommodate the special needs of the child with a chronic illness. The needs of the chronically ill child, including finding appropriate child care, may be a barrier to employment of the mother, who is most often the full-time caregiver. The need to maintain health insurance and manage the financial cost of medications and

changes to the home environment presents challenges for the families of children with a chronic health problem (Mansour et al., 2000). Families may also struggle with discrimination toward children with a chronic health problem, which comes from a variety of sources including peers, schools, organizations, and institutions (Turner-Henson, Holaday, Corser, Ogletree, & Swan, 1994).

How a parent defines the situation will influence behaviors that will be used to manage the chronic illness on a daily basis (Knafl, Breitmayer, Gallo, & Zoeller, 1996). The chronic stressor of the illness may affect normal childhood developmental tasks as well as relationships in the family system (Hamlett, Pellegrini, & Katz, 1992). Increased parental distress in parents of children with chronic illness has been found to be related to the level of functional impairment for the child (Canning, Harris, & Kelleher, 1996). However, on the other hand, other findings have identified that parental distress is associated with hope, social support, and perceived caregiver stress related to caring for a child with a disability rather than objective measurement of functional impairment (Horton & Wallander, 2001).

FAMILIES AND THE HEALTH CARE SYSTEM

In the 1980s, the separation of infants, children, and adolescents from their family during hospitalization was recognized as highly stressful for all concerned. Subsequently, visiting policies changed markedly. As a result of experiences in neonatal intensive care units, separation of mothers from their newborns was demonstrated to affect bonding, even many years after the experience (Pinch, 2002). In a critical review of the studies on children's experiences in critical care, Giganti (1998) found that children in intensive care report higher stress levels when separated from their parents, and some parents report symptoms of post-traumatic stress disorder (PTSD) (Melnyk & Alpert-Gillis, 1998).

The presence and active involvement of parents during a child's acute or critical illness is crucial in today's health care system. Their ongoing involvement facilitates better decision making, enhances clinical care, and facilitates the child's adjustment and builds parents' skills in caregiving for post-hospital care (Ahmann, Abraham, & Johnson, 2003). Yet the inevitable responses of parents to the threats posed by separation, invasive procedures, pain, and isolation from support networks usually experienced during an acute or critical illness require active intervention and support by health professionals in order to successfully adapt and negotiate the illness experience. These interventions should clearly build on existing evidence that documents the positive responses of parents and other family members, as well as the child, and should be tailored to the families' unique context and existing strengths.

Health insurance coverage and cultural implications are important components of access to health care for families with a child with special needs. An estimated 1.3 million children with special needs are uninsured, with the majority of the children in families living at poverty level. Cultural and language barriers can impede understanding of eligibility and insurance enrollment processes (Newacheck, McManus, Fox, Hung, & Halfon, 2000).

In addition to financial needs for access to health care services, families identify continued need for information from health care providers. A study of mothers and fathers of children with a chronic health problem identified agreement between the two parents that over 70% of the families have unmet needs for information, with the most specific need in the area of future planning for the needs of the child (Perrin, Lewkowicz, &

Young, 2000). Parents identified education for the child and social needs of the child as more significant needs than financial information or direct care assistance (Perrin et al., 2000).

INTERVENTION RESEARCH WITH ILL CHILDREN

Theoretical Perspectives

Theoretically, interventions in this area have hypothesized that if parents were provided with information about their child's behavior, including what experiences and events they could expect, ways to support and protect their child, and adaptive ways of coping with the stress of the illness, they would be less stressed, less anxious, provide higher levels of support for their child, and use effective strategies to adapt. Several assumptions, supported by research, have guided the development and implementation of the interventions for families of an ill child:

1. Hospitalization, surgery, and invasive procedures are viewed as threatening by both children and their parents;

2. A child's acute or critical illness affects all members of a family;

3. Parents want to be present, involved, and supportive during a child's or adolescent's illness;

4. Parental emotions and behavior have a direct impact on the child's ability to cope with acute illness and/or hospitalization; and

5. Procedural and sensory information about an impending threatening event during hospitalization will facilitate the child's and family's coping and reduces distress.

Table 27.1 outlines selected examples in intervention studies with families with a child who suffers an acute or chronic condition.

Table 27.1 Selected examples of intervention studies with families of children with an acute or chronic illness

Author	Sample	Intervention	Findings
Interventions: Acute/Critical illness			
Melnyk, et al., 1997	30 mothers of critically ill 1–6-year-old children randomly assigned to experimental or control groups	COPE: 1) descriptive information about their child's responses 2) instruction in parental activities specific to situation	Mothers in COPE group: 1) provided more support to child during intrusive procedures 2) reported less negative mood state and parental stress 3) less PTSD symptoms and less parental role change 4 weeks after hospitalization
Chronic Illness Interventions: Support strategies to enhance coping			
Burke, et al., 2001	115 children & family Child's age 7 to 15 years. Two groups 1) Intervention 2) Usual care control group	Intervention: Stress-Point Intervention by Nurses (SPIN) psychosocial and educational intervention focuses on parents' issues and concerns relating to child's hospitalization	Intervention parents had better parental coping and were more satisfied with family functioning than usual care parents.
Williams, et al., 2003	Siblings and parents 252 families Ages 7 to 15 years Random assignment to three groups 1) full intervention 2) partial intervention 3) wait list control group	Intervention for Siblings: Experience Enhancement (ISEE) includes illness information, psychosocial sessions, 5-day residential summer camp, and two follow up sessions.	Siblings in intervention group demonstrated greater disease knowledge, mood improvement, and declines in behavior problems. Greatest amount of change for social support was in the partial treatment group. Self esteem scores improved for the full and partial intervention groups.

Author	Sample	Intervention	Findings
Wysocki, et al., 2000; Wysocki, et al., 2001	119 families Ages 12 to 16.75 years randomized to three groups 1) Behavioral Family Systems Theory (BFST) 2) Education and support 3) Current therapy	Behavioral Family Systems Therapy (BFST) 10 sessions with licensed psychologist and detailed therapy manual with session outlines, educational handouts and homework assignments.	Improvement in parent-adolescent relations and reduced diabetes-specific conflict in BFST group.
Chronic Illness Interventions: Disease Management			
Bonner, et al., 2002	430 families contacted by phone: 223 families agreed to participate, 119 families returned signed consent forms; 100 families were available for follow up interviews at 3 months. 4 to 19 years of age two groups; random assignment 1) Intervention group 2) Usual care control group	Family education program teaches basic asthma care, use of diary of asthma symptoms and use of peak flow meters.	Intervention group improved communication with health care providers leading to better pharmacological control of asthma symptoms.
Georgiou, et al., 2003	401 randomly selected households Ages 5 to 13 years	Educational mailings, reminder aids, videos, peak flow meters and telephone case management.	Intervention group had reduction in lost work days for adult caregivers, decreased asthma symptoms, and decreased activity restricted days for the child.

Much of the intervention literature with families of children with an acute or critical illness in the acute care system area is based on broad conceptual frameworks that reflect a focus on stress, coping, support, self-regulation, and anxiety reduction. Mothers provide the majority of care during and after hospitalization, so most of the intervention studies that have focused on a family member other than the child have targeted the mother.

Knafl and colleagues (1996) described the varying ways families respond to a child's chronic illness with the development of the Family Management Style (FMS) model. Five different family management styles were identified: thriving, accommodating, enduring, struggling, and floundering. The thriving family has a focus on normalcy for their child and their family goals. Normalcy was a key theme for families identified as accommodating, but some component of their response to the illness was more negative than those identified as thriving. The enduring family had a theme of difficulty in their descriptions of their families' management of the care of the child with a chronic illness. A key difference between parents who thrive and parents who endure is the meaning the parents attach to their proactive management behaviors (Knafl et al., 1996).

Interventions: Acute or Critical Illness

Previously tested interventions with families of a child with an acute or critical illness have primarily focused on two areas: (1) psychoeducational preparation of the child and parent for hospitalization, surgery, and procedures, including cognitive-behavioral strategies for the child and parent to reduce anxiety, pain, and distress; and (2) education and support strategies for parents to enhance their coping and reduce distress and to increase their ability to care for the child during and after hospitalization.

Psychoeducational Interventions. The purpose and intent of these interventions are to provide the child and parent with information about experiences they can anticipate during hospitalization or treatment for an illness (Broome & Huth, 2001). Studies have targeted mothers of low birth weight infants (Melnyk, Feinstein, & Fairbanks, 2002), mothers of preschool and school-age children prior to surgery (Nelson & Allen, 1999; Seid & Varni, 1999), parents of children and adolescents with cancer prior to procedures (Reeb & Bush, 1997), and mothers of children in intensive care units (Melnyk & Allpert-Gillis, 1998). The findings from these studies suggest that psychological preparation is beneficial for many children and their parents. That is, preparation can increase their understanding of impending events, decrease anxiety, increase parental satisfaction, and ultimately increase parental participation in care during hospitalization. Increased parental participation has been found to decrease anxiety in children who are hospitalized.

Research has consistently documented that the majority of parents want to be present when their child experiences an invasive or painful procedure (Boudreaux, Francis, & Loyacono, 2002). Early research focused on the effects of parental presence as a comfort intervention when children underwent minor painful procedures such as a blood draw or immunization (Broome, 2000). Even in more invasive and highly distressing situations, such as lumbar punctures and intensive care unit procedures, research has demonstrated that when parents are emotionally available to the child and perceived as supportive, the child's distress level decreases dramatically. Research has supported the effectiveness of parents being taught how to use physical support (stroking), distraction, and relaxation across settings (e.g., neonatal intensive care units, emergency departments).

Studies testing the effectiveness of cognitive-behavioral interventions (CBT) have occasionally focused on parent's response as well as those of the child. These interventions are designed to provide the child with the ability to distract him or her during distressing procedures or pain using a variety of behaviors such as distraction, relaxation, and so on. The research over the past 15 years has supported the effectiveness of these interventions on reducing a child's distress level (Kleiber & Harper, 1999). However, given the reliance of the child and adolescent on the parent when under stress associated with hospitalization and procedures, many researchers have attempted to include parents in their interventions (Broome, 1998). Parents have primarily been used as "coaches" for their child who is implementing the CBT. Unfortunately, the research has been mixed on their effectiveness (Kleiber & Harper, 1999), and more research, using larger samples and more controlled conditions, needs to be done. To date, the coach model has not addressed how the parent's interaction and support of the child reduces their own distress, and studies should consider testing interventions designed to directly alleviate the parent's distress while also using the parent to facilitate the child's coping.

Parental Coping Interventions

Melnyk, Feinstein, and Fairbanks (2002) recently summarized and critiqued interventions tested with mothers of low birth weight infants. Most of the studies provided mothers with anticipatory guidance about neonatal and infant behavior and skills to enhance their ability to parent. Positive outcomes were found related to infant mental development, parent satisfaction, maternal confidence, maternal-infant interaction, and lower stress. In further intervention studies with mothers of children in an intensive care unit, researchers tested the Creating Opportunities for Parental Empowerment (COPE) program, designed to help mothers to increase

their confidence and role certainty, thereby increasing their ability to cope with and participate in their child's care during a critical illness (Melnyk & Alpert-Gillis, 1998; Melnyk, Alpert-Gillis, Hensel, Cable-Beiling, & Rubenstein, 1997; Melnyk et al., 2001). The COPE program consists of a psychoeducational component in which the mother is provided information about typical responses of children to a hospitalization, as well as activities to engage in with her child throughout the hospitalization, which build on her parenting skills. When the program was evaluated, mothers who had been randomly assigned to the COPE program provided their children with more support during painful procedures and reported less stress and negative mood state, less parental role change, and fewer PTSD symptoms four weeks after hospitalization.

The death of a child has been found to be one of the most stressful life events for any parent. Interventions of families of a child who is terminally ill have focused on testing supportive strategies with parents and siblings primarily after the child has died. These bereavement interventions variably focus on (1) individual parents, (2) couple counseling, (3) family counseling, and (4) bereavement support groups (Worden & Monahan, 2001). Parents' acceptance of the type of intervention varies, and research has reported that the timing of the intervention was as important as the type of intervention itself (Worden & Monahan, 2001). Research evaluating support groups found that although parents who participated changed their attitudes about bereavement, their mental health status or marital functioning was not affected.

Interventions: Chronic Health Problems

An abundance of descriptive studies identify the many special needs of families with a child with a chronic health problem. However, intervention research in this area is limited. Deatrick (1998), in an integrative review of nursing family intervention research, identified eight studies that tested interventions. Miles (2003) identified seven programs of nursing research focused on parents and parenting of children with a chronic illness. Although not a comprehensive analysis, an expansion of previous reviews of intervention studies was completed to develop an interdisciplinary description of intervention studies with families of a child with a chronic health problem. Most intervention studies with families of a child with a chronic health problem are interdisciplinary, in contrast to many studies evolving from nursing for the child with an acute health problem. Nurses historically have had more access to the acutely ill child and their family members than other disciplines. Focus areas of intervention studies with families of children with chronic illnesses address similar needs to families providing care to children during an acute illness. The most significant difference in the needs identified are reflected in education programs to prepare families for a lifetime of care of a child with a chronic health problem. Two topic areas emerge as focus areas of education programs for families of children with a chronic health problem: (1) interventions to enhance coping, and (2) disease management.

Interventions to Enhance Coping. Providing care to a child with a chronic health problem creates unique demands on the family system. Challenges include difficulty establishing and maintaining social support systems for the child and the family and dealing with health care needs during developmental transition periods from childhood to adolescence. Intervention studies have utilized education programs to teach parents the skills needed to cope with the multiple daily tasks.

Adolescents with chronic health problems have a dual challenge of managing their illness during periods of normal growth and development and developing autonomy from their family. Programs targeting parent-adolescent communication to assist with the developmental process and maintain compliance with treatment protocols have been effective for diabetes management (Anderson, Brackett, Ho, & Laffel, 1999; Laffel et al., 2003; Wysocki et al., 2000; Wysocki, Greco, Harris, Bubb, & White, 2001).

Nontraditional interventions are being tested to provide assistance to families. Mothers' anxiety symptoms were reduced in a community-based program that matched experienced mothers of older children—over the age of 18—with a chronic health problem and mothers of younger children with chronic health problems (Ireys, Chernoff, DeVet, & Kim, 2001). A total of 39 experienced mothers were trained in communication skills and later joined child life specialists to develop a team intervention. Another unique study employed a three-day retreat format to enhance coping skills for families and children with juvenile rheumatic disease (Hagglund et al., 1996). The utilization of a retreat format for the intervention permits a more intensive intervention package than might be available in separate classes.

Parents and nurses describe hospitalization for a child with a chronic health problem to be different from that of a child who is acutely ill (Burke, Handley-Derry, Costello, Kauffmann, & Dillon, 1997). A stress point intervention by nurses (SPIN) to improve coping with repeat hospitalization of the child with a chronic health problem was compared to families receiving traditional care (Burke, Harrison, Kauffmann, & Wong, 2001; Burke et al., 1997). Different levels of nurse educational backgrounds and roles were tested with the SPIN intervention to assist parents in the development of problem-focused coping skills. The studies included children with cerebral palsy, spina bifida, congenital genitourinary defects, cancer responding to treatment, chronic renal disease, cystic fibrosis, congenital hip defects, other orthopedic conditions, cardiac defects, gastrointestinal conditions, muscular dystrophy, cleft palate, diabetes, and epilepsy. The findings from these studies suggest family needs are consistent among different types of chronic illnesses, and the intervention moderates the impact of the hospitalization on family functioning.

The importance of including siblings in education programs for families with a child with a chronic health problem was supported by an intervention using the Intervention for Siblings: Experience Enhancement (ISEE) program, which provides illness information, psychosocial sessions, a five-day residential summer camp, and two follow-up sessions with siblings and their parents (Williams et al., 2003). The study included 252 families with children with chronic health problems such as cystic fibrosis, diabetes, spina bifida, cancer, and developmental disabilities. The siblings participating in the full intervention developed significantly greater knowledge about the illness, an improvement in mood, and declines in behavior problems. The greatest amount of change for social support was in the partial treatment group. At the final data collection point, self-esteem scores improved for both the intervention group and the partial intervention group.

A particular challenge to researchers planning interventions with families of children with chronic health problems is the identification of effective times to meet with families. The importance of participation for families in interventions focused on developing family coping skills was addressed by changing group meeting times to multiple weekend sessions (Goldbeck & Babka, 2001), single sessions on a weekend day (Kazak et al., 1999), and the use of a three-day family retreat (Hagglund et al., 1996). Weekend formats requiring multiple weekend sessions achieved participation of only 50% of eligible families (Goldbeck & Babka, 2001).

Complications, such as the availability of family members and the travel distance to tertiary care centers, influence the structure and frequency of interventions (Kazak et al., 1999).

Disease Management Interventions. As health care systems have evolved from inpatient hospital systems to outpatient systems, parents of children with a chronic health problem have assumed progressively more responsibility for the management of complex daily health care treatments. Compliance with the treatment protocols reduces health care visits, absences from school, and missed work days for parents. Education programs have assisted parents with improved compliance with treatment protocols and the development of effective communication skills with their health care provider. Examples of such programs have included interventions for asthma management (Bonner et al., 2002; Georgiou et al., 2003) and teamwork development with adolescents for diabetes management (Anderson et al., 1999; Laffel et al., 2003).

The difficulty of effecting change and the many variables associated with a family intervention surfaced in an intervention designed to reduce exposure of asthmatic children to tobacco smoke. The study included 87 caregivers and children with asthma between the ages of 3 and 12 years (Wilson et al., 2001). Three structured counseling sessions were completed with parents by a nurse-educator to provide education relating to asthma care and the effect of environmental tobacco smoke (ETS). Children were included in the counseling sessions if they were at a developmental age to participate. The complexities of such an intervention were demonstrated in the findings, with no significant difference in cotinine levels between the intervention and control groups. The intervention group did demonstrate a decrease in the number of acute medical visits.

Efficacy of a family intervention for sickle cell disease management was evaluated (Kaslow et al., 1997) and further tested in a pilot study for effectiveness (Kaslow et al., 2000). Kaslow and colleagues (1997) noted that cultural sensitivity can be taught; however, the time necessary to establish an effective rapport with the participants can be reduced by the participation of African American therapists conducting the intervention. Families assigned to the intervention group met with an African American therapist weekly (Kaslow et al., 2000). Families were encouraged to include all family members; however, most sessions were attended only by the female caregiver and the child. Significant differences were identified between children and their families who completed the intervention and those who dropped out of the study (Kaslow et al., 2000). Noncompleter children were older, were in a higher grade, had lower IQ scores, and caregivers had less disease knowledge. Evaluation of knowledge of the management of the disease process was significant for the child and the parent; however, no difference was identified for family functioning scores.

Similarities in family needs for education relating to the management of chronic diseases are found in descriptions of the modules of interventions for cystic fibrosis, diabetes, and sickle cell disease education. The Cystic Fibrosis Family Education Program, a self-management program, is based on social cognitive theory and presents instructional modules for respiratory care, nutrition and malabsorption, communication, and coping (Bartholomew et al., 1997). Manuals to provide consistency in program instruction were also used in a diabetes teamwork study and included modules for communication, glycemic control and teamwork, response to blood sugars and blame/shame cycle, and sharing the burden of care (Laffel et al., 2003). A manual for instruction in management and coping for a sickle cell disease education

program included modules for education, preventive health strategies, coping/cognition, feelings/communication, and interpersonal relationships (Kaslow et al., 1997).

CHALLENGES AND FUTURE DIRECTIONS IN CONDUCTING RESEARCH WITH FAMILIES OF AN ILL CHILD

We have learned a great deal over the past four decades about how children respond to hospitalization and acute or critical illness. Over the last decade, researchers have tested interventions for families to reduce stress and anxiety and support coping. Yet, studies to date have been somewhat limited by a number of methodological and logistical issues that have impacted the ability of researchers to extend knowledge in this area. These include (1) the almost exclusive focus on Caucasian, middle-class mothers; (2) the inability to examine pre-existing characteristics of families that would predict their coping and adaptation; (3) the lack of theories and models that would provide direction for programs of research in the area; and (4) environmental and illness factors that can restrict access to families during hospitalization.

Focus on Mothers

The continued focus on mothers, most often Caucasian, as the target for interventions is both understandable and problematic. The reality is that mothers are the primary caregivers of young children when acutely ill or hospitalized, and are therefore easier to access and collect data from. However, past research has demonstrated that both fathers and siblings are affected by the child's illness and that interventions directed at these family members are critical to expanding our understanding about how to best support them. The hospital environment has limited access, open mostly to physicians, nurse researchers, and occasionally to psychologists and child life specialists. This access to these families will become even more challenging given the Health Information and Portability Act of 1996, which prevents staff members from screening children and families and referring them to researchers to approach for participation in their study. Researchers will no longer be allowed to approach families on acute care units. Even if interested, families will have to work very hard to enroll in studies that are posted on units. This is unlikely—especially for families from minority populations. In addition, cultural barriers in some minority groups are significant and go beyond simple language differences. In fact, during a child's critical illness the clash of cultural beliefs about health and illness can not only produce stress for both family and caregivers but also affect outcomes.

Pre-existing Characteristics

The ability of researchers to study preexisting characteristics of families is hampered by the usually sudden, and often unexpected, nature of acute or critical illness. Unlike other phenomena of interest to family researchers, the family is often unknown to the researchers until they find themselves in the middle of what they consider to be a catastrophic event. It is highly likely then that their behavior and responses are not reflective of their usual patterns. Therefore, even though one may be able to assess the effectiveness of an intervention on selected variables, it will be much more difficult to determine whether a particular family would benefit from a specific intervention. For example, certain families are more cohesive and might respond better to certain interventions. However, when their child becomes acute or critically ill, that level of cohesiveness can change. Families vary considerably in their past experiences, styles of coping and support, response to and

perception of illness as a stressor, and how much support they get from the community. Each of these variables could serve as strong mediators or moderators of the effectiveness of the intervention. Yet, how and when to assess these, as well as the validity of the assessment when a family is under such stress, is not yet known.

Theories and Models

With few exceptions, most interventions are not grounded in a clear conceptual framework (Melnyk, 2000). This lack of theoretical grounding makes it difficult to interpret or explain results. Even when an intervention is found to be effective, without some pre-existing theoretical model one is never sure what the underlying mechanism was by which the intervention was successful. More substantive theories and models would guide when it might be most effective to intervene and what the most effective outcome might be in terms of family adaptation (Gillis & Knafl, 1999).

Institutional, Environmental, and Family Constraints

Researchers must constantly be aware of issues of sensitivity and burden for families of an acute or critically ill child. The period after an unplanned or unexpected hospitalization is chaotic for most families, and parents report heightened levels of anxiety and distress. So although, ideally, interventions designed to increase family coping should begin as soon as possible after admission, this may not be possible. The burden of designs with multiple self-report measures or interviews, videotaping, or even physiologic measures of stress may be viewed as very intrusive by family members during this time (Broome, 1998).

Intervention studies are notoriously complex and costly to evaluate. Traditional research designs call for randomization of families to experimental or control groups, blinding of interventionists and data collectors, repeated measures over time, and large samples. Each of these, when implemented, is problematic in the acute or critical care setting. Yet, even when found to be effective in ameliorating stress and improving coping, the translation of these interventions has been disappointing (Melnyk et al., 2002). The translation can remain costly in terms of staff time, materials, and continued evaluation. However, some of the interventions discussed in this chapter are less expensive than others, and given the consistency in findings across many, it might be more fruitful to evaluate how to reduce cost while maintaining quality and positive effects. For instance, adapting some of the informational programs into CDs parents can listen to, or view on the computer, might be feasible alternatives.

Descriptive research provides a starting point for future intervention research, especially in children with a chronic health condition. Ray (2002) describes one model, Parenting and Childhood Chronicity (PACC), which evolved from a qualitative study with 43 parents of children with chronic health problems. The parents identified the intensity of the work associated with providing care to a child with a chronic health problem, including the difficulty of gaining benefit from respite care and the invisible work associated with receiving assistance (Ray, 2002). A study of a three-year respite program for families with chronically ill children identified benefits for siblings and reductions in mother's somatic symptoms as well as trends of lower numbers of hospitalizations (Sherman, 1995). As increasing numbers of children with chronic health problems receive care within communities, a better understanding of the benefits and problems associated with respite care is needed. Future research is also needed to address the needs of caregivers using an

expanded definition of family. Many grandparents and foster parents have assumed roles as caregivers of chronically ill children. Interventions are needed to assist nonparental caregivers of chronically ill children. In addition, interventions are beginning to explore some of the diversity of cultural differences among families. However, further studies are needed with families of chronically ill children to identify culturally appropriate interventions. Siblings of children with a chronic health problem may experience wide ranges of responses to changes in the family. It is difficult to differentiate which responses may relate to the presence of the child with a chronic health problem and which responses may be part of developmental issues which would present in any circumstance. A review of 43 studies of siblings of children with a chronic health problem found 60% of the studies reported increased risk of emotional, social, and academic problems (Williams, 1997). Findings were consistent across different types of chronic illness, supporting a noncategorical approach to future interventions (Williams, 1997). A later review found that studies with siblings are evolving to identify variables which may be modifiable (Van Riper, 2003). There have been a limited number of intervention studies to assist siblings of children with a chronic health problem in their modified family role.

Future research with families of an ill child should focus on testing multifocal interventions across several sites. Few institutions or agencies serving these children have access to the numbers of families required to meaningfully assess how individual, family, and environmental factors differentially influence how any intervention improves child and family outcomes over time. If investigators work across sites, they will be better able to examine, for instance, how interventions must be tailored based on the ethnicity of a child, or the age of siblings, or the support inherently available in a particular family system. Of course, this requires that more theoretical work be done. That is, models that would guide these interventions must be developed, and most importantly, they must reflect the interdisciplinary perspectives of those who work with these families. And one of the more important perspectives will be that of the families themselves. It is only after these models are conceptualized that interventions can be developed and tested with families.

REFERENCES

AAP. (1993). Psychosocial risks of chronic health conditions in childhood and adolescence. *Pediatrics, 92*(6), 876–878.

Ahmann, E., Abraham, M., & Johnson, B. (2003). *Changing the concept of families as visitors: Supporting family presence and participation.* Bethesda, MD: Institute for Family-Centered Care.

Anderson, B. J., Brackett, J., Ho, J., & Laffel, L. (1999). An office-based intervention to maintain parent-adolescent teamwork in diabetes management. *Diabetes Care, 22*(5), 713–721.

Bartholomew, L. K., Czyzewski, D. I., Parcel, G. S., Sockrider, M., Mariotto, M. J., Schidlow, D. V., et al. (1997). Self-management of cystic fibrosis: Short-term outcomes of the cystic fibrosis family education program. *Health Education & Behavior, 24*(5), 652–666.

Bonner, S., Zimmerman, B. J., Evans, D., Irigoyen, M., Resnick, D., & Mellins, R. B. (2002). An individualized intervention to improve asthma management among urban Latino and African American families. *Journal of Asthma, 39*(2), 167–179.

Boudreaux, E., Francis, L., & Loyacono, T. (2002). Family presence during invasive procedures and resuscitation in the emergency department: A critical review and suggestions for future research. *Annals of Emergency Medicine, 40*(2), 193–205.

Broome, M. (1998). Acutely Ill children and their families. In M. Broome, K. Knafl, K. Pridham, & S. Feetham (Eds.), *Children and families in health and illness* (pp. 163–174). Thousand Oaks, CA: Sage.

Broome, M. (2000). Helping parents to support their child in pain. *Pediatric Nursing, 26*(3), 315–317.

Broome, M., & Huth, M. (2001). Preparation for hospitalization, surgery, and procedures. In M. Craft-Rosenberg & J. Denehy (Eds.), *Nursing interventions for infants, children and adolescents* (pp. 281–298). Thousand Oaks, CA: Sage.

Burke, S. O., Handley-Derry, M. H., Costello, E. A., Kauffmann, E., & Dillon, M. C. (1997). Stress-point intervention for parents of repeatedly hospitalized children with chronic conditions. *Research in Nursing & Health, 20*, 475–485.

Burke, S. O., Harrison, M. B., Kauffmann, E., & Wong, C. (2001). Effects of stress-point intervention with families of repeatedly hospitalized children. *Journal of Family Nursing, 7*(2), 128–158.

Canning, R., Harris, E., & Kelleher, K. (1996). Factors predicting distress among caregivers to children with chronic medical conditions. *Journal of Pediatric Psychology, 21*(5), 735–749.

Centers for Disease Control (CDC). (2001). *Summary health statistics for U.S. children: National Health Interview Survey, 2001* (Series 10, Number 216).

Washington, DC: Center for Disease Control and Prevention, National Center for Health Statistics.

CDC. (2003). *America's children 2003*. Centers for Disease Control and Prevention, National Center for Health Statistics. Retrieved December 26, 2003, from www.childstats.gov/ac2003

Deatrick, J. (1998). Integrative review of intervention research with children who have chronic conditions and their families. In M. E. Broome, K. Knafl, K. Pridham, & S. Feetham (Eds.), *Children and families in health and illness* (pp. 221–235). Thousand Oaks, CA: Sage.

Garwick, A. W., Patterson, J. M., Meschke, L., Bennett, F. C., & Blum, R. W. (2002). The uncertainty of preadolescents' chronic health conditions and family distress. *Journal of Family Nursing, 8*(1), 11–31.

Georgiou, A., Buchner, D. A., Ershoff, D. H., Blasko, K. M., Goodman, L. V., & Feigin, J. (2003). The impact of a large-scale population-based asthma management program on pediatric asthma patients and their caregivers. *Annals of Allergy, Asthma, & Immunology, 90*(3), 308–315.

Giganti, A. W. (1998). Families in critical care: The best option. *Pediatric Nursing, 24*(3), 261–265.

Gillis, C., & Knafl, K. (1999). Nursing care of families in non-normative transitions: The state of the science and practice. In A. Hinshaw, S. Feetham, & J. Shaver (Eds.), *Handbook of clinical nursing research* (pp. 231–249). Thousand Oaks, CA: Sage.

Goldbeck, L., & Babka, C. (2001). Development and evaluation of a multi-family psychoeducational program for cystic fibrosis. *Patient Education and Counseling, 44*(2), 187–192.

Hagglund, K. J., Doyle, N. M., Clay, D. L., Frank, R. G., Johnson, J. C., & Pressly, T. A. (1996). A family retreat as a comprehensive intervention for children with arthritis and their families. *Arthritis Care and Research, 9*(1), 35–41.

Hamlett, K. W., Pellegrini, D. S., & Katz, K. S. (1992). Childhood chronic illness as a family stressor. *Journal of Pediatric Psychology, 17*(1), 33–47.

Hanson, J. L., Johnson, B. H., Jeppson, E. S., Thomas, J., & Hall, J. H. (1994). *Hospitals: Moving forward with family-centered care*. Bethesda, MD: Institute for Family-centered Care.

Horton, T. V., & Wallander, J. L. (2001). Hope and social support as resilience factors against psychological distress of mothers who care for children with chronic physical conditions. *Rehabilitation Psychology, 46*(4), 382–399.

Ireys, H. T., Cernoff, R., DeVet, K., & Kim, Y. (2001). Maternal outcomes of a randomized controlled trial of a community-based support program for families of children with chronic illnesses. *Archives of Pediatrics and Adolescent Medicine, 155*, 771–777.

Kaslow, N. J., Collins, M., Loundy, M., Brown, F., Hollins, L. D., & Eckman, J. (1997). Empirically validated family interventions for pediatric psychology: Sickle cell disease as an exemplar. *Journal of Pediatric Psychology, 22*(2), 213–227.

Kaslow, N., Collins, M. H., Rashid, F. L., Baskin, M. L., Griffith, J. R., Hollins, L., et al. (2000). The efficacy of a pilot family psychoeducational intervention for pediatric sickle cell disease (SCD). *Family, Systems, and Health, 18*(4), 381–404.

Kazak, A. E., Simms, S., Barakat, L., Hobbie, W., Foley, B., Golomb, V., et al. (1999). Surviving cancer competently intervention program (SCCIP): A cognitive-behavioral and family therapy intervention for adolescent survivors of childhood cancer and their families. *Family Process, 38*(2), 175–191.

Kleiber, C., & Harper, D. (1999). Effects of distraction on child pain and distress during medical procedures: A meta-analysis. *Nursing Research, 48,* 44–49.

Knafl, K., Breitmayer, B., Gallo, A., & Zoeller, L. (1996). Family response to childhood chronic illness: Description of management styles. *Journal of Pediatric Nursing, 11*(5), 315–326.

Laffel, L., Vangsness, L., Connell, A., Goebel-Fabbri, A., Butler, D., & Anderson, B. J. (2003). Impact of ambulatory, family-focused teamwork intervention on glycemic control in youth with type I diabetes. *Journal of Pediatrics, 142,* 409–416.

Mansour, M. E., Lanphear, B. P., & DeWitte, T. (2000). Barriers to asthma care in urban children: Parent perspective. *Pediatrics, 106*(3), 512–519.

Melnyk, B. (2000). Intervention studies involving parents of hospitalized young children: An analysis of the past and future recommendations. *Journal of Pediatric Nursing, 15*(1), 4–13.

Melnyk, B. M., & Alpert-Gillis, L. J. (1998). The COPE program: A strategy to improve outcomes of critically ill young children and their parents. *Pediatric Nursing, 24*(6), 521–527.

Melnyk, B., Alpert-Gillis, L., Feinstein, N., Fairbanks, E., Schulltz-Czarniak, J., Hust, D., et al. (2001). Improving cognitive development of low birth weight premature infants with the COPE program: A pilot study of the benefit of early NICU intervention with mothers. *Research in Nursing and Health, 24,* 373–389.

Melnyk, B., Alpert-Gillis, L., Hensel, P., Cable-Beiling, R., & Rubenstein, J. (1997). Helping mothers cope with a critically ill child: A pilot test of the COPE intervention. *Research in Nursing and Health, 20,* 3–14.

Melnyk, B., Feinstein, N., & Fairbanks, E. (2002). Effectiveness of informational/behavioral interventions with parents of low birthweight (LBW) premature infants: An evidence base to guide clinical practice. *Pediatric Nursing, 28*(5), 511–516.

Miles, M. S. (2003). Parents of children with chronic health problems: Programs of nursing research and their relationship to developmental science. In J. J. Fitzpatrick (Ed.), *Annual review of nursing research 2003: Research on child health and pediatric issues* (Vol. 21, pp. 247–277). New York: Springer.

Miles, M., & D'Auria, J. (1994). Parenting the medically fragile infant. *Capsules and Comments in Pediatric Nursing, 1*(1), 2–7.

National Institutes of Health (NIH). (2003, August 6). *Chronic illness self-management in children.* National Institute of Health. Retrieved December 21, 2003, from www.grants1.nih.gov/grants/guide/pa-files/PA-03–159.html

Nelson, C., & Allen, J. (1999). Reduction of healthy children's fears related to hospitalization and medical procedures: The effectiveness of multimedia computer instruction in pediatric psychology. *Children's Health Care, 28,* 1–13.

Newacheck, P. W., & Halfon, N. (1998). Prevalence and impact of disabling chronic conditions in childhood. *American Journal of Public Health, 88*(4), 610–617.

Newacheck, P. W., McManus, M., Fox, H. B., Hung, Y. Y., & Halfon, N. (2000). Access to health care for children with special health care needs. *Pediatrics, 105*(4), 760–767.

Perrin, E. C., Lewkowicz, C., & Young, M. H. (2000). Shared vision: Concordance among fathers, mothers, and pediatricians about unmet needs of children with chronic health conditions. *Pediatrics, 105*(1), 277–285.

Perrin, E. C., Newacheck, P., Pless, I. B., Drotar, D., Gortmaker, S. L., Leventhal, J., et al. (1993). Issues involved in the definition and classification of chronic health conditions. *Pediatrics, 91*(4), 787–793.

Pinch, W. J. (2002). *When the bough breaks: Parental perception of ethical decision-making in the NICU*. New York: University Press of America.

Ray, L. D. (2002). Parenting and childhood chronicity: Making visible the invisible work. *Journal of Pediatric Nursing, 17*(6), 424–438.

Reeb, R., & Bush, J. (1997). Preprocedural psychological preparation in pediatric oncology: A process oriented study. *Children's Health Care, 25*(4), 265–280.

Seid, M., & Varni, J. (1999). Pediatric day surgery outcomes management: The role of preoperative anxiety and a home management protocol. *Journal of Clinical Outcomes Management, 6*(2), 24–30.

Sherman, B. R. (1995). Impact of home-based respite care on families of children with chronic illnesses. *Children's Health Care, 24*(1), 33–45.

Thompson, R. H. (1985). *Psychosocial research on pediatric hospitalization and health care: A review of the literature*. Springfield, IL: Charles C. Thomas.

Todres, I. D., Earle, M. R., & Jellinek, M. S. (1994). Enhancing communication. The physician and family in the pediatric intensive care unit. *Pediatric Clinics of North America, 41*(6), 1395–1404.

Turner-Henson, A., Holaday, B., Corser, N., Ogletree, G., & Swan, J. H. (1994). The experiences of discrimination challenges for chronically ill children. *Pediatric Nursing, 20*(6), 571–577.

Van Riper, M. (2003). The sibling experience of living with childhood chronic illness and disability. In J. J. Fitzpatrick (Ed.), *Annual review of nursing research 2003: Research on child health and pediatric issues* (pp. 279–302). New York: Springer.

Vernon, D. T., Foley, J., Sipowicz, R., & Schulman, J. (1965). *The psychological responses of children to hospitalization and illness*. Springfield, IL: Charles C. Thomas.

Williams, P. D. (1997). Siblings and pediatric chronic illness: A review of the literature. *International Journal of Nursing Studies, 34*(4), 312–323.

Williams, P. D., Williams, A. R., Graff, J. C., Hanson, S., Stanton, A., & Hafeman, C., et al. (2003). A community-based intervention for siblings and parents of children with chronic illness or disability: the ISEE study. *Journal of Pediatrics, 143*, 386–393.

Wilson, S. R., Yamada, E. G., Sudhakar, R., Roberto, L., Mannino, D., Mejia, C., et al. (2001). A controlled trial of an environmental tobacco smoke reduction intervention in low-income children with asthma. *Chest, 120*(5), 1709–1722.

Worden, J. W., & Monahan, J. R. (2001). Caring for bereaved parents. In M. Armstrong-Dailey & S. Zarbok (Eds.), *Hospice care for children* (pp. 137–156). New York: Oxford University Press.

Wysocki, T., Greco, P., Harris, M., Bubb, J., & White, N. H. (2001). Behavior therapy for families of adolescents with diabetes. *Diabetes Care, 24*(3), 441–446.

Wysocki, T., Harris, M. A., Greco, P., Bubb, J., Danda, C. E., Harvey, L. M., et al. (2000). Randomized, controlled trial of behavior therapy for families of adolescents with insulin-dependent diabetes mellitus. *Journal of Pediatric Psychology, 25*(1), 23–33.

End Note: Interdisciplinary Perspectives of Families and Health

ELAINE S. MARSHALL AND D. RUSSELL CRANE

TEN NEXT STEPS

This work represents a beginning effort to bring together the works of scholars and practitioners to consider issues related to families and health from a broad range of disciplines. Obviously, no such work can be comprehensive in its coverage of specific topics, methods, or implications. It does provoke thinking about the current state of knowledge and practice among professionals whose work is to help families. The preparation of the work has provided an enriching experience in dialogue among professionals from a variety of areas of expertise. The review of the work provides the opportunity to reflect on next steps for family health scholars. Here, we refer to the "ten next steps."

1. *Family and health scholars, practitioners, and families must continue to come together in truly integrated and collaborative ways.*

This work is an effort to bring together the work of thinkers from a broad range of disciplines. Even at its best, it is a compilation and not an integration. As scholars and practitioners interested in the health of families, we must continue to learn how to speak the language of each other, value the work and methods of each other, include families in our teams and communities, and forge new areas of scholarship and practice. At the same time, we must continue our efforts

to include families in genuine partnerships in health care and policy. It is important that we document and share our efforts in both professional and public literature. This needs to be done not only across disciplines but across nations and cultures. A variety of authors of this work, as well as some other impressive groups, are already in these endeavors, but there is still much work to be done.

2. *Family and health scholars must continue our work in theory building and refinement of methods that meet the needs of the complex endeavor of family health scholarship.*

This means expanding our thinking and practice in creative and evidence-based ways to develop knowledge. This means embracing qualitative and quantitative methods as well as discovering new methods to address the family unit. For example, in this work, William Griffin outlines agent-based modeling as an example of one method that may replace or expand our practice in structural equation modeling and other forms of sophisticated methodologies.

3. *Our study and practice among specific ethnic and cultural groups need to be intensified.*

In this volume, we only sampled some work with a few cultural and ethnic groups.

467

We need to know more about effective interventions, differences, and commonalities in a broad range of ethnic, cultural, and religious groups across the world.

4. *We need to be prepared to deal with health conditions of the future.*

The advent of new infectious diseases in the last couple of decades has opened our awareness to a need to learn about effective care for families dealing with illnesses that we may have not even identified. There is much to learn about biohazards, new infectious diseases, and conditions related to public safety and national security. Recent world events in armed conflict to reports from the Institute of Medicine point to our need to address issues of safety and national security. These events and issues have an effect on families physically and emotionally. These are new arenas for study and practice.

5. *We need to continue efforts to practice according to evidence.*

The current focus on evidence-based practice has implications for all areas of health care scholarship and practice with families. It also provides opportunities to work with families to understand, evaluate, and make effective decisions based on appropriate evidence.

6. *We need to be able to help families negotiate health care systems.*

Health care systems continue to become more complex. Family scholars and practitioners have opportunities to study and implement ways to help families negotiate the complex and sometimes intimidating systems of care, finance, and policy. Families are often required to confront policy issues and health care systems at times when they are most vulnerable.

7. *We need to know more about home and family as the center of caregiving.*

There is a need for clear understanding of the meaning of home and family as the center of health care. How do professionals recognize and practice according to this reality? How do professionals help families to provide the most effective and meaningful care within the home and family environment?

8. *We need to study and integrate issues of religion and spiritual implications of health challenges in families.*

There is growing evidence for the powerful influence of religion and spirituality in the lives of families dealing with health and illness. There is a need for systematic examination of such issues and subsequent integration into practice. This has broad implications for the study of family roles and relationships; perspectives of partnerships, marriage, and children; meanings of cure and healing; family caregiving; the place for clergy in health care practice; and a variety of other topics.

9. *We need to systematically study and revise how we educate health care professionals.*

There is a need for analysis, planning, and change in the educational preparation of health care professionals to include topics on the complexity of family study, practice in collaborative ways, understanding of interdisciplinary perspectives, and effective practice in new local and global environments.

10. *Family and health care scholars and practitioners need to contribute to decisions in health care policy and finance.*

Decision makers in family health policy and financing of health care are in need of the best evidence and practice as we move into the future. It is important that family scholars and practitioners, as well as experts in health care practice, are included in this process. This has implications for the quality and usefulness of our research and capacity and facility in communication in areas not usually familiar to scholars.

We are confident that as soon as this volume comes off the press, we will think of other important steps toward the future of interdisciplinary scholarship, practice, and policy related to families and health. Like this entire book, these are beginning thoughts toward coming together for a better future for families.

Author Index

Subject Index

About the Editors

D. Russell Crane, Ph.D., is Director of the Family Studies Center and Associate Director for Research in the School of Family Life and Professor of Marriage and Family Therapy at Brigham Young University. His research focuses on families and health issues, with a particular interest in the influence of marital and family therapy on health care use. His research team was the first to document decreases in health care use following marital and family therapy. He is on the editorial board of three journals and is the author of numerous articles and the book *Fundamentals of Marital Therapy* (1996), published by Taylor Francis (Brunner/Mazel). He and his wife Eileen are the parents of eight children.

Elaine S. Marshall, R.N., Ph.D., is Professor and Dean of the College of Nursing at Brigham Young University. Her research is on families and health, with particular recent focus on families with children with disabilities. She is the author of the book *Children's Stress and Coping: A Family Perspective* (1993), published by Guilford, for which she was awarded the New Professional Book Award by the National Council on Family Relations. She has been designated a Distinguished Writer by Sigma Theta Tau, the International Honor Society for Nursing, and is the winner of several awards for writing. She is the author of dozens of refereed journal articles and book chapters. She and her husband John are the parents of nine children.

About the Contributors

Melissa A. Alderfer, Ph.D., conducts research and works clinically with families of children with cancer. Dr. Alderfer's research centers on adjustment to childhood chronic illness, specifically post-traumatic stress responses and adjustment to childhood cancer. Her research is based on a social ecology model and examines multiple social systems of importance to child development, including families and peer networks. She is particularly interested in developing intervention protocols aimed at improving adjustment by intervening on multiple levels (e.g., individual child, parental couple, family system, peer system).

Jenny Altschuler is a systemic psychotherapist and consultant clinical psychologist whose work has focused on families facing illness and migration. The author of *Working With Chronic Illness: A Family Approach* (Macmillan, 1997), she has worked in inpatient and outpatient settings and has been involved in the training of systemic psychotherapists and clinical and educational psychologists at the Tavistock Clinic, where she established a multidisciplinary course for professionals working with illness. She helped establish counseling centers in Kosova and retains a consultative and training role in the Kosovan project, works as an independent psychotherapist, and is engaged in research on migration and racialization.

Jacqueline L. Angel, Ph.D. (Rutgers University, 1989) is an associate professor at the LBJ School of Public Affairs and Sociology at The University of Texas at Austin. Her research focuses on health policy with a special emphasis on minority populations. She has published numerous articles, as well as three books, *Health and Living Arrangements of the Elderly* (Garland Publishing, 1991), and with Ronald J. Angel, *Painful Inheritance: Health and the New Generation of Fatherless Families* (University of Wisconsin Press, 1993) and *Who Will Care for Us? Aging and Long-Term Care in Multicultural America* (New York University Press, 1997).

Ronald J. Angel, Ph.D. (Wisconsin, 1981), is professor of sociology at the The University of Texas at Austin. His research focuses on social welfare, health policy, and the health risks faced by Hispanic and other minority populations. He is the author of numerous articles and with Jacqueline Angel he is author of *Painful Inheritance: Health and the New Generation of Fatherless Families* (University of Wisconsin Press, 1993) and *Who Will Care for Us? Aging and Long-Term Care in Multicultural America* (New York University Press, 1997). He served as editor of the *Journal of Health and Social Behavior* from 1994 to 1997.

Lee L. Bean received his Ph.D. from Yale University in 1961. He is professor emeritus, Department of Sociology, University of Utah. He previously served as chair, Department of Sociology and director, The Middle East Center, University of Utah. His major research interest has focused on historical demography based on the development of and utilization of the Utah Population Database. The central thrust of much of his research has been fertility change of the Utah population during the later 19th and early 20th century. Much of this research is summarized in *Fertility Change on the American Frontier* (1992), published by the University of California Press and co-authored with Geraldine P. Mineau and Douglas L. Anderton. Recent journal articles (co-authored) include studies of infant mortality, mortality, and longevity.

Marion E. Broome, Ph.D., RN, is professor and University Dean at Indiana University School of Nursing. She received her master's in family nursing from the University of South Carolina, and her Ph.D. in Child and Family Development from the University of Georgia. Dr. Broome is best known for her research with ill children funded by the National Institutes of Health, the American Cancer Society, and Pfizer, Inc. She has published over 80 articles, chapters, and books. She is currently editor-in-chief of *Nursing Outlook,* the official journal of the American Academy of Nursing.

Lynn Clark Callister, RN, Ph.D., is a professor in the College of Nursing at Brigham Young University. Her research has focused on cross-cultural studies of women and the lived experiences of childbearing families. She is a Fellow in the American Academy of Nursing and was a 2004 Fulbright Scholar to the Russian Federation. She serves on the editorial board of four professional journals and has received several national research awards for her work. She is the author of dozens of refereed journal articles and book chapters.

Thomas L. Campbell, M.D., is the William Rocktaschel Professor and chair of Family Medicine at the University of Rochester School of Medicine and Dentistry and associate director of the University's Center for Primary Care. His expertise is in the role of the family in medical practice and the

influence of the family on health. His NIMH monograph, *Family's Impact on Health,* has been an influential review of the research in this area. Other books he has co-authored include *Families and Health* and *Family-Oriented Primary Care* (2nd edition). He co-edits *Families, Systems & Health: The Journal of Collaborative Family Healthcare.*

John S. W. Carpenter, AcSS, holds the chair of Social Work and Applied Social Science at the University of Bristol, England. He was previously professor and director of the Centre for Applied Social and Community Studies, University of Durham. His research concerns the organization, outcomes, and costs of health and welfare services for people with severe mental illness, and for children and families. He is a registered social worker, chartered psychologist, and family therapist. In 1999 he was elected as a founding academician of the Academy of the Social Sciences in the United Kingdom.

Barbara J. Dale is a consultant systemic psychotherapist working in the Tavistock Clinic, where she has been a major contributor to the development of the multi-disciplinary program of systemic training to doctoral level. Between 1989 and 2001, she worked with colleagues in Zimbabwe to establish the Zimbabwe Institute of Systemic Therapy, which provides systemic training at all levels. Her clinical interests and publications have focused on the impact of parents' serious addictions on family life and child development and the effect that a parent having a life-threatening illness has on parenting patterns, with particular interest in the role of gender.

Janet A. Deatrick, Ph.D., RN, teaches in the pediatric acute-chronic care nurse practitioner and the doctoral programs at the University of Pensylvania School of Nursing.

Her areas of expertise are qualitative research and children with chronic conditions and their families. She completed a year's sabbatical study (2001) in pediatric oncology at The Children's Hospital of Philadelphia to refocus her research and clinical practice to families whose children have cancer.

Peggye Dilworth-Anderson, Ph.D., is professor of Health Policy and Administration/School of Public Health and director of the Center for Aging and Diversity in the Institute on Aging (NIA). She is the principal investigator of two projects on health disparities pertaining to Alzheimer's disease and related dementias. A KO7 leadership grant from the NIA allows her to develop a research and academic training structure on ethnic minority aging at the University of North Carolina at Chapel Hill. She also serves in a number of consulting and advisory positions related to health issues in later life, and she has served in a number of leadership roles in the field of aging.

Todd M. Edwards, Ph.D., is associate professor and director of the Marital and Family Therapy program at the University of San Diego. His research is on family interventions for diabetes management and medical family therapy supervision. He works with individuals, couples, and families at Metro Family Physicians in San Diego.

V. Jeffery Evans earned a Ph.D. in economics from Duke University in 1973 and a J.D. from the University of Maryland School of Law in 1978. Since 1975, he has been employed at the National Institutes of Health (NIH) in the National Institute of Child Health and Human Development (NICHD). He is part of the extramural program at NICHD and has long been associated with funding research dealing with issues involving families and children, health disparities, and mind-body influences on health.

Thomas E. Finucane, M.D., is professor of Medicine at Johns Hopkins and chair of the Ethics Committee at the Johns Hopkins Bayview Medical Center. He is a busy clinician and teacher and has published widely on problems concerning life-sustaining treatment late in life. His wife and he have five children.

Agatha M. Gallo, Ph.D., APN, CPNP, is a professor in the Department of Maternal-Child Nursing at the University of Illinois at Chicago. Dr. Gallo has focused her research on family response to childhood chronic illness, more recently families where there is a child with a genetic condition. She has been especially interested in parents' approaches to information management in the context of a childhood chronic genetic condition. Dr. Gallo has strong expertise in caring for children with chronic conditions and their families as a pediatric nurse practitioner and nurse educator.

Kelly M. Glazer, M.S., is a doctoral student in the Graduate Training Programs in Clinical and Health Psychology at the University of Utah.

Dannie Hoffman, M.A., has been directing research projects at UCLA since 1991. She currently manages several protocols for Dr. Debra Murphy, including two multi-site projects through the Adolescent Trials Network, a national consortium of researchers exploring the impact of HIV on adolescent populations.

William A. Griffin, Ph.D., founded the marriage and family therapy program at Arizona State University (ASU) in 1988 and served as its director until 1997. He also directs ASU's Marital Interaction Lab, conducting studies of interaction patterns in couples and families. Dr. Griffin is the author of *Family Therapy: Fundamentals of Theory and Practice*. He also co-authored

Models of Family Therapy: The Essential Guide. Research interests include the analysis of interaction patterns among distressed, non-distressed, and post-divorce couples, and the computer modeling and simulation of the micro-social interactions found in married dyads and in children forming playgroups.

Harvey H. Hillin, Ph.D., is a policy analyst for Kansas Medicaid and an instructor in statistics for Baker University. He has Ph.D. (Kansas State University) and MSW (University of Kansas) degrees. He is author of *Better Living Through Chemistry? What You Should Know About Addiction* (2002) and with his wife (Mary Hillin, Ph.D., Kansas Division of Children and Family Policy) he has a forthcoming book, *Drugs and Youth: What Parents, Teachers, and Helping Professionals Can Do* (2005).

Gene A. Kallenberg, M.D., serves as the chief of the Division of Family Medicine and vice-chair for Clinical Affairs, Dept. of Family and Preventive Medicine. He is currently working with colleagues from the Marriage and Family Therapy Program at University of California San Diego (UCSD) to establish a truly collaborative practice within his Division's family medicine offices that will serve as a teaching model for medical students and family medicine residents at UCSD.

George Knafl, Ph.D., serves as biostatistician, consulting with faculty and students on their research. He is also professor emeritus of computer science at DePaul University where he founded and directed the Software Engineering Program. He has a Ph.D. in mathematics, specializing in statistics, from Northwestern University (1978). His research interests include applications of statistics to nursing research, modeling and analysis of the impact of dioxin exposure, heuristic methods for statistical model selection, adaptive modeling of electronic monitoring data, statistical evaluation of survey instruments, and software reliability.

Kathleen Knafl, Ph.D., is a professor at Yale University School of Nursing where she teaches family and research design courses in the doctoral and pediatric nurse practitioner programs. Her research focuses on family management of childhood chronic illness. Her work sets the stage for developing and testing nursing interventions that meet the needs of diverse families and support optimal family and child functioning. She is widely published and her work has been funded by both private and public sources. Additionally, she serves as a consultant to the National Institutes of Health as well as to other universities and researchers.

Margo D. Maine, Ph.D., is a clinical psychologist specializing in eating disorders. She is author of *Body Wars: Making Peace With Women's Bodies* (2000), *Father Hunger: Fathers, Daughters, and the Pursuit of Thinness* (2004), and *The Body Myth: The Pressure on Women to Be Perfect* (Wiley, 2005), and senior editor of *Eating Disorders: The Journal of Treatment and Prevention*. A founding member and fellow of the Academy for Eating Disorders and a founder of the National Eating Disorders Association, she serves on the boards of the Eating Disorders Coalition for Research, Policy, and Action, and Dads and Daughters.

William D. Marelich, Ph.D., is an assistant professor of psychology at California State University, Fullerton. He is also a lecturer at the University of California at Los Angeles (UCLA), and a consulting statistician with the Health Risk Reduction Projects (affiliated with UCLA's Integrated Substance Abuse Programs). His research interests include decision-making strategies in health and organizational settings, patient/provider interactions, interpersonal relationships, and statistical/methodological approaches in experimental and applied research. His work has been published in journals such as *AIDS Care, Journal of Personality and Social Psychology,* and the *Journal of Studies on Alcohol.*

Susan H McDaniel, Ph.D., is professor of psychiatry and family medicine and director of family programs and the Wynne Center for Family Research in Psychiatry, and associate chair of family medicine at the University of Rochester School of Medicine & Dentistry. She is known for her publications in the areas of mental health and primary care, medical family therapy, and family systems medicine. Her special areas of interest are genetic testing, assisted reproductive technologies, somatization, and gender and health. She is a frequent speaker at meetings of both health and mental health professionals.

Geraldine P. Mineau, Ph.D., is a research professor in the Department of Oncological Sciences and director of population sciences for Huntsman Cancer Institute at the University of Utah. She has almost 30 years of experience with the Utah Population Database, a research resource with over 8 million records. Her research includes co-authoring a book, *Fertility Change on the American Frontier: Adaptation and Innovation* (1990), and publishing over 40 articles and chapters. In 2003 she co-authored an article titled "Biomedical Databases: Protecting Privacy and Promoting Research." She holds research grants from the National Institutes of Health, "Rocky Mountain Cancer Genetics Network" and from the Centers for Disease Control, "Development of a Genealogical Database to Support Genetic Disease."

Kim T. Mueser, Ph.D. is a licensed clinical psychologist and a professor in the Departments of Psychiatry and Community and Family Medicine at the Dartmouth Medical School in Hanover, New Hampshire. Dr. Mueser's clinical and research interests include the psychosocial treatment of severe mental illnesses, family therapy, dual diagnosis, and post-traumatic stress disorder. He has published extensively and given numerous lectures and workshops on psychiatric rehabilitation.

Debra A. Murphy, Ph.D., is a research psychologist and director of the Health Risk Reduction Projects, Department of Psychiatry, University of California, Los Angeles. She has conducted HIV/AIDS behavioral research with children, adolescents, adults, and families over the past 14 years. Her research areas include the effect of maternal HIV/AIDS on children and young adolescents, family-based HIV risk reduction programs, and secondary prevention for HIV-infected adolescents. She is a member of the NICHD Adolescent Trials Network, which is investigating behavioral, therapeutic, and vaccine strategies for adolescents. She has first-authored over 30 papers on HIV/AIDS, and co-authored over 60 other papers and chapters.

Lynn B. Myers, Ph.D., is a senior lecturer in Health Psychology and director of the master's program in health psychology at Surrey University in the United Kingdom. Her research interests include adherence/compliance to medical treatment, repressive coping style, inhibition of emotion and disease, risk perception for health-related events, stress and dentists, social cognition models and health-related behaviors, romantic adult attachment styles, and inhibitory processes in memory.

Robert J. Parsons, Ph.D., is a professor of economics in the George W. Romney Institute of Public Management at Brigham Young University (BYU) where he teaches managerial economics, economic development, and process management. Dr. Parsons' administrative duties at BYU have included director of the Master of Public Administration Program, chair of the Managerial Economics Department, assistant Dean of the Marriott School, and director of the Survey Research Center. His research interests have been in the areas of health care economics, strategic planning, and urban economic development.

Jo Ellen Patterson, Ph.D., is a professor in the marriage and family therapy (MFT) program at the University of San Diego. She is also a clinical instructor in psychiatry and family medicine at the University of California, San Diego (UCSD). She supervises MFT interns and family medicine residents in the UCSD Department of Family Medicine Residency Program. In addition, she is the author of three books, *Essential Skills in Family Therapy* (Guilford), *Mental Health Professional in Medical Settings* (Norton), and *Psychopharmacology Simplified, Collaborative Care Clarified: Essential Skills for the Contemporary Therapist* (forthcoming, Guilford Press).

Mary Politi, M.Phil., is a doctoral candidate in the Clinical Psychology program at The George Washington University. Her research is on individual and family coping in response to cancer and the effects of psychological distress on physiological functioning. She is particularly interested in evaluating acceptance-based clinical interventions for the treatment of psychological distress during the chronic illness experience.

Wilma Powell Stuart, RN, M.A., is the vice president, chief nursing officer of Shannon Medical Center, a doctoral student at the University of Alabama in Birmingham, and the assistant editor of the journal *Nursing Outlook*. Her research interest is adolescent weight management. She is a member of

Sigma Theta Tau International, the North American Association for the Study of Obesity (NAASO), and the Southern Nursing Research Society. Her work with children with a chronic illness includes employment as an endocrinology research data coordinator, as a staff nurse in a children's hospital, and as a pediatric nurse manager.

Jonathan G. Sandberg, Ph.D., is an associate professor in the Department of Marriage and Family Therapy at Syracuse University. He completed his doctoral work in marriage and family therapy at Kansas State University in 1998. He is interested in the relationship between emotional and physical health problems and marital dynamics. Dr. Sandberg has authored or co-authored numerous papers on marital quality, depression, and health, particularly in later life. His recent collaborative work centers on spousal supportive behavior as a means of improving adherence to diabetes treatment.

Mark A. Schuster, M.D., Ph.D., is professor of Pediatrics and Public Health at the University of California at Los Angeles (UCLA), senior natural scientist at RAND, and co-director of the RAND Center for Maternal, Child, and Adolescent Health Research. He is the founder and director of the UCLA/RAND Center for Adolescent Health Promotion, a community-based participatory research center funded by the Centers for Disease Control. Dr. Schuster conducts research primarily on child, adolescent, and family issues. Currently, he is conducting a study funded by the National Institute of Child Health and Development examining HIV-infected parents and their children. He practices pediatrics at Mattel Children's Hospital at UCLA.

William J. Sieber, Ph.D., is an assistant clinical professor in the Department of Family and Preventive Medicine at the

University of California, San Diego. Dr. Sieber earned his Ph.D. from Yale University and as a clinical health psychologist has focused his research on quality of life and outcomes assessment, chronic pain, and the impact of psychological well-being on both perceived and actual health status. Dr. Sieber also serves as a consultant to the biotechnology and pharmaceutical industry on research design and outcomes assessment issues, and speaks nationally to health care professionals on issues of stress, health, and optimizing performance.

Ken R. Smith, Ph.D., is professor of Human Development and Family Studies, co-leader, Program in Cancer Control and Population Sciences, Huntsman Cancer Institute, University of Utah. He is a demographer and social epidemiologist interested in familial aspects of health, aging, and longevity. He is investigating the socio-environmental and genetic origins of exceptional longevity in families. Another area of interest is the psychosocial and behavioral factors in cancer prevention and control as well as a long-standing interest in genetic testing for adult-onset illnesses and how genetic tests may affect the psychosocial well-being and demographic outcomes of families and their members.

Timothy W. Smith, Ph.D., is a professor of psychology at the University of Utah, a member of the faculty of the Graduate Training Program in Clinical Psychology, and coordinator of the Graduate Training Program in Health Psychology. He received his doctorate in clinical psychology from the University of Kansas, and completed a pre-doctoral internship and post-doctoral fellowship in clinical psychology and behavioral medicine at the Brown University Program in Medicine. He is a past president of the Division of Health Psychology of the American Psychological Association.

Marcia Van Riper, RN, Ph.D., is an associate professor at the University of North Carolina at Chapel Hill. She has a joint appointment in the School of Nursing and the Carolina Center for Genome Sciences. She received a B.S. in Nursing from De Pauw University, a M.S. in Nursing from the University of Wisconsin-Milwaukee, a M.A. in Bioethics (with an emphasis on genetic issues) from Case Western Reserve University, and a Ph.D. in Nursing and Psychology from the University of Wisconsin-Madison. Her research is on the family experience of being tested for and living with a genetic condition.

Beth Vaughan-Cole, Ph.D., APRN, is professor and chair of the Division of Acute and Chronic Care in the College of Nursing at the University of Utah. In addition, she is the director of Caring Connections: A Hope and Comfort in Grief Program, sponsored by the University of Utah Hospitals and Clinics and the University of Utah College of Nursing. Her primary research has been on children and families with her current interest in grieving children and families. She co-authored a textbook, *Family Nursing Practice*. Also, she co-authored *Dealing with Sudden and Unexpected Death: A Handbook for Survivors*.

Arlene L. Vetere, Ph.D., is deputy director of the Clinical Psychology Doctorate at Surrey University in the United Kingdom. She is a chartered clinical psychologist and systemic psychotherapist registered with the UKCP. Dr. Vetere was recently elected as president of the European Family Therapy Association, and is an academician of the UK Academy of the Learned Societies in the Social Sciences.

Sharon Wallace Williams, Ph.D., is an assistant professor in The Department of Allied Health Sciences, Division of Speech and Hearing Sciences, at the University of North Carolina at Chapel Hill (UNC-CH). She is also a research scientist with UNC-CH's Center on Aging and Diversity. Dr. Williams received a Ph.D. in Human Development and Family Studies and completed a gerontology postdoctoral fellowship. Her research examines disabilities, caregiving, and disease management at the family level. Current funding extends her research to include end-of-life experiences of older adults and family caregivers. Her work has appeared in *The Journals of Gerontology, The Gerontologist, Aging and Mental Health,* and *Family Relations.*

Karen Weihs, M.D., is associate professor of psychiatry and a comprehensive member of the National Cancer Center–designated Arizona Cancer Center in the College of Medicine in Tucson, Arizona. She graduated from the University of Iowa College of Medicine and is board certified in Family Practice and General Psychiatry. Her research is on family, social, and emotional factors that influence disease control in breast cancer patients. She has published and lectured widely in peer-reviewed venues, focusing on psycho-oncology, family adjustment to stressful events, and psychopharmacology.

Sven E. Wilson holds a Ph.D. in economics (1997) from the University of Chicago. He is currently an associate professor and director of the Graduate Program in Public Policy at Brigham Young University, visiting co-director of the Center for Population Economics at the University of Chicago, and research economist at the National Bureau of Economic Research. He has published several articles and a book on the economics and demography of health and the family, and he is a senior investigator on a project funded by the National Institutes of Health, titled *Early Indicators of Later Work Levels, Disease, and Death.*

Barbara A. Zsembik, Ph.D., is associate professor and associate chair of the Department of Sociology at the University of Florida. Her research interests lie at the intersection of race/ethnic studies and medical demography. Her current research focuses on Latino child health and health disparities among adult Latinos.